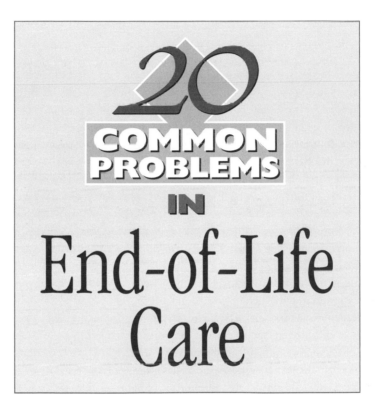

20
COMMON
PROBLEMS
IN
End-of-Life
Care

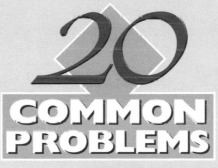

20 COMMON PROBLEMS IN

End-of-Life Care

EDITORS

BARRY M. KINZBRUNNER, M.D.
Vitas Healthcare Corporation, Miami, Florida

NEAL J. WEINREB, M.D.
Vitas Healthcare Corporation Broward, Ft. Lauderdale, Florida

JOEL S. POLICZER, M.D.
Vitas Healthcare Corporation–Dade, Miramar, Florida

SERIES EDITOR

BARRY D. WEISS, M.D.
Professor of Clinical Family and Community Medicine
University of Arizona College of Medicine, Tucson, Arizona

McGraw-Hill
Medical Publishing Division

New York   Chicago   San Francisco   Lisbon   London   Madrid   Mexico City
Milan   New Delhi   San Juan   Seoul   Singapore   Sydney   Toronto

McGraw-Hill

A Division of The McGraw·Hill Companies

20 COMMON PROBLEMS IN END-OF-LIFE CARE

4 5 6 7 8 9 0 DOC DOC 0 9 8 7 6 5 4

ISBN 0-07-034883-9

This book was set in Garamond by V&M Graphics, Inc.
The editors were Susan R. Noujaim and Andrea Seils.
The production supervisor was Richard C. Ruzycka.
Project management was provided by Andover Publishing Services.
The cover designer was Marsha Cohen/Parallelogram.
The index was prepared by Angie Wiley.

R. R. Donnelley & Sons was printer and binder.

This book is printed on acid-free paper.

Library of Congress Cataloging-in-Publication Data

20 common problems in end-of-life care / editors: Barry M. Kinzbrunner, Neal J.
    Weinreb, Joel S. Policzer.
        p. ; cm.
    Includes bibliographical references and index.
    ISBN 0-07-034883-9
    1. Terminal care.
    2. Terminally ill—Care.   3. Hospice care. I. Title: Twenty common problems in
end-of-life care. II. Kinzbrunner, Barry M. III. Weinreb, Neal J. IV. Policzer, Joel S.
[DNLM: 1. Terminal Care—psychology. 2. Advance Directives. 3. Palliative
Care—methods. 4. Palliative Care—psychology. 4. Terminal Care—methods.
WB 310 Z999 2002]
R726.8. A15 2002
362.1'75—dc21   2001030452

This book is dedicated to my wife, Anita, and to my parents, Norbert and Thelma, who have provided me with the love, help, and support that led me to where I am today and which resulted in the opportunity to complete this book.

—*BMK*—

Contents

Contributors

Jeanne Micklich Ash, R.N., B.S.N.
VITAS Healthcare Corporation
Orange, California

Michael Bozeman
Chaplain
VITAS Healthcare Corporation–Broward
Ft. Lauderdale, Florida

Michael Clark, Pharm.D.
Director of Pharmacy
VITAS Healthcare Corporation
Miami, Florida

Richard Fife, M. Div., D. Min.
Vice President of Bioethics and Pastoral Care
VITAS Healthcare Corporation
Miami, Florida

Domingo Gomez, M.D.
Team Physician
VITAS Healthcare Corporation–Dade
Miramar, Florida

Barry M. Kinzbrunner, M.D.
Vice President/National Medical Director
VITAS Healthcare Corporation
Miami, Florida

Judith Ann Haythorne Macurda, M.D., M.P.H.
Medical Director
VITAS Healthcare Corporation
Orange, California

Tina Maluso-Bolton, M.S.N., R.N., O.N.P.
VITAS Healthcare Corporation–San Gabriel
Covina, California

Elizabeth A. McKinnis, M.D.
Medical Director
VITAS Healthcare Corporation–Dallas
Dallas, Texas

Sarah E. McKinnon, M.A.
Performance Consultant
VITAS Healthcare Corporation
Miami, Florida

Melanie P. Merriman, Ph.D.
Consultant
Touchstone Consulting
North Bay Village, Florida

Bob Miller, M. Div.
Director of Education and Training
VITAS Healthcare Corporation
Miami, Florida

Vincent D. Nguyen, D.O.
Medical Director
VITAS Healthcare Corporation–Coastal
Orange, California

Joel S. Policzer, M.D.
Medical Director
VITAS Healthcare Corporation–Dade
Miramar, Florida

Bruce Schlecter, M.D.
Medical Director
VITAS Healthcare Corporation–San Gabriel
Covina, California

Richard A. Shapiro, M.D.
Team Physician
VITAS Healthcare Corporation–Chicago Central
Lincolnwood, Illinois

Neal J. Weinreb, M.D.
Medical Director
VITAS Healthcare Corporation–Broward
Ft. Lauderdale, Florida

Michael Wohlfeiler, M.D.
Private Practice
Miami Beach, Florida

James B. Wright, M.D.
Medical Director
VITAS Healthcare Corporation–Ft. Worth
Ft. Worth, Texas

Introduction

"No problem is more distressing than that presented by the patient with an incurable disease, particularly when premature death is inevitable. . . . The physician also must be prepared to deal with guilt feelings on the part of the family when a member becomes gravely or hopelessly ill."

These statements can be found in the introductory chapter of *Harrison's Principles of Internal Medicine,* in the opening paragraphs of a section on "incurability and death." Clearly, the goal of this section in what many consider to be the bible of internal medicine is to assist medical students and physicians-in-training in better understanding how to approach the care of patients who are terminally ill. And therein lies the challenge.

On the surface, these statements would seem perfectly reasonable. After all, facing an incurable or terminal illness is certainly distressing. The question is, though, distressing for whom? A careful reading reveals that the subject of the distress is not the person who is dying; rather, it is the individual "presented by the patient with an incurable disease," namely the physician.

Should the physician be distressed? Certainly, taking care of a patient when that patient is near the end of life is a formidable task, and the physician should be empathetic to the patient's and family's distress. However, the physician's professional obligation to the patient and family requires that distress be avoided in favor of providing support, guidance, and continued hope during this most difficult and challenging time. It is this obligation,

especially as it relates to providing continued hope, which raises additional issues with the statement above. For how can a physician give a patient and family hope when the patient is thought to be "hopelessly ill"?

The above analysis is not meant to suggest that either the authors of these statements or physicians in general focus more on their own distress than that of the patient and family or intentionally view their patients as hopeless, even in the face of a terminal illness. Far from it! However, the statements do suggest that these issues are subtly woven into the attitudes that physicians carry with them when caring for patients who are near the end of life.

The goals of this book, *20 Common Problems in End-of-Life Care*, are to assist physicians and other clinicians in overcoming their "distress" and in providing the patients they care for who are near the end of life with hope in the face of apparent "hopelessness." To help accomplish these goals, the book is divided into four major sections that logically walk clinicians through the perceived complexities of providing patients and families with quality end-of-life care.

Part 1: Preparing Patients for End-of-Life Care

The opening section, *Preparing Patients for End-of-Life Care*, attempts to answer some of the fundamental questions related to the "who, what, and where" of care at the end of life. The first problem, who needs to receive this care, is addressed in Chapter 1, which discusses the various clinical guidelines and criteria that, when combined with the physician's clinical judgment, will assist clinicians in identifying patients who require end-of-life care. Chapter 2 then follows with a discussion of how and where this care can be obtained, including a detailed examination of the Medicare Hospice Benefit, as well as a look at other forms of end-of-life care that are available in various communities.

Once the patients and the type of care they need have been identified, clinicians must then confront the challenge of sharing this information with their patients and families. Communication techniques to assist clinicians in accomplishing this formidable task are discussed in Chapter 3. Chapter 4 then provides an overview of how end-of-life care interdisciplinary teams function to care for terminally ill patients, with specific attention on the multiple roles that physicians play in working with these teams. Chapter 5 examines the various ways that outcomes and quality of life can be measured, giving the clinician confidence that the providers of patient end-of-life services are doing what they say they will, improving the quality of care and life of the patients and families they serve.

Part 2: Common Symptoms Near the End of Life

Having solved the logistical problems of getting patients cared for near the end of life, the clinicians' next task is to meet the physical, emotional, and spiritual needs of their patients and families. To accomplish this, Part 2 discusses the management of many of the common symptoms experienced by patients who are nearing the ends of their lives.

It is fitting that the management of pain is addressed first (Chapter 6), as the challenges associated with controlling pain near the end of life have been and continue to be for many the raison

d'etre of hospice and palliative care. Following the discussion on pain management, Chapters 7 through 9 review the management of respiratory, gastrointestinal, and neurological symptoms that cause challenges for the terminally ill. Chapter 10 then examines disorders that affect the skin and mucous membranes, and Chapter 11 addresses depression, as well as a number of other end-of-life symptoms not previously discussed. The uniqueness of the dying experience is addressed in Chapter 12, which examines the challenges that clinicians face when managing symptoms of patients who are in their last several days of life.

Although clinicians tend to focus on the physical symptoms experienced by patients who are approaching life's end, it is important that these clinicians have a working knowledge of the psychosocial and spiritual concerns that patients experience during their last weeks and months. Chapter 13 provides this overview in a somewhat unique way, by looking at these issues as opportunities by which these patients, with the help of the clinicians caring for them, can grow and progress even as life draws to a close.

One of the cardinal principles of end-of-life care is that the patient and family together represent the unit of care, and that care therefore does not end when the patient takes his or her final breath. How those that the patient has left behind deal with their loss is every bit as important a part of hospice and palliative care as is the management of pain during the remaining life of the patient. Therefore, Chapter 14 addresses the subject of bereavement care and the role that clinicians may play in recognizing the signs and symptoms of and providing appropriate interventions for both normal and abnormal grief reactions.

Part 3: Ethical Issues and Controversies Near the End of Life

There are four major principles that comprise medical ethics: autonomy, beneficence, nonmale-

Table 1

Cardinal Principles of Medical Ethics

PRINCIPLE	DEFINITION
Autonomy	Self-determination by choosing among available treatment options.
Beneficence	Taking action for the patient's benefit.
Nonmaleficence	Avoiding harm.
Justice	
a. Societal justice	Doing what is good for society as a whole.
b. Distributive justice	Allocating resources justly.

SOURCE: Lo B: Ethical issues in clinical medicine. In: Isselbacher KJ, Braunwald E, Wilson JD, et al, eds: *Harrison's Principles of Internal Medicine,* 13th ed. New York: McGraw-Hill, 1994.

ficence, and justice, which are defined in Table 1. As end-of-life care has evolved over the last several decades, medical ethics has had an ever-increasing influence in assisting clinicians, as well as patients and families, in making many of the difficult decisions during this challenging final period of life. Therefore, Part 3 of this book examines some of the ethical dilemmas that clinicians and the patients and families they care for face when life is approaching its end.

First and foremost in addressing medical ethical issues at the end of life is the need to respect a patient's wishes by having advanced knowledge of the care that a patient would or would not want to receive if those desires could not be expressed. Hence, Chapter 15 examines the issues (both ethical and legal), around advance directives, as well as the appropriateness of providing cardiopulmonary resuscitation to patients who are near the end of life from both the medical and ethical perspectives.

As patients near the end of life, their desire to ingest food and fluid often diminishes voluntarily, or they may become physically unable to eat and drink. Physicians and family members often become concerned that these patients who do not eat or drink are succumbing to malnutrition or dehydration, rather than to the natural processes associated with dying. These concerns often lead to the decision to provide the patient with food and fluid by artificial means, even at the expense of increased patient discomfort. To address these concerns, Chapter 16 discusses the medical and ethical issues that surround the provision of hydration and nutritional support for terminally ill patients.

Chapter 17 attempts to answer one of the questions that has always plagued providers of hospice and palliative care: the place, if any, of invasive diagnostic studies and therapies for patients near the end of life. Primarily using the ethical principles of beneficence and nonmaleficence, potential benefit versus harm, this chapter evaluates the potential palliative indications of such invasive interventions as chemotherapy, radiation therapy, surgery, endoscopy, blood transfusions, and parenteral antibiotics.

Chapter 18 presents a discussion of what is probably the most difficult ethical dilemma facing clinicians today, the role, if any, of physician-assisted suicide and euthanasia. While recognizing that this book has an editorial bias against these practices, the authors of the chapter have attempted to present both sides of this debate, which today rages throughout organized medical societies across the globe, so that readers can form their own opinions.

Part 4: Special Groups

No book on end-of-life care would be complete without discussing some of the special needs that certain groups of patients have when life is almost at an end. Chapter 19 examines the special needs of patients with acquired immunodeficiency syndrome (AIDS), who may suffer from more complex physical symptoms secondary to opportunistic infections and may have more challenging psychosocial problems due to their younger average age and, for many, alternative life-styles.

Last, but certainly not least, Chapter 20 discusses the special needs of terminally ill pediatric patients. Among the issues discussed are the challenges of working with grieving parents and siblings, the differing approaches to care and support of terminally ill children based on age and developmental level, and the need for adjusting pharmacologic interventions based on the different metabolic needs of children as opposed to adults. Despite the emotional difficulty that many health care providers experience when acknowledging that children may need end-of-life care, these children, as well as their siblings and parents, need this support just as much as the elderly, when the acceptance that life is approaching its end is somewhat more palatable

Whether you are a clinician in training or have been in practice for twenty years, whether you provide primary care or practice a subspecialty, whether you are in the community setting or in academic medicine, you will, at least from time to time, need to deal with the distress and the feelings of hopelessness expressed by your patients who are near the end of life. Therefore, you should find the material outlined above and contained in *20 Common Problems in End-of-Life Care* of great utility. By understanding the principles of hospice and palliative care, clinicians can look to those who provide end-of-life care as patient-care partners, assisting them in providing their patients and families with the care that they need in a positive atmosphere of hope. As stated by Dame Cicely Saunders, considered the "mother" of hospice and end-of-life care, and, having been trained as a doctor, nurse, and social worker, an interdisciplinary team all rolled into one: "You matter because you are you, and you matter until the last moment of your life. We will

do all we can, not only to help you die peacefully, but also to live until you die."

Acknowledgments

I would like to take this opportunity to thank all the chapter authors who devoted the time and energy necessary to contribute to this book. I would especially like to thank my co-editors, Dr. Neal Weinreb and Dr. Joel Policzer, whose additional editorial support was crucial to the completion of this project. Thanks are also extended to Dr. Barry Weiss, series editor of *20 Common Problems*, for his editorial comments, and to my secretary, Cecilia Serrano, for her assistance in preparing the final manuscripts and figures. Finally, I want to give special thanks to Susan Noujaim, Senior Developmental Editor of the Medical Publishing Division of McGraw-Hill. Without her patience and, ultimately, without her setting of firm deadlines, this book would not be in existence today.

BMK

References

Isselbacher KJ, Braunwald E, Wilson JD, et al: Chapter 1, The practice of medicine. In Isselbacher KJ, Braunwald E, Wilson JD, et al, eds: *Harrison's Principles of Internal Medicine,* 13th ed. New York: McGraw-Hill, 1994.

Kinzbrunner BM: The terminally ill patient. In: Abeloff MD, Armitage JO, Lichter, AS, Niederhuber JE, eds: *Clinical Oncology,* 2nd ed. New York: Churchill Livingstone, 2000, p. 597.

Lo B: Ethical issues in clinical medicine. In: Isselbacher KJ, Braunwald E, Wilson JD, et al, eds: *Harrison's Principles of Internal Medicine,* 13th ed. New York: McGraw-Hill, 1994.

Stoddard S: *The Hospice Movement: A Better Way of Caring for the Dying,* revised ed. New York: Vintage, 1991.

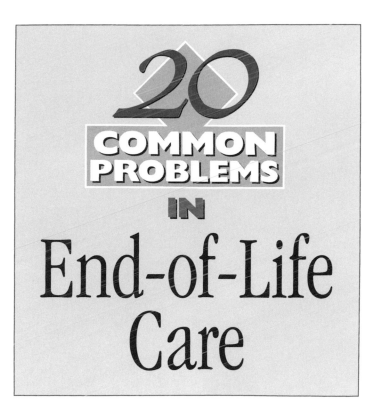

20 COMMON PROBLEMS

IN

End-of-Life Care

Preparing Patients for End-of-Life Care

Barry M. Kinzbrunner

Chapter

1

Predicting Prognosis: How to Decide When End-of-Life Care Is Needed

Introduction

One of the major problems that physicians must address as they plan care for their patients near the end of life is to determine when, based upon a prediction of the patient's prognosis, such care should be initiated. The ability of the physician to make a reasonable estimate of how long a patient is likely to live is critical, whether one is considering referral to a hospice program (which, as discussed in Chapter 2, requires the physician to certify that the patient has a prognosis of 6 months or less) or to an alternative end-of-life care program if the patient's prognosis is somewhat longer.

Prognostic Accuracy

Studies assessing the ability of physicians to accurately predict prognosis have reported varying results, making it difficult to draw any conclusions. For example, while a 1972 study suggested that physicians and other caregivers were overly optimistic when asked to predict the patient survival, the more recent Study to Understand Prognoses and Preferences for Outcomes and Risks of Treatment (SUPPORT) reported that physicians tend to be pessimistic when predicting patient prognosis near the end of life. Interestingly, and in sharp contrast to both of these studies, review of SUPPORT data also suggests that for certain subgroups of patients, physician accuracy in predicting patient prognosis may actually be quite good. In one published report, 85 percent of patients who were identified by their physicians as having an 85 percent probability of dying during the next 6 months (which would be the group of patients most likely in need of hospice and end-of-life care), actually died during that period. In a second report specifically devoted to patients with

cancer diagnoses, the SUPPORT investigators drew the conclusion that "physicians estimated prognosis quite accurately."

Hospice data does little to shed light on the accuracy of physicians in predicting survival. A study based on 1990 Medicare claims data reported that over 85 percent of patients admitted to hospices during a 3-month period died within 6 months, indicating that physicians were fairly accurate in predicting the prognosis of this group of individuals. On the other hand, these same patients had a median survival of only 36 days. This short median survival may be explained by the fact that, with so much uncertainty in the medical literature surrounding this subject of predicting prognosis, physicians are understandably reluctant to consider hospice or other end-of-life care services for their patients until death is certain.

Utilizing Guidelines to Predict Prognosis

To assist physicians in predicting prognosis near the end of life, the development of guidelines has been suggested. These guidelines would aid physicians in identifying when patients are likely in need of hospice or other end-of-life care services. Such guidelines, both formal and informal, can be found in the medical literature, and information about them will be presented in this chapter. It should be noted that these guidelines were developed primarily for identification of patients who have a prognosis of 6 months or less, which is required for eligibility for the Medicare/Medicaid Hospice Benefit (see Chapter 2). Although this may be perceived as a limiting factor in the utility of guidelines, the continued uncertainty surrounding the prediction of prognosis near the end of life suggests that the guidelines may have applicability for determining patient need for end-of-life care programs outside the confines of the Medicare Hospice Benefit as well.

Guidelines for predicting patient prognosis near the end of life are not intended to be used in a dogmatic fashion, and should not be converted into a scored checklist with some magic number of items required to consider a patient ready for hospice or palliative care. When the guidelines recommend the use of objective studies, such as pulmonary functions, diagnostic x-rays, or laboratory tests, these studies should not be used to rule in or rule out a patient's need for end-of-life care. Specifically, patients should not be compelled to undergo testing to qualify for hospice or palliative care; nor should they be barred from receiving such care, if clinically indicated, because they choose to avoid further such testing. What is recommended is that these guidelines and associated tests be used in a thoughtful fashion, with each specific criterion representing a piece of information that should be evaluated in the context of a patient's clinical condition and clinical course at the time of assessment. When the assessment is completed, the information obtained should be combined with other clinical and psychosocial information, making the decision to recommend that a patient receive end-of-life care one of CLINICAL JUDGEMENT, based on the needs of that specific patient.

General Guidelines

When the concept of hospice first began to take hold in Great Britain, Canada, and the United States, there was an implicit understanding that the primary intent was to care for terminally ill patients suffering from cancer. Cancer patients, after all, tend to show a steady decline in health as the illness progresses, making the ability to predict when a patient's life is nearing its end seemingly straightforward. However, as the 1980s came to a close, it became clear that patients with nonmalignant end-stage condition, such as congestive heart failure, chronic lung disease, and dementia,

would also benefit from end-of-life care. A major reason for the inclusion of patients with nonmalignant diagnoses was that physicians and others working in hospice and palliative care observed that patients who were terminally ill, regardless of the primary diagnosis, had convergence of their symptoms and treatment approaches as the time of death became closer. For example, the shortness of breath experienced by a patient who is dying of a malignancy with lung involvement is much the same as shortness of breathing in a patient who has severe COPD. The approach to therapy in these patients will likewise be similar.

The concept of similarity in presentation also extends itself to the determination of when patients require end-of-life care. Whether patients are dying of a neoplastic process, or of a long-standing nonmalignant illness, there are some characteristics shared by all patients that can be expressed in a set of general guidelines for determining prognosis, as set forth in Table 1–1, and discussed in detail in the next sections.

Clinical Progression of Disease

Crucial to determining prognosis is the demonstration that the patient's primary disease process is progressing over time. There are a number of sources of important information that can help the clinician recognize when the patient's condition is worsening. As an illness progresses, patients may find themselves more frequently in need of health care services, causing them to spend increasing amounts of time in hospitals, emergency rooms, or the doctor's office. Serial office visits demonstrating persistent or increasing symptoms, such as fatigue or weight loss, may be a marker of progressive illness. Abnormal physical findings and diagnostic studies, including x-rays and blood work, show progressive abnormalities in blood gases, liver function, elevated tumor markers, renal function, or cardiac ejection fraction (to name a few examples). For patients living in long-term care facilities, deterioration in parameters measured serially as part of the Minimal Data Set (MDS),

Table 1–1
General Criteria

CLINICAL PROGRESSION OF DISEASE
Multiple hospitalizations, emergency department visits, or increased use of other health care services Serial physician assessments, laboratory or x-ray studies consistent with progressive illness Changes in minimal data set (MDS) for patients in Long-Term Care Facilities Progressive deterioration of the patient while receiving home health care
DECLINING FUNCTIONAL STATUS AS DEFINED BY:

For patients with malignant diseases:
   Karnofsky performance status (KPS) ≤ 50 or ECOG ≥ 3
   KPS ≤ 60 or ECOG ≥ 2 with symptoms
   Decline in KPS of at least 20 units in 2–3 months
 	
For patients with nonmalignant diseases:
   Dependence in at least 3/6 activities of daily living
   KPS or palliative performance scale (PPS) score ≤ 50

DECLINING NUTRITIONAL STATUS AS DEFINED BY:
Unintentional weight loss ≥ 10% of normal body weight and/or BMI < 22 kg/m^2
INTANGIBLE FACTORS
Patient's personal goals, approach to his or her disease, treatment Burden of investigation and treatment versus potential gain for the patient

especially those related to functional status, provide important clues to the clinician regarding changes in the patient's status. Another important source of information is the home health care nurse, who while visiting the patient on a regular basis at home, may note that the patient has

reached a point in the illness when home health nursing visits alone will no longer suffice.

Declining Performance Status

KARNOFSKY PERFORMANCE STATUS (KPS) AND RELATED MEASURES

It was recognized during the earliest phases of cancer chemotherapy development that patients with an imparied functional status would have a poorer prognosis and would not respond as well to chemotherapy as patients with the same malignancy who had better functional status. This led to development of measures of functional status, such as the Karnofsky Performance Status index (KPS), designed in the late 1940s as an adjunctive tool to evaluate the activity levels of patients with cancer who were participating in cancer chemotherapy trials.

The KPS, assessing ambulation, self-care ability, activity level, and evidence of disease, is described in Table 1–2. Studies have demonstrated that there is a rapid fall in KPS of at least 20 to 30 points during the last 2 to 3 months of life and that the median survival of patients with advanced cancer was found to correlate with the KPS rating. It was also demonstrated that patients with active symptoms, including dyspnea, anorexia, weight loss, dry mouth, and difficulty swallowing, have shorter survivals than patients with the same KPS rating who are not symptomatic.

In the field of oncology, other, less complex measures of performance have been developed by such organizations as the Eastern Cooperative Oncology Group (ECOG) and the World Health Organization (WHO). These scales were designed to simplify the rated levels of patient functional status from the 0 to 100 scale of the KPS to a 1 to 4 scale. Because many clinicians are more comfortable with ECOG and WHO scales, while the studies involving performance status as a marker involve the KPS, the ECOG scale is superimposed on the KPS in Table 1–2 for comparison purposes.

One of the limitations of the KPS and the other measures discussed is that they are primarily

Table 1–2

Measures of Performance Status: KPS and ECOG

KPS	KPS-SPECIFIC CRITERIA	ECOG
100	Normal, no complaints or evidence of disease	0
90	Able to carry on normal activity, minor disease symptoms	
80	Normal activity with effort, some disease symptoms	1
70	Cares for self; unable to do normal activity or work	
60	Requires occasional assistance, able to care for most needs	2
50	Requires considerable assistance and frequent medical care	
40	Disable, requires special care and assistance	3
30	Severely disabled, death not imminent	
20	Very ill, active care and attention required continuously	4
10	Moribund	
0	Death	

SOURCE: Adapted from MacDonald N: Principles governing the use of cancer chemotherapy in palliative medicine. In: Doyle D, Hanks GWC, MacDonald N, eds: *Oxford Textbook of Palliative Medicine.* Oxford, Oxford University Press, 1993; p. 105.

designed as an indicator of performance status for patients with malignant disease. To help overcome this limitation, a modification of the KPS, called the palliative performance scale (PPS), has been proposed (Table 1–3). In addition to the activities already measured in the KPS, the PPS assesses the patient characteristics of food/fluid intake and level of consciousness. The utility of the PPS as an indicator of prognosis requires further study, but an initial report did suggest that, in a group of hospice patients admitted to an inpatient setting, PPS ratings directly correlated with short-term prognosis for terminally ill patients with and without cancer.

Based on clinical experience and the information mentioned, it is generally accepted that a KPS or PPS score of 50 or less, or an ECOG score of 2 or higher, is predictive that the patient may have a prognosis of 6 months or less.

ACTIVITIES OF DAILY LIVING

The most common method of assessing the functional status of patients with diagnoses other than cancer is by the evaluation of what are called the activities of daily living (ADLs). The original six activities as described by Katz in the 1960s were bathing, dressing, toileting, transfer, continence, and feeding. A patient's ability to perform each of these activities, with modifications from Katz's original work, continues to be measured routinely in hospitals as well as in long-term care facilities as part of the minimal data set (MDS).

The evaluation of ADLs on a serial basis has been found to be an important indicator of patient prognosis. In a group of elderly patients receiving residential care in Great Britain, patients who had significant ADL deficits had a median survival of 6 months, with a 2-year mortality rate of 80 percent. In a study evaluating various factors as predictors of prognosis in hospitalized elderly patients, regression analysis showed ADL deficits were the most important predictor of 6-month mortality, outranking diagnosis, mental status, and even whether or not the patient required intensive care. Comparison of ADL deficits with Karnofsky performance status (KPS) ratings has shown that patients with a KPS score of 50 typically have dependence in at least three of the six ADLs.

Declining Nutritional Status

Another key indicator of poor prognosis is a decline in a patient's nutritional status. This is best expressed as an *unintentional* weight loss of 10 percent of normal body weight over a period of about 6 months, with the loss of weight usually due to the patient's life-limiting condition. Reversible causes of weight loss, such as depression and metabolic disturbances (diabetes, thyroid disease), should be excluded prior to assuming that

Table 1–3
Palliative Performance Scale (PPS)

PPS RATING	AMBULATION	SELF-CARE	INTAKE	LOC	ACTIVITY	EVIDENCE OF DISEASE
100	Full	Full	Normal	Full	Normal	No evidence of disease
90	Full	Full	Normal	Full	Normal	Some evidence of disease
80	Full	Full	Normal or reduced	Full	Normal with effort	Some evidence of disease
70	Reduced	Full	Normal or reduced	Full	Unable to do normal work	Some evidence of disease
60	Reduced	Occasional assistance	Normal or reduced	Full or confusion	Unable to do hobby or housework	Significant disease
50	Mainly sit/lie	Considerable assistance	Normal or reduced	Full or confusion	Unable to do any work	Extensive disease
40	Mainly in bed	Complete assistance	Normal or reduced	Full, drowsy, or confusion	Unable to do any work	Extensive disease
30	Bed confined	Total care	Reduced	Full, drowsy, or confusion	Unable to do any work	Extensive disease
20	Bed confined	Total care	Minimal sips	Full, drowsy, or confusion	Unable to do any work	Extensive disease
10	Bed confined	Total care	Mouth care only	Drowsy or coma	Unable to do any work	Extensive disease
0	Death					

SOURCE: Adapted from Anderson F, Downing GM, Hill J, et al: Palliative Performance Scale (PPS): A new tool. *J Palliat Care* 12:5, 1996.

the weight loss is due to the terminal illness and a true indicator of the patient's prognosis. (Remember, terminally ill patients may still have reversible causes of weight loss.) For terminally ill patients with reversible cause of weight loss, weight loss will be less helpful in determining prognosis.

Corroborating evidence that a weight loss of 10 percent or more is associated with a poor prognosis can be found in a key study (Murden and Ainsley, 1994) that examined the predictability of weight loss in a group of patients living in a long-term care facility. Of 53 elderly patients who had unintentionally lost 10 percent or more of body weight over 6 months, 62 percent died in the next 6 months, while only 9 percent of 190 patients who had not lost weight died during the same period. In patients with advanced cancer, weight loss has been shown to negatively effect median survival regardless of the primary site of the neoplasm.

Body mass index (BMI) is another useful way to evaluate a patient's nutritional status near the end of life. BMI is a reflection of body weight in relationship to height, and therefore might give a truer picture of the patient's nutritional status than body weight alone. The formula for BMI is:

$$\text{BMI in kg/m}^2 = \frac{703 \times \text{Weight in pounds}}{(\text{Height in inches})^2}$$

(The factor 703 converts lb/in^2 into kg/m^2)

A recent study demonstrated that BMI values less than 22 kg/m² correlated with dependence in Activities of Daily Living as well as with increased mortality rates in elderly patients. It has also been reported that in seriously ill hospitalized patients, those with BMI values less than 20 kg/m² had the highest risk of mortality in the 6 months following hospitalization.

Anthropomorphic measures such as triceps skin fold thickness may be useful indicators of poor nutritional status for patients who are unable to be weighed, and are used by some hospice providers as surrogate measures of weight loss. Studies correlating these measures with patient survival have not been published to date.

Low serum albumins levels have been found to have prognostic significance as well. However, the utility of serum albumin in determining patient prognosis is limited, due that fact that there are nonterminal medical conditions associated with low serum albumin levels, such as nephrotic syndrome and alcoholic liver disease.

Intangible Factors

With the current emphasis on the ethical value of autonomy in health care decision making, it is critical to consider the desires of the patient and/or family when thinking about referring a patient to a hospice or palliative care program near the end of life. In fact, some might consider these factors relatively more important in determining the need of a patient for end-of-life care then the more objective criteria more commonly used to determine prognosis and the need for hospice care.

The physician should consider the potential benefits versus potential burdens of disease evaluation and treatment when discussing therapeutic options with a patient and or family. The physician should work with each patient/family to set realistic and achievable goals, based on the wishes of the patient/family. By approaching patients with advanced illness in this fashion, clinicians, as well as patients and families, will have a better sense of when end-of-life care is the most appropriate therapeutic option.

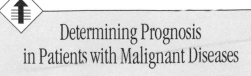

Determining Prognosis in Patients with Malignant Diseases

In spite of the common signs and symptoms that patients demonstrate near the end of life, the differences are significant enough between various illnesses that disease-specific guidelines are necessary to assist clinicians in determining when patients require end-of-life care. For patients with cancer, interest in developing such guidelines has not been particularly great, as there is a sense that physicians who care for cancer patients have a fairly good sense of when a patient is terminally ill. As already noted, the SUPPORT study suggested that physicians predict prognosis of patients with cancer with a relatively high degree of accuracy. That physicians are comfortable referring cancer patients for end-of-life care would also seem to be supported by data from the National Hospice Organization (NHO), which stated that in 1995, 50 percent of patients dying of cancer received hospice care prior to death.

A closer look at the data, however, suggests that all is not as it seems. In its recent position paper entitled "Cancer Care During the Last Phase of Life," the American Society of Clinical Oncology stated that "hospice is a widely available and excellent model for managing of end-of-life care and should be better utilized." To back up that impression, a recent study of data compiled by a large nationwide hospice organization demonstrated the median hospice length of stay of cancer patients was extremely short and getting shorter, falling from 19 days in 1995 to 17 days in 1998. One is, therefore, forced to conclude that although the majority of patients with terminal neoplastic disease are receiving end-of-life care, most are receiving it so late in their clinical course that the full benefits of such services cannot possibly be realized. Therefore, guidelines that would help oncologists and other physicians caring for cancer patients direct those patients to a hospice or palliative care program earlier would seem to be most beneficial.

Guidelines to help clinicians specifically identify when patients with malignant disease are in need of end-of-life care must take several factors into account. These factors include the stage of disease, natural history of the illness, and potential responsiveness of the specific malignancy to the multiple modalities of antineoplastic therapy available today.

Stage of disease as a prognostic factor is fairly straightforward. Cancer patients who require hospice or palliative care generally suffer from advanced disease, which is defined as metastatic spread of the malignancy from the primary site to other areas of the body and/or massive tumor growth at the primary site.

To define the prognostic factors of natural history and responsiveness to antineoplastic therapies is much more complex, as there is a wide spectrum of variation in these factors between different neoplasms as well as between subtypes of the same malignant illness. To address this, a classification system of common neoplastic diseases has been proposed, dividing the malignancies into five categories based upon their natural history and responsiveness to treatment in patients with advanced (stage IV) disease. This classification system will be presented next, with the cancers in each category listed in tabular form, and with a short discussion of the characteristics that neoplasms within each category share. More detailed descriptions of specific neoplasms and their applicable therapies are beyond the scope of this chapter, and the interested reader is referred to any up-to-date oncology text for further information.

Category I

The malignancies in category I are listed in Table 1–4. These diseases represent some of the greatest successes in medical oncology, curable in the majority of patients, even when they present with advanced metastatic disease. Treatment of these illnesses, even when far advanced at the time of patient presentation, should be strongly encouraged.

The only exception to this might be the elderly patient with multiple comorbid conditions that would preclude intensive therapy. Patients who require end-of-life care with one of these illnesses will generally have a lengthy medical history inclusive of extensive antineoplastic therapy, and will be suffering from advanced metastatic disease that is now resistant to further disease-directed treatment.

Table 1–4
Category I: Treatable, High or Moderate Expectation of Cure

MALIGNANCIES	CHARACTERISTICS
Testicular carcinoma Choriocarcinoma and trophoblastic malignancy Childhood acute lymphoblastic leukemia Other pediatric malignancies Acute promyelocytic leukemia Hodgkin's disease	Stage IV Cure potential high to moderate End-of-life care indicated when there is disease progression after extensive anti-neoplastic therapy

SOURCE: Adapted from Kinzbrunner BM: The terminally ill patient. In: Abeloff MD, Armitage JO, Lichter AS, Niederhuber JE, eds: *Clinical Oncology.* New York, Churchill Livingstone, 2nd ed., 2000, p. 597.

Category II

The category II malignancies listed in Table 1–5 share the characteristic of being relatively sensitive to antineoplastic therapy, with complete remission rates, even in the face of stage IV disease, of 60 percent or higher. Although many of the patients who attain a complete remission relapse within 1 to 2 years of treatment, approximately 20 percent of patients remain without evidence of disease on a long-term basis, and are possibly considered cured. With the potential for cure, or of substantial improvement in both quality of life and length of life even if cure is impossible, treatment in most circumstances should be encouraged (providing that therapy is not contraindicated by comorbid medical conditions). For patients who do not achieve a complete remission from first-line antineoplastic therapy, or who develop recurrent cancer following a complete remission, there may be benefits to second-line therapy, especially in ovarian carcinoma, the acute leukemias, and the aggressive lymphomas. In general, however, cure is not possible once the illness has recurred. End-of-life care may be appropriate for patients with one of these malignancies when there is evidence of progressive metastatic disease following first or second-line therapy (depending upon the illness).

Table 1–5
Category II: Treatable, High Probability of Complete Remission, Low Probability of Cure

MALIGNANCY	CHARACTERISTICS

Ovarian carcinoma
Adult acute myeloblastic leukemia and
   acute lymphoblastic leukemia
Intermediate and high-grade non-Hodgkin's
   lymphoma
Small cell (oat cell) bronchogenic carcinoma
	Stage IV
	Cure potential low
	Remission potential high to moderate
	Antineoplastic therapy in stage IV disease improves
	   quality and length of life
	End-of-life care indicated when there is disease
	   progression following first or second-line therapy
	   (depending upon the illness)

SOURCE: Adapted from Kinzbrunner BM: The terminally ill patient. In: Abeloff MD, Armitage JO, Lichter AS, Niederhuber JE, eds: *Clinical Oncology.* New York, Churchill Livingstone, 2nd ed., 2000, p. 597.

Category III

The malignancies in category III (Table 1–6) present the most challenges in deciding when end-of-life care is necessary. For patients who develop one of these diseases, while cure is generally not an option once the illness has spread beyond the confines of the primary site, there are numerous effective antineoplastic treatment options available. Hormonal agents such as tamoxifen in breast cancer and luprolide in prostate cancer, and oral chemotherapeutic agents such as chlorambucil and alkeran in the hematologic malignancies listed in Table 1–6, are efficacious, easily administered to patients, and are generally well tolerated, even by the elderly and infirm. Some clinicians would even advocate not treating stage IV patients until symptoms occur, as there is no strong evidence that treatment in the absence of symptoms improves survival. The life expectancy of patients with these illnesses is generally measured in years, and varies based upon the specific disease.

Therefore, end-of-life care for patients with one of the malignancies in this category is indicated in the face of disease progression only after the patient has been treated with at least one or more often with several different antineoplastic therapeutic regimens (dependant upon the specific diagnosis), and the malignancy has become resistant to further antineoplastic therapy.

Category IV

The malignancies in category IV (Table 1–7) consist of the majority of adult solid tumors. However one chooses to interpret the current state of the art in the treatment of these cancers, the sobering facts are that once these diseases have metastasized they are incurable. Additionally, although some patients who suffer from a malignancy in this category will benefit from systemic antineoplastic therapy, for the fewer than 50 percent of patients who do have a response to treatment, that response is generally short lived and has little effect on long-term survival.

It is proposed that for these patients, end-of-life care be considered not when available treatment has been exhausted, but as an initial therapeutic option, focusing on symptom control and quality of life rather than on disease control. Viewing hospice and palliative care as a therapeutic option is not meant to exclude antineoplastic treatments. Rather, this approach is meant to reframe

Table 1–6

Category III: Treatable, Incurable when Metastatic, Favorable Prognosis

MALIGNANCY	CHARACTERISTICS
Prostate carcinoma	Stage IV
Breast carcinoma	Incurable
Chronic lymphocytic leukemia	Remission potential high to moderate
Chronic mylocytic leukemia and the myeloproliferative disorders	Indolent course with a long prognosis
Low-grade non-Hodgkin's lymphoma	Antineoplastic therapy may be relatively side-effect free (e.g., oral hormonal therapy)
Multiple Myeloma and the immunoproliferative disorders	End-of-life care indicated when there is evidence of disease progression after one or multiple regimens
Myelodysplastic syndrome	(dependent upon specific disease) of standard
Thyroid carcinoma (except anaplastic)	antineoplastic therapy

SOURCE: Adapted from Kinzbrunner BM: The terminally ill patient. In: Abeloff MD, Armitage JO, Lichter AS, Niederhuber JE, eds: *Clinical Oncology*. New York, Churchill Livingstone, 2nd ed., 2000, p. 597.

Table 1–7
Category IV: Treatable in a Minority of Patients with Metastatic Disease, Less Favorable Prognosis

MALIGNANCY	CHARACTERISTICS
Bladder carcinoma	Stage IV
Primary brain tumors	Incurable
Glioblastoma	
Grade III astrocytoma	Responses to therapy in < 50% of patients
Gynecological malignancies other than ovary	Short prognosis even after response to first-line chemotherapy
Colorectal carcinoma	End-of-life care should be presented as a therapeutic
Non-small-cell bronchogenic carcinoma	option to patients alongside second-line
Squamous-cell carcinoma	chemotherapy and for patients with poor
Adenocarcinoma	performance status (KPS ≤ 50 or EKOG ≤ 2),
Large-cell carcinoma	alongside first-line chemotherapy
Bronchoalveolar carcinoma	
Head and neck carcinomas	
Esophageal carcinoma	
Gastric carcinoma	
Pancreatic carcinoma	
Soft-tissue sarcomas	

SOURCE: Adapted from Kinzbrunner BM: The terminally ill patient. In: Abeloff MD, Armitage JO, Lichter AS, Niederhuber JE, eds: *Clinical Oncology*. New York, Churchill Livingstone, 2nd ed., 2000, p. 597.

end-of-life care in a more positive light. By allowing patients (and their physicians) to view hospice and palliative care as a treatment choice, *hope* of symptom control and quality of life can replace the perception that end-of-life care should be reserved only for those patients for whom there is no longer effective antineoplastic treatment available.

Category V

The illnesses listed in Table 1–8 are among the most frustrating to oncologists. Standard antineoplastic therapy for patients with advanced stages of these malignancies is ineffective in virtually all patients treated. Some of these patients, especially those who are relatively young and have good

Table 1–8
Category V: Generally Unresponsive to Standard Therapy

MALIGNANCY	CHARACTERISTICS
Renal cell carcinoma	Stage IV
Malignant melanoma	Incurable
Hepatobiliary and gall bladder carcinoma	Generally unresponsive to standard therapy
Adrenal carcinoma	Patients who qualify may consider investigational therapy
AIDS-associated high-grade lymphoma	End-of-life care may be the treatment of choice for this group of patients, unless they qualify for and desire investigational therapy

SOURCE: Adapted from Kinzbrunner BM: The terminally ill patient. In: Abeloff MD, Armitage JO, Lichter AS, Niederhuber JE, eds: *Clinical Oncology*. New York, Churchill Livingstone, 2nd ed., 2000, p. 597.

performance status, may be interested in and should be considered for investigational treatment. However, for the vast majority of patients suffering from one of these neoplasms, end-of-life care should be considered as a treatment option at the time metastatic disease is identified. Some would even suggest that hospice and palliative care would be the treatment of choice in this group of individuals.

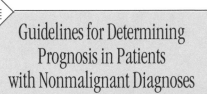

Guidelines for Determining Prognosis in Patients with Nonmalignant Diagnoses

Although hospice and palliative care originated with the cancer model, it became apparent toward the end of the 1980s that patients with diagnoses other than cancer had special end-of-life needs that could be met by the interdisciplinary care that hospices provide. Elderly patients with relatively common chronic debilitating illness such as chronic obstructive pulmonary disease, congestive heart failure, and Alzheimer's disease, as well as younger patients with AIDS, began to find their way onto hospice programs in ever-increasing numbers. As hospice programs began caring for these patients, it became clear that the clinical course of these patients differed from their counterparts with malignant disease. For while cancer patients generally had a progressive downhill course, patients with nonmalignant diagnoses were observed to have much more variable disease progression, with periods of severe symptoms intermingled with periods of relative stability.

The variable clinical course of patients with nonmalignant disease was, not surprisingly, perceived as a major challenge to predicting when these patients would require hospice or palliative care. Detailed analysis of 1990 Medicare claims data cited earlier showed that of the 15 percent of patients surviving on hospice programs more than 6 months, the majority had noncancer diag-

noses. Although, as already noted, the SUPPORT study demonstrated that physicians did a good job predicting the prognosis of patients with malignant disease, the same could not be said for the ability of physicians to estimate when patients with illnesses other than cancer were likely to die.

The heightened degree of uncertainty in predicting when patients with nonmalignant diseases require end-of-life care mandated the development of clinical guidelines in this area. Articles attempting to delineate such guidelines began to appear in the medical literature toward the end of the 1980s and into the 1990s. Crystallizing the information contained in these and other articles led, in 1995, to the development by the National Hospice Organization of "Medical Guidelines for the Determining Prognosis in Selected Non-Cancer Diseases." The document included "General Guidelines," which in large part form the basis of the general guidelines discussed earlier, and specific guidelines for determining when patients with heart disease, lung disease, and dementia would be in need of end-of-life care. A second edition of this document published in 1996 added other non-cancer illnesses, including stroke and coma, renal disease, liver disease, amyotrophic lateral sclerosis, and HIV.

The criteria for determining when patients with the various nonmalignant diseases require end-of-life care will be reviewed. As with the earlier discussion of malignant disease, a list of the disease-specific criteria will be presented in tabular form, and also a short discussion of the criteria, with corroboration from the medical literature where appropriate.

End-Stage Lung Disease

Knowing when patients with COPD, pulmonary fibrosis, or other forms of end-stage lung disease require end-of-life and hospice care can be exceedingly challenging. This is because the clinical course of patients with advanced pulmonary disease usually consists of periods of relatively stable disease punctuated by episodic acute decompensation. It is clear, however, that as time progresses, the acute episodes become more frequent and the periods of stability become the exception rather than the rule. At such a time in the course of illness of a patient with advanced pulmonary disease, interventions by a hospice or palliative care interdisciplinary team can be invaluable. Guidelines that help determine when it is time to consider end-of-life care for patients with COPD and other forms of end-stage pulmonary disease are listed in Table 1–9 and are described next.

DISABLING DYSPNEA

Studies in the pulmonary literature have identified many factors that affect the mortality of patients with COPD, with the most important being

Table 1–9
Criteria for Hospice Care in End-Stage Lung Disease

DISABLING DYSPNEA DEFINED BY THE FOLLOWING:
Dyspnea at rest or with minimal exertion
Dyspnea poorly responsive or unresponsive to bronchodilator therapy
Dyspnea results in other debilitating symptoms such as decreased functional activity, fatigue, and cough
FEV-1 < 30% predicted post-bronchodilator, if available

PROGRESSION IN PULMONARY DISEASE AS MANIFESTED BY:
Multiple hospitalizations, emergency department visits, or doctor's office visits.
Cor pulmonale

OTHER INDICATORS OF POOR PROGNOSIS:
Body weight ≤ 90% of ideal body weight, or ≥ 10% loss of weight
Resting tachycardia > 100/min
Abnormal blood gases, if available
po_2 ≤ 55 mm Hg or o_2 saturation ≤ 88%
pco_2 ≥ 50 mm Hg
Continuous oxygen therapy

SOURCE: Stuart B, Connor S, Kinzbrunner BM, et al: *Medical Guidelines for Determining Prognosis in Selected Non-cancer Diseases.* Arlington, National Hospice Organization, 2nd ed., 1996.

age, postbronchodilator FEV-1, total lung capacity, maximal work capacity of the patient, and resting heart rate. Age and resting heart rate (Table 1–9) are both easy to measure and correlate directly with patient mortality, while decreases in total lung capacity, maximal work capacity, and postbronchodilator FEV-1 are associated with a poor prognosis. Measures of total lung capacity and maximal work capacity that specifically predict a poor prognosis have not been reported. However, it has been demonstrated that postbronchodilator FEV-1 values consistently under 30 percent of predicted values are associated with the highest mortality rate in COPD patients.

As stated in the introduction to the general guidelines, it is not appropriate to force patients to undergo objective testing in order to ensure that they receive needed end-of-life care. Therefore, it was necessary to translate these specific objective parameters into more easily accessible clinical terms. Hence, a poor total lung capacity may be represented by the criterion of disabling dyspnea at rest or with minimal exertion, a postbronchodilator FEV-1 value less than 30 percent of that predicted reflects unresponsiveness or poor responsiveness to bronchodilators, and a highly impaired maximal work capacity may be manifested by decreased functional activity and fatigue. The importance of the clinical interpretation of these objective parameters in assessing patient prognosis is underscored by a study (Aida, et al, 1994) that demonstrated that patients with higher degrees of subjective dyspnea, regardless of pulmonary function studies, had significantly shorter survival times than patients who were less symptomatic.

PROGRESSION IN PULMONARY DISEASE

Progression of disease is an important parameter of poor prognosis. This may be manifested objectively, as it has been demonstrated that persistent and significant decreases in FEV-1 measured serially over several years portends a poor prognosis. More importantly, on a clinical level, as patients with COPD worsen, they generally develop more frequent episodes of acute bronchitis and pneumonia, requiring more attention from health care providers. Therefore, as already mentioned in the general criteria, an increase in the frequency of doctor's office visits, emergency room trips, and hospital admissions is highly indicative that the patient's illness is progressing and that end of life care interventions may be beneficial.

COR PULMONALE

The development of pulmonary hypertension resulting in failure of the right side of the heart, termed cor pulmonale, is associated with increased mortality in patients with COPD. Studies have shown that 50 percent of patients with COPD and cor pulmonale succumb to their illness in 1 to 3 years, and that patients with cor pulmonale and COPD are 50 percent more likely to die in a 2½-year period than COPD patients without cor pulmonale.

OTHER INDICATORS OF POOR PROGNOSIS

There are several other important characteristics of patients with advanced pulmonary disease that may be predictive of a poor prognosis. Patients with COPD who weigh less than 90 percent of ideal body weight have a shorter overall survival than patients with similar levels of pulmonary function impairment whose weight is either at or exceeds ideal body weight. The presence of a resting tachycardia above 100/min is another important sign that the patient's COPD may be at an end stage, and the measurement of po_2, oxygen saturation, and pco_2 may be helpful as well. Generally, patients with a poor prognosis have po_2 levels of 55 mm Hg or less, and/or an oxygen saturation as measured by pulse oximetry of 88 percent or less. It is also generally accepted that patients who chronically have pco_2 levels greater than 50 mm Hg have a poor prognosis, although patients with primarily emphysematous disease may have a poor prognosis in the absence of hypercapnea (discussed next).

Patients with advanced COPD often require continuous or long-term oxygen therapy. Patients on continuous oxygen therapy who are unable to elevate their po_2 above 65 mm Hg despite the oxygen therapy have a poor prognosis. Other clinical indicators of a poor prognosis in this group of patients include patients with severe bronchial obstruction, increasing age, and the presence of chest wall abnormalities. Finally, as alluded to earlier, patients who require continuous oxygen therapy and have normal or low pco_2 levels have the highest mortality among this group of patients.

End-Stage Cardiac Disease

DISABLING DYSPNEA OR CHEST PAIN

The principles for determining when patients with end-stage cardiac disease require end-of-life care, found in Table 1–10, are actually similar to those for determining prognosis of patients with advanced pulmonary disease. In other words, these are patients who have symptoms of either con-

Table 1–10

Criteria for Hospice Care in End-stage Cardiac Disease

DISABLING DYSPNEA OR CHEST PAIN AS DEFINED BY:
Dyspnea or chest pain with rest or minimal exertion (NYHA class IV)   Ejection fraction ≤ 20%, if available   Persistent symptoms despite optimal medical management with vasodilators and diuretics, or   Inability to tolerate optimal medical management due to hypotension and/or renal failure
OTHER COMORBID CONDITION ASSOCIATED WITH A POOR PROGNOSIS
Symptomatic arrhythmias resistant to antiarrhythmic therapy   History of cardiac arrest and resuscitation   History of syncope, regardless of etiology   Cardiogenic brain embolism   Concomitant HIV disease

SOURCE: Stuart B, Connor S, Kinzbrunner BM, et al: *Medical Guidelines for Determining Prognosis in Selected Non-cancer Diseases*. Arlington, National Hospice Organization, 2nd ed., 1996.

gestive heart failure or unstable angina pectoris at rest or with minimal exertion, and can therefore be classified as New York Heart Association class IV. Additionally, these patients are so severely ill that they either no longer respond to optimal medical management, including diuretics and vasodilators, or can no longer tolerate the medications due to intolerable side effects such as hypotension and renal failure.

For patients with end-stage congestive heart failure, corroborating objective evidence of a terminal prognosis would be an ejection fraction of 20 percent or less, based upon a study that demonstrated that such patients had a median survival of 12 weeks, and a 75 percent mortality rate at 6 months. However, as already noted, clinical evidence of persistent disease far outweighs the importance of ejection fraction, as demonstrated in a study (Marantz, et al, 1992) showing that the presence of clinical congestive heart failure was a more sensitive predictor of mortality than the numerical value for ejection fraction.

OTHER COMORBID CONDITIONS ASSOCIATED WITH A POOR PROGNOSIS

Patients with end-stage cardiac disease who either suffer from or have experienced one or more of the comorbid conditions listed in Table 1–10 are likely candidates for a hospice or palliative care program.

End-Stage Neurologic Diseases

For the purpose of determining patient prognosis near the end of life, end-stage neurologic diseases have been divided into three major subgroups: Alzheimer's disease and other dementias, cerebrovascular disease, and amyotrophic lateral sclerosis (ALS) and related motor neuron disorders.

ALZHEIMER'S DISEASE AND OTHER DEMENTIAS

COGNITIVE DISORDER CONSISTENT WITH FAST 7 Guidelines for determining when patients with

Alzheimer's and other dementias require end-of-life care can be found in Table 1–11. Recognition that patients with Alzheimer's disease and other dementias required hospice and/or palliative care services near the end of life was first recognized in the 1980s. It was proposed that patients be stratified into one of five levels of care based

Table 1–11

Criteria for Hospice Care in End-Stage Alzheimer's Disease and Other Dementias

PATIENT HAS A COGNITIVE DISORDER CONSISTENT WITH FAST 7, AS MANIFESTED BY:
Inability to ambulate without assistance Inability to speak or communicate meaningfully with speech limited to approximately a half-dozen or fewer intelligible or different words Loss of ADL functions including bathing and dressing (Stage 6) Incontinence of bowel and bladder (Stage 6)
PATIENT HAS HAD ONE OR MORE OF THE FOLLOWING COMORBID CONDITIONS IN LAST 3–6 MONTHS:

Aspiration pneumonia
Pyelonephritis or upper urinary tract infection
Septicemia
Decubitus ulcers, usually multiple and stages III or IV
Fever, recurrent after antibiotics
An altered nutritional status as manifested by:
    Difficulty swallowing or refusal to eat such that sufficient fluid or caloric intake cannot be maintained and the patient refuses artificial nutritional support
    OR
    If the patient is receiving artificial nutritional support (NG or G tube or parenteral hyperalimentation), there must be evidence of an impaired nutritional status as defined in the General Guidelines (≥ 10% loss of body weight)

SOURCE: Stuart B, Connor S, Kinzbrunner BM, et al: *Medical Guidelines for Determining Prognosis in Selected Non-cancer Diseases.* Arlington, National Hospice Organization, 2nd ed., 1996.

upon the stage of patient's illness, and upon the wishes of the patient and family regarding future care. The various levels of care proposed represented points on a continuum, with levels 4 and 5, and perhaps at times level 3, all being consistent with needing some degree of hospice and palliative care. The challenge for the clinician caring for such patients was, not surprisingly, knowing when a patient's dementia was severe enough to warrant a shift in the philosophy of care to that of palliation.

Enter the functional assessment staging classification (FAST), published by Reisberg in 1986. This classification of Alzheimer's dementia defines seven stages, paralleling normal human development in reverse, with a spectrum ranging from patients with no perceptible mental status changes (stage 1) to patients who are so severely demented that they lose their ability to ambulate, speak, sit up, and even smile (stage 7). It was believed that a patient who exhibited the characteristics defined as FAST stage 7-C, the loss of ambulatory ability in a patient who was unable to communicate meaningfully and who required assistance in all activities of daily living, was a good candidate for hospice services. These criteria were formally adopted by the NHO in 1995, and are listed in Table 1–11.

It should be emphasized that inability to ambulate without assistance appears to be the key functional deficit that identifies patients who are in need of end-of-life care. Inability to ambulate should not be confused with a bed-bound status, and includes patients who can be lifted into and sit in a chair with support, or who can even walk short distances with support from caregivers. The other important criteria are those that define stages 7-A and 7-B, namely loss of intelligible speech and meaningful communication. However, it should be noted that some patients do not progress consecutively through the substages of stage 7, and may on occasion lose the ability to ambulate prior to the loss of their communication skills. These patients should still be considered eligible for hospice or palliative care services, although, as will be discussed, their prognosis is somewhat more variable than patients who progress ordinally through the stage 7 substages.

ONE OR MORE COMORBID CONDITIONS IN LAST 3 TO 6 MONTHS   It is well known from clinical experience that patients with advanced dementia, even those far advanced enough to quality as FAST 7-C, may live for many months or even years. What usually determines mortality in this group of patients is the presence of one or more comorbid conditions, especially those related to the loss of functional status, namely infection and decubitus ulcers, or related to a deteriorating nutritional status.

Patients with advanced dementias are highly susceptible to a number of infectious illnesses. Aspiration pneumonia, either due to the difficulty swallowing or the presence of a feeding tube (either NG or gastrostomy), is a common problem, and is associated with an increase in patient mortality at 6 months. These patients are also more likely to develop recurrent upper urinary tract infections and episodes of septicemia requiring antibiotic therapy on an intermittent but recurring basis. Such recurrent febrile episodes in this population are not only associated with an increased mortality rate, but studies have shown that the mortality is unaffected by the decision to treat such patients with antibiotics. Based on this and follow-up studies, it has been suggested, because patients have been shown to be more comfortable and less distressed when not treated with antibiotics, that they be avoided in this group of patients.

Decubitus ulcers are another significant comorbid factor in this group of patients. Fifty percent of patients admitted to nursing homes with multiple stage III and/or stage IV decubiti, and 38 percent of patients who develop such decubiti within 3 months of nursing home admission, die within 1 year.

Altered nutritional status is a significant comorbid condition in this group of patients as well. Patients who lose the ability to eat secondary to dementias and/or other neurologic conditions have a higher mortality rate whether or not they receive nutritional support via artificial means. Patients who have elected, based either upon advance directives or the instructions of durable powers of attorney, not to receive artificial nutritional support have an increased mortality rate either secondary to the inability to sustain themselves calorically or due to the increased risk of aspiration pneumonia if oral feedings are continued. For patients who have elected artificial nutritional support, studies have demonstrated increased morbidity and increased mortality as well, especially if they continue to lose weight following initiation of the feedings. (For a full discussion of this topic, see Chapter 16.) Therefore, patients with advanced dementia who are losing weight and either do not elect artificial nutritional support or are losing weight in spite of artificial nutritional support are likely candidates for end-of-life care. (The reader should be reminded that these comorbid factors are not mutually exclusive. For example, patients who are being artificially fed and are maintaining weight, may be eligible for hospice and palliative care if they suffer from frequent infections and/or multiple decubiti.)

PROGNOSTIC ACCURACY OF DEMENTIA GUIDELINES   A study designed to test the accuracy of the guidelines for determining the prognosis of patients with end-stage dementia was published in 1997. This study validated the importance of comorbid factors, especially related to nutritional status, in determining prognosis in these patients. The subgroup of patients who presented with classical FAST 7-C or beyond had a median survival of significantly less than 6 months whether or not they received traditional medical interventions for acute illnesses (such as antibiotics for febrile episodes). Patients who were more cognitively intact than stage 7-C had a median survival of almost 2 years. A third subgroup of patients identified in this study, and alluded to earlier, were patients who did not progress consecutively through the substages of stage 7, losing, for example, the ability to ambulate prior to the loss of their communication skills. Interestingly, these patients succumbed to their illness in a median time of less than 6 months if they did not receive traditional medical interventions for acute illnesses,

while they survived a median of almost 15 months if they did receive such intervention. Therefore, in addition to confirming the importance of stage 7-C and the presence of comorbid conditions in determining the need for end-of-life care in patients with Alzheimer's disease and other dementias, the study suggests that patients who exhibit some, but not all, characteristics of stage 7-C might be appropriate for hospice and palliative care, especially if they elect comfort measures rather than traditional medical interventions for intercurrent illnesses.

CEREBROVASCULAR DISEASE

Guidelines for determining when patients with advanced cerebrovascular disease require end-of-life care are listed in Table 1–12. There have been two distinct categories of patients identified: those who have recently suffered a severe acute neurologic event, and those who are experiencing the debility and aftereffects of chronic cerebrovascular disease.

ACUTE CEREBROVASCULAR DISEASE AND COMA   In considering the question of when a patient who has just experienced an acute cerebrovascular event, or has become comatose due to another cause, might need hospice or palliative care, it is important to first allow such patients some time for recovery. It is well known that patients who appear moribund or comatose during the first few hours or first day following an acute neurologic insult, may often, with proper support and rehabilitation, go on to a meaningful recovery. Based on a report from the SUPPORT investigators, it would appear that patients who suffered from acute cerebrovascular attacks or became comatose from other causes (such as cardiac arrest) had a high mortality rate if they did not show signs of recovering neurologic function within 3 days of the acute insult. Persistent neurologic deficits associated with the highest risk of mortality after day 3 included a decerebrate response to external stimuli, absent verbal response, and absent withdrawal response to pain. Older patients

Table 1–12

Criteria for Hospice Care in Cerebrovascular Disease

ACUTE CEREBROVASCULAR DISEASE AND COMA
Patient has one of the following conditions for at least *3 days* duration: 　Coma 　Persistent vegetative state 　Severe obtundation accompanied by myoclonus 　Postanoxic stroke Other factors associated with a high risk of mortality after 3 days (Hamel et al, 1995) 　Abnormal brainstem response 　Absent verbal response 　Absent withdrawal response to pain 　Serum creatinine ≥ 1.5 mg/dL 　Age ≥ 70 years
CHRONIC CEREBROVASCULAR DISEASE, COMA, AND PERSISTENT VEGETATIVE STATE (PVS)
Poststroke or multi-infarct dementia consistent with FAST 7, if patient not comatose or in PVS Patient has had one or more of the following comorbid conditions in the last 3–6 months: 　Aspiration pneumonia 　Pyelonephritis or upper urinary tract infection 　Septicemia 　Decubitus ulcers, usually multiple and stages III or IV 　Fever, recurrent after antibiotics 　An altered nutritional status as manifested by: 　　Difficulty swallowing or refusal to eat such that sufficient fluid or caloric intake cannot be maintained and the patient refuses artificial nutritional support 　　OR 　　If the patient is receiving artificial nutritional support (NG or G tube or parenteral hyperalimentation), there must be evidence of an impaired nutritional status as defined in the General Guidelines (≥ 10% loss of body weight)

SOURCE: Stuart B, Connor S, Kinzbrunner BM, et al: *Medical Guidelines for Determining Prognosis in Selected Non-cancer Diseases.* Arlington, National Hospice Organization, 2nd ed., 1996.

(age ≥ 70 years) and patients with renal function impairment (serum creatinine ≥ 1.5 mg/dL) were also associated with a poor prognosis. In fact, patients who exhibited four of the five factors after day 3 had a 97 percent probability of succumbing to their illnesses within 2 months.

CHRONIC CEREBROVASCULAR DISEASE　For patients with chronic cerebrovascular disease, long-standing coma, or persistent vegetative state (PVS), criteria that assist in determining that end-of-life care is necessary closely resemble those for dementia, as outlined in Table 1–12. Patients who are not in coma or in a PVS will usually have signs of multi-infarct dementia, with deficits in functional activity that closely resemble FAST 7. For all patients, comorbid conditions such as recent infections, decubiti, or a deteriorating nutritional status, the same criteria described for patients with long-standing terminal dementia, would serve as additional indicators for a poor prognosis.

AMYOTROPHIC LATERAL SCLEROSIS AND OTHER FORMS OF MOTOR NEURON DISEASE

Predicting the prognosis of patients with amyotrophic lateral sclerosis (ALS) (also known as Lou Gehrig's disease) and other forms of motor neuron disease may be very challenging. Patients tend to be younger and, with nutritional and/or ventilatory support, can live for extended periods of time, measured in years, even in the face of severe neurologic dysfunction. In today's high-tech society, patients who can do little more than blink their eyelids communicate and lead productive lives with computer aids and other technologic supports.

Despite these great scientific advances, however, there are patients afflicted with ALS who, as their neurologic condition deteriorates, would not choose to become dependent on feeding tubes, ventilators, or computers. For these patients, end-of-life care would become a serious option, especially when the ability of such patients to either swallow or breathe independently becomes significantly impaired.

Clinical characteristics of ALS make the timing of decisions regarding end-of-life care somewhat difficult. It has been shown that, although ALS does progress over time, the rate of neurologic deterioration varies markedly from patient to patient. Additionally, the location of the first muscles involved has not been shown to correlate with survival.

What seems to correlate most with short survival of patients with ALS is the development of "rapid progression," which is outlined in Table 1–13 and basically defined as the development of severe neurologic disability within a 12-month period. In addition to rapid progression, patients who have a limited prognosis and are in need of hospice or palliative care generally will have a critically impaired ventilatory status, significant nutritional impairment, or other life-threatening complications that bear a striking resemblance to the comorbid conditions compatible with poor

Table 1–13

Criteria for Hospice Care in Amyotrophic Lateral Sclerosis (ALS) and other Motor Neuron Diseases

RAPID PROGRESSION OF ALS
Development of severe neurologic disability over a 12-month period. Examples include:
Progression from independent ambulation to wheelchair or bed bound
Progression from normal to barely intelligible or unintelligible speech
Progression from normal to blenderized diet
Progression from independence in most or all ADLs to needing major assistance in all ADLs
CRITICALLY IMPAIRED VENTILATORY CAPACITY
Vital capacity < 30% predicted
Significant dyspnea at rest
Supplemental oxygen needed at rest
Refusal by patient of intubation, tracheostomy, other forms of mechanical ventilatory support
Note: If patient is already on some form of ventilatory support, he or she may still be appropriate for hospice or palliative care management if he or she exhibits one or more comorbid conditions as delineated below.
CRITICAL NUTRITIONAL IMPAIRMENT
Difficulty swallowing or refusal to eat such that sufficient fluid or caloric intake cannot be maintained and the patient refuses artificial nutritional support
OR
If the patient is receiving artificial nutritional support, the patient should be experiencing continued weight loss despite the feedings.
COMORBID CONDITIONS
Aspiration pneumonia
Pyelonephritis or upper urinary tract infection
Septicemia
Decubitus ulcers, usually multiple and stages III or IV
Fever, recurrent after antibiotics

SOURCE: Stuart B, Connor S, Kinzbrunner BM, et al. *Medical Guidelines for Determining Prognosis in Selected Non-cancer Diseases.* Arlington, National Hospice Organization, 2nd ed., 1996

prognosis of patients with dementias and cerebrovascular disease.

End-Stage AIDS

Access to end-of-life care for patients suffering from HIV infection and AIDS has been variable throughout the years since the syndrome was first described in the early 1980s. During the decade of the 1980s, due in part to the relative youth of the majority of patients infected with HIV virus, it was unusual to see patients with AIDS in hospice programs except during the last week or two of life. As a better understanding of AIDS was acquired, markers for poor prognosis became available. Hospices, sensing the fact that patients with AIDS tended to avoid end-of-life care because of their relative youth, developed end-of-life care programs that deemphasized the terminal nature of the illness, while giving such patients the same compassionate interdisciplinary care that patients with more traditional advanced illnesses were receiving. These two factors led to increasing numbers of patients with AIDS accessing hospice and palliative care programs for significantly longer periods of time prior to death.

At the start of the new century, the nature of HIV infection and AIDS has shifted once again. The development of new antiretroviral agents, specifically the protease inhibitors, and the ability to better control opportunistic infections, has shifted AIDS from a terminal illness to a chronic one. Patients are now living for years, as contrasted to several years ago when they would have only survived months. This has significantly decreased the number of patients who use hospice and other palliative care services, albeit for the right reasons. Nevertheless, there are patients with advanced AIDS who still require end-of-life care, hence, and guidelines are needed to determine when this is necessary.

The guidelines for determining when patients with AIDS require end-of-life care can be found in Table 1–14. Unlike most of the other illnesses discussed, where laboratory studies are helpful but not required, measurements of CD4$^+$ count and HIV RNA (viral load) are crucial to determining when patients with AIDS require end-of-life care. Patients with either CD4$^+$ counts below 25 cells/μL, especially during periods free of acute illness, or persistent HIV RNA levels above 100,000 copies, are likely to have a prognosis of less than 6 months. Conversely, patients with CD4$^+$ counts above 50 cells/μL clearly have a prognosis much longer than 6 months unless they have a non-HIV illness that is life threatening or terminal. Patients who have viral loads of below 100,000 may be candidates for end-of-life care only if they elect to forego antiretroviral therapy, other forms of prophylactic therapy, have a declining functional status, and suffer from an HIV-related illness or exhibit one or more poor prognostic factors as listed in Table 1–14.

There are a number of life-limiting infections and malignancies associated with HIV infection that may dictate a need for a palliative plan of care. These illnesses, as well as their approximate prognoses, are delineated in Table 1–14. Other factors that predict a poor prognosis in patients with AIDS include low serum albumin, advancing age, persistent diarrhea, and concomitant heart disease.

End-Stage Renal Disease

Criteria indicating terminal prognosis for patients with end-stage renal disease can be found in Table 1–15. Patients with chronic renal failure who should be considered for end-of-life care include those who are candidates for hemodialysis, peritoneal dialysis, and/or renal transplant but choose not to be dialyzed or receive a transplant. Another subset of patients with renal failure that might benefit from hospice and palliative care would be those who have been undergoing dialysis and either decide to stop or become too ill to tolerate dialysis any longer. Patients who are still being dialyzed, but are considering stopping due to a perceived poor quality of life, pose an interesting dilemma for hospice programs. Clearly,

Table 1–14

Criteria for Hospice Care in AIDS

CD4+ COUNT < 25 CELLS/μL IN PERIODS FREE OF ACUTE ILLNESS
OR
HIV RNA (VIRAL LOAD) > 100,000 COPIES ON A PERSISTENT BASIS
HIV RNA (VIRAL LOAD) < 100,000 COPIES IN THE PRESENCE OF:
Patient refusal to receive antiretroviral or prophylactic medications Declining functional status One or more "other factors" listed below

HIV-RELATED OPPORTUNISTIC ILLNESSES	
Disease	**Prognosis**
CNS lymphoma	2.5 months
Progressive multifocal leukoencephalopathy	4 months
Cryptosporidiosis	5 months
AIDS wasting syndrome (loss of ⅓ lean body mass)	< 6 months
MAC bacteremia, untreated	< 6 months
Visceral Kaposi's sarcoma, unresponsive to treatment	50% 6-month mortality
Renal failure, refuses dialysis	< 6 months
Advanced AIDS dementia complex	6 months
Toxoplasmosis	6 months

OTHER FACTORS ASSOCIATED WITH A POOR PROGNOSIS FOR PATIENTS WITH AIDS
Chronic persistent diarrhea for 1 year Persistent serum albumin < 2.5 g/dL Concomitant substance abuse Age > 50 Decision to forego antiretroviral therapy, chemotherapy, and prophylactic drug therapy related to HIV disease and related illnesses Congestive heart failure, symptomatic at rest

SOURCE: Stuart B, Connor S, Kinzbrunner BM, et al: *Medical Guidelines for Determining Prognosis in Selected Non-cancer Diseases.* Arlington, National Hospice Organization, 2nd ed., 1996.

these patients would benefit from the additional psychosocial and spiritual support that a hospice can provide while considering their options. However, such patients could not be considered terminally ill and admitted to a hospice program until they make the decision to stop dialysis.

Laboratory criteria compatible with end-stage renal failure are compatible with values estab-lished by HCFA (form #2728) and include a cre-atinine clearance less than 10 mL/min (<15 mL/min in patients with diabetes) and a serum cre-atinine greater than 8.0 mg/dL (> 6.0 mg/dL in patients with diabetes). One must be careful not to use blood urea nitrogen (BUN) levels to deter-mine whether a patient meets guidelines for end-stage renal disease, as BUN elevations can

Table 1–15

Criteria for Hospice Care in End-Stage Renal Disease

PATIENT MEETS CRITERIA FOR DIALYSIS AND/OR RENAL TRANSPLANT AND REFUSES
PATIENT WITH RENAL FAILURE ON DIALYSIS WHO CHOOSES TO DISCONTINUE DIALYSIS
LABORATORY CRITERIA
Creatinine clearance < 10 mL/min (< 15 mL/min with diabetes) Serum creatinine > 8.0 mg/dl (> 6.0 mg/dL with diabetes)
SIGNS AND SYMPTOMS OF PROGRESSIVE UREMIA
Confusion and obtundation Intractable nausea and emesis Generalized pruritis Restlessness Oliguria: Urine output < 400 mL/24 hrs Intractable hyperkalemia: Serum potassium > 7.0, not responsive to medical management Pericarditis Intractable fluid overload Hepatorenal syndrome
ACUTE RENAL FAILURE: COMORBID ILLNESSES ASSOCIATED WITH A POOR PROGNOSIS

Mechanical ventilation	Malignancy
Chronic lung disease	Advanced cardiac disease
Advanced liver disease	Sepsis
Immunosuppression/AIDS	Serum albumin < 3.5 g/dL
Cachexia	Platelet count < 25,000
Age > 75 years	Disseminated intravascular coagulation (DIC)
Gastrointestinal bleeding	

SOURCE: Stuart B, Connor S, Kinzbrunner BM, et al: *Medical Guidelines for Determining Prognosis in Selected Non-cancer Diseases.* Arlington, National Hospice Organization, 2nd ed., 1996.

be elevated due to prerenal azotemia from volume depletion.

As patients develop progressive renal failure and their prognosis worsens, various symptoms of uremia occur. The onset of such symptoms may assist the clinician in determining the appropriate time to institute end-of-life care in a patient with borderline renal failure who is not a candidate for dialysis or transplant. These symptoms are listed in Table 1–15.

The development of acute renal failure may be associated with a poor prognosis, especially when it occurs in relationship to acute illness. Condi-

tions that, when accompanied by acute renal failure, tend to predict early patient mortality are listed in Table 1–15 as well.

End-Stage Liver Disease

The guidelines for patients suffering from hepatic failure due to nonmalignant causes may be found in Table 1–16. In essence, patients with liver disease requiring hospice or palliative care are those who suffer from persistent symptoms of hepatic failure, such as ascites, hepatic encephalopathy,

Table 1–16

Criteria for Hospice Care in End-Stage Liver Disease

PROGRESSIVE SYMPTOMS NOT RESPONSIVE TO MEDICAL MANAGEMENT OR PATIENT NONCOMPLIANCE, INCLUDING:
Ascites, refractory to sodium restriction and diuretics, especially with associated spontaneous bacterial peritonitis
Hepatic encephalopathy refractory to protein restriction and lactulose or neomycin
Recurrent variceal bleed despite therapeutic interventions
Hepatorenal syndrome
LABORATORY INDICATORS OF END-STAGE LIVER DISEASE
Protime ≥ 5 seconds more than control
Serum albumin ≤ 2.5 g/dL
OTHER FACTORS ASSOCIATED WITH A POOR PROGNOSIS IN PATIENTS WITH END-STAGE LIVER DISEASE
Progressive malnutrition
Muscle wasting with reduced strength and endurance
Continued active ethanol intake (> 80 g ethanol per day)
Hepatocellular carcinoma
HbsAg positivity

SOURCE: Stuart B, Connor S, Kinzbrunner BM, et al: *Medical Guidelines for Determining Prognosis in Selected Non-cancer Diseases.* Arlington, National Hospice Organization, 2nd ed., 1996.

and/or recurrent variceal bleeding, despite adequate medical management. They generally have multiple liver function abnormalities, with the most sensitive laboratory indicators of severe hepatic impairment being a prothrombin time that is at least 5 seconds over control, and a serum albumin less that 2.5 g/dL.

Other Nonmalignant Terminal Disease

Patients suffering from advanced illnesses other than the ones described will sometimes also need end-of-life care. These patients should be assessed for end-of-life care on an individual basis. In many instances, the guidelines for the various illnesses discussed can be applied to other patients. For example, for other advanced neurologic illnesses, such as Parkinson's disease, functional status deterioration, weight loss, and comorbid conditions such as defined in the criteria for end-stage Alzheimer's disease may be helpful determinants for directing patients with these conditions to hospice or palliative care programs.

Debility, Unspecified or Adult "Failure to Thrive"

There are elderly patients who appear to be approaching the end of life for whom a definitive terminal illness is not evident. These patients usually suffer from multiple medical illnesses or may be experiencing multiple comorbid conditions or progressive disabilities, such as declining functional status or weight loss. The combination of multiple chronic illnesses and a declining condition often prompt the patient, family, or attending physician to realize that the patient's clinical situation is irreversible, and a hospice or palliative treatment plan is sought.

Attempts to develop a standard diagnostic nomenclature for this group of patients have been challenging. One diagnostic term that would accurately characterize this group of patients is adult "failure to thrive." In fact, this term has been appearing with increasing regularity in the geriatric literature since the 1970s. However, when attempts were made to admit patients with this diagnosis to hospice programs in the 1980s, the fiscal intermediaries refused to reimburse services provided for such patients due to the fact that they perceived "failure to thrive" as a pediatric diagnosis, inappropriate for use in adult patients.

An alternative diagnosis was sought, and found in Section 16 of the ICD-9 code book, "Symptoms, signs, and ill-defined conditions (780-799). In the subsection "ill-defined and unknown causes of morbidity and mortality" (797-799), is code 799.3, "Debility, unspecified," which by its nature would characterize elderly, debilitated patients who are ill (morbidity) and have a high risk of dying (mortality).

In 1996 a retrospective analysis of 53 hospice patient charts was performed in an attempt to identify the characteristics of patients admitted for terminal care with the diagnosis "Debility, unspecified." The study demonstrated that these patients had severe functional deficits, a variety of comorbid medical illnesses most commonly involving the central nervous system or the cardiorespiratory system, but did not meet any of the illness-specific criteria that would determine a specific diagnosible terminal illness. These patients had a median survival in the hospice program of less than 3 weeks, and average survival of about 2 months.

Based on this study, it is clear that patients without a specific terminal diagnosis do constitute a population of terminally ill patients and should have access to end-of-life care. Criteria for considering patients for hospice or palliative care services when a definitive terminal diagnosis is not apparent are presented in Table 1–17. In some respect, these patients represent a population of elderly individuals who meet the general criteria for a terminal prognosis such as severe functional impairment and weight loss (see Table 1–1), but do not meet any of the illness-specific criteria defined earlier. They generally suffer from one, or more often multiple, comorbid conditions, and it is unclear which condition will prove to be fatal. In some cases, the patient and/or family will elect not to pursue aggressive medical evaluation or treatment due to either the patient's advanced age or overall deteriorating medical condition.

Whether the diagnosis of "Debility, unspecfied" or a similar diagnosis, such as adult "Failure to Thrive," is utilized is unimportant. What is critical is for the clinician to recognize that elderly patients with multiple medical illnesses and/or showing signs of rapid decline who either refuse medical evaluation or are found to have irreversible conditions, should be given the opportunity to receive appropriate end-of-life care.

Table 1–17

Criteria for Hospice Care in Debility, Unspecified or Adult Failure to Thrive

PATIENT MEETS GENERAL CRITERIA AS OUTLINED IN TABLE 1–1
Declining Functional Status Declining Nutritional Status especially BMI < 22 kg/m² Multiple hospitalizations over the last several months
PATIENT HAS ONE OR MORE COMORBID MEDICAL CONDITIONS INCLUDING, BUT NOT LIMITED TO:
Heart disease   COPD Dementia   Diabetes mellitus Cerebrovascular disease   Sepsis and/or Multiple decubiti   frequent infections Patient does not meet guidelines for a terminal prognosis based on any one of the comorbid illnesses from which they suffer AND/OR It is unclear which comorbid condition is most likely to result in death. Patient and/or family may have chosen not to pursue further evaluation of an undiagnosed medical condition or acute care treatment of one or more comorbid medical conditions due to advanced age and/or overall deterioration of patient health

References

Aida A, Miyamoto K, Nakano T, et al: Dyspnea grade as a prognostic factor in patients with chronic obstructive pulmonary disease. *Nippon Kyobu Shikkan Gakkai Zassi* 32:9, 1994.

Alexander HR, Norton JA: Pathophysiology of cancer cachexia. In: Doyle D, Hanks GWC, MacDonald N, eds. *Oxford Textbook of Palliative Medicine.* Oxford, Oxford University Press, 1993, 316.

American Society of Clinical Oncology Task Force on Cancer Care at the End of Life: Cancer care during the last phase of life. *J Clin Oncol* 16:1986, 1998.

Anderson F, Downing GM, Hill J, et al: Palliative Performance Scale (PPS): A new tool. *J Palliative Care* 12:5, 1996.

Anthonisen NR: Prognosis in chronic obstructive pulmonary disease. Results from multi-center clinical trials. *Am Rev Respir Dis* 140:S95, 1989.

Arkes HR, Dawson NV, Speroff T, et al: The covariance decomposition of the probability score and its use in evaluating prognostic estimates. *Med Decis Making* 15:120, 1995.

Brandeis GH, Morris JN, Nash DJ, Lipsitz LA: The epidemiology and natural history of pressure ulcers in elderly nursing home patients. *JAMA* 264:2905, 1990.

Campbell-Taylor I, Fisher RH: The clinical case against tube feeding in palliative care of the elderly. *J Am Geriatr Soc* 35:1100, 1987.

Christakis NA: Predicting patient survival before and after hospice enrollment. *Hospice J* 13:71, 1998.

Christiakis NA, Escarce JJ: Survival of medicare patients after enrollment on a hospice program. *N Engl J Med* 335:172, 1996.

Ciocon JO, Silverstone FA, Graver LM, Foley CJ: Tube feeding in elderly patients. Indications, benefits, and complications. *Arch Intern Med* 148:429, 1988.

Corti M, Guralnik JM, Salive ME, Sorkin JD: Serum albumin level and physical disability as predictors of mortality in older persons. *JAMA* 272:1036, 1994.

Cowcher K, Hanks GW: Long-term management of respiratory symptoms in advanced cancer. *J Pain Symptom Manag* 5:320, 1990.

Clark LP, Dion DM, Barker WH: Taking to bed. Rapid functional decline in an independently mobile older population living in an intermediate-care facility. *J Am Geriatr Soc* 38:967, 1990.

Dewys WD, Begg C, Lavin PT, et al: Prognostic effect of weight loss prior to chemotherapy in cancer patients. *Am J Med* 69:491, 1980.

Donaldson LJ, Clayton DG, Clarke M: The elderly in residential care: Mortality in relation to functional capacity. *J Epidemiol Community Health* 34:96, 1980.

Dubois P, Jamart J, Machiels J, et al: Prognosis of severely hypoxemic patients receiving long-term oxygen therapy. *Chest* 105:469, 1994.

Fabiszewski KJ, Volicer B, Volicer L: Effect of antibiotic treatments on outcome of fecers in institutionalized Alzheimer's patients. *JAMA* 263:3168, 1990.

Galanos AN, Pieper CF, Kussin PS, et al: Relationship of body mass index to subsequent mortality among seriously ill hospitalized patients. *Crit Care Med* 25:1962, 1997.

Hamel MB, Goldman L, Teno J, et al: Identification of comatose patients at high risk for death or severe disability. *JAMA* 273:1842, 1995.

Hurley AC, Volicer B, Mahoney MA, Volicer L: Palliative fever management in Alzheimer patients: Quality plus fiscal responsibility. *Adv Nurs Sci* 16:21, 1993.

Hurley AC, Volicer BJ, Volicer L: Effect of fever management strategy on the progression of dementia of the Alzheimer's type. *Alzheimer Dis Assoc Disord* 10:5, 1996.

Karnofsky SA, Abelmann WH, Craver LF, Burchenal JH: The use of nitrogen mustard in the palliative treatment of carcinoma. *Cancer* 1:634, 1948.

Katz S, Ford AB, Moskowitz RW, et al: Studies of illness in the aged, the index of ADL: A standardized measure of biological and psychosocial function. *JAMA* 185:914, 1963.

Kawakami Y: Prognostic factors in COPD: The importance of pulmonary hemodynamic variables. *Practical Cardiol* 11:124, 1985.

Kinzbrunner BM: Utilization of hospice services by terminally ill cancer patients. *Proc ASCO* :2226, 1999.

Kinzbrunner BM: Hospice 2000: 15 years and beyond in the care of the dying. *J Palliat Med* 1:127, 1998.

Kinzbrunner BM: The terminally ill patient. In: Abeloff MD, Armitage JO, Lichter AS, Niederhuber JE, eds. *Clinical Oncology.* New York, Churchill Livingstone, 2nd ed, 597.

Kinzbrunner BM: Hospice: What to do when anticancer therapy is no longer appropriate, effective, or desired. *Semin Oncol* 21:792, 1994.

Kinzbrunner BM: Non-malignant terminal diseases: Criteria for hospice admission. *Hospice Update* 3:3, 1993.

Kinzbrunner BM, Weinreb NJ, Merriman MP: Debility unspecified: A terminal diagnosis. *Am J Hospice Palliat Care* 13: 1996.

Knaus WA, Harrell FE, Lynn J, et al: The SUPPORT prognostic model. Objective estimates of survival for seriously ill hospitalized patients. *Ann Intern Med* 122:191, 1995.

Landi F, Zuccala G, Gambassi G, et al: Body mass index and mortality among older people living in the community. *J Am Geriatr Soc* 47:1072, 1999.

Likoff MJ, Chandler SL, Kay HR: Clinical determinants of mortality in chronic congestive heart failure secondary to idiopathic dilated or to ischemic cardiomyopathy. *Am J Cardiol* 59:634, 1987.

Luchins DJ, Hanrahan P, Murphy K: Criteria for enrolling dementia patients in hospice. *J Am Geriatr Soc* 45:1054, 1997.

Lynn J, Harrell F, Cohn F, et al: Prognoses of seriously ill hospitalized patients on the days before death: Implications for patient care and public policy. *New Horiz* 5:56, 1997.

Lynn J, Teno JM, Harrell FE: Accurate prognostications of death. Opportunities and challenges for clinicians. *West J Med* 163:250, 1995.

MacDonald N: Principles governing the use of cancer chemotherapy in palliative medicine. In: Doyle D, Hanks GWC, MacDonald N, eds. *Oxford Textbook of Palliative Medicine*. Oxford, Oxford University Press, 1993; p. 105.

Marantz PR, Tobin JN, Wasserthell-Smoller S, et al: Prognosis in ischemic heart disease. Can you tell as much at the bedside as in the nuclear laboratory? *Arch Intern Med* 152:2433, 1992.

Mor V, Laliberte L, Morris JN, et al: The Karnofsky performance status scale. An examination of its reliability and validity in a research setting. *Cancer* 53:2002, 1984.

Murden RA, Ainslie NK: Recent weight loss is related to short-term mortality in nursing homes. *J Gen Int Med* 9:648, 1994.

Narain B, Rubenstein LZ, Wieland GD, et al: Predictors of immediate and 6-month outcomes in hospitalized elderly patients. The importance of functional status. *J Am Geriatr Soc* 36:775, 1988.

National Hospice Organization: *Hospice Fact Sheet*, June 1, 1997.

Parkes CM: Accuracy in predictions of survival in later stages of cancer. *Br Med J* 2:29, 1972.

Patrick H, Schrogie JJ, Nadipelli VR, Vaccaro J: Staging disease severity and predicting prognosis in patients with end-stage COPD. A preliminary unstudy. Unpublished data.

Postma DS, Burema J, Gimeno F, et al: Prognosis in severe chronic obstructive pulmonary disease. *Am Rev Resp Dis* 119:357, 1979.

Reisberg B: Dementia: A systematic way to identifying reversible causes. *Geriatrics* 41:30, 1986.

Reuben DB, Mor V, Hiris J: Clinical symptoms and length of survival in patients with terminal cancer. *Arch Intern Med* 148:1586, 1988.

Rosenthal MA, Gebski VJ, Kefford RF, Stuart-Harris RC: Prediction of life-expectancy in hospice patients: Identification of novel prognostic factors. *Palliat Med* 7:199, 1993.

Rudman D, Mattson DE, Nagraj HS, et al: Antecedents of death in men of a Veteran's Administration nursing home. *J Am Geriatr Soc* 35:496, 1987.

Sarkisian CA, Lachs MS: "Failure to thrive" in older adults. *Ann Intern Med* 124:1072, 1996.

Stuart B,Connor S, Kinzbrunner BM, et al: *Medical Guidelines for Determining Prognosis in Selected Non-cancer Diseases*. Arlington, National Hospice Organization, 2nd ed., 1996.

Stuart SP, Tiley EH, Boland JP: Feeding gastrostomy. A critical review of its indications and mortality rates. *South Med J* 86:169, 1993.

SUPPORT Principal Investigators: A controlled trial to improve care for seriously ill hospitalized patients. The study to understand prognoses and preferences for outcomes and risks of treatment. *JAMA* 274:1591, 1995.

Volicer BJ, Hurley A, Fabiszewski KJ, et al: Predicting short-term survival for patients with advanced Alzheimer's disease. *J Am Geriatr Soc* 41:535, 1993.

Volicer L, Rheaume Y, Brown J, et al: Hospice approach to the treatment of advanced dementia of the Alzheimer type. *JAMA* 256:2210, 1985.

Von Gunten CF, Twaddle ML: Terminal care for non-cancer patients. *Clin Geriatr Med* 12:349, 1996.

Weeks JC, Cook EF, O'Day SJ, et al: Relationship between cancer patients' predictions of prognosis and their treatment preferences. *JAMA* 279:1709, 1998.

Wilson DO, Rogers RM, Wright EC,Anthonisen NR: Body weight in chronic obstructive pulmonary disease. The National Institutes of Health intermittent positive-pressure breathing trial. *Am Rev Respir Dis* 139:1435, 1989.

Yates JW, Chalmer B, McKegney FP: Evaluation of patients with advanced cancer using the Karnofsky performance status. *Cancer* 45:2220, 1980.

Barry M. Kinzbrunner

Chapter 2

How to Help Patients Access End-of-Life Care

Introduction

As the end of life approaches, patients, and the families who care for them, have many needs. Patients require expert management of pain and other physical symptoms. Patients and their families need a wide variety of emotional, social, and spiritual supports, and they also face significant financial and bureaucratic burdens.

The responsibility for ensuring that patients and families receive the treatments and services they need at the end of life falls in large part to the clinician responsible for the patient's care. Unfortunately medical school and postgraduate medical education on pain and symptom management near the end of life is limited, leaving many physicians without the expertise necessary to provide appropriate pain and physical symptom management. Even when physicians are comfortable managing the physical ailments of their terminally ill patients, most physicians lack both the expertise and time commitment required to provide for the nonphysical needs of the patient and family.

Fortunately, however, help is available, with almost 3000 hospice programs caring for terminally ill patients in virtually all parts of the United States, and with nonhospice end-of-life care programs being developed with increasing frequency. With the ever-growing availability of end-of-life care, the major dilemma facing physicians is not finding assistance for their terminally ill patients. Rather, the challenge is determining what type of provider of end-of-life care is best for their patients.

Aiding physicians in deciding whether a patient should be referred to a hospice program or to a nonhospice provider of palliative care near the end of life is the focus of this chapter. Hospice in the United States as defined by the Medicare Hospice Benefit will be reviewed, followed by a discussion of alternative end-of-life care programs that have been and are being developed. Issues that physicians should consider when choosing an appropriate end-of-life care program for ter-

minally ill patients and families under their care will then be discussed.

Hospice in the United States and the Medicare Hospice Benefit

History

Historically, hospice had its origins in the Middle Ages. Derived from the Latin term *hospes*, meaning host or guest, hospices served as way stations for travelers between Europe, Africa, and the Middle East. One can speculate that the association between hospices and the care of the sick and dying may have come from the fact that during the Crusades, wounded soldiers would often stop at hospices on the way home, and many would not survive their injuries.

The modern concept of hospice as an interdisciplinary approach for providing comprehensive care to patients near the end of life had its origins in Great Britain during the 1960s. Dame Cicely Saunders, using the vast health care experience she had gained as a physician, nurse, and social worker (a modern hospice team rolled into one), established the first hospice facilities in London, England, initially at St. Joseph's Hospice, and then at St. Christopher's Hospice. Drawing on the British experience, hospices began to develop in Canada in the 1960s and in the United States during the 1970s. Unlike the British model of hospice that revolved around providing care in designated inpatient facilities, however, the hospice model developed in the United States emphasized providing services to patients in the home environment, with inpatient care reserved for patients with specific needs that could not be managed at home.

As the hospice movement grew in the United States, specific funding was sought, leading to the establishment of the Medicare Hospice Benefit as part of the Tax Equity and Fiscal Responsibility

Act (TEFRA) of 1982. The benefit defined a patient's eligibility for hospice services based on life expectancy, defined the services that the hospice was to provide, and established reimbursement rates for these services on a per diem basis. This hospice benefit has continued to the present with only minor modifications over the years, and its provisions have formed the basis of the hospice model of end-of-life care in the United States. The Medicare Hospice benefit has also served as a model for the provision and reimbursement of end-of-life care services to patients receiving Medicaid, and for increasing numbers of managed care and private insurance medical plans.

Provisions of the Medicare Hospice Benefit

Patient Eligibility

The basic features of the Medicare Hospice Benefit are listed in Table 2–1. For a patient to receive the Medicare Hospice Benefit, the patient must be entitled to Medicare Part A benefits and must be certified as terminally ill, defined by the Medicare hospice regulations as having "a medical prognosis that his or her life expectancy is six months or less if the illness runs its normal course." At the time of referral and admission to the hospice program, the patient must be certified as terminally ill by two physicians, the patient's attending physician and the hospice medical director or the physician member of the hospice interdisciplinary team. The clinical characteristics that help identify patients who meet this requirement are the subject of Chapter 1. The hospice benefit has two defined periods of 90 days, covering a total 180 days or 6 months of care. For patients who unexpectedly survive beyond 6 months after services begin (as discussed in Chapter 1, predicting prognosis is not an exact science), the Medicare Hospice Benefit provides for continued hospice services

past the 6-month point with coverage divided into 60-day benefit periods. Prior to the beginning of the second 90 day period within the first 180 days, and any subsequent 60-day period, the hospice

Table 2–1

Basic Features of the Medicare Hospice Benefit

The patient must be terminally ill
    Life expectancy is 6 months or less if the illness runs its normal course
    Certified by two physicians: attending physician, hospice medical director
The hospice benefit is a Part A Medicare Benefit. It replaces all other Part A and Part B Medicare Benefits except:
    Professional services of the attending physician
    All services for illnesses unrelated to the terminal illness
The benefit is divided into distinct periods
    Two benefit periods of 90 days each followed by unlimited number of benefit periods of 60 days each
    Prior to the start of any new benefit period patients require recertification of their terminal prognosis by the Hospice Medical Director
A patient can choose to revoke the Medicare Hospice Benefit at any time, leaving the hospice program. Regular Medicare benefits are immediately restored (without any waiting period)
Reimbursement is on a per-diem basis (fixed daily rate) for a defined group of services (see Table 2–2), and for four levels of care:
    Routine home care
    Continuous home care
    General inpatient care
    Respite inpatient care
No more than 20% of a hospice's days of care may be at the general inpatient level of care
An annual payment cap is placed on each hospice program based on the number of patients enrolled

medical director or the physician member of the hospice interdisciplinary team is required to recertify that the patient continues to have a terminal illness with a "a medical prognosis that his or her life expectancy is six months or less if the illness runs its normal course."

Patients who are no longer certifiable as terminally ill are discharged from the hospice program with an extended prognosis, and their regular Medicare benefits are immediately restored. Patients may, at any time, voluntarily choose to revoke the hospice benefit and leave the hospice program. Such patients, similar to those discharged with an extended prognosis, have their regular Medicare benefits immediately reinstated.

Reimbursement and Covered Services

Reimbursement for care rendered to patients covered by the Medicare Hospice Benefit is made to hospice programs on a per-diem basis. Hospices receive a fixed sum per day per patient to provide whatever services are required to care for the patient. There are four distinct payment rates, based upon the patient's level of care (see "Levels of Hospice Care," later in the chapter).

Hospices are responsible to cover all services that are needed to care for "the terminal illness as well as related conditions." A list of these services may be found in Table 2–2. The care and treatment of conditions "unrelated" to the terminal illness are not covered by the Medicare Hospice Benefit and are not the responsibility of the hospice. In such circumstances, patients have access to regular Medicare Part A and Part B benefits. In addition to the hands-on care provided by the various members of the hospice interdisciplinary team, hospices provide all medications, durable medical equipment, and medical supplies that are required by the patient, relieving patients and families of significant financial burdens. Therapeutic modalities less commonly associated with hospice care, such as chemotherapy, radiation therapy, and transfusion of blood products, are also covered

Table 2–2

Hospice Services Included in Per-Diem Reimbursement

Nursing services
Medical direction and physician participation in the development of the plan of care
Medical social services
Counseling services
   Pastoral or spiritual counseling
   Bereavement counseling: provided to the family for up to 1 year following the death of the patient
   Dietary counseling
   Other counseling by qualified professionals as required
Home health aide services
Homemaker services
Drugs and biologicals
Durable medical equipment
Other medical supplies
Laboratory and diagnostic studies for care related to the terminal illness
Physical therapy, occupational therapy, and speech therapy if indicated

when indicated for the treatment of symptoms related to the terminal illness (see Chapter 17 for further discussion).

A unique service provided by hospice programs is bereavement counseling, offered by the hospice to surviving family members for at least one year following the death of the patient. Hospices provide this service despite the fact that there is no additional reimbursement for bereavement services after the patient has died (see Chapter 14 for further discussion).

An important exception to the per diem reimbursement program is related to physician services. Included in the per diem are such physician activities as administrative medical direction and physician participation in the development and modification of each patient's individualized plan of care. Professional physician services, including visits made by either hospice physicians or consultant physicians under contract to the hospice, are paid for by the hospice. However, these activities may be billed for and are reimbursed by Medicare Part A on a fee-for-service basis. Visits made to a patient by an attending physician are not considered hospice services, and are reimbursed as usual by Medicare Part B, unless the physician is also under contract with the hospice (in which case the hospice would pay the physician and bill Part A as described). A more detailed discussion of this issue can be found in Chapter 4.

Levels of Hospice Care

As previously stated, as hospice care evolved in the United States, it was intended to deliver the comprehensive services required to care for patients near the end of life in the most familiar and comfortable environment possible, the patient's own home. It was recognized, however, that there were times when the patient's clinical condition required care that was beyond the scope of services defined by the basic Medicare Hospice Benefit. An additional concern was that, because the Medicare Hospice Benefit is a Part A Medicare benefit (which covers all inpatient services, as contrasted with Medicare Part B, which primarily covers outpatient and physician services), patients who elect to receive hospice services no longer had hospitalization coverage under Medicare Part A. To address these issues, the Medicare Hospice Benefit provides for alternative levels of care, reimbursed at different per-diem rates, that reflect the intensity of services provided by the hospice to meet the needs of the patient. There are four distinct levels of care: routine home care, continuous home care, general inpatient care, and inpatient respite care.

ROUTINE HOME CARE

Home care is the basic hospice care provided in the patient's home. It incorporates the services

outlined in Table 2–2 and discussed earlier. For patients who live in a long-term care facility (a nursing home), the facility is considered their home for the purpose of the Medicare Hospice Benefit, and the care received is considered routine home care (see "Hospice and Long-Term Care," later in the chapter).

CONTINUOUS HOME CARE

Continuous home care may be indicated for patients who develop acute medical or psychosocial symptoms in the home environment, or elect to remain at home, and require more intensive, often around-the-clock, care and support than can be provided under the routine home level of care. Clinical indications for continuous care can be found in Table 2–3. The care provided to the patient must be primarily (more than 50%) nursing, and must be for a minimum of 8 hours a day (not necessarily consecutively) to a maximum of 24 hours a day. Rather than a daily per diem, reimbursement for continuous care is based upon a fixed hourly rate.

GENERAL INPATIENT HOSPICE CARE

During the course of a terminal illness, some patients will experience symptoms that cannot be effectively managed even under a continuous home care level of care. Other patients, when faced with severe symptoms, will not be comfortable remaining in the home environment. For these patients, an inpatient hospice environment is indicated. However, as noted earlier, patients who elect the Medicare Hospice Benefit no longer have Medicare Part A benefits to cover hospitalization. Therefore, the Medicare Hospice Benefit requires that all hospices provide patients access to general inpatient hospice care for the management of pain and other symptoms (both physical and psychosocial) that cannot be managed in the home environment. Clinical criteria for general inpatient care parallel those for continuous care as outlined in Table 2–3.

Table 2–3

Clinical Indicators for Continuous Care and General Inpatient Hospice Care

Uncontrolled pain
    Sudden onset or new manifestation of pain
    Ongoing pain management, regardless of
        route of administration or type of analgesia:
        When modalities used under a routine
            home care plan of care have proven
            unsuccessful
        When frequent adjustments in the dose of
            analgesia require constant monitoring
            and evaluation
    Alternative modalities of pain control that
        cannot be managed under a routine home
        care plan of care
Intractable nausea, emesis, or other major
    gastrointestinal symptoms
Respiratory distress
Severe decubiti or other skin lesions/wounds
Any other physical symptom defined by the
    interdisciplinary team that cannot be man-
    aged under a routine home care plan of care
Psychosocial problems and uncontrolled
    symptoms that can create significant psycho-
    social pathology in the patient and/or family
    Behaviorial or cognitive abnormalities that do
        not appear to have neurological or organic
        etiology
    Severe depression, anxiety, or both, dictating
        increased supervision (continuous care) or
        a change in environment (inpatient care)
    Acute breakdown or disruption in family
        dynamics, preventing family members
        from functioning as adequate caregivers
        for reasons that can either be physical or
        emotional

Hospices provide general inpatient care in a variety of venues. Free-standing hospice inpatient units are dedicated facilities owned and operated by the hospice. Inpatient hospice units may also occupy a wing in a hospital or long-term care facility, usually leased by the host facility to the hospice and operated either by the hospice or jointly by both organizations. Some hospices have entered into contractual agreements with local hospitals and/or long-term care facilities to provide inpatient beds on an individual patient basis. In hospitals, these beds are most commonly located either on the general medical/surgical floor or the oncology floor, while in the long-term care facility (LTCF), such patients should be cared for on the skilled nursing floor. Table 2–4 reviews some of the advantages and disadvantages that hospice programs must weigh when considering the various locations in which general hospice inpatient care can be provided in their community.

Differences in the quality of hospice inpatient care provided in the various venues have never been formally evaluated. However, anecdotal experience suggests that dedicated hospice inpatient units, whether free-standing or in a hospital or LTCF, have significant advantages over contract beds. In the former, patient care is provided by hospice-employed and trained personnel in a home-like atmosphere and is consistent with palliative care standards. In the latter, patients receive most of their care from hospital or facility staff in an acute care or skilled care setting, with the care being only supplemented by hospice personnel. Therefore, the environment and the care provided to hospice patients in contract beds is much less in keeping with the goals of hospice and palliative care than when care is provided in a hospice inpatient unit or free-standing facility.

RESPITE CARE

The fourth defined level of care under the Medicare Hospice Benefit is respite inpatient care. This level of care is indicated when patients do not meet the requirements for the general inpatient level of care, but are placed in an inpatient environment to allow caregiver family members

Table 2–4

Comparison of Locations for Hospice General Inpatient Care

LOCATION	ADVANTAGES	DISADVANTAGES
Free-standing facility	Owned, operated by hospice Hospice-trained staff Community identity and visibility Home-like environment	Need to provide ancillary support services Cost of operation Limitation of location may negatively affect patient or physician access
Inpatient unit in hospital or LTCF leased by hospice	Hospice-trained staff Community identity and visibility Home-like environment Partnership with other community health care providers Avoids duplication of ancillary support services	Limitation of location may negatively affect patient or physician access (but less than free-standing facility) Perception as a nursing home if located in LTCF
Contract bed in hospital or LTCF	Partnership with many community health care providers Greater patient, physician accessibility	Hospital staff not as familiar with hospice and palliative care principles Acute care or LTCF environment

needed respite from the day-to-day care they are providing to the patient at home. Respite care is limited to 5 consecutive days at any time.

DETERMINING THE LEVEL OF CARE

When patients are admitted to a hospice program, they may be admitted to any of the four levels of care, based upon their needs at the time of initial assessment. Once in the hospice program, patients may be transferred from one level of care to another within the program. For example, if a patient on a routine home care level of care experiences uncontrolled pain requiring more intensive management than can be provided in the home setting, they could be transferred, rather than admitted, to a general inpatient level of care. Once the pain is brought under control, the patient would be transferred, rather than discharged, back to a routine home care level of care.

Limitations on Reimbursement to Hospices

To ensure the proper use of hospice services and prevent excessive costs, certain safeguards have been built into the Medicare Hospice Benefit. A global cap on payment, limiting the average reimbursement that a hospice can receive per patient admitted during a year, was established to ensure that hospice costs would not exceed what Medicare would otherwise spend on health care for a patient during the last 6 months of life. The cap amount is based upon a figure equivalent to 95% of the average Medicare expenditures per patient during the last 6 months of life and is adjusted annually to account for inflation and hospice rate increases. To determine whether a hospice program has exceeded the global cap, total Medicare reimbursement for services provided (which includes per-diem payments for the various levels of care as well as physician services billed outside the per diem) is divided by the number of individual beneficiaries admitted to the hospice during the year. If the calculated amount exceeds the global cap amount, then the hospice's reimbursement for that year is limited to the global cap amount multiplied by the number of patients admitted during the year.

In addition to the global cap, a second reimbursement limitation was placed on hospice services provided at a general inpatient care level of care. As previously discussed, when hospice was established in the United States, the goal was that it should be home based, rather than centered around an institution. To encourage Medicare-certified hospices to provide care primarily in the home, the Medicare benefit limited reimbursement for the general inpatient level of care to no more than 20% of its total days of care.

By instituting these caps on reimbursement, use of higher levels of care, the numbers of long-stay patients, and using of physician services billed outside the per diem, cost can be controlled without denying care to any specific patient who needs care.

Hospice and Long-Term Care

In the early years following the passage of the Medicare Hospice Benefit, it was recognized that there was a group of patients who were in need of end-of-life care who could not receive it, because they were considered ineligible for the hospice benefit. These were patients who were residents of long-term care facilities (LTCFs) and primarily receiving custodial care (as opposed to those patients receiving skilled nursing care under Medicare Part A, who were, and continue to be ineligible for the Medicare Hospice Benefit, which is a mutually exclusive Part A benefit). Legislation subsequently modified the hospice benefit, allowing patients residing in an LTCF to receive hospice services, with the LTCF being considered as the patient's home for purpose of the hospice benefit. Reimbursement for hospice services provided to patients living in LTCFs is the same as the reimbursement provided for those patients living in their own homes, with one exception. For patients who are receiving Medicaid benefits for custodial nursing home care and who are receiving hospice care under the Medicare Hospice Benefit, the hospice program is reimbursed at a "unified rate," consisting of 95 percent of the sum of the Medicaid nursing home room and board rate and the hospice home care per diem rate. The hospice is then responsible to pay the LTCF for the patient's room and board.

Hospices must have contractual agreements with each LTCF in which they care for patients, while the hospice maintains the professional management responsibility for facility patients enrolled in the hospice program. To ensure that patients' needs are appropriately met and are consistent with a palliative plan of care, hospices and LTCFs are mandated to develop "coordinated plans of care" for the patients who are jointly served by the two health care organizations.

The hospice experience in serving patients residing in LTCFs has been positive. Terminally ill patients require a complexity of care that staffing levels in LTCFs are not designed to provide. Hospice programs provide such patients with supplementary nursing and nursing aide support that assists the LTCF staff in ensuring that patients receive the necessary palliative symptom management, optimal skin care, nutritional assistance, and psychosocial and spiritual support. Hospice social workers and chaplains provide support to family members of LTCF patients, who often have strong feelings of guilt about having placed a loved one in long-term care, especially when death is near. Long-term care facility staff, considered members of the patient's extended family, greatly benefit from the psychosocial and bereavement support that a hospice program provides.

Hospice Coverage Under Managed Care and Other Health Care Plans

Medicare patients who are terminally ill and are being cared for by a managed care organization (MCO) can receive hospice services covered by the Medicare Hospice Benefit, under what is termed a "Medicare carve-out." Rather than mandate that the MCO provide hospice services as part of its covered services, under the provisions of the "carve-out" the hospice is reimbursed directly by Medicare at the standard per-diem rates, for services provided to the patient. The MCO, however, is reimbursed at a reduced rate, as it is still responsible to provide health care to the patient for conditions unrelated to the terminal illness.

For terminally ill patients who are not covered by the Medicare program, hospice is also becoming increasingly accessible. State Medicaid programs in most states have hospice benefits that parallel the Medicare benefit. MCOs and private health insurance plans are covering hospice services with increasing frequency, with most commercial plans also following the Medicare model, albeit frequently with lifetime dollar limits on benefits. Some plans, in an effort to be "cost effective," have asked hospice providers to "unbundle" their services, allowing the plan, for example, to purchase only nursing and home health aide care for patients. (See "How to Choose an End-of-Life Care Provider" later in the chapter for a further discussion of "unbundling.")

Alternative End-of-Life Care Programs

Based on the description given, hospice, as defined by the Medicare Hospice Benefit, would appear to be an excellent program, providing comprehensive end-of-life care services to patients who are terminally ill. And it is! Statistics show that the growth of hospice programs throughout the 1990s has been at a record pace, with more than 500,000 terminally ill patients and families now receiving hospice care annually.

Unfortunately, there is also a sobering side to these statistics. The 500,000 patients who use hospice annually only account for 17 to 20 percent of the individuals who die each year. Additionally, patients are spending less time under hospice care, suggesting that they are not receiving hospice services until very late in the terminal phase of their illnesses. During the last several years, average lengths of stay have decreased by about 2 weeks, from 60 days to 45 days, and median lengths of stay have fallen from a little over 1 month to less than 3 weeks.

Physician discomfort with predicting that a patient has 6 months or less to live (see Chapter 1), lack of open communication between patients, families, and physicians regarding end-of-life care issues (see Chapter 3), and the lack of inpatient relationships between hospices and hospitals have been cited among the reasons that hospice remains underutilized by terminally ill patients and families. Although increasing physician and patient education and growing numbers of relationships between hospitals and hospices are helping to make hospice care more accessible, the recognition that patients and families require more comprehensive services near the end of life has led to the development of a growing number of alternate nonhospice "palliative care programs" throughout the United States. These alternative programs, either hospital based or home-care based, will be described next. Some key features of these programs are listed in Table 2–5 and compared with those provided by hospice programs under the Medicare Hospice Benefit.

Hospital-Based Palliative Care Programs

The primary goal of the increasing number of palliative care programs being developed is to provide for "unmet patient and family needs by extending hospice-like, interdisciplinary, primary care and consultative services to inpatients . . . and to many terminally ill outpatients who would benefit from such services but do not meet formal hospice eligibility requirements." A secondary goal is to "create important opportunities for training health professionals about end-of-life care."

Patient eligibility for palliative care services, which has been a major impetus for the evolution of these programs, is by design less limited than required for the Medicare Hospice Benefit. While patients cared for by palliative care programs generally require life-limiting illnesses, most programs will accept patients with life expectancies of 1 year or less (rather than 6 months or less). In some circumstances, patients with chronic, incurable, debilitating illnesses with indeterminate life expectancies are being cared for as well.

The typical inpatient palliative care consultation team is multidisciplinary and consists of, at minimum, a physician, nurse, and social worker. Other health care professionals who would be involved in the care of the patient on an as-needed basis would include a pastoral counselor and consultants from various services in the hospital including nutritional, physical, and occupational therapy, psychiatry, and pharmacy. Most palliative care programs provide outpatient services by working with one or more affiliated home health agencies that have palliative care expertise as well as local hospice programs. (See the next section for a further discussion of home-based palliative care.)

Table 2–5

Comparison of Hospice and Nonhospice Palliative Care Services

	HOSPICE	NONHOSPICE PALLIATIVE CARE
Eligibility	Prognosis of < 6 months	Determined by program

Professional services	Interdisciplinary team
	    Physician
	    Nurse
	    Social worker
	    Pastoral counselor
	    Certified nursing assistants
	    Others as needed
		Multidisciplinary team
		    Physician
		    Nurse
		    Social worker
		    Others as needed

Other services	Medications
	DME
	Bereavement care
	Others (see Table 2–2)
		No required services. Services
		    provided are determined by
		    program

Location of services	Comprehensive
	    Home care
	    LTCF
	    Inpatient
		Based on primary location.
		    Requires networking and
		    partnering between hospital-
		    based and home-based
		    programs.

Funding	Medicare Hospice Benefit
	Most state Medicaid programs
	Many HMOs and commercial
	    insurers
	Charity (not-for-profit hospices)
		No defined palliative care
		    coverage
		Traditional hospitalization
		Traditional home care
		Grants
		Charity

Referral of patients to these programs is usually for palliative care consultations, and most often occurs while patients are hospitalized, in contrast to hospice, where referral may occur while patients are either in the inpatient or outpatient setting. Patients may be cared for either on the acute care wards they occupy at the time of consultation or, if available, in specially designated palliative care units developed by the institution. These units, similar to their hospice counterparts, are decorated in a more home-like fashion than an acute care hospital ward, and are staffed with personnel who have special training in palliative care.

The greatest challenge facing these new palliative care services is, not surprisingly, funding. At present, there is no specific funding for palliative care services. HCFA is currently evaluating the merits of a Palliative Care DRG (ICD-9 code V66.7), which would allow for additional reimbursement above that provided for the standard principal diagnosis if palliative or "comfort" care was delivered to a terminally ill patient in an acute care hospital setting. Although HCFA was due to make a final decision on the feasibility of a palliative care DRG in October 1998, a lack of understanding on how to properly utilize the code has postponed any decision for the immediate future. Meanwhile, fledgling palliative care programs are forced to rely on traditional acute care reimbursement and fee-for-service billing for financial support, which does not take into account the extra services needed and provided to patients and families near the end of life. What has allowed these programs to evolve and offer the comprehensive services required is additional funding provided by grants from organizations such as the Robert Wood Johnson and Soros Foundations, which are currently focusing research efforts on increasing the access to and improving the quality of end-of-life care for terminally ill patients and families.

Home-Based Palliative Care

The desire to reach patients sooner in the course of terminal illness has prompted some hospice providers to create home-based palliative care programs. Such "prehospice" or "bridge" programs are designed to provide hospice-like services to patients who do not meet hospice eligibility requirements, are not yet ready to accept the implications of hospice regarding their prognosis, and/or are receiving life-prolonging therapy that is not consistent with a hospice plan of care. The "prehospice" program parallels the hospice regarding the interdisciplinary approach to care. If the prehospice and hospice programs are part of the same agency, continuity of care, at least in theory, may be enhanced as the same team members may care for patients from the time of admission to death, regardless of whether they are on the prehospice or the hospice.

Much like for inpatient palliative care, the key challenge for home-based palliative care programs is financial. At present, these programs are funded primarily from basic home health benefits, which provide reimbursement for skilled nursing care to a patient who is *confined* to the home. These restrictions place limits on patients, who cannot receive services if they go out of the house, and on the agencies, which must provide nonreimbursed services if they are to be true to the interdisciplinary nature of palliative care. Again, supplementary funding from outside organizations is helping to make these programs a reality.

How to Choose an End-of-Life Care Provider

With a better understanding of the end-of-life care options available to terminally ill patients, the physician is faced with the challenge of helping patients and families determine which palliative care provider will best serve their needs. This challenge is compounded by the fact that in most medium and large-sized communities several hospice programs are likely to be available, and more and more hospitals and home health agencies are beginning to offer end-of-life care and palliative care programs outside the Medicare Hospice Benefit.

In order to assist patients and families in accessing the end-of-life care services they need, the physician needs to determine what services are most important to the patient and family being treated, and compare these to the services that the various end-of-life care providers in the community have to offer. While patient/family needs are, to some extent, unique, there are some basic services that, based upon a survey of physicians, were deemed to be important for all patients who are in need of palliative care. These services are listed in Table 2–6, and discussed below.

Demonstrated Effective Pain Management, with Written Guidelines and Protocols

A quality end-of-life care provider, whether a hospice or a palliative care program, should be able to demonstrate that patients under its care have

Table 2–6

Important Features for an End-of-Life Care Program

Demonstrated effective pain management, with written guidelines and protocols

Ability to treat the patient in the home, an LTCF, or an inpatient setting

Involvement of the attending physician, with satisfactory communication and support

Family counseling provided by skilled professionals on issues related to death and dying during the patient's illness and the bereavement period that follows

Interdisciplinary care from a team of professionals trained in end-of-life care, including:
  Physician
  Registered nurse
  Certified nursing assistant
  Social worker
  Chaplain

pain (and other symptoms) effectively managed. The provider should have pain management guidelines and/or protocols that are comparable with the standards set in the medical literature, and the nurses and physicians who work for the hospice or palliative care provider should endorse and use those guidelines. The provider should also be able to demonstrate, through outcomes management and performance improvement activities, that patients under its care actually have pain well controlled.

Ability to Treat Patient in the Home, LTCF, or Inpatient Setting

End-of-life care providers should be able to serve, or at least coordinate service, for patients in whatever setting is required to care for them. Medicare-certified hospices are, in general, best equipped to do this, as the Medicare Hospice Benefit requires that patient care be provided not only in the home environment (which may also be an LTCF) but in an inpatient setting as well. Most hospices also have relationships with multiple LTCFs in their communities, allowing terminally ill patients who live in that environment to obtain palliative care.

Coordination of services may not be as simple, however, for the nonhospice providers of palliative who are not affiliated with a hospice. Inpatient palliative care programs, by design, are centered around services provided in the hospital setting, making it imperative that nonhospice programs have working relationships with hospices or home-care-based palliative care programs to insure that patients who leave the inpatient setting receive appropriate end-of-life care. Likewise, home care programs that provide palliative care should have inpatient partners to provide appropriate end-of-life care to patients who require hospitalization. Home care palliative programs are also limited in that they may not serve patients living in long-term care facilities.

The location of inpatient services is another factor that can be of great importance in choosing an end-of-life care provider. As shown in Table 2–4, hospice inpatient care can be delivered in a number of settings, each of which has advantages and disadvantages. For most patients, families, and clinicians, the preferred sites of hospice or nonhospice palliative inpatient care would be either a free-standing inpatient facility or a designated inpatient unit within a hospital. For some patients and families, as well as their physicians, however, geographic constraints may create challenges in using these facilities and units, which are limited in number. Under such circumstances, flexibility is required. Hospices, for example, could make contract beds available in almost all hospitals in the community, while inpatient palliative care programs could provide consultation services in hospitals other than the ones in which they are based. Accommodations such as these will allow patients and families the convenience of more familiar surroundings closer to home, and allow physicians to follow their patients at a time when they are most needed.

Involvement of the Attending Physician, with Satisfactory Communication and Support

The attending physician is generally recognized as being the most knowledgeable physician regarding any patient's medical condition. In recognition of this important relationship, the Medicare Hospice Benefit provides for attending physician reimbursement through normal Part B channels, as opposed to via a contract with the hospice, and considers the attending physician an integral member of the hospice interdisciplinary team. Therefore, whether the patient is receiving end-of-life care from a hospice or from a nonhospice end-of-life care provider, communication between that provider and the attending physician is key to successful care of the terminally ill patient and family. (For a more thorough discussion of the role of the attending physician, see Chapter 4.)

The members of the interdisciplinary team must be able to communicate in an appropriate professional manner with the attending physician. Active involvement of the hospice or palliative care medical director in patient care and physician communications provides the attending physician with consultation, advice, and expertise in the areas of pain and symptom control. The ability of the hospice staff to provide the attending physician with accurate information about a patient's condition, in a succinct and professional manner, allows for prompt and appropriate interventions. Coupled with the confidence that attending physicians will develop in the end-of-life care program when the staff communicates accurately and professionally, this ultimately results in improved patient care.

Family Counseling

One of the features that makes end-of-life care unique is the fact that the patient and family together make up the unit of care. Therefore, it is vital that the hospice or palliative care program has adequate family support services. For Medicare-certified hospice programs, family counseling responsibilities are generally shared by psychologists, social workers, clergy, and others. The same professionals will usually serve this function for nonhospice palliative care programs as well. Physicians should be aware of the qualifications of these professionals employed by their hospice or palliative care provider of choice, and should also be certain that the number of social workers and chaplains is adequate to meet patient and family needs.

In hospice and palliative care, support for the family does not cease at the time of patient death. Bereavement services are another integral component of a quality end-of-life care program. Under the Medicare Hospice Benefit, bereavement support to surviving family members is mandated and considered part of the per diem reimbursement rate that the hospice receives while the patient is alive and under its care. Whether the patient is cared for on the hospice for one day, one week, one month, or one year, the hospice must provide bereavement support for at least one year following the death of the patient. As there is no traditional health care reimbursement for bereavement support, nonhospice palliative care programs must use outside funding sources to provide family counseling after patient death. The importance of quality bereavement care should not be underestimated. Studies have been published suggesting that appropriate bereavement support improves the health of surviving family members, as demonstrated by a decrease in use of health care resources and reduced absenteeism from work. (A full discussion of bereavement services in end-of-life care can be found in Chapter 14.)

Interdisciplinary Care from a Team of Professionals Trained in end-of-life Care

The provision of end-of-life care requires a special expertise that usually requires special training and experience. Therefore, a quality end-of-life care program will be one that has a majority of full-time trained staff in each of the key disciplines: nursing, medicine, social work, and pastoral counseling. It should be noted that the hospice benefit allows the option of contracting for these services under certain circumstances, and many end-of-life care providers (both hospice and nonhospice) have found that contracting for certain services is more cost effective than hiring and training staff. However, for most patient care needs, it is important to select hospice and palliative care services that employ trained professionals.

Full-time and properly trained end-of-life care staff is apt to be more responsive than contracted staff to patient and family needs, extending from prompt and efficient admission to the hospice or palliative care program to a sense of urgency when a patient is experiencing an uncontrolled symptom. Committed staff will also be more sensitive to the needs of patients and families on weekends, holidays, and other emotionally challenging times. None of this is meant to question the clinical expertise of staff from a contracted agency. However, one would have to wonder whether such staff, if usually functioning in an acute care and curative environment, would be as sensitive to the unique needs of terminally ill patients and families

as properly trained, full-time members of a hospice or palliative care interdisciplinary team.

Determining if End-of-Life Care Provider Meets the Needs of Patients and Families

With proper elucidation of the services that patients and families require as described, it is incumbent upon the clinician to determine whether the end-of-life care organization of choice provides those services at an appropriate level of quality. An algorithm to assist the clinician in choosing the proper end-of-life care provider is provided in Figure 2–1.

Although it might be thought that all end-of-life care providers provide similar services at similar levels of quality, the facts are that, until recently, there has been little in the way of standardization in the field of hospice and palliative care. Eighty percent of hospices operating in the United States are Medicare certified, meaning that 20 percent of hospices are not. In addition, nonhospice palliative care providers are not certified by Medicare, and they are not compelled by regulation to provide the scope of services that a Medicare-certified hospice is obligated to offer. Therefore, although the services provided by a noncertified end-of-life care provider may appear similar to those of hospice programs that are certified, it would be prudent for a referring physician to consider whether a noncertified hospice, or nonhospice palliative care program, at least meets Medicare hospice standards. It is also incumbent for the physician to consider whether a Medicare patient referred to a non-Medicare-certified end-of-life care program will incur out-of-pocket expenses, such as the cost of oral medication, that would be covered by the Medicare Hospice Benefit if the patient were enrolled in a Medicare-certified hospice program.

Although the Medicare benefit dictates what services must be provided, it does not adequately address the standards that define quality end-of life-care. The issue of quality is being taken up by accrediting bodies such as the Joint Commission

Figure 2–1

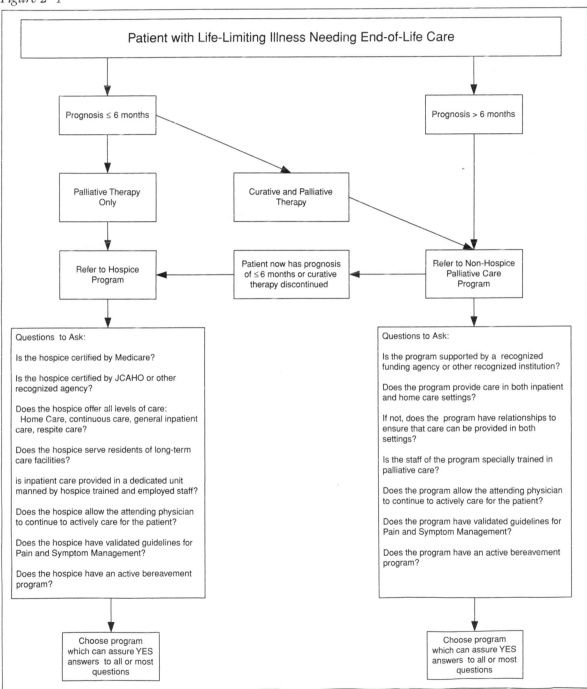

Algorithm for choosing the proper end-of-life care provider

on Accreditation of Healthcare Organizations (JCAHO), which now provides accreditation for hospice programs. In fact, JCAHO has recently been granted "deemed status" with the Medicare program, meaning that a hospice that is accredited by JCAHO will be "deemed" to be Medicare certified as well. With increasing numbers of hospice and palliative care providers available to patients and families, the array of services defined by the Medicare Hospice Benefit and accreditation by the JCAHO or similar accrediting body that attests to the quality of care provided should be considered by physicians seeking end-of-life care for terminally ill patients under their care.

Conclusion

It is clear from the information given that choosing the appropriate end-of-life care provider for a patient and family can be daunting task. With improved knowledge of the services that are available and should be expected from an end-of-life care provider, and of the Medicare Hospice Benefit and other forms of end-of-life care reimbursement, this task will, hopefully, be a little less complex.

Bibliography

ASCO Task Force on Cancer Care at the End of Life: Cancer care during the last phase of life. *J Clin Oncol* 16:1986, 1998.

Bascom PB: A hospital based comfort care team: Consultation for seriously ill and dying patients. *Am J Hospice Palliat Care* 14:57, 1997.

Bayer R, Feldman E: Hospice under the Medicare wing. *Hastings Cent Rep* 12:5, 1992.

Beresford L: Does hospice have a role in palliative care? *Hospice Manager's Monograph* 3(4):1, 1998.

Billings JA: What is palliative care? *J Palliat Med* 1:73, 1998.

Billings JA: Proposal for an MGH palliative care service. Executive summary. 1996.

Billings JA, Block S: Palliative care in undergraduate medical education. Status report and review. *JAMA* 278:733, 1997.

Capello CF, Meier DE, Cassel C: Payment code for hospital-based palliative care: Help or hindrance? *J Palliat Med* 1: 155, 1998.

Cassel CK, Vladeck BC: Sounding board. ICD-9 code for palliative or terminal care. *N Engl J Med* 335:1232, 1996.

Christakis NA, Escarce JJ: Survival of Medicare patients after enrollment on a hospice program. *N Engl J Med* 335:172, 1996.

Coluzzi PH, Grant M, Doroshow JH, et al: Survey of the provision of supportive care services at National Cancer Institute-designated cancer centers. *J Clin Oncol* 13:756, 1995.

Coor CA, Coor DM, eds. *Hospice Care: Principles and Practice*. New York, Springer, 1983.

Criteria for inpatient care. Policy 5:22. In: *Vitas Policy Manual*. Miami, Vitas Healthcare Corporation, 1993.

Editorial Board: New diagnosis code will track palliative care in hospitals. *Network News* 5:1, 1996.

Evans LK, Yurkow J, Siegler EL: The CARE program: A nurse-managed collaborative outpatient program to improve function of frail older people. *J Am Geriatr Soc* 43:1160, 1995.

Ferrell BR, Virant R, Grant M: Improving end of life care education in home care. *J Palliat Med* 1:11, 1998.

42 Code of Federal Regulations, Part 418, Medicare Hospice Regulations, 1993.

Grantmakers Concerned with Care at the End of Life: Paying for Care at the End of Life. Implications for Individuals and Families, Health Care Providers, and Society. New York, 1998.

Hanson LC, Tulsky JA, Danis M: Can clinical interventions change care at the end of life: *Ann Intern Med* 126:381, 1997.

Hospice Fact Sheet. National Hospice Organization, 1997.

Institute of Medicine End of Life Care Committee: *Approaching Death: Improving care at the end of life*. Washington: National Academy Press, 1997.

JervisMark Associates, Inc.: *Evaluation of Market for Hospice Care*. Miami, Vitas Healthcare Corporation, 1992.

Kinzbrunner BM: Hospice: 15 years and beyond in the care of the dying. *J Palliat Med* 1:127, 1998.

Kinzbrunner BM: The terminally ill patient. In Abeloff MD, Armitage JO, Lichter AS, Niederhuber JE, eds. *Clinical Oncology*. New York, Churchill Livingstone, 2nd ed., 2000, p. 597

Lynch-Schuster J: Palliative care programs help people with CHF/COPD stay home and stay healthy. *ABCD Exchange* 1(2):1, 1997.

Lynn J: An 88 year old woman facing the end of life. *JAMA* 277:1633, 1997.

Lynn J: Caring at the end of our lives. *N Engl J Med* 335:201, 1996. Editorial.

Mahoncy JJ: A new diagnosis-related group for palliative care. *N Engl J Med* 336:1029, 1997. Correspondence.

McKeen E, Billings JA: Reimbursement for physician services under the Medicare benefit. *Hospice Update,* December 1991.

Meier D, Morrison S, Cassel CK: Improving palliative care. *Ann Intern Med* 127:225, 1997.

Miller FG, Fins JJ: Sounding Board. A proposal to restructure hospital care for dying patients. *N Engl J Med* 334:1740, 1996

1997–1998 Comprehensive Accreditation Manual for Home Care, Chicago, Joint Commission on Accreditation of Healthcare Organizations, 1996.

Palmetto Government Benefit Administrators: *Medicare Advisory Hospice 97-11,* Hospice provisions enacted by the balanced budget act (BBA) of 1997. September, 1997.

Rhymes J: Hospice care in America. *JAMA* 264:369, 1990.

Smith DH, Granbois JA. The American way of hospice. *Hastings Cent Rep* 11:8, 1992.

Stoddard S: The Hospice Movement. A Better Way of Caring for the Dying (revised). New York, Vintage, 1991.

SUPPORT principal investigators: A controlled trial to improve care for seriously ill hospitalized patients. *JAMA* 274:1591, 1995.

Tierney J, Wilson D: Hospice care versus home health care: Regulatory distinctions and program intent. *Am J Hospice Palliat Care* 11:14, 1994

U.S. Department of HHS: *Medicare: Hospice Manual.* Springfield, U.S. Department of Commerce, January 1992.

U.S. Department of HHS: *Medicare: Hospice Manual,* Section 230.1 E (revised). Springfield, U.S. Department of Commerce, December 1992.

U.S. Department of HHS: *Medicare: Hospice Manual,* Section 306.1 (revised). Springfield, U.S. Department of Commerce, November 1993.

Von Gunten CF, Neely KJ, Martinez J: Hospice and palliative care: Program needs and academic issues. *Oncology* 10:1070, 1996.

Walsh D: The Medicare Hospice Benefit: A critique from palliative medicine. *J Palliat Med* 1:147, 1998.

Weissman DE: Palliative medicine education at the Medical College of Wisconsin. *Wis Med J* 94:505, 1995.

Welch HG, Wennberg DE, Welch WP: The use of Medicare home health care services. *N Engl J Med* 335:324, 1996.

Wilson SA, Daley BJ: Attachment/Detachment: Forces influencing care of the dying in long-term care. *J Palliat Med* 1:21, 1998.

Vincent D. Nguyen
Neal J. Weinreb

Chapter
3

How to Inform the Patient: Conveying Bad News

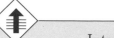

Introduction

The practice of medicine is science applied to the art of caring. To be truly competent, physicians must demonstrate an ability to listen, a willingness to acknowledge a patient's fears and concerns, an aptitude to empathize and to explain, a capability to assess and marshal social support, and a commitment to never abandon hope for the betterment of a patient's life.

Conveying bad news is one of the most difficult, and all too frequent, responsibilities for a physician in clinical practice. This task is stressful, even when the focus of decision-making is on curative or life-prolonging therapeutic options. How much more unpleasant the experience, and greater the level of discomfort, when the message to be given is the worst news a patient and loved ones can get: the disease process is incurable, life-prolonging treatment will most likely be ineffective, and the end of the patient's life is near. It is tempting for the physician to evade, or even to totally deny the issue, especially because physicians receive little if any formal training or effective mentoring in how to discuss end-of-life issues with patients and their families. Furthermore, the push for ever-increasing physician productivity in managed care settings has introduced constraints that do not favor the time-intensive efforts that are required to address these issues with clarity, sensitivity, and compassion. Nevertheless, the substantial attention that physician communication is attracting in the medical literature, in the lay press, and in the media, tells us that there is no excuse for us to continue to neglect this crucial clinical skill.

Although there have been few scientifically designed studies of the best way to convey bad news, a number of books and computer programs have become available to help clinicians improve and perfect their communication techniques. Medical schools and house officer training programs are beginning to include these methods in their curricula. Nonetheless, although methodology can provide useful tools, and knowledge of principles of medical ethics is an important framework, successful communication is ultimately not a technological *tour de force*. Rather, it depends on motivation, dedication, and a hearty helping of common sense and decency. This chapter will highlight some of the major barriers to conveying bad news, particularly in the context of end-of-life care, and will provide some practical guidance on how to do it effectively. It is hoped that the suggestions offered here, when adapted to each unique clinical situation, will increase physician confidence in the ability to communicate, and will enhance the physician–patient relationship.

The Difficulties in Conveying Bad News

Why is this task so difficult? Consider the following scenario, quoted from a newspaper article by Jane E. Brody entitled "Bad News Well Delivered: A Prescription for Doctors" (1999):

> Breathing difficulties prompted Frank to return to the hospital days before he was to receive his next chemotherapy treatment for lung cancer. When Frank asked if he'd be getting his treatment as scheduled, a doctor neither he nor his family had ever seen before replied bluntly: "We can't give you another treatment. It would kill you." To Frank, who knew his life depended on the drugs, those 10 words were a death sentence, delivered in the cruelest possible fashion. Frank's shaken family members were left on their own to try in vain to rekindle some slim hope for his survival.

The author correctly notes the inadequacies of the above communication process. However, she misses the main point. Identifying with the patient's unrealistic expectations of the chemotherapy regimen, she finds it hard to accept that which seems medically evident. Frank's prospects for survival are not merely slim, but virtually nil, yet she criticizes

Table 3–1

Implications of Life-Threatening Illness: The Patient's Perspective

TYPE OS LOSS	EXAMPLE
Loss of control	"My body has betrayed me."
Loss of identity as a normal, healthy person	"I am no longer the person I used to be."
Loss of relationships and roles	"I am afraid of losing everybody and everything."
Loss of life	

the physician for giving the patient what he perceived as a "death sentence." What she failed to recognize was that the physician should have focused his discussion with the patient, not on preserving a modicum of false hope for survival as she suggests. Rather, he should have concentrated on helping the patient and family confront an end-of-life situation realistically, with assurance that care would be continued or even intensified with a concentration on palliation of symptoms and optimization of all dimensions of the quality of remaining life. The denial displayed by this highly informed and well-intentioned columnist demonstrates one of the reasons why breaking bad news, particularly as related to end-of-life care, is so challenging.

As pointed out by Dr. Robert Buckman in "How to Break Bad News" (1992), we live in a society that values the young, the healthy, and the wealthy. Those that do not belong to this group, such as the elderly, the sick, and the poor, are often "marginalized" outside the mainstream of society. Patients with debilitating or terminal diseases are frequently left isolated from family and friends who cannot cope with the personal implications of these conditions. Therefore, it is natural that people do not want to be told that they have a life-threatening illness. They find it difficult to deal emotionally with impending losses, such as loss of control, the loss of identity as a normal, healthy person, the loss of relationships and roles, and ultimately, the loss of life itself (Table 3–1). Serious illness is frequently perceived by patients as

eroding their lifestyle, limiting choices, eliminating opportunities that healthier people enjoy, and threatening their physical and mental well-being.

For physicians, having to deliver bad news may cause great distress as well (Table 3–2). Physicians may experience a sense of professional inadequacy for having "failed" the patient, and these feelings may be compounded by a sense of ineptness in performing such tasks, particularly when they have not been properly trained to do so. Bad news usually elicits strong reactions from the recipient that may sometimes be expressed with histrionics or even graphic physical behavior. Physicians may be intimidated or be "put off" by even a potential patient outburst, especially when they are poorly prepared to defuse such emotional and/or physical reactions. To further complicate matters, even nonhostile but nevertheless strong adaptive reactions by the patient may cause

Table 3–2

Implications of Delivering Bad News: The Physician's Reactions

Feelings of ineptness in performing such tasks
Feelings of inadequacy in dealing with the emotions involved
Feelings of intimidation in being blamed for the patient's illness
Feelings of professional impotence for "failing" the patient

physicians to express their own emotions (anger, panic, sadness that may lead to tears). Although debatable, this is often perceived as weak and unprofessional behavior. However, keeping in mind that the patient is the one with the disease, why is it wrong for physicians to share in their pain and distress, provided that they can simultaneously retain professional objectivity?

Physicians are trained not to inflict pain without offering anesthesia or sedation. Bad news certainly causes pain to the person receiving it. Unfortunately, when presenting bad news, there is no place for anesthetics or sedatives. The physician must deliver it while the patient is awake, alert, and mentally competent to understand the situation, which only magnifies the degree of physician discomfort.

Besides distaste for inflicting pain, physicians also fear being blamed for delivering bad news. Commonly, the bearer of bad tidings is inappropriately perceived as the cause of the circumstance. Anger that is misdirected at the physician should be directed at the underlying disease process or at "the slings of outrageous fortune." Nevertheless, after a good outcome, the physician usually is happy to take the credit! Thus, when things go wrong, even when out of one's control, it should be anticipated that there might be an element of unspoken or even overt hostility. The physician must be prepared to deal with this in a way that promotes the patient's best interests.

Physicians have been trained to believe that there is an effective treatment for every illness, a pill for every ill, an ideal solution for every problem. The concept of therapeutic impotence is difficult to accept because every judgment is constantly scrutinized. One is always asking whether there was something else that could have been done, some additional test or procedure that could have been performed, or some drug(s) that could have been tried. It often feels professionally degrading to have to say "I don't have an answer." Remember, however, that although this blow to a physician's ego may be troubling, what the doctor feels pales in comparison to what the patient, faced with his or her own mortality, must endure.

How to Break Bad News Well

An aphorism in the Book of Proverbs states: "There are those that speak like the piercing of a sword; but the tongue of the wise heals." Breaking bad news may be difficult, but it can be and should be done.

As part of the physician's duty and responsibility to the patient, being able to convey bad news in an appropriate fashion is a basic skill comparable to history-taking or physical examination. The latter tools are essential to reaching a correct diagnosis and initiating treatment. Similarly, when the task of conveying bad news is done with honesty and compassion, enhanced trust strengthens the patient–doctor relationship and increases the likelihood that the patient will choose an appropriate treatment approach. Conversely, bad news delivered badly can cause needless emotional pain and lead to a loss of confidence in the doctor's recommendations and plan of treatment.

Not only does it benefit patients when physicians are capable of conveying bad news properly, but it is in the best interest of the physician to have these skills finely tuned as well. A patient rightfully expects to be spoken to in a caring and professional manner. A physician is unlikely to have a successful community practice if he or she is cold, impersonal, and insensitive. In addition, more malpractice litigation results from poor communication than from actual medical negligence. Finally, developing these skills and appropriately applying them enhances professional satisfaction in a job well done.

Delivering bad news successfully requires the physician to adequately prepare for this encounter, to relay the message in a clear and concise manner that the listener(s) can understand, and to take time tending to the patient's physical and emotional needs. Bad news will forever change the patient's reality, whether the illness is life threatening or life altering. Thus, it is important to note that the way the news is presented sets the tone for the patient, the family, and the doctor for the entire illness experience together.

"SPIKES"

S P I K E S is an acronym used by Dr. Buckman and his colleagues (1992) to represent a six-step protocol for breaking bad news. It stands for setting, perception, invitation, knowledge, empathy, and summation. These steps are summarized in Table 3–3 and discussed next.

Setting

Preparation is the essential concept in this step. Review medical notes and laboratory results beforehand. The more prepared you are for the meeting with the patient, and the more knowledgeable you are about the case, the more you will feel in control. The patient and family will have greater assurance that your assessment and recommendations are based on forethought and total knowledge of the case. The more that you know about the patient's family and cultural and religious background, the better you will be able to help that patient. There are significant cultural differences that influence what and how much a patient wishes to know. In an ever-increasingly multicultural society, we must be aware of and respect these varying attitudes.

Breaking bad news is done best in a face-to-face encounter. There is a great sense of rapport and humanness conveyed by a live presence that is lost in a telephone call. If, due to distance or other circumstance, it is impossible to meet face to face, then make a point of mentioning to the patient/family that you are sorry that a personal meeting was not feasible.

Unless it is absolutely unavoidable, meetings about bad news should be done in privacy. A

Table 3–3

"SPIKES"—Six Practical Considerations in Delivering Bad News

	STEP	CHARACTERISTICS
S	Setting	Prepare in advance
		Face-to-face visit
		Choose a private or quiet environment
		Family/loved one/confidante
		Provide an interpreter, if necessary
P	Perception	Ask the patient what he or she knows or perceives
I	Invitation	Seek the patient's invitation to break news
		Ask how much the patient wants to know
		Share information clearly and directly
		Listen and be patient
K	Knowledge	Listen to the patient's response
		Listen to the patient's emotions
E	Empathy	Respond by identifying and validating patient's emotions
S	Summation	Summarize the delivered news
		Review the patient's treatment options
		Schedule follow-up visits

noisy public setting does not allow the parties to fully pay attention to what is being discussed, and, at worst, may be embarrassing or even insulting. Therefore, choose a quiet place and minimize any distractions.

If at the bedside, close the door or draw the curtain in a nonprivate room to maintain a sense of privacy. Set yourself in a position of comfort relatively close to the patient, and try to be at the patient's eye level. This is a sign to the patient that you would like to engage in a nonpatronizing conversation. Always try to make the patient feel at ease. In your office, pull up a chair, and try to sit on the same side of the desk rather than opposite the patient. Maintain a comfortable distance, but close enough that holding a hand, touching an arm, or offering a facial tissue can be easily accomplished. Be conscious that your body language conveys your interest and dedication to the task at hand. Avoid interruptions as much as possible. If at all possible, turn off your pager and divert all incoming telephone calls. Apologize for even the briefest interruption.

Use the patient's family and friends as a resource. Studies have shown that strong family and social bonds alleviate sickness and enhance patient cooperation with medical treatments. Furthermore, many patients, on hearing bad news, tune the doctor out, and may not understand or remember what was actually said or discussed. Ask if the patient wants to invite a confidante, and in fact urge that the patient come with someone who they trust. The patient will likely require emotional and psychosocial support from this relative or friend. Remember, however, that the bad news may be as upsetting for the loved one as it is for the patient. Be sure that you introduce yourself and anyone else who may be present.

If the patient does not speak English, and you are not fluent in the patient's language, try not to use a family member or friend as an interpreter. Rather, find a professional interpreter, if available, and ask the interpreter to translate as accurately as possible the thought as well as the verbiage.

Perception

Before blurting out and divulging the bad news, it is wise to find out what the patient suspects or already knows. The responses from the patient will serve as a guide, particularly when the patient is prompted with open-ended questions to which the replies are usually more revealing than simple yes-or-no answers. The patient's level of comprehension and the vocabulary used will further set the stage for what the physician should say. For example, referring to the scenario at the start of the chapter:

> Frank, before I can answer your question about the chemotherapy, let me ask you a question. Where do you think things stand with your illness?

Depending on the answer, the physician might follow up with a question about Frank's worsening dyspnea in terms of the extent it is worrisome to the patient, its import and implications. By so doing, the doctor should have a better idea as to whether Frank suspects or understands that he likely has disease that has progressed despite chemotherapy, and whether he has made the connection between his worsening shortness of breath and the refractoriness of his lung cancer. Of course, if the worsening dyspnea is related to a reversible, intercurrent infection rather than to progressive disease, an immediate direct answer that chemotherapy could be resumed when the infection is resolved would be appropriate. Nevertheless, even in that circumstance, this is a propitious moment to attempt to learn what Frank understands about his disease process and course to date. In this way, the doctor shows the patient that he or she is interested in the patient's perceptions and input.

Invitation

In this step, the physician finds out how much the patient wants to know about his or her condition, and seeks the patient's invitation to break the news. How much the patient wishes to know depends on personality, religion, ethnicity, and culture. The patient most likely knows at this stage that good news is unlikely, but some patients still prefer not to actually hear bad news themselves. In some cultures, there is the belief that relating bad news actually hastens or guarantees the event. Thus, before disclosure, the doctor should always offer the patient a true choice, and exhibit the sensitivity to ask.

> Frank, I have looked at your chest x-rays a few minutes ago. Would you like to talk about the results?

Depending on his response, the physician can probe further.

> It sounds as if you don't wish to talk about it. Are you afraid that the results might not be good? Would you prefer that I discuss the results with your wife?

If the patient does not want to know or does not wish to hear the full details at that moment, the physician must not cut off all lines of communication.

> I sense that you are uncomfortable at this moment. Is there anything that I can do for you, Frank? If you prefer, let's reschedule our meeting later today or tomorrow morning.

Being sensitive to the patient's desire for realism and to his readiness for acceptance is crucial at this moment, because you are about to deliver news that may confirm his worst fears. Denial is quite common at this stage. Some patients consciously or unconsciously regularly use denial as an adaptive technique to buffer themselves from distress, while others merely need to buy time to acclimatize themselves to their worsening condition.

Most often, the patient will wish to continue the discussion, at which time the physician should proceed by foreshadowing the bad news in simple language. Gauge his reaction. Be careful not to give the patient more information than he is ready to hear because the patient may not be prepared for all of the details at this time.

> Frank, I'm sorry to have to tell you that the x-ray doesn't look good. I'm afraid that the cancer has begun to grow again.

After stating the bad news, it's a good idea to stop talking and to listen. Silence at this time may be uncomfortable or even unbearable for the physician. However, a pause from speaking is essential to allow patients to collect their thoughts, and for you to watch their reaction. Observe the impact on the patient of the news you have conveyed. Various reactions by the patient are possible: from rage to withdrawal, from screaming to silence, from crying to anger. These first reactions can give significant insight into the patient's personality. With the passage of time, it will become clear whether the patient's responses are adaptive or maladaptive. Accepted and even useful defense mechanisms for dealing with bad news include limited denial, anger (either abstract or directed at the disease), crying, fear, and sometimes, humor. Oftentimes, patients will engage the doctor in a type of bargaining or channel their energy towards a realistic future goal such as a key holiday or family event. On the other hand, morbid guilt; pathologic denial often associated with inappropriate behavior; anger directed at caregivers, family, or physicians; profound despair; overtly manipulative behavior; and unrealistic hope associated with "the impossible quest" are maladaptive responses that may sometimes require professional intervention. Some of these problems may be anticipated based on the patient's initial reaction to the bad news.

Listening allows the doctor to learn and understand what the illness means to the patient. Patients may often give clues or express what matters most to them. Empathy, like attentive listening, requires patience, which is a virtue that requires practice. Unfortunately, patience is rarely an inherent physician character trait, and is seldom taught. However, patience and empathy promote trust. Only with establishment of a trusting relationship will the physician be granted access to the patient's deeper feelings, values, and ideas.

Knowledge and Empathy

Empathy is defined by Block and Coulehan (1988) as

> a type of understanding. It is not an emotional state of feeling sorry for someone. Nor is it the same virtue as compassion. Although compassion may well be your motivation for developing empathy with patients, empathy is not compassion. In medical interviewing, being empathetic means listening to the total communication—words, feelings, and gestures—and letting patients know that you are really hearing what they are saying. The empathetic physician is also the scientific physician because understanding is at the core of objectivity.

The two steps of knowledge and empathy occur consecutively as the doctor follows a statement of fact (knowledge) with a response to the patient's reaction (empathy). Empathetic behavior requires you to identify the emotion that the patient is experiencing as well as the origin of that emotion. It also requires you to respond in a kind way that tells patients that you understand them.

> Frank, I feel that I must have knocked you over with this report. You certainly have every reason to be upset, sad, and angry. I appreciate that not knowing exactly what the future holds in store is frightening, and I share your concern.

Remaining silent after an empathetic remark, perhaps by counting slowly and silently to 10 before saying anything else, is often recommended by numerous authors. This pause allows the patient to absorb the feeling of being understood, and permits the physician to consider how and what the patient is thinking and feeling. Avoid the temptation to continue the conversation in order to fix the situation or to assuage the patient. It is hard to overcome the urge to quickly turn to a treatment plan so as to divert the patient from the painful news just delivered. Eventually, an appropriate action plan will need to be proposed and agreed to by the patient/family, but at this point it is premature.

The manner of breaking bad news is not a "one size fits all" approach. Truthfulness is important, but even the truth sometimes needs to be tailored to match individual patient needs. Sometimes it may be wise to temper the burden of complete knowledge. However, if due to poor understanding about the diagnosis, the prognosis, or the therapeutic options, the patient may make a poor choice about proposed interventions, the physician is medically, legally, and ethically obligated to give patients or their designated surrogates sufficient information to make appropriate informed choices.

A patient's feelings of hopelessness can further exacerbate sickness and deterioration, and even lead to a premature death. Even near the end of life, hope may be preserved in various ways. Studies reveal that few patients abandon hope for a cure, even when highly improbable. Other patients find hope by exercising control of their choices and ensuring that they will not suffer a lingering death complicated by prolonged tube feedings, ventilator support, or cardiopulmonary resuscitation. Even in the case of a terminal illness, a doctor's offer of hope, when presented as a commitment to ensure a comfortable, peaceful, and dignified dying experience, free of pain and suffering, is not a deception.

In the era of managed care, some physicians may believe that they do not have sufficient time for empathetic communication. However, research has shown that an up-front "investment" in good communication ultimately saves enormous amounts of time—time the patient will otherwise spend asking repetitive questions. Empathetic communication is one of the few panaceas in medicine. It predictably generates improved patient and physician satisfaction, fewer malpractice suits, better patient adherence to therapy, and improved clinical outcomes including the often-sought "good death."

Summation

The last task in the six-step SPIKE protocol requires the physician to summarize the delivered news and review the potential treatment options. These may include combinations of therapeutics such as chemotherapy, radiation therapy, surgery, or experimental treatment for malignant illnesses. When faced with an incurable disease for which definitive treatment options are lacking or futile, physicians should offer hospice care to assist in palliation of symptoms, to focus on the relief of total suffering, and to help patients die with comfort and dignity. Pay attention to identifying caregivers, ensuring proper living arrangements, and establishing contact with support groups and/or community agencies. The patient and family need to leave the meeting with a clear understanding of what has happened to date and what is planned for the future. End by inviting future questions, scheduling follow-up visits, and planning an agenda for the next meeting. When the patient concludes this session with you, he or she should leave with assurance as to your continued availability, with a clear understanding of a mutually acceptable plan of care open to future revision as needed, with the knowledge that his or her wishes will be respected, and with reasonable hope that pain and suffering will be alleviated.

Conclusion

Breaking bad news can be a grueling mental and emotional experience. It is easy to do it poorly due to haste, anxiety, guilt, or insensitivity. Although desiring in principle to be supportive to patients and families, many doctors, aware of their own discomfort and lack of ease during such emotionally charged patient encounters, deliver a rapid-paced, fact-filled monologue without stopping to elicit any response from the listener. Delivering bad news in a rushed, thoughtless, uncaring manner can cause unnecessary harm to patients and to their families, and can often make the bad news worse. Studies clearly demonstrate that the way bad news is communicated leaves an indelible, long-lasting impression on patients and their loved ones.

The suggestions and ideas offered in this chapter can help clinicians convey bad news more effectively and compassionately. The manner in which bad news is delivered can have a major effect on your patient's attitude and compliance. It also reflects on your image as a caring and empathetic clinician. The ability to communicate well is not inborn. It is a learned behavior. With practice, this skill can be artfully polished and become one of the most important elements of the care that you render.

In the final analysis, think how you would wish to be treated if you (as will inevitably occur) were the patient. You would hope that your experience would match that of Dr. Deborah Young Bradshaw (1999):

> I recognized that what had happened in that examination room was simply an act of love. Love in any relationship, including that between doctor and patient, requires the courage to risk revealing oneself unedited, the willingness to notice and to listen, the willingness to surrender one's own ease or comfort, the willingness to share the suffering of another and the courage to risk and accept gentle confrontation. In this way, any loving relationship can heal. Any relationship hoping to heal without love falls short.
>
> That day, I learned what it is to be in need and to be taken care of. That day, I felt healing hands upon me and was left breathless with new awareness of the awesome gift and profound responsibility I had been given as a physician.

Bibliography

Annunziata MA: Ethics of relationship. From communication to conversation. *Ann N Y Acad Sci* 809:400, 1997.

Annunziata MA, Foladore S, Magri MD, et al: Does the information level of cancer patients correlate with quality of life? A prospective study. *Tumori* 84:619, 1998 (in English).

Block MR, Coulehan JL: A taxonomy of difficult physician–patient interactions. *Fam Med* 20:221, 1988.

Bradshaw DY: A visit to the doctor. *Ann Intern Med* 131:627, 1999.

Brody J: Personal Health: Bad News. *New York Times,* 24 August 1999, Health and Fitness.

Buckman R: *How to Break Bad News: A Guide for Health Care Professionals.* Baltimore, Johns Hopkins, 1992, pp. 65–171.

Landro L: Patient–physician communication: An emerging partnership. *Oncologist* 4:55, 1999.

Lintz KC, Penson RT, Cassem, et al: A staff dialogue on aggressive palliative treatment demanded by a terminally ill patient: psychological issues faced by patients, their families, and caregivers. *Oncologist* 4:70, 1999.

Lo B, Snyder L, Sox HC: Care at the end of life: Guiding practice where there are no easy answers. *Ann Intern Med* 130:772, 1999.

Nowak TV: The ritual. *Ann Intern Med* 130:1025, 1999.

Petrasch S, Bauer M, Reinacher-Schick A, et al: Assessment of satisfaction with the communication process during consultation of cancer patients with potentially curable disease, cancer patients on palliative care, and HIV-positive patients. *Wien Med Wochenschr.* 148:491, 1998 (in English).

Poulson J: Bitter pills to swallow. *N Engl J Med* 338: 1844, 1998.

Quill TE, Townsend P. Bad news: delivery, dialogue, and dilemmas. *Arch Intern Med* 151:463, 1991.

Suchman AL, Markakis K, Beckman HB, Frankel R: A model of empathetic communication in the medical interview. *JAMA* 277:678, 1997.

Joel S. Policzer

Chapter 4

How to Work with an Interdisciplinary Team

Introduction

American society has become more aware of the need to adequately provide for the needs of people near the end of life, and to this end there has been a growth in the system of hospices. There are now estimated to be more than 3000 hospices in the United States, and most communities have one, if not many. Therefore, it will be common for a practicing physician to have contact with a hospice when caring for patients during the final stage of life.

American physicians tend not to be comfortable with the care of dying patients, as the necessary skills are often not taught during medical education and training. Rather, physician training revolves around the care of the living and the battle against disease. Disability and death are perceived as failures of medical care, and often failure of the physician. Traditional training of physicians has rarely included end-of-life issues, and it should therefore not be surprising that training in the functioning of hospice is lacking as well. In addition, the widely held attitude that death is equivalent to failure, the medicolegal climate that holds that death is suspect and may be due to physician error, and the view that hospice care is best delayed for those who are actively dying all serve to delay physician acceptance of the true role of hospice as a facilitator of end-of-life care.

In caring for patients near the end of life, addressing physical symptoms alone is not sufficient to achieve adequate comfort. Patients require comprehensive care from professionals who recognize and can help with the psychological and spiritual causes of distress. From the recognition that quality end-of-life care comes from the coordinated efforts of individuals from various disciplines, the Medicare Hospice Benefit has mandated that certified hospice programs meet patient and family needs by providing care via an interdisciplinary team. The importance of the interdisciplinary team approach to care is further underscored by the

fact that it has been adopted by many nonhospice palliative care programs.

The interdisciplinary team consists of, at the minimum, a registered nurse, physician, social worker and chaplain. Other professionals often added to the team include home health aides, homemakers, pharmacists, and volunteers. With the patient, family, and attending physician, who are considered core members of the team, it is the responsibility of the entire interdisciplinary team to develop and implement a comprehensive plan of care. With multiple disciplines offering insight into patient-identified problems from different viewpoints, individualized and innovative solutions to these problems will lead to more successful patient care outcomes.

The team approach to end-of-life care is unique among health care services offered in the United States. For physicians caring for terminally ill patients, therefore, it is important to understand how the interdisciplinary team functions, how each member contributes to the whole, and how they, as physicians, may effectively participate with the team to optimize care for their patients at the end of life.

The Physician's Role in Hospice and End-of-Life Care

The physician who works with hospices and other end-of-life care programs will need to learn how to function, as do other members of a team. This team approach is somewhat foreign to most physicians, who have been trained to work independently and autonomously, as well as to be "the captain of the ship," holding ultimate responsibility for the outcome of care provided. This traditional view, that the physician knows best, directly challenges the basic tenet of hospice and palliative care—that the patient is the center of the team's focus and that the patient knows best.

There are distinct roles that a physician can play when caring for patients enrolled in an end-

Table 4–1

Physician Roles in Hospice Care

PHYSICIAN ROLE	DEFINITION
Attending physician	The physician who is identified by the patient as having the most significant role in the determination of that patient's medical care
Long-term care medical director	The physician who is responsible to oversee the medical care provided to all patients residing at all care levels in the facility
Managed care medical director	The physician employed by a managed care organization who is responsible to oversee the medical care provided to patients on the plan
Consulting physician	A physician contracted by the hospice to provide a specific medical service to a patient that cannot be provided by the attending physician or the hospice medical director
Hospice medical director	A physician, usually employed by the hospice, who is primarily responsible for oversight of the medical care rendered to patients cared for by the hospice
Hospice team physician	A physician, usually employed by the hospice, who is responsible for providing hands-on medical care to patients cared for by the hospice.

of-life care program. These roles are most clearly defined by the Medicare Hospice Benefit and the hospice approach to care. The hospice model will be used as the template for this discussion, with the understanding that, in many respects, similar physician activities will occur in nonhospice palliative programs as well.

Physician roles are either outside or inside the hospice organization. Physicians may interact with hospices as attending physicians, long-term care medical directors, managed care medical directors, or consulting physicians. Physicians working with hospice programs may function as hospice medical directors or as hospice team physicians. Table 4–1 lists each role with a brief description, and more detailed discussion is provided next.

Attending Physician

By federal regulation, the attending physician is a physician of medicine or osteopathy who "is identified by the individual, at the time he or she elects to receive hospice care, as having the most sig-

nificant role in the determination of the individual's medical care." The continued involvement and participation of this physician as a member of the interdisciplinary team in all phases of a patient's care near the end of life is vital.

Table 4–2 summarizes the responsibilities of the attending physician in relationship to a hospice program. The first obligation of the attending physician is to determine that a patient is entering into the final stage of life. Although the argument is often made that no one knows exactly when any given person will die, guidelines published by the National Hospice and Palliative Care Organization, as well as by other reputable sources, can be helpful to the physician in assessing patient prognosis. Combining these guidelines with sound clinical judgment, physicians can better identify when patients are approaching the end of life and in need of hospice and palliative care. (See Chapter 1 for a detailed discussion of this topic.)

The next step for the attending physician is to communicate the need for end-of-life care to patients and caregivers. This is never an easy task and there are many tools available to the physi-

Table 4–2
Role of the Attending Physician

Key member of the interdisciplinary team
Certifies that the patient has a limited life
  expectancy
Discusses need for end-of-life care with patient
  and family
Actively participates in the care of the patient
  on the hospice program
Professional services are reimbursable under
  Medicare Part B
    Office, home, and long-term care facility
      visits
    Care planning (30–60 minutes per month)

cian to illustrate how this type of information is best communicated. The goal is to have patients understand where in their illness they find themselves and what forms of treatment have been used and are available. As the patient's treatment options become more limited, the options of hospice and palliative care become of more value. If making the underlying disease better cannot relieve symptoms, then symptom relief via expert palliative and hospice care is of real benefit. With appropriate counseling it is possible to have the majority of end-of-life patients accept hospice-type care early in the course of their terminal phase, not just prior to the moment of death. (See Chapter 3 for a detailed discussion of this topic.) Once the patient and caregiver have agreed to a referral to a hospice, the attending physician refers the patient to an appropriate hospice agency and certifies that the patient indeed has a limited life span, expected to be less than 6 months if the disease follows its natural course.

Once the patient is admitted to the hospice program, the attending physician should be directly involved in all medical decision making, working together with the hospice medical director as well as the other members of the interdisciplinary team. The attending physician is likely to know the

patient better than the hospice caregivers, and be aware of the patient's goals, preferences for treatment, and how the patient perceives the reality that his or her life is ending.

Ideally, all attending physicians would continue to work closely with the hospice interdisciplinary team, but this is sometimes not the case. Some physicians are uncomfortable caring for patients near the end of life, either for personal reasons or, more often, due to lack of formal training and expertise in palliative care. Fortunately, with the expertise of the hospice personnel, and with an open attitude of cooperation and willingness to learn, physicians who do not have a background in palliative medicine can become comfortable and proficient in the care of their end-of-life patients. This serves not only their patients, but will add to the physician's own personal sense of accomplishment.

As a member of the interdisciplinary team, the attending physician will be kept informed of a patient's course of illness, verbally by various members of the hospice interdisciplinary team, and less often, in writing. The attending physician may attend the hospice interdisciplinary team meeting, if not in person then by conference call, and directly participate in the care planning of common patients. Medication orders and orders to change a patient's hospice level of care are usually provided to the hospice nurse by the attending physician, unless the attending physician is either unavailable or has asked that the hospice medical director accept that responsibility.

In recognition of the fact that the attending physician is a fully active and vital member of the hospice interdisciplinary team, the Medicare Hospice Benefit has made special provisions to ensure that attending physicians are compensated for their continued care and support to patients and families at the end of life. Under the Medicare Hospice Benefit, the hospice is responsible to provide all health care services related to the terminal illness for patients under its care. (See Chapter 2 for a more detailed discussion of the Medicare Hospice Benefit.) However, the patient's attending physician may also receive Medicare reimbursement for professional services provided to patients via normal Medicare Part B reimbursement means. This allows the attending physician to be compensated for visiting patients either at their places of residence (home or long-term care facility), inpatient hospice, or in the physician's office. Medicare also provides reimbursement to attending physicians for care planning services, so that physicians may be compensated for their active participation in care for their patients who are receiving hospice care near the end of life.

Long-Term Care Facility Medical Director

One of the goals of end-of-life care is to allow patients to be cared for at home, if that is their wish. Home is defined as where the patient lives, and does not need to be a house or apartment. As patients weaken and are not able to receive adequate care in a private residence, some become residents of long-term care (LTC) facilities (nursing homes). The LTC facility becomes the patient's place of residence or home, and care is rendered there.

The LTC facility medical director is the physician primarily charged with overseeing the medical care

Table 4–3
Role of the Long-Term Care Medical Director

Serve as attending physician
Collaborate with hospice medical director
Coordination of patient care planning
Development of treatment guidelines
Education of LTC and hospice staffs
Oversight of patient care in LTC facility
Identify patients who may need end-of-life care
Ensure hospice patients are receiving appropriate end-of-life care

provided to all patients residing in the facility. In relationship to a hospice program, the LTC facility medical director interacts in a number of ways, summarized in Table 4–3, and discussed next.

First, in many LTC facilities, the medical director will have primary care responsibilities for some or all of the patients living in the home; and for those patients receiving hospice services, the medical director will function as the attending physician. (See Table 4–2 and the earlier discussion.)

Second, as the overseer of the medical care provided to patients in the LTC facility, the medical director is responsible for making certain that patients receive the care that they need, including hospice and palliative care when appropriate. For patients near the end of life, the LTC facility medical director can accomplish this by collaborating directly with the hospice medical director(s) from hospice organization(s) with which the LTC facility holds contracts. Joint activities between the respective medical directors may include ensuring that there are coordinated plans of care for common patients; developing palliative care treatment guidelines that meet patient needs while meeting safety, efficacy, and regulatory standards of both organizations; and educating LTC facility and hospice staff on how to better serve patients who are near the end of life.

Interaction between the respective medical directors may also occur when there is a conflict between the hospice plan of care and the LTC facility's plan of care. With both physicians properly communicating about the nature of the potential conflict, a solution that meets the needs of the patient and family, as well as of both the LTC and the hospice, is more likely to be developed.

Finally, the LTC facility medical director may provide needed oversight for patients being cared for by other facility attending physicians. The medical director can assist in identifying facility patients who might need hospice or palliative care, as well as verify that the care rendered meets both the needs of the patient and family, and the safety, efficacy, and regulatory needs of the LTC facility and the hospice.

Managed Care Medical Director

The managed care medical director is a physician employed by a managed care organization whose primary responsibility is to oversee the medical care provided to patients who receive insurance benefits from the plan. Unlike the LTC facility medical director, a managed care medical director rarely, if ever, carries a significant patient care role. Hence, in their interaction with hospice programs, it is much less common for the managed care medical director to function as an attending physician to a hospice patient.

Interactions between hospices and managed care medical directors are primarily administrative in nature. Examples of these interactions are listed in Table 4–4.

Much like the LTC medical director, the managed care medical director should work with his or her hospice counterpart to ensure that hospice guidelines and treatment protocols meet the standards of the managed care organization. Educating staff is also crucial, and for the managed care medical director this means assisting the hospice in communicating with managed care case managers and attending physicians, regarding identification of patients who need end-of-

Table 4–4
Role of the Managed Care Medical Director

Collaborate with hospice medical director
    Coordination of case management and patient care planning
    Development of treatment guidelines
    Education of managed care case managers and hospice staffs
Oversight of patient care
    Identify patients who may need end-of-life care
    Ensure hospice patients are receiving appropriate end-of-life care
    Determine relationship of interventions to terminal illness

life care, as well as disseminating palliative care treatment guidelines.

The managed care medical director must also work with the hospice medical director to ensure that patients are cared for in a comprehensive fashion. For Medicare patients cared for by a managed care organization this can be a challenge. Medicare regulations have determined that when a Medicare patient enrolls on a hospice program, Medicare will reimburse the hospice for services related to the terminal illness, just as for a fee-for-service Medicare patient, adjusting reimbursement to the managed care organization to reflect its responsibility for care that is unrelated to the terminal illness. This may create conflict between the hospice and the managed care organization around whether a particular patient need is the responsibility of the hospice program or the managed care organization. It is the responsibility of the managed care medical director, together with the hospice medical director, to determine which organization should be required to provide the particular service, based upon its relationship to the terminal illness.

For commercially insured patients, the most common arrangement between hospices and managed care organizations is a per-diem contract that mirrors the Hospice Medicare Benefit. Here, the hospice provides the clinical service under contract (and with payment from) the managed care organization; under such circumstances the managed care medical director and the hospice medical director need to work together to ensure that common patients receive appropriate services and appropriate levels of care.

Consulting Physician

The role of the consulting physician may at first glance seem unnecessary for patients who are nearing the end of life. Principles of palliative care, after all, suggest that invasive therapies should be avoided or at the very least kept to a minimum. To best meet patient needs, however, there will be occasions when invasive therapies will be the best

Role of Consulting Physicians

Consultant	Example of Indication
Orthopedics	Pathologic fracture
Urologist	Suprapubic stent placement
Pulmonologist	Therapeutic thoracentisis
Radiologist	Biliary stent placement
Gastroenterologist	PEG tube placement

approach to providing patient comfort. (A full discussion of invasive treatments that may be necessary for patients near the end of life can be found in Chapter 17.) On occasion, expert advice about a patient's condition will be required that is outside the expertise of both the attending physician and the hospice medical director. In either of these circumstances, consulting physicians may be required.

Examples of the services that consulting physicians provide to terminally ill patients can be found in Table 4–5. What is important when considering whether or not a patient requires care from a consulting physician is to evaluate the need for the consultation in the face of the patient's current condition, the symptom or symptoms being treated, and the chances of a successful outcome.

For patients being cared for by hospice programs under the Medicare Hospice Benefit, consulting physician services are to be provided by the hospice program. Therefore, the hospice must have a contract with the consulting physician for the physician to provide services to a patient, and the hospice is responsible to compensate the physician directly. It may also bill the hospice Medicare Part A intermediary and be reimbursed for the professional services of the consultant.

Hospice Medical Director

The Medicare Hospice Benefit requires a certified hospice to have a medical director who is primarily responsible to oversee the medical care rendered to patients cared for by the hospice. The various responsibilities of the hospice medical director are outlined in Table 4–6, and discussed next.

QUALITY MEDICAL CARE IN CONSONANCE WITH PRINCIPLES OF PALLIATIVE CARE

The hospice medical director is responsible for ensuring that patients receive care that is both necessary and appropriate. This responsibility begins by ensuring that patients who are receiving hospice services are in need of hospice services. This is accomplished by either directly certifying (together with the attending physician) that the patients have life-limiting illnesses with a predicted survival of 6 months or less, or if the patient is certified by another hospice physician, providing oversight to make certain that the hospice physician is exercising proper judgment.

Table 4–6
Roles of the Hospice Medical Director

Ensure that patients receive quality medical
care in consonance with principles of
palliative care
Ensure patients who receive care are
terminally ill
Development of treatment guidelines,
protocols, and standards
Participate in interdisciplinary team care
planning conferences
Provide expert advice to attending physicians, hospice physicians, and hospice staff
Assume administrative and management roles
within the hospice
Supervise hospice team physicians
Pharmacy utilization management
Strategic and business planning
Survey and regulatory compliance
Assist in education and training of hospice staff
Engage in community professional education
and liaison activities
Develop medical education and palliative care
research programs

(See Chapter 1 for a discussion of guidelines that help determine patient prognosis.) If prognosis requires reevaluation, it is the hospice medical director's responsibility to ensure that the hospice physician assesses the patient properly. (See Chapter 2 for further discussion of the Medicare Hospice Benefit.)

Once the patient is admitted to the hospice program, the hospice medical director must make certain that care being rendered to patients meets hospice and palliative care standards. This is accomplished in a variety of ways, including the development of treatment guidelines, protocols, and standards, and participation in hospice care planning meetings. Participation in hospice quality improvement functions and audits is a vehicle by which the medical director can monitor how well treatment guidelines, protocols, and standards, as well as other aspects of the quality of patient care are being followed.

Ensuring that patients receive treatment consistent with palliative care principles also entails frequent interaction with attending physicians, especially when there is uncertainty surrounding a patient's diagnosis or prognosis or when there is question regarding the optimal care to be rendered. In these circumstances, the hospice medical director can function as an expert consultant, providing the patient's attending physician with advice regarding, for example, optimal approaches to relieve a patient's pain, or whether the patient is eligible for hospice services. Due to lack of understanding by many physicians regarding the principles of hospice and palliative care, disagreements between attending physicians and hospice medical directors sometimes occur. Although this should be expected in the normal course of patient care, the relationship between the hospice medical director and attending physician should be viewed as cooperative, with the best interests of the patient always being paramount.

In addition to serving as a palliative care expert for attending physicians, hospice medical directors may function in a similar capacity for hospice team physicians and other hospice staff. Being available to provide expertise to hospice nurses and physicians can go a long way to making sure patients receive optimum care in a timely and efficient manner.

ADMINISTRATIVE AND MANAGEMENT ROLES WITHIN THE HOSPICE

The hospice medical director should be the medical leader of the hospice program. Working together with other clinical and administrative leaders, the medical director should play a major role in all facets of the operation of the hospice program.

Supervision of hospice team physicians is an important medical director function. The hospice medical director provides medical leadership to hospice physicians, assisting them in participating in the interdisciplinary team environment. Hospice medical directors ensure that the other hospice physicians are, for example, actively involved in the team care planning conferences. They encourage the hospice physicians to follow hospice treatment guidelines and protocols, making certain that appropriate palliative care interventions are being provided to patients and families. They also review hospice physicians' prognosis certification and recertification decisions to ensure that patients receiving hospice services are and remain eligible for the hospice benefit.

As palliative care has become more complex, and as resources have become less available, the appropriate use of pharmaceutical products has become a major challenge for many hospices. By understanding the efficacy of various interventions available for patients near the end of life, the medical director can, by the development of formularies and ongoing utilization monitoring, assist hospice physicians and management in providing appropriate palliative interventions in a cost-effective manner.

As the medical leader of the hospice program, the hospice medical director should be actively involved in all aspects of the hospice's strategic and business planning efforts This includes setting goals and objectives for all aspects of the hospice operation, specifically involving areas in which the medical director is directly involved, such as quality improvement and pharmacy utilization.

Another important task for the medical director is participation in survey and regulatory compliance activities. Understanding the hospice regulations and conditions of participation will allow the medical director to respond to surveyor concerns about aspects of the care provided to patients and families. Increasing regulatory scrutiny regarding patient eligibility for hospice services has led Health Care Financing Administration (HCFA) fiscal intermediaries to develop "Local Medical Review Policies" (LMRPs) that better define patient eligibility criteria for hospice services. When reimbursement of hospice services to a patient is retrospectively denied, it is the medical director, with his or her knowledge of the patient's clinical course, who will be in the best position to successfully argue with the fiscal intermediary as to why the patient was, in fact, eligible for hospice services.

EDUCATION AND TRAINING OF HOSPICE STAFF

The medical director needs to be actively involved in educating and training hospice staff members, including physicians, nurses, and other staff members. Palliative care treatment guidelines, pharmacy utilization management issues, and new developments in palliative care are among the key topics that the medical director must continually bring to the attention of interested staff to maintain high standards of patient care.

COMMUNITY PROFESSIONAL EDUCATION AND LIAISON ACTIVITIES

Education of hospice staff is not enough. The hospice medical director should be viewed as an end-of-life care expert in the community, providing education to health care providers throughout the hospice program's service area. Medical conferences and grand rounds programs are an effective approach to reaching physician colleagues, as are one-on-one or small group meetings. In-service presentations at hospitals and long-term care facilities are other educational activities in which the hospice medical director may participate.

MEDICAL EDUCATION AND PALLIATIVE CARE RESEARCH PROGRAMS

As palliative medicine evolves as a specialty, medical education and research will become increasingly important. Hospices are an excellent resource to assist medical schools and residency programs, as they have a ready source of patients for students or residents, and palliative care experts for trainees to learn from. Leading the effort for the hospice program should be the medical director, working directly with his or her academic colleagues to ensure that the training experience is a meaningful one.

In regard to research, the hospice program provides the highest concentration of patients to enroll in trials to study the effectiveness of end-of-life interventions. Observational and retrospective analysis, and reporting of effective palliative care protocols, are also valuable in helping improve care for patients near the end of life.

Hospice Team Physician

The hospice physician is considered a core member of the interdisciplinary team, alongside the nurse, social worker, and chaplain. In smaller hospices, the hospice medical director may also fill this role, while in larger hospices, multiple hospice physicians in addition to the medical director are usually required. The physician fulfills many important roles that are necessary for the proper care of the patient, outlined in Table 4–7, and discussed next. (The hospice physician may at times also serve as a patient's attending physician.)

As the physician from the hospice primarily responsible for direct patient care, the hospice physician's responsibilities begin at the time of patient admission, by certifying, together with the patient's attending physician, that the patient has a prognosis of 6 months or less. (See Chapter 1 for a discussion of guidelines that help determine patient prognosis.) The goal of certification, of course, is to make certain that patients receive hospice services at an appropriate time in their illness and life.

Table 4–7

Roles of the Hospice Team Physician

Patient certification and recertification of
terminal prognosis
Patient home visits and inpatient visits
Medical intervention to treat patient symptoms
Resource as expert in palliative care to other
members of interdisciplinary team
Liaison with attending physicians on the current
status of their patients
Staff education and support at interdisciplinary
team meetings

Once in the hospice program, the Medicare Hospice Benefit periodically requires that the patient's prognosis be reevaluated. (See Chapter 2 for further discussion of the Medicare Hospice Benefit.) These reviews, commonly termed recertification, are meant to assess whether, due to changes in a patient's clinical condition, the patient continues to have a prognosis of 6 months or less and to remain eligible for hospice services. If a patient's medical condition has improved and the patient no longer meets the hospice eligibility criteria, the hospice physician will not recertify the patient as terminally ill. The hospice physician will work with the interdisciplinary team, including the patient, family, and attending physician, to provide appropriate planning prior to discharging the patient from the hospice and back to the care of the attending physician.

Although hospice visits at home are typically from nurses, home health aides, social workers, or chaplains, physician visits to patients in their homes can also be invaluable. These visits provide patients, who often are too ill to leave the house and visit their attending physicians in the office, with a sense of belonging and connection, and also assure them that a doctor genuinely cares about them. By visiting the patient, the hospice physician can medically assess the patient and provide direct information to assist the team in planning care. The team physician, after making a home visit, can communicate with the attending physician to make palliative care recommendations, thereby providing patients with better symptom control. Additionally, patients are comforted in the knowledge that their attending physicians have up-to-date and professionally derived information about their current status.

In addition to the direct benefits to the patient provided by the physician visit, once the physician has seen the patient, ongoing care planning is more efficient, because the physician now has a live reference to associate with the verbal information shared by other team members. Follow-up physician visits are often indicated if patients develop acute problems or as deterioration and death approach. When continuous home care (see Chapter 2) is indicated, a periodic physician visit can provide invaluable assistance in helping control patient symptoms.

For patients receiving inpatient hospice care, a physician visit should occur on a daily basis. Just as in the traditional acute care hospital setting, these patients are typically very ill, too ill to remain at home. The need for daily care is mandated by the need to assure better control of the clinical symptoms. When the patient's attending physician elects to supervise patient care in the inpatient setting, the hospice physician may fill the role of an expert consultant, providing palliative care expertise if necessary. However, if the attending physician does not or cannot follow the patient, the hospice physician will provide the care.

The hospice physician serves as a palliative care expert, assisting the attending physician when the patient is at home as well as when the patient is on an inpatient hospice unit. Although attending physicians are encouraged to remain actively involved in the care of their patients, when this is not feasible or not desired, or when the attending physician is not available, the hospice team physician becomes primarily responsible for medical decision making. Hospice team physician are well equipped to fill this role, as they are knowledgeable about all the patients on their team from discussions held at the team care planning conferences, and in many cases from having visited the patients at home. When the hospice team physician directly intervenes, it is important to communicate with the attending physician to ensure continuity of care. Hospice physicians should also communicate with attending physicians whenever patients have changes in status or when a change in patient prognosis prompts the consideration of patient discharge from the hospice program.

The hospice physician, much like the hospice medical director, functions as an educator as well. During the interdisciplinary team conference, ample opportunities for the hospice physician to teach staff present themselves. As an educational forum, the team conference is particularly valuable, as it allows the physician to associate specific subjects with real examples—the patients and families being cared for by the team.

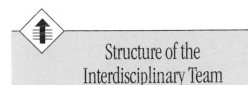

Structure of the Interdisciplinary Team

The overwhelming majority of physicians practicing today were trained in some variation of the teaching hospital model of care, with its emphasis on vertical integration of the staff (Figure 4–1).

At the top of the ladder was the physician, the captain of the ship, in charge of managing patient care. Just below the physician, but very clearly subordinate, were the nurses, who were traditionally viewed as providing care ordered by the physician, usually without independent thought, question, or challenge. Below the nurses in this health care hierarchy were various ancillary personnel, including social workers, dieticians, physical and occupational therapists, pharmacists, and others whose job it was to ensure that patient care was provided smoothly and efficiently. Supporting this structure were those considered less skilled, such as nurses' aides, porters, and dietary workers.

This hierarchical structure has evolved to some degree in traditional hospital and medical practices, but the physician continues to be the primary driver

of health care for patients and families. However, in the hospice model of care, this structure has been vastly altered. As illustrated in Figure 4–2, the hierarchical structure with the physician at the top has been replaced by the interdisciplinary team, which has the patient and family as the unit of care at its center. All care providers, from the doctor to the nurse to the home health aide, are all on an equal level, with the goal being for each care provider to use their special skills and expertise to provide expert end-of-life care as needed and directed by the patient and family.

As one reflects on the model of "suffering" or "total pain" that has been well accepted as a major dynamic in care near the end of life, the purpose of the interdisciplinary (ID) team becomes clear. It is only by combining the expertise of professionals from multiple disciplines, working together collegially, and focused on meeting the patient needs as determined by the patient and family, that the outcomes of end-of-life care can be successful. To paraphrase Orwell, "All are equal, but *none are more equal* than others."

As a member of a team, it is important for physicians to not only understand their role, but to understand the role of the other members of the team as well. What follows, therefore, is an overview of the role of each individual who par-

Figure 4–1

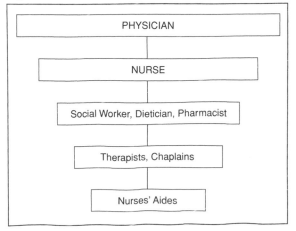

Traditional hierarchical structure of the health care team

Figure 4–2

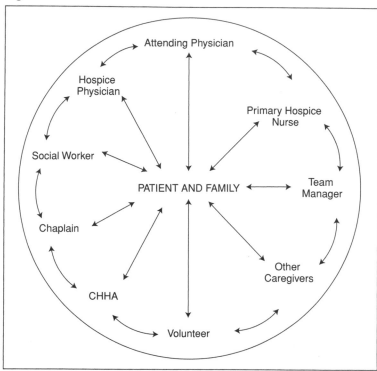

Structure of hospice interdisciplinary team

ticipates in providing end-of-life care to patients as members of the ID team.

Nurse

Nurses play two distinct roles in the care of the hospice patient: management and patient care. Any group of individuals acting in concert to perform a task needs a leader to make certain that the job is done correctly and efficiently. The ID team is no exception. Although many of the health care professionals who participate in the ID team would be capable of leading the team, that task has traditionally fallen to a registered nurse (RN), usually called the team manager or patient care coordinator. These nurse managers have multiple tasks, not directly related to hands-on patient care, but related to ensuring that the professionals on the team do their jobs in an efficient and coordinated fashion.

Among the tasks of the team manager are to assign patients to the primary care nurses and make sure that all the nurses on the team have a reasonable number of patients to care for. The team manager makes certain that scheduling of visits by all disciplines is appropriate to meet patient needs, and facilitates the team care planning conferences, often referred to simply as team meetings, during which time the care plans of patients are reviewed and updated. The team manager functions as the primary supervisor of all ID team members (including the physician), resolving conflicts, ensuring that all team members perform their tasks properly and efficiently, and being responsible for allocating of resources.

Nurses also play a major role in the hands-on care of patients and families. In most hospice programs, each patient is assigned a primary nurse, who is responsible for case management and primary patient care. At the time of hospice admission, it is the primary nurse who assesses the patient to develop together with other ID team members individualized care plans for patients. This nurse visits the patient on a regular basis (generally one to three times per week based on patient need) to evaluate the effectiveness of the plan of care and to coordinate any changes or additions if indicated. If changes in the care plan require a physician's order, it is the primary nurse who is responsible for contacting either the attending physician or hospice physician, to explain what is occurring, and often to suggest possible palliative interventions to the physician. The nurse is the primary educational resource for the patient and family, reviewing all medications, teaching the patient and family how to properly administer the medications, and monitoring to ensure appropriate medication use. The nurse will also instruct families on other aspects of care, such as wound and decubiti care, and on how to avoid these and other problems if the patient is at further risk. The great emphasis on teaching caregivers is due to the fact that hospice programs are not meant to provide 24-hour hands-on care, but to assist the family caregivers in providing much of the basic custodial support that patients require near the end of life.

Primary nurses function as case managers, overseeing patient care, interacting with family, aides, physicians, and other members of the interdisciplinary team to provide optimal care. They need to know their patients in depth; have the skills to recognize how specific patient illnesses affect the course of care; possess knowledge of the physical, psychosocial, and spiritual realities near the end of life; and be proactive in making certain that needs and potential complications of the patients under their care are anticipated and treated.

Social Worker

The role of the social worker is varied and diverse, as there are few aspects of the patients' care in which a social worker does become involved. Every patient admitted to a hospice or nonhospice palliative care program needs a psychosocial

evaluation to assess the nonphysical needs of the patient and family, and this evaluation is typically performed by a social worker. Social workers may provide patients and families with assistance accessing community services such as Meals-on-Wheels, or facilitating application for Medicaid, if the patient is eligible to obtain LTC facility room-and-board coverage. Social workers may also work more directly with patient and families as well, providing counseling and support throughout the course of the terminal illness, helping patients and families to better cope with their current situation, and/or having the patients and families understand what options are open to them. Social workers provide psychological support as patient lives draw to a close, and often support families by attending a patient's death. Following a patient's death, the social worker assists the chaplain in providing grief and bereavement support to families (see Chapter 14 for a discussion of bereavement services).

Finally, social workers provide counseling and support to the other members of the ID team as well as to other caregivers, such as the staff of LTC facilities who work with the hospice program.

Chaplain

Pastoral care has always been viewed as a core hospice service. Even though society currently has a secular orientation and many patients are not actively practicing any religion, imminent death often leads even nonreligious people to a search for meaning and/or for a greater involvement in spiritual or religious matters. Although it would be ideal to receive pastoral care from one's own minister, rabbi, or priest, the majority of Americans are unaffiliated with formal religious institutions and therefore are not able to directly access this vital function.

Fortunately, hospices are able to offer pastoral care, and do so by employing clergy of various religious affiliations. This allows for the multiple variations in religious practice in society to be represented, so that most specific patient requests can be met. The focus of pastoral end-of-life care is spiritual, not formally religious; hence the individuals are seen as "generic" chaplains rather than as a member of a particular religious group, sect, or order. For chaplains working for a hospice, this means having the flexibility to serve the spiritual needs of patients who may not be of their own religious denomination and to do so without being judgmental or attempting to proselytize. At times, therefore, a priest may be asked to counsel Jewish patients, while a rabbi may serve Methodist patients, and so on. In recognition of patient autonomy, on the other hand, if a patient requests a chaplain of a particular faith, the hospice has the obligation to attempt to fulfill the request, and to not try to force the "generic" chaplain on the patient.

Chaplains may assist the social worker by providing additional support in the psychosocial realm. They are generally capable of performing psychosocial as well as a spiritual assessments, and at times provide psychosocial counseling. The chaplain generally has the responsibility to coordinate grief and bereavement programs that are provided by the hospice, including one-on-one counseling, support groups, and memorial services. (See Chapter 14 for a discussion of bereavement services.)

Certified Home Health Aide

Often perceived as "just" a maid or cleaning lady, the certified home health aide (CHAA) performs a core function on the interdisciplinary team and has been described as a "saint from God." Unlike nurses' aides who work in hospitals and long-term care facilities, the CHHA must function under the direct visual supervision of a registered nurse. CHHAs possess a high level of skill, receive ongoing training, and hence are able to function in a patient's home independent of the RN's presence.

Patients who are near the end of life present complicated and challenging personal hygiene needs that often overwhelm families. It takes the expertise of a trained CHHA to safely see patients into a shower, bathe them in bed if they cannot walk, clean them when they have been inconti-

nent, and/or give them gentle touch when others may be afraid of physical contact. In view of the intimate relationship between the patient and the CHHA, strong bonds often form. The CHHA, therefore, may be the member of the ID team who best knows what the patient truly needs, and may provide the most valuable input as the ID team plans care for the patient. It is not uncommon for the family to offer their greatest thanks to the CHHA after the patient's death; and conversely, the CHHAs may experience a great deal of grief after the death of a patient in their charge for a long time.

Volunteers

Volunteers in many respects were the backbone of the early hospice movement. Before the creation of the Medicare Hospice Benefit, most hospice care was provided by volunteers. In keeping with that spirit, the Medicare Hospice Benefit requires that volunteers provide services to hospice programs equivalent in hours to 5 percent of all patient care hours. Volunteer services are appreciated by patients and families, the hospice programs they serve, and by the volunteers themselves.

By visiting with patients, volunteers can provide patients with additional human contact, especially when the patients are home bound. They allow the patients to be distracted from the realities of their illness and to feel "normal" again. Volunteers can also provide caregivers with needed respite time. As most patients cannot be left alone, volunteers can stay with a patient while the caregiver can tend to personal needs, family needs, or just take a needed break to refresh and recharge. For patients who are able to get out of the house, volunteers can participate by taking patients out for rides, to the mall, and for other nonmedical experiences.

Volunteers may also work administratively in the hospice program office. Activities from filing of records and reports, to stuffing envelopes, to making phone calls can help lighten the clerical burden of hospice personnel and allow them to focus on more direct patient care activities. Whether hospice volunteers work directly with patients or in an administrative capacity, they are usually motivated individuals, often with a prior personal hospice experience, who derive personal satisfaction from sharing of themselves with others.

A special volunteer for patients near the end of life is the "pet therapist." This is a domesticated animal, most often a dog, that has been carefully evaluated and trained to function in a health care environment, such as an LTC facility or a hospice inpatient unit. The animals are placid, not afraid of strangers, and do not startle with the sudden noises that come from wheelchairs, trays, and so on. It has been shown that animals bring a sense of calm to patients and caregivers and can often serve to defuse crisis situations. The gentle stroking of an animal's fur is a tactile experience that often brings back pleasant childhood memories. The right animal can be a very useful member of the team.

Ancillary Members

PHARMACIST

The pharmacy consultant provides periodic review of the medications that patients on the hospice program are receiving. Often, patients are receiving multiple medications for their various symptoms, some of which will interact with one another. The pharmacist can advise clinicians on potential drug–drug interactions, suggest alternative therapeutic approaches to difficult symptom management problems, and educate the staff on the newer medications and therapies available for use.

OTHER MEMBERS OF THE TEAM

Dieticians can be helpful in advising patients and families on the various alternatives that might assist in optimizing caloric intake for patients. Physical therapists and occupational therapists may assist hospice staff in figuring out ways of maximizing patient function, while wound specialists may provide alternative approaches to difficult-to-heal wounds. Alternative

therapies such as massage therapy, therapeutic touch, and aromatherapy are being used with increasing frequency, and hospices will often engage the assistance of practitioners in these areas as well.

Conclusion

As was stated at the outset, the role of the physician as a member of an end-of-life care interdisciplinary team is not the traditional one that physicians are used to. Physicians must view themselves as team players, which requires a greater level of cooperation and interaction with other health care professionals than is seen in other aspects of the physician's professional life. It requires a change of vision, from that of being "right" to accepting that death will occur, and recognizing that what is "correct" is that which optimizes the quality of the patient's life rather than prolonging life. It requires regular discussions with the other professional members of the ID team, with physicians caring for patients, and with physicians in management roles.

Physicians have to be prepared to have their actions questioned, and to be able to justify how what they propose for the patient is not only accepted medical practice, but is necessary and beneficial. At times, they may have to deal with being told "No, this is not best for the patient nor what the patient wants. Therefore, it will not happen."

The relationship between the various physicians and other members of the ID team need not be confrontational. The field of hospice and palliative medicine is still relatively new and there is still a divergence between what the average physician in practice understands regarding the care of the dying and what the palliative medicine physicians or other health care professionals in the field know. Physicians who are open to cooperation and primarily concerned about the welfare of patients under their care will see working with hospice and palliative care providers as a way of improving their knowledge and skill in caring for terminally ill patients, while providing their patients with optimal care near the end of life.

Bibliography

Academy of Hospice Physicians, Hospice Medical Practice Committee: Role definitions for Hospice Medical Director, Associate Medical Director, and Hospice Physician. St. Petersburg, FL, Academy of Hospice Physicians, 1993.

Cummings I: The interdisciplinary team. In: Doyle D, Hanks GWC, MacDonald N, eds. *Oxford Textbook of Palliative Medicine,* 2nd ed. Oxford, Oxford University Press, 1998, pp. 19–30.

Hoy T: Hospice chaplaincy in the caregiving team. In Corr CA, Coor DM, eds. *Hospice Care: Principles and Practice.* New York, Springer, 1983, p. 177.

Kinzbrunner BM: The role of the physician in hospice. *Hospice J* 12:49, 1997.

Kurtz ME: The dual role dilemma. In: Curry W, ed: *New Leadership in Health Care Management: The Physician Executive.* Tampa, Lithocolor, 1988, p. 66.

Medical Director job description, policy 9:04. In: *Vitas Policy Manual.* Miami, Vitas Healthcare, 1997.

Medicare Hospice Regulations, *42 Code of Federal Regulations,* Part 418, 1993.

Registered nurse job description, policy 9:14. In: *Vitas Policy Manual.* Miami, Vitas Healthcare, 1997.

Storey P: What is the role of the hospice physician? *Am J Hospice Palliat Care* 10:2, 1993.

Team physician job description, policy 9:13. In: *Vitas Policy Manual.* Miami, Vitas Healthcare, 1997.

Melanie P. Merriman

Chapter

5

Measuring Outcomes and Quality of Life

Introduction

How can we know if end-of-life care has been a success? Ultimately, success will be defined by the patient and the close family or friends involved in the patient's care. Nevertheless, professional caregivers who participate in or refer patients for hospice or palliative care have a responsibility to define goals of end-of-life care and to assure that care is evaluated based on how well these goals are met. Quality in health care is determined both by what is done (or not done) by caregivers and by the results or outcomes of interventions for patients and families. According to the Institute of Medicine, creating desired outcomes for patients is paramount to delivering quality care. Specifically, the Institute has defined health care quality as "the degree to which healthcare services for individuals and populations increase the likelihood of desired health outcomes and are consistent with current professional knowledge."

Outcomes Measurement

Outcomes measurement is concerned with what happened for the patient and family. Obviously, for the terminally ill patient it is inappropriate to expect that the major outcome is for the patient to be made well. One can expect, however, that the patient and family could be made "better" in several ways. Patients should experience symptom relief, enhanced quality of life, and emotional and spiritual support. Families should experience relief of anxiety, and improved coping skills. Therefore, at the end of life, the focus of outcomes measurement needs to be based on what the patient and family have experienced as a result of the health care providers' actions.

The collection of outcomes data serves many synergistic purposes. For individual patients and clinicians, outcomes measurement provides information concerning clinical utility and quality of care. Did the patient benefit from the treatment provided? Is more or different treatment advisable? In a research context, outcomes data contribute to the evidence base for medicine by revealing which treatments are the most efficacious, safe, and cost efficient. From both the industry and consumer viewpoints, outcomes data also can be used for accountability. When providers document outcomes, consumers can compare providers on the basis of quality and price. All providers then become accountable for offering efficient and effective care.

Outcomes Measurement Challenges Near the End of Life

End-of-life care is subject to both internal (quality improvement, evidence-based development) and external (accountability) forces that drive how outcomes measurement is implemented. Measurement of outcomes near the end of life, therefore, offers some unique challenges. Health care outcomes for nonterminal patients are typically measured in the context of an episode of illness or an episode of treatment from which the patient will emerge changed by the health care encounter. Health status (defined and measured in a variety of ways) is often evaluated prior to the health care encounter or encounters and then after an episode is over (following hospital discharge, or the completion of outpatient or rehabilitative care). Patients being cared for near the end of life, however, do not emerge from this episode of care and, during the episode, their physical and functional status will decline inexorably. Hence "typical" measures rarely provide meaningful data for end-of-life care.

Therefore, the first critical question that one has to consider is what to measure in evaluating end-of-life care. Other questions that require asking include which patient should have outcomes measured and when these measures should be applied. Although certain diagnoses are clearly life limiting, the prospective identification of those who are at the end of life may be difficult. And because patients cannot offer outcomes data after they are dead, when can evaluation be done? A related question is whether family or caregivers can report accurately on the effect of interventions for patients.

What, who, when, and how to measure outcomes of end-of-life care are thorny issues and have become the topic of many national initiatives. Relying on research studies, national discussion, and practical experience, this chapter will provide some guidelines for evaluating outcome measures applied to end-of-life care. In general, these outcome measures will be applied in hospice or palliative care settings. Appropriate measures of end-of-life care, however, should be applicable in any settings where patients receive care. In fact, outcome measures and resultant reports should be among the parameters that clinicians use when choosing providers or partners for end-of-life care.

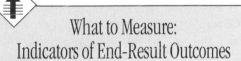

What to Measure: Indicators of End-Result Outcomes

In the same way that time can be defined as that which is measured by a clock, end-of-life care will, at least in part, be defined by the ways that it comes to be measured. Meaningful outcomes must be based on the goals of care for patients with terminal illness. If measures focus on physical symptoms and acute medical intervention, then end-of-life care will become defined as a period to address and alleviate physical suffering. If the measures focus on psychological, psychosocial, or spiritual problems, then end-of-life care will become defined as a period to address and alleviate psychospiritual and psychosocial suffering. The challenge, therefore, has been to define a group of measures that address the range of issues faced by patients and families at the end of life—the "problems" addressed elsewhere in this volume—and the opportunities that are presented to those who are living at the end of life.

The prevailing wisdom in evaluation of end-of-life care is that outcomes must be both meaningful and valuable to the patient and family, who together comprise the unit of care. Additionally, outcomes need to be meaningful to the providers and payers of care, and it is critical that outcomes measurement be manageable in the context of that care. As is often the case, the outcomes themselves may not be directly measurable. Therefore, as individuals and local and national groups define outcomes of care, they need to also identify indicators of these outcomes that are measurable. Some of these indicator measures are being implemented currently and others are being tested for feasibility as this chapter is being written.

American Geriatric Society Framework for Quality of Care Near the End of Life

Following the publication in late 1995 of the SUPPORT study, which revealed shortcomings in the outcomes of end-of-life care in major medical centers, numerous providers, national forums, health care associations, and funding agencies began developing initiatives aimed at improving care of the dying. In an effort led by Dr. Joanne Lynn, the American Geriatric Society (AGS) drafted "Suggested Domains for Measuring Quality at the End of Life" (Table 5–1). Several organizations have endorsed this list, which provides a convenient framework for defining outcome measures for end-of-life care. As specific outcome measures and the challenges in their implementation are discussed throughout the chapter, reference will be made to this framework.

End-Result Outcomes Defined by Hospice Groups

In its "Pathway for Patients and Families Facing Terminal Illness," the National Hospice and Palliative Care Organization (NHPCO) has identified three primary end-result outcomes for terminal care. Although the NHPCO represents hospice providers,

Table 5–1

Suggested Domains for Measuring Quality Near the End of Life

1. Physical and emotional symptoms such as pain, shortness of breath, fatigue, depression, fear, anxiety, and skin breakdown.
2. Support of function and autonomy, including maintaining personal dignity and self-respect.
3. Advance care planning so that decisions can reflect patients' preferences and circumstances rather than be responses to crises.
4. Aggressive care near death: site of death, CPR, and hospitalization when the short-term outcome is very likely to be death.
5. Patient and family satisfaction—particularly with the decision-making process, care given, outcomes achieved, and the extent to which opportunities were provided to complete life in a meaningful way. The goal is that the time near the end of life be especially precious, not merely tolerable.
6. Global quality of life, which can be good despite declining physical health.
7. Family burden, including financial and emotional effects.
8. Survival time, with measures that illuminate priorities and tradeoffs within each care system.
9. Provider continuity (including the achievement of sustained relationships with the health care givers based on trust, reliability, and effective communication) and relevant skills including rehabilitation, symptom control, and psychological support.
10. Bereavement services for survivors.

SOURCE: Lynn J: Measuring quality of care at the end of life: A statement of principles. *J Am Geriatr Soc* 45:526, 1997.

and the pathway draws on care experience with hospice patients, the pathway and the outcomes were designed to be applicable in any care setting. In late 1998, the National Hospice Work Group (NHWG) and NHPCO Outcomes Taskforce developed and began pilot testing several indicators or measures of quality care near the end of life (Table 5–2).

COMFORTABLE DYING

The first of the four end-result outcomes identified by the NHPCO Pathway is comfortable dying. This outcome encompasses the goals of pain and symptom management, preservation of independence, ability to perform activities of daily living in ways that do not endanger the patient or caregivers, and education of family members to be confident and competent caregivers. The comfortable dying indicator is patient-reported pain management, and data are gathered from the patient during the first week of care.

SAFE DYING

As an indicator of safe dying, the NHWG/NHPCO Outcomes Taskforce has drafted a measure of family reported confidence in their ability to care for the dying patient safely at home. The data are gathered as part of an after-death survey of families. This measure is based on literature describing self-efficacy that links confidence in one's ability to perform various tasks to competence in actual performance. Another appropriate indicator of safe dying would be "reportable incidents," which include falls, medication errors, and skin tears/lacerations.

SELF-DETERMINED LIFE CLOSURE

The second end-result outcome from the NHPCO Pathway is self-determined life closure. This outcome encompasses the goals of autonomy and advance-care planning. The indicator drafted by the NHWG/NHPCO Outcomes Taskforce measures the frequency with which the choices of the patient (or legal representative) with respect to hospitalization and CPR were honored. The measure tracks the preferences, as expressed by the patient or legal representative, over the course of care and uses the patient record to determine if and how often these preferences were honored.

Table 5–2

National Hospice Work Group/ National Hospice and Palliative Care Organization Proposed Outcome Measures

END-RESULT OUTCOME	INDICATOR	MEASURE
Comfortable dying	Pain relief in the first 72 hours of care	Patient report on admit and 72 hours later
Safe dying	Family confidence in ability to care for patient safely at home	Family survey 1 to 3 months after death
Self-determined life closure	Adherence to patient (or legal representative) preferences regarding hospitalization and CPR	Patient/legal representative report of preferences and chart review to determine adherence
Effective grieving	Family ability to cope with changes following loss	Family survey 13 months after death

Another appropriate indicator of self-determined life closure is the percentage of patients who have documented conversations regarding preferences and advance-care planning, including but not limited to the presence of a formal advance-directive document. The latter is a measure of process, not outcome, but may be considered as one prerequisite to self-determined life closure.

EFFECTIVE GRIEVING

The third end-result outcome identified in the NHPCO Pathway is effective grieving. This outcome encompasses the grieving of the family and the patient, both of whom experience loss. The focus, however, is on the family and the goal of healthy bereavement for families following the death of the patient. Indicators for this outcome include return to work and to one's social role. For the NHWG/NHPCO Outcomes Taskforce measure, family members report on coping with changes following the loss of a loved one. The data are collected via an after-death survey of family. The Grief Experience Inventory by Sanders and associates (1991), and the Grief Resolution Index by Remondet and Hanson (1987), are among the excellent tools available for evaluating the impact of grief on individuals and their "recovery" from grieving. To evaluate effective patient grieving during the dying process, indicators that may be looked for

would include documented opportunities for life closure, what Ira Byock calls the landmarks and tasks of end of life (Table 5–3). Again, the latter is a measure of process, not of outcome, and is an indicator of an environment where effective grieving is possible.

Other Indicators for End-of-Life Care

While indicator development by the NHPCO taskforce is at a nascent stage, the end-result outcomes are fairly comprehensive. Referring to the AGS framework of suggested domains (Table 5–1), the end-result outcomes would seem to comprise portions of nearly all domains. Three additional areas that are implicit in, but not specifically addressed by, the end-result outcomes are continuity of care, patient and family satisfaction, and quality of life.

CONTINUITY OF CARE

Continuity of care refers to both continuity between care settings within one provider or institution (an integrated delivery system) and continuity between or among providers. The AGS framework suggests that continuity of care includes "sustained relationships with health care providers based on trust, reliability, and effective communication."

Other elements of continuity are systems and processes that foster care coordination and cut down on duplicative data gathering and diagnostic or treatment procedures. Indicators of continuity of care include both process measures and outcome measures. Process indicators might include (1) the presence of an electronic patient record accessible by various providers or a paper-based care plan that stays with the patient throughout care, or (2) the number of duplicative laboratory tests. The best outcome indicator would be the patient's and/or family's perception of continuity assessed via a sur-

Table 5–3

Developmental Landmarks and Tasks for the End of Life

- Sense of completion with worldly affairs
  Transfer of fiscal, legal, and formal social responsibilities
- Sense of completion in relationships with community
  Closure of multiple social relationships (employment, commerce, organizational, congregational).
    Components include: expressions of regret, expressions of forgiveness, acceptance of gratitude and appreciation
    Leave-taking: the saying of goodbye
- Sense of meaning about one's individual life
  Life review
  The telling of "one's stories"
  Transmission of knowledge and wisdom
- Experienced love of self
  Self-acknowledgement
  Self-forgiveness
- Experienced love of others
  Acceptance of worthiness
- Sense of completion in relationships with family and friends
  Reconciliation, fullness of communication and closure in each of one's important relationships.
    Component tasks include: expressions of regret, expressions of forgiveness and acceptance, expressions of gratitude and appreciation, *acceptance* of gratitude and appreciation, expressions of affection
  Leave-taking: the saying of goodbye
- Acceptance of the finality of life—of one's existence as an individual
  Acknowledgement of the totality of personal loss represented by one's dying and experience of personal pain of existential loss
  Expression of the depth of personal tragedy that dying represents
  Decathexis (emotional withdrawal) from worldly affairs and cathexis (emotional connection) with an enduring construct
  Acceptance of dependency
- Sense of a new self (personhood) beyond personal loss
- Sense of meaning about life in general
  Achieving a sense of awe
  Recognition of a transcendent realm
  Developing/achieving a sense of comfort with chaos
- Surrender to the transcendent, to the unknown—"letting go"

SOURCE: Byock IR: The nature of suffering and the nature of opportunity at the end of life. *Clin Geriatr Med* 12:2, 1996.

Figure 5–1

```
┌─────────────────────────────────────────────────────────┐
│  Have the doctors and nurses talked with you, in a way    │
│  that you can understand, about treating your pain?       │
│                                                           │
│            □ YES                 □ NO                      │
│                                                           │
│                                                           │
│  Have you and your doctor made plans to ensure that your  │
│  wishes for medical treatment will be followed?           │
│                                                           │
│            □ YES                 □ NO                      │
└─────────────────────────────────────────────────────────┘
```

Examples of patient-centered report questionnaire items. Two items that might be used to evaluate the patient's experience and perception of care. Note that the items do not ask patients to rate their care or express satisfaction or dissatisfaction. Instead, respondents simply indicate whether certain activities took place.
Modified from the "Patient Interview," Toolkit of Instruments to Measure End-of-Life Care, www.chcr.brown.edu/pcoc/toolkit.htm.

vey that asks whether the patient (or family) always knew who was the physician responsible for the patient's care, and whom to call about a care issue. In their book *Through the Patient's Eyes,* Gerteis and coworkers (1993) have provided excellent descriptions of several continuity measures.

PATIENT AND FAMILY SATISFACTION

Satisfaction is perhaps the most fundamental and critical outcome measure of terminal care; it is also uniquely challenging to assess in a reliable manner. Satisfaction is closely linked to expectations, and with respect to end-of-life care (specifically) and all health care (more generally), patient and family expectations tend to be relatively uninformed. Hence, satisfaction scores tend to be high even when the health care experience included less than optimal interventions and/or service components. For example, several studies have shown that individuals who report that they are "satisfied" or "very satisfied" with a health care encounter will often describe aspects of the encounter that providers recognize as substandard care.

Because patient and family expectations, goals, and needs with respect to end-of-life care differ widely, the more accurate indicator to measure is patient or family experience, rather than satisfac-

tion. Gerteis and coworkers (1993) have described the use of patient-centered "reports" that allow the provider to measure how often preset standards of care are met (Fig. 5–1). Typical satisfaction surveys would, for example, ask whether the patient and family were satisfied with pain management. This type of question requires that respondents (1) know what can be expected with respect to pain relief, and (2) make a judgement about how well the provider implemented available treatments. A patient-centered report item would ask whether the patient experienced pain, and if so, how often and how bothersome it was. In this way the provider learns whether pain was managed without asking the patient or family to make a judgment about the quality of care and without assuming what the expectation was.

QUALITY OF LIFE

Quality of life measures have become increasingly popular in health care, particularly as a way of evaluating the burdens and benefits of experimental therapies. For terminal patients, when quantity of life is known to be limited, quality of life becomes a primary goal of care. It is incumbent on all end-of-life care providers to have some way of assessing quality of life for patients. Although quality of life is difficult to define, many researchers, including Anita Stewart, Ira Byock, Robin Cohen, and Balfour Mount, have identified components of quality of life for patients with life-limiting illness, and several instruments have been developed to quantify health-related quality of life. Table 5–4 outlines the elements that would characterize a valid and reliable quality of life assessment scale. Two of these elements—subjectivity (report by the patient) and inclusion of a patient rating of the importance of various domains of quality of life—are critical.

Quality of life at the end of life has unique characteristics that must be reflected in outcome measures. Typically health-related quality of life measures are designed to assess the impact of ill-ness and/or treatment on the patient's role and functioning. In fact, many health-related quality of life instruments are constructed with the underlying assumption that functionality (physical, emotional, and social) and quality of life are directly proportional. For patients whose physical health and functional status are inexorably declining, quality of life becomes defined by other domains of living. In the case of the McGill Quality of Life Index, for example, research has shown that the spiritual dimension is a major determinant of overall quality of life near the end of life. Appropriate tools for this population will measure multiple dimensions of quality of life.

The Missoula-VITAS Quality of Life Index (MVQOLI) was designed specifically for use with terminally ill patients. It is based on Ira Byock's theoretical framework of lifelong growth and development (1998). Byock has described the concept of landmarks and tasks to be completed before dying (Table 5–3) and posits that quality of life increases when these landmarks are reached. Results from the use of the instrument with hospice patients support the notion that quality of life for a terminal patient is not determined primarily by physical or functional status. Data from the use of this instrument, in fact, suggest that the important construct to measure for these patients may be "quality of life closure."

Table 5–4

Critical Features of a Quality of Life Assessment Tool

- A well-defined construct that has clinical applicability.
- Self-reported rather than observer-rated; a subjective assessment.
- Multidimensional, assessing relevant spheres of personhood including those related to health and function, as well as psychological, emotional, and spiritual dimensions of self.
- Scoring of the instrument provides for weighting of dimensions by the person.
- The tool measures changes experienced by the person in both negative and positive directions from pre-illness status ('baseline') within each dimension.
- Both the total score and the component dimensional cores are meaningful.
- "Sensibility," which includes measures of validity as well as "real-world" applicability and utility, including ease of administration and scoring.
- Use as both a discriminative tool, measuring differences between groups, and an evaluative tool, measuring changes in an individual over time.

SOURCE: Byock IR, and Merriman MP: Measuring quality of life for patients with terminal illness: The Missoula-VITAS quality of life index. *Palliat Med* 12:231, 1998.

Who and When to Measure during End-of-Life Care

To Whom Should Measures Be Applied?

A significant challenge in measuring the outcomes of end-of-life care is identification of the patients for whom the measures should be applied. Teno and Coppola (1999) have referred to this as the denominator problem—how do we prospectively identify patients who are in the last months of life? While much has been written about the difficulty in determining prognosis, particularly for non-cancer patients, the fact is that hospices have a good record of admitting patients with 6 months or less to live, suggesting that accurate criteria exist to identify this population. But delineation of these criteria may lead to definitions that are too exclusive, partly because the relevant criteria are not exclusively medical or physical.

Joanne Lynn, of the Center to Improve Care of the Dying, has suggested (1997) that providers, particularly physicians, think of end-of-life care as applicable not to individual patients for whom a specific and limited prognosis can be made, but rather to the group of patients "who are sick enough that you would not be surprised if they died in the next several months to a year." Surely providers who care for the sickest patients—hospitals, hospices, and nursing homes—should consider measuring self-determined life closure, safe and comfortable care (if not dying), opportunities for life closure, continuity of care, experience of care (satisfaction), and quality of life for any patient who fits this description. Then at any point in time, one can analyze the data for patients who were in fact in the dying phase, after they have died, and without having to be sure how close they were to dying prospectively.

For the purpose of measuring outcomes and quality of life, it seems wise to cast a wide net for prospective measurement, and then conduct data analysis and reporting on only that portion of those measured who actually died within a defined period (1, 3, 6, or 12 months) prior to the analysis date. Even though we are interested in measures crafted to evaluate end-of-life care, there would seem to be little downside in applying these measures to a slightly larger population, some of whom may not die, especially because many of the measures reflect excellence in outcomes even for patients who are not dying.

When Should Measures Be Applied?

Because patients cannot complete measures of end-of-life care following completion of care, measurement must be conducted during the treatment phase. Fortunately ongoing measurement has advantages that outweigh the burdens of continuous data collection. Elements appropriate for measure-

ment during the course of care are those that are most meaningful when they are patient reported. These include pain and symptom relief, patient/family preferences and conformance to those preferences, quality of life, patient experience of care, and "reportable incidents." These elements can and should be measured through a repetitive assessment process, and collection of such data also permits the analysis of intermediate outcomes that allow the provider to document and improve outcomes for individuals.

In the same way that regular measurement of vital signs provides an indicator of the patient's overall clinical condition and drives choice of interventions, measurement of symptom relief, preferences (goals), quality of life, and patient experience of care provides an indicator of the success of end-of-life care and guides adjustment in the care plan. Some providers are, in fact, implementing pain measurement as a "fifth vital sign" (Fig. 5–2A), and tracking patient-reported pain severity on a graph similar to that used for blood pressure. Such data when used daily to inform clinicians regarding the care of individuals, can be aggregated monthly or quarterly to determine overall success with end-of-life care. Patient experience must also be measured during care, but at less frequent intervals than the measures that are used in an ongoing assessment.

Family experience of end-of-life care is best assessed following the death, usually between 1 and 3 months after, and should be an integral part of the outcomes measurement program of any end-of-life care provider. Measures of effective grieving, including specific evaluation of any bereavement care provided, are typically assessed at 13 and 24 months following the death.

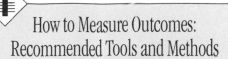

How to Measure Outcomes: Recommended Tools and Methods

For most outcomes of end-of-life care, patient self-reported indicators are the preferable method of data collection whenever possible. After-death

Figure 5–2

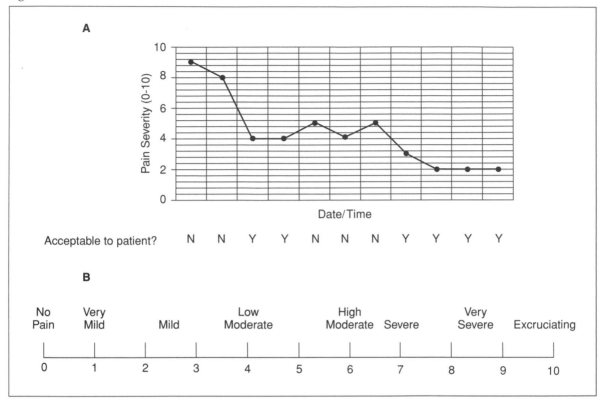

Pain as the fifth vital sign. **A.** An example of how pain might be recorded in the patient chart as a fifth vital sign. Like other vital signs, patient-reported pain severity is elicited at least daily, and the date and time are recorded along with the pain severity on a specified scale. In addition, the patient may be asked whether the current pain severity is acceptable. This answer is recorded beneath the date and time using **Y** for yes and **N** for no. **B.** An example of one pain severity scale. This one uses a 0–10 scale; others use a 0–5 scale. Other scales are available from the Agency for Healthcare Policy and Research, the American Pain Society, and the medical literature.

surveys are typically used to assess family experience and satisfaction. If the same tools are widely used (by many providers), opportunities increase to assure consistency of care quality across settings and to compare outcomes (benchmark) among providers.

As discussed, pain and symptom relief, quality of life, conformance to preferences, and experience of care (satisfaction) are examples of measures that should be patient reported. Data regarding the reliability of surrogate reporting are sparse but tend to suggest that few surrogate reports are concordant with patient self-reports. When patients cannot report, family caregivers who

spend a lot of time with the patients are probably the best surrogates.

Pain and Symptom Measures

There are several good methods for evaluating pain and symptom relief. Any of these methods are acceptable measures of pain and symptom management. The American Pain Society (APS) has recommended that pain measurement, as a fifth vital sign, consist of a patient-reported pain severity on a scale from 0 (no pain at all) to 10 (worst pain imaginable) and a patient report of the acceptability of the current pain level (Fig. 5–2). Data collected using this measure can be used to determine the mean pain severity (and relief) over time for patients whose initial pain was mild (1 to 3), moderate (4 to 6), or severe (7 to 10).

The NHWG/NHPCO outcomes task force is testing a measure that asks patients whether they are uncomfortable because of pain on an initial visit. They then are later asked whether their pain was brought to an acceptable level within the first 72 hours of care.

The patient survey from the Toolkit of Instruments to Measure End-of-Life Care (TIME), which is available on the Internet from www.chcr.brown.edu/pcoc/toolkit.htm, suggests another measurement strategy. Patients identify their two most bothersome symptoms, and then are asked three questions about these symptoms: (1) how often the symptom occurs, (2) the severity of the symptom, and (3) how much distress the symptom generates. The TIME survey also includes several other items concerning pain management.

Quality of Life Measures

As already mentioned, there are several instruments designed to measure health-related quality of life. At least three instruments have been developed specifically for patients in the terminal phase of illness. These are the Missoula-VITAS Quality of Life Index (MVQOLI), the McGill Quality of Life Index, and the Hospice Quality of Life Index (HQOLI). These instruments measure similar domains and all are designed for patient self-report; they differ in the type of items and scoring protocols used. The MVQOLI is administered by leaving the questionnaire with patients for completion on their own. The McGill Index is typically administered via an in-person "interview." The HQOLI has not been reported to be used in day-to-day practice; in a research setting it was administered in person by staff.

The MVQOLI, which is being used in several hospices and other palliative care centers, has the advantage over other end-of-life care instruments in that it can also serve as an assessment instru-

ment to guide care directed at enhancing quality of life. The instrument generates a quality of life "profile" that reveals the magnitude to which each dimension contributes or detracts from quality of life (Fig. 5–3). Use of the instrument will be discussed further later.

Satisfaction, Continuity of Care, and Performance Measures

Patient experience (satisfaction), which includes perception of continuity of care, is best measured via survey. Ideally, patient interviews by individuals not involved in care would be conducted, but this is rarely feasible for many providers or for large numbers of patients. Typically providers use a confidential survey conducted by mail. The TIME patient survey is in use across several settings of care and includes numerous items relating to the experience of care and continuity. The TIME survey also includes items concerning advance care planning that indicate whether patients have had the opportunity to discuss preferences and to collaborate in planning care.

Care consistency with preferences can be measured via chart review, assuming that preferences are documented. Retrospective chart review can, for example, evaluate proper use of the comprehensive pain assessment, care coordination and continuity, documented conversations regarding advanced care planning, and the number and nature of "reportable incidents." In an attempt to measure care consistency with preferences prospectively, the NHWG/NHPCO Outcomes Taskforce is recommending a measure that documents patient preferences, including those voiced by a legal representative if the patient cannot communicate regarding care, and then evaluates the actual care for conformance to the stated preferences. Whether outcomes are measured retrospectively or prospectively, providers might choose a well-constructed chart review tool, such as the one developed for TIME to assess several other critical outcomes of end-of-life care, or develop one of their own. The chart review tool should be able to assess whether

Figure 5–3

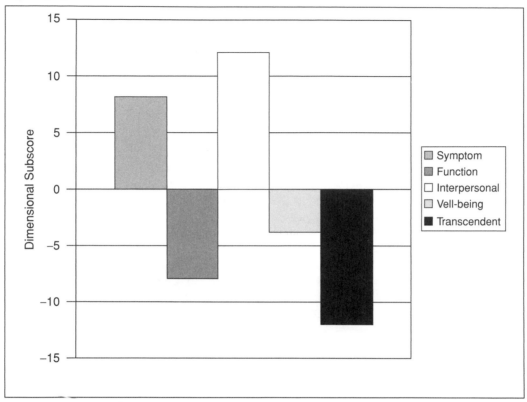

Missoula-VITAS Quality of Life Profile. The profile generated by graphing dimensional scores from the Missoula-VITAS Quality of Life Index. The longer bars indicate dimensions that are contributing the most to the patient's overall quality of life; generally, these are the domains that are most important to the patient. Positive bars (above zero) are adding to good quality of life; negative bars (below zero) are detracting from good quality of life.

care was consistent, whether patient and family preferences were met, whether opportunities were provided for life closure (were the patient's spiritual concerns addressed, and were there conversations about life closure?) and whether all of this was appropriately documented.

Family experience, like patient experience, is best measured via in-person interviews, after the death of the patient. Most typically, however, families are surveyed by mail 1 to 3 months following the death of a loved one. The NHPCO has developed a Family Satisfaction Survey that has been used by more than 300 hospices nationwide. With slight revision, the survey could be used by other end-of-life care providers and it is available from the organization (National Hospice and Palliative Care Organization, 1700 Diagonal Road, Suite 300, Alexandria, VA 22314). An after-death survey developed for TIME is comprehensive and offers items that have been used by providers from various settings. The entire instrument is long (over 100 items), lending itself better to research settings; however, it has been excerpted or modified for routine use in practice. The TIME survey contains items that report family experience and surrogate (family) perception of the patient experience. This survey, and others being developed by the same group, make extensive use of the concept of patient-centered reports discussed earlier and avoid the pitfalls of other satisfaction surveys.

Examples: Outcomes and Quality of Life Measurement in Practice

In looking at a provider's strategy for measuring outcomes and quality of life in the context of end-of-life care, simplicity should be seen as a plus. Successful programs have featured a small number of measures chosen because they are both meaningful—to patients, families, and professional caregivers—and actionable, providing information that will facilitate better care. As noted, a provider's choice of measures will be based on the primary goals of the end-of-life care program under evaluation, and thus reveal the program's underlying values. In addition, because one of the principles of outcomes management (the use of outcome data in managing patient care) is the *standardized* collection of outcomes data, the provider should have a detailed protocol for outcomes data collection.

The examples, given next, of outcomes measurement being used for terminally ill patients, serve as models for hospice, palliative care, and other settings. They represent the efforts of individuals and groups of providers that have made a commitment to measuring outcomes of end-of-life care and designed successful strategies for collecting and using data.

Hospice Providers

Several hospice providers began measuring outcomes related to clinical status, quality of life, and satisfaction in the mid-1990s. As a measure of clinical status, providers have typically used patient-reported pain severity and/or patient satisfaction with pain management. As a quality of life measure, versions of the Missoula-VITAS Quality of Life Index have been favored, although several other instruments are in use as well. Satisfaction or perception of care measures tend to differ from provider to provider.

In two different groups of hospices, protocols were designed to assure that all competent patients report on pain management in the same way and at the same points following admission. Staff have been taught language to use in asking the pain management question, and primary nurses inform patients about the measures when they are first admitted. At one group of hospices, patient-reported pain severity (on the 0 to 10 scale recommend by the World Health Organization) can be entered into a central database daily using a telephone voice-response data entry system. With telephone data entry into a computer, information on individual patents can be available instantly to all staff, including those who may hear from the patient via phone on nights or weekends (Fig.5–4). At the second group, pain was reported by having patients use the 10-point scale, and an additional item that asked whether pain relief was acceptable. The data were collected by nurses in the course of their usual visits to patients, and in the context of their routine assessment process. Scannable forms were used to record the data, and these were sent to a contracted firm for data input, storage, and analysis services. For both hospice groups, the data can be analyzed for the entire patient population quarterly in order to determine how well pain is managed overall. Clinical managers can use this quarterly performance measure data to determine whether performance improvement efforts are required. In the case of data collection by a contracted firm, the reports can be used to set benchmarks for performance and allow individual providers who participate in data collection to compare their performance with one another.

These same two hospice groups have also implemented the Missoula-VITAS Quality of Life Index to measure quality of life during end-of-life care. The index is administered to patients who can complete it on admission, and then at approximately one-month intervals thereafter. If patients are unwilling or unable to complete the index, this information is also recorded. The index is designed to be administered in the course of routine visits to patients. Anecdotally, irrespective of patient responses to various items on the instrument, discussions that have arisen during and following patient completion of the index have led to important psychosocial and spiritual interventions that have significantly benefited patients and families (see Chapter 13).

The two hospice groups have used different versions of the MVQOLI. One group chose a shortened version that generates a single overall quality of life score. This group then analyzes data on the entire patient population on a quarterly basis. The other hospice group uses a longer version of the MVQOLI that generates sub-scores for five domains of quality of life. The score in each domain is weighted according to how important that domain is to overall quality of life. Then the scores can be

plotted on a bar graph called the quality of life profile (Fig. 5–3) that shows which of the five domains are most important to the patient and which are detracting from or adding to quality of life. The hospice care team can use this information for care planning, an example of outcomes management for individual patients. The profile helps to prioritize interventions. Domains that are most negative present the best opportunities to improve quality of life. If caregivers can change or help the patient adapt to a situation that is detracting from quality of life, a domain that is important may be made positive and add considerably to quality of life. The longer version of the MVQOLI also generates a total score that can be used to

Figure 5–4

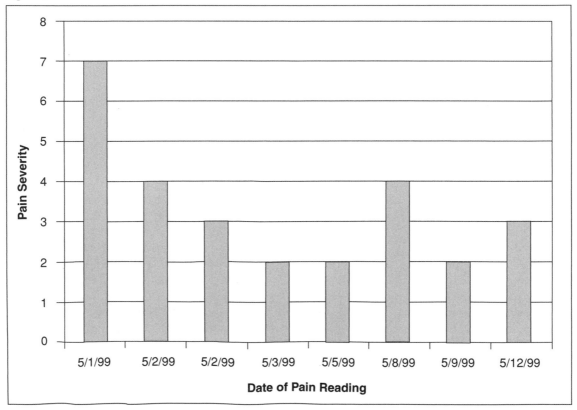

Individual patient's pain severity graph. Patient-reported pain scores that have been entered into a database can be displayed in a graph such as this one. The graph shows the pattern of pain and allows the care team to identify factors that contribute to increasing pain severity. When a graph like this is available in real time to all care staff, they are better able to respond to current patient pain reports.

analyze data on the entire population of respondents quarterly or annually for use in performance improvement activities.

For measuring satisfaction or perception of care, both hospice groups chose surveys that were mailed to family members after the patient's death. In one group, the surveys were printed on scannable forms and were returned by mail to a central processing department. Survey scanning hardware and software were used to produce monthly and quarterly summaries of results. The data were used to provide feedback to staff and for performance improvement.

Not all palliative care providers, including hospices, need outcomes measurement programs of this complexity, but all should be measuring outcomes relevant to end-of-life care. From 1998 to 1999, the NWHG/NHCPO Outcomes Taskforce implemented the alpha and beta tests of the four new end-of-life care outcomes measures discussed earlier (Table 5–2). Although the measures were tested in hospices, they are intended for use in any care setting. They are based on the end-result outcomes identified in the NHCPO Pathway for Patients and Families Facing Terminal Illness, and include two that are patient focused and measured during care, and two that are reported by family after the patient's death. The two patient-focused measures, acceptability of pain relief (or patient comfort) in the first 48 hours following admission and adherence to patient preferences regarding hospitalization and cardiopulmonary resuscitation, are designed to be recorded on a data collection form by a nurse in the routine course of care. Data from the form can be collated manually or via a computerized spreadsheet or database. Family measures of (1) confidence in their ability to care for the patient and (2) grief resolution are designed to be assessed via a survey mailed out after the patient dies.

Hospitals and Medical Centers

In an impressive national effort to improve palliative care for terminally ill patients, one national group of medical centers included palliative care

indicators in its quality performance measures beginning in 1997. Most of these measures evaluated processes (Was there an advance care planning document in the file? Was there evidence of a pain management care plan?), but the focus was on processes that drive desired outcomes.

Additionally, as more hospitals develop palliative care units, outcome measures such as pain severity scores as a fifth vital sign, quality of life, advance care planning, or conformance to patient preferences are becoming more commonplace, and will eventually become standard end-of-life care outcome measures.

Conclusion

As has often been said, death is not the only outcome of end-of-life care. Even when disease cannot be cured, and the prognosis for improvement is limited, much can be done for patients and the family and friends involved in the care of the terminally ill. Professionals providing end-of-life care have an obligation to help patients and families set realistic goals and then assess how well those goals are achieved. Despite the many challenges discussed, it is possible to measure quality of life and other outcomes of terminal care in a variety of health care settings. Critical outcomes include pain management, advance care planning, conformance to patient preferences, and satisfaction with the experience of care. Several quality of life measures have now been validated for use with a terminal population, and other measures are in use and being refined for end-of-life care. Widespread implementation of these measures will serve many purposes. The data will assure the best course of care for individual patients, and will provide the means to demonstrate it to referral sources and payers. It will also contribute to the evidence base for palliative care and the identification of best practices. Finally, there is a potential for impact at a societal level. As more patients get better care at the end of life, defined as care that meets their individual needs and contributes to quality of life as they define it, the next generation of the dying may develop increased confidence in the ability of the medical community to deliver excellent end-of-life care.

References

Bandura A: Self-efficacy determinants of anticipated fears and calamities. *J Pers Soc Psych* 45:464, 1983.

Byock IR: *Dying Well.* New York, Riverhead Books, 1997.

Byock IR: The nature of suffering and the nature of opportunity at the end of life. *Clin Geriatr Med* 12:2, 1996.

Byock IR: Growth: The essence of hospice. *Am J Hospice Care* Nov/Dec 1986, 16.

Byock IR, Merriman MP: Measuring quality of life for patients with terminal illness: The Missoula-VITAS quality of life index. *Palliat Med* 12:231, 1998.

Cleary PD, et al: Patients evaluate their hospital care: A national survey. *Health Affairs* 10:254, 1991.

Cohen SR, Mount B: Quality of life in terminal illness: Defining and measuring subjective well-being in the dying. *J Palliat Care* 8:40, 1992.

Cohen SR, Mount BM, Tomas JJN, Mount LF: Existential well-being is an important determinant of quality of life. *Cancer* 77:576, 1996.

Fowler FJ, Barry MJ, Lu-Yao G, et al: Outcomes of external beam radiation therapy for prostate cancer: A study of Medicare beneficiaries in three surveillance, epidemiology and results areas. *J Clin Oncol* 14:2258, 1996.

Fowler FJ, Coppola KM, Teno JM: Methodological challenges for measuring quality of care at the end of life. *J Pain Symptom Manage* 17:93, 1999.

Gerteis M, Edgeman-Levitan S, Daley J, et al: *Through the Patient's Eyes.* San Francisco, Jossey-Bass, 1993.

Gill TM, Feinstein AR: A critical appraisal of the quality of quality-of-life instruments. *JAMA* 272:619, 1994.

Hearn J, Higginson IJ: Outcome measures in palliative care for advanced cancer patients: A review. *J Public Health Med* 19:193, 1997.

IOM (Institute of Medicine), KN Lohr, ed: *Medicare: A Strategy for Quality Assurance.* Washington, DC, National Academy Press, 1990.

Lynn J: Measuring quality of care at the end of life: A statement of principles. *J Am Geriatr Soc* 45:526, 1997.

MacMillan SC, Mahon M: Measuring quality of life in hospice patients using a newly developed hospice quality of life index. *Qual Life Res* 3:437, 1994.

Remondet JH, Hanson RO: Assessing widow's grief—a short index. *J Gerontol Nurs* 13:30, 1987.

Sanders CM, Nauger PA, Strong PA: *A Manual for the Grief Experience Inventory.* Palo Alto, CA: Consulting Psychologists Press and Charlotte, NC: Center for the Study of Separation and Loss, 1991 (originally published 1985).

Stewart AL, Teno JM, Patrick DL, Lynn J: The concept of quality of life of dying persons in the context of health care. *J Pain Symptom Manage* 17: 93, 1999.

SUPPORT Principal Investigators: A controlled trial to improve care for seriously ill hospitalized patients. *JAMA* 274:1591, 1995.

Teno JM, Coppola KM: For every numerator, you need a denominator: A simple statement but key to measuring the quality of care of the "dying." *J Pain Symptom Manage* 17:109, 1999.

Williams SJ, Callan M: Convergence and divergence: Assessing criteria of consumer satisfaction across general practice, dental, and hospital settings. *Soc Sci Med* 33:707, 1991.

Part

Common Symptoms
Near the End of Life

Neal J. Weinreb
Barry Kinzbrunner
Michael Clark

Chapter

6

Pain Management

Introduction

The effect of uncontrolled pain during the last 6 to 12 months of life is substantial. Studies reveal that the prevalence of "important pain problems" is as high as 50 percent among community-dwelling older people near the end of life, and that the prevalence of "substantial pain" ranges from 45 to 80 percent among nursing home residents. One in four elderly cancer patients in nursing homes receives no treatment at all for daily pain. One in three outpatients with cancer pain indicated that it interfered with the way they lived, and up to 90 percent of patients with advanced cancer suffer from pain that they describe as "significant." About 40 percent of cancer patients have undertreated pain. Based on such statistics, it is not surprising that proper pain relief is among the top five concerns that patients have about the quality of end-of-life care.

Although cancer is the illness that is most often associated with pain near the end of life, patients with nonmalignant terminal illnesses including AIDS; end-stage cardiac, pulmonary, and cerebrovascular diseases; and Alzheimer's and other neurodegenerative diseases often suffer from pain as well. With demographic analyses projecting a progressive "graying" of the American population, the prevalence of these illnesses will inevitably increase. Primary care physicians will therefore need to assume a growing and formidable responsibility for the adequate management of pain near the end of life.

Recently, the problem of pain near the end of life and the associated increased interest in legalizing assisted suicide have prompted legislative and other regulatory remedies. Starting in January 2001, the Joint Commission on Accreditation of

Healthcare Organizations has enforced new standards in hospitals, nursing homes, and outpatient clinics ensuring that "patients have the right" to proper pain assessment and treatment, and that a patient's pain be measured and recorded regularly from the time the patient checks in. Numerous other health care organizations have developed national and international pain treatment guidelines and published position and policy statements. However, it remains to be seen whether these efforts will succeed in altering the current state of affairs, in which pain is still the most feared and often the most undertreated symptom in terminally ill patients.

Barriers to Effective Pain Management Near the End of Life

Although valid pain treatment guidelines are widely available, there are several recognized barriers to pain management near the end of life (Table 6–1).

Table 6–1

Barriers to Effective Pain Management

Inadequate pain assessment by clinicians
Inadequate education and training in pain
　management
Patient reluctance to report pain
Patient reluctance to take opioid analgesics
Physician reluctance to prescribe opioids
Undertreatment of specific populations of patients
　　Minorities 3:1 compared to nonminorities
　　Nonsurgical patients 2:1 to surgical patients
　　Women 1.5:1 to men
　　Elderly 2.4:1 to younger patients
Fear of addiction
Premature death due to the respiratory
　depressant effects of opioids

Patient Reluctance to Report Pain

Patients are sometimes reluctant to inform physicians that they are in pain for fear of being regarded as complainers or malingerers. Patients also often recognize that pain is a sign that their illness is becoming worse and/or that the treatment they are receiving is not effective. In these circumstances, some patients use denial as a defense mechanism to avoid confronting the prognostic implications of the increasing pain.

Patient Reluctance to Use Opioid Analgesics

Patients often associate opioid analgesics (especially morphine) with approaching and proximate death. Many patients and their families associate opioids with a high risk of addiction and, particularly in light of the antidrug ("Just say no!") campaigns of the last two decades, fear the social implications of taking medications that are akin to "street drugs." Many patients also believe that opioid use is associated with unpleasant or unmanageable side effects, and that if opioids are started "too soon," there will be no other medication to help them when the pain becomes "really bad."

Inadequate Physician Education and Training

Studies and surveys of physicians indicate a pervasive conviction that education and training, beginning with medical school and extending through residency and continuing medical education curricula, have failed to adequately address techniques for pain assessment and treatment. A recent review of leading medical textbooks for end-of-life care information concluded that little helpful information was offered on the topic of pain management (Carron et al, 1999). Medical oncologists have repeatedly expressed dissatisfaction with their lack of expertise in controlling pain. Primary care physicians, whose training emphasizes a "whole patient" perspective, should be particularly qualified to manage pain in the terminally ill. Evidence suggests that by applying the pain management techniques described in this chapter, clinicians should be able to relieve or substantially reduce pain for at least 90 percent of patients at the end phase of life.

Inadequate Pain Assessment by Clinicians

It is well known that 80 to 90 percent of all information about a patient can be obtained via a thorough assessment (history and physical examination). Evaluating pain is no exception. A proper pain assessment provides the baseline data that will determine selection of treatment, medication dosage and intervals, and the need for adjunctive interventions. Unfortunately, an increased reliance on technologically sophisticated diagnostic studies has degraded the importance of the face-to-face patient encounter and eroded the clinical skills necessary for physicians and other health care professionals to perform adequate assessments for pain and other subjective symptoms that are not quantifiable by machine. Time-intensive in-person assessments are also not encouraged by a medical system that increasingly values patient volume over the quality and comprehensiveness of the patient visit.

Undertreatment of Specific Patient Populations

Medical literature demonstrates that certain patient groups are at a higher risk for poor pain control than the general population. Unfortunately, the most cogent explanation for this phenomenon is overt or subliminal stereotyping by physicians, nurses, and other caregivers. For example, minority patients are three times more likely to have uncontrolled pain than non-minority patients, perhaps reflecting a bias associating minorities with drug abuse and addictive behavior. Because postoperative patients have a more obvious basis for pain than patients with medical pain syndromes, the latter are twice as likely to have uncontrolled

pain as the former. Gender biases—which assume that women exaggerate pain more than men, and that men complain only when pain is very severe—account for the fact that women are 1.5 times more likely to have uncontrolled pain than men. This bias holds true whether the caregivers questioned are male or female. Elderly patients are almost 2.5 times more likely to have uncontrolled pain compared to younger patients, in part because elderly patients are often believed to be less credible, and partly because of concerns that elderly patients will not tolerate analgesics as well as younger patients.

Physician Reluctance to Prescribe Opioids

Many physicians still have a poor understanding of opioid pharmacology and are fearful of causing addiction, respiratory depression, or premature patient death, despite the fact that these concerns have been scientifically disproved. An exaggerated fear of the development of analgesic tolerance often prompts physicians to withhold opioids from patients with severe pain until the patients are near death, thinking that premature use of opioids will obviate their efficacy near the end of life when patients need them most. The heightened regulatory scrutiny surrounding opioids and other controlled substances has also discouraged the prescription of these agents, especially in states with expensive and burdensome triplicate prescription programs. Repeated official statements of reassurance that practitioners who appropriately prescribe opioids for pain control will not be subject to special examination and punitive review have been received with skepticism. Physicians remember incidents such as occurred in Florida in 1998 when a medical examiner accused a hospice program of routinely killing patients with what turned out to be normal therapeutic doses of morphine.

Fear of Addiction

Fear of addiction is overemphasized by patients and physicians despite the obvious conclusion that addiction should be an irrelevant concern for terminally ill patients. Many physicians continue to confuse physical dependence with addiction. Physical dependence is the universal, unavoidable altered physiologic adaptation to opioid use that requires continued use of the opioid to avoid withdrawal reactions. It usually occurs within days to weeks of starting the chronic use of opioids. For patients in whom the source of pain is removed, opioids may be rapidly and safely tapered without any residual need for continued use of the medication.

In contrast, addiction represents a state of psychological dependence in which the patient exhibits a behavioral pattern that is characterized by craving for the drug and an overwhelming involvement in obtaining and using the drug for reasons other than pain relief. The life-style of the addicted patient is geared to acquisition of the desired drug despite the legal, financial, and psychosocial difficulties entailed. Psychological dependence is a rare phenomenon among patients who have a medical need for opioid analgesics, with studies showing that it occurs in less than 0.1 percent of patients. Patients at highest risk for psychological dependence usually have a history of alcoholism or other substance abuse, and/or a history of mental illness, especially depression. Even these patients, although requiring careful and sometimes specialized management, should NOT be deprived of needed analgesia especially when the experienced pain occurs near the end of life.

Fear of Opioid-Induced Respiratory Depression and Premature Death

Although opioids have suppressant effects on the respiratory center, tolerance to the respiratory depressant effects of opioid analgesics develops rapidly and early in the course of treatment. Within a few days of initiation of opioid therapy, the threshold dose for respiratory depression far exceeds the analgesic threshold. In fact, opioids have traditionally been used to treat cardio-

pulmonary problems such as acute pulmonary edema, due to their vasodilatory and preload reduction effects on the heart and circulatory system. Opioids are also effective in reducing subjective dyspnea in patients with severe chronic obstructive lung disease without increasing the risk of respiratory depression in this high-risk population. Furthermore, patients with uncontrolled dyspnea who are receiving chronic opioid therapy for pain management require doses equivalent to 1.5 to 2.5 times their regular dose of analgesia to control symptoms of breathlessness. Therefore, there is no evidence that chronic opioid use negatively affects respiratory status, and there is no basis for the fear that giving the next scheduled opioid dose even to an actively dying patient will cause or hasten death.

Effective Pain Management Near the End of Life

Despite the barriers to good pain control discussed earlier, and despite the daunting challenge posed by the high prevalence of pain in patients with advanced illnesses, the pain that patients experience near the end of life can be effectively managed even when concurrent medical conditions are present. Suggested guidelines for effective pain management are outlined in Table 6–2, which will also serve as the organizational chart for the remainder of this chapter. Using these guidelines, the clinician should be able to abolish or significantly reduce pain, prevent its return, and positively influence quality of life even as that life draws to a close.

Definitions

The first step in understanding how to manage pain effectively is to develop a common language. To accomplish that, it is important to clearly define

Table 6–2

Guidelines for Effective Pain Management

1. Always perform a thorough assessment of the patient's pain to identify and differentiate the various types and degrees of pain the patient may be experiencing.
2. Use medication and dosage schedules based on the characteristics of the patient's pain.
   a. Follow the World Health Organization (WHO) stepladder approach (see the section on the Selection of the Appropriate Analgesic) to choose the right drug for the appropriate degree of pain severity.
   b. For acute, intermittent pain, the appropriate dose of an analgesic with a rapid onset of action should be used, with dosing on an as-needed or prn basis.
   c. For chronic, continuous pain, the appropriate dose of analgesic, individually titrated for the patient's needs, should be used. A long duration of action is preferred and should be given on an around-the-clock basis to prevent pain return. Use breakthrough medication where appropriate to treat incident pain or acute exacerbation of chronic pain.
   d. Use appropriate adjunctive analgesics for specific types of pain, such as bone pain or neuropathic pain.
   e. Consider appropriate nonpharmacologic forms of intervention, when indicated.
3. Choose the appropriate, least invasive route of therapy to meet the patient's needs. According to the literature, more than 90 percent of patients with chronic pain may be managed with oral medications.
4. Reassess the patient frequently. Routine monitoring and reassessment is the best way to maintain good pain control.

the various terms that are used when assessing and treating patients with pain.

DEFINITION OF PAIN

The International Association for the Study of Pain (IASP) defines pain as "an unpleasant sensory and emotional experience associated with actual or potential tissue damage or described in terms of such damage." Clarifying this definition further, the IASP notes that pain is subjective, and that individuals create their own definition of pain based on their own experiences. This means that the way a patient defines or expresses pain may be very different from how family members or professional caregivers perceive the patient's pain. This inherent subjectivity leads to a simpler and more practical definition:

> Pain is whatever the experiencing person says it is, existing whenever the experiencing person says it does.

Believing the patient, accepting the patient's pain for what it is, and abstaining from superimposing one's own definition of pain upon the patient are the first steps the clinician must take to effectively manage pain. With those steps accomplished, methodic assessment of the cause of the pain will lead the clinician, with the help of the patient, family, and other members of the end-of-life care team, to the development of the plan of care and interventions necessary for effective treatment.

NOCICEPTIVE AND NEUROPATHIC PAIN

Using pathophysiology to categorize pain helps to better understand the etiology of a patient's symptoms and to choose the most appropriate interventions. Pain is divided into two major physiologic types, nociceptive and neuropathic. Nociceptive pain is further subdivided into somatic and visceral subtypes. Table 6–3 presents differential characteristics of somatic and visceral nociceptive pain and neuropathic pain.

SOMATIC NOCICEPTIVE PAIN   Somatic nociceptive pain is caused by tissue injury that results in direct

Table 6–3

Characteristics of Nociceptive and Neuropathic Pain

| | NOCICEPTIVE | | NEUROPATHIC |
	SOMATIC	VISCERAL	
Pathophysiology	Tissue injury resulting in direct stimulation of intact afferent nerve endings. A subset of somatic pain is caused by direct cancerous infiltration of the bone mediated by prostaglandins	Activation of nociceptors resulting from stretching, distension, or inflammation of the internal organs of the body	Injury to peripheral nerves or central nervous system structures
Description	Usually well localized, and may be described as sharp, dull, aching, throbbing, or gnawing in nature	Poorly localized and may be described as deep, aching, crampy, or a sensation of pressure	May be described as burning, shooting, tingling, stabbing, or like a vise or electric shock. It may be constant or paroxysmal and it is often associated with paresthesias or dysesthesias
Affected organs	Typically affected parts of the body include bones, joints, and soft tissues	Internal organs	Brain, central nervous system, nerve plexi, nerve roots, peripheral nerves
Examples	Metastatic cancer to bone, fractures, tumors or erosive ulcers invading soft tissues, arthritis	Periumbilical pain of bowel obstruction. Shoulder pain secondary to liver or lung metastases. Jaw and/or left arm pain secondary to coronary insufficiency	Brachial or lumbosacral plexopathy, herpes zoster, diabetic neuropathy, alcoholic neuropathy
Pharmacologic management	NSAIDs, opioids	Opioid	Less responsive to opioids. Requires adjuvant medications: Tricyclic antidepressants, Steroids, Anticonvulsants (See Table 6–20)

stimulation of intact afferent nerve endings. Somatic pain is usually described in the following terms: sharp, dull, aching, throbbing, gnawing in nature. It occurs in bones, joints, and soft tissues and tends to be relatively well localized. Causes for somatic pain include fractures, arthritis, burns, abrasions, abscesses, and tumor invasion of soft tissue. Somatic nociceptive pain responds well to opioid analgesics. Bone pain due to tumor metastases is a subcategory of somatic nociceptive pain that is largely mediated by prostaglandins, and therefore amenable to treatment not only with opioids but also with nonsteroidal anti-inflammatory drugs (NSAIDs).

VISCERAL NOCICEPTIVE PAIN   As with somatic pain, visceral nociceptive pain is caused by tissue injury, inflammation, or stretching that results in direct stimulation of intact afferent nerve endings. Visceral pain affects internal organs, is poorly localized, and is often referred to various somatic sites. Visceral pain is usually described as a deep ache, cramp, or sensation of pressure. Examples of referred visceral pain include shoulder pain caused by liver metastases or cholecystitis, and the left arm and jaw pain that is classical for coronary insufficiency. An example of poorly localized visceral pain is the periumbilical discomfort that may be associated with multiple inflammatory or obstructive gastrointestinal conditions. Visceral nociceptive pain also tends to respond well to opioid analgesics.

NEUROPATHIC PAIN   Neuropathic pain is caused by direct injury to peripheral nerves and/or the central nervous system resulting in aberrant neural discharges unrelated to external noxious stimuli. Neuropathic pain is usually described with the following terms: burning, shooting, tingling, vice-like, electric. The pain may be constant or paroxysmal, and it is often associated with paresthesias, dysesthesia, and allodynia. Causes of neuropathic pain include spinal cord compression, plexopathy, neurotoxicity secondary to cancer chemotherapy, chemical and metabolic neuropathies such as diabetes mellitus, postherpetic neuralgia, tic douloureux, postmastectomy syndrome, and phantom limb pain. Unlike nociceptive pain, neuropathic pain is relatively unaffected by opioid analgesics and optimal treatment requires the prescription of adjuvant agents such as corticosteroids, tricyclic antidepressants, and anticonvulsants in addition to opioid analgesics (see Table 6–20).

ACUTE AND CHRONIC PAIN

Pain is also categorized as acute or chronic based on the nature of its onset and its duration. The characteristics of acute and chronic pain are summarized in Table 6–4.

Acute pain is defined as a pain that occurs suddenly, usually with an identifiable cause. The acuity

Table 6–4

Characteristics of Acute and Chronic Pain

	ACUTE PAIN	CHRONIC PAIN
Onset	Usually sudden	Usually of long duration
Characteristics	Generally sharp, localized, may radiate	Dull, aching, persistent, diffuse
Signs and symptoms	Physiologic response:	Physiologic response:
	Increased blood pressure and heart rate, sweating, pallor	Often absent
	Emotional response:	Emotional response:
	Increased anxiety and restlessness	Patient may be depressed, withdrawn, expressionless, and exhausted
Therapeutic goals	Relief of pain	Prevention of pain
	Sedation often desirable	Sedation not desirable
Timing	As needed (prn) or upon request	Regular preventive schedule
Dosing	Generally standard	Individualized based upon patient needs
Route of administration	Parenteral/oral	Oral preferred

SOURCE: Adapted with permission from: Kinzbrunner BM: *Vitas Pain Management Guidelines*. Miami: Vitas Healthcare, 1995.

of onset causes the patient to develop subjective and objective physical signs associated with hyperactivity of the autonomic nervous system, such as tachycardia, hypertension, and diaphoresis. The patient usually exhibits overt signs of pain including facial grimacing, groaning, crying, or even screaming. Classical examples of acute pain include that associated with a fracture immediately after a fall, and postoperative pain.

Chronic pain is best defined as a pain that has been persistent and unremitting for some time. Although the literature typically refers to a time frame of 6 months, this seems unnecessarily restrictive and unrealistic in the context of end-of-life care. Unlike patients with acute pain, patients with chronic pain do not exhibit the typical autonomic or physical signs commonly associated with pain. Rather, they often seem apathetic, withdrawn, and depressed, leading the untrained or insensitive observer to doubt that the patient is experiencing pain at all. It is precisely this large group of patients, whose credibility is so easily questioned, that is at the greatest risk for poor pain management.

Distinguishing acute from chronic pain is important because of differences in the therapeutic approach to each problem (Table 6–4). Acute pain should be treated with analgesia as needed, with the expectation that the painful stimulus will remit over time. In contrast, chronic pain must be treated with regular, around-the-clock, dosing to prevent recurring pain that will persist or even worsen. Sedation is usually desirable when patients are having acute pain as this will alleviate anxiety, promote rest, and allow healing to occur. Sustained sedation is undesirable for patients with chronic pain, because one of the major goals of pain relief is to allow resumption of a maximum number of activities of daily living. Because treatment for acute pain is expected to be transient, standard, "one size fits all," analgesic doses are common, and parenteral routes of administration are not objectionable. For patients with chronic pain, treatment is likely to be sustained for the duration of the underlying illness. Analgesic doses must be titrated to the needs of the individual patient and should be administered by the least invasive route possible, preferably by mouth.

Terminally ill patients with chronic pain often have acute exacerbations, particularly as the disease process progresses and new complications ensue. When this occurs, the clinician must be careful not to overlook a potential new painful stimulus as a cause of the acute event. Every new flare-up of pain is a legitimate reason to initiate a new pain assessment, and if indicated, adjust or modify the treatment plan.

The Pain Assessment

The principal components of a thorough pain assessment are outlined in Table 6–5. The importance of developing and exercising good assessment

Table 6–5

Performing a Thorough Pain Assessment

1. Always obtain a complete history, preferably from the patient, paying specific attention to:
   a. Full pain history (see Table 6–6)
   b. Psychosocial, spiritual, and family history
   c. Medication history, including over-the-counter medications
2. Perform a physical examination focused on:
   a. Painful areas
   b. A thorough neurologic examination
3. Establish a pain diagnosis or diagnoses
4. Institute an appropriate plan of care based on the pain assessment
5. Directly involve the patient and/or primary caregivers
   a. Explain your findings to the patient (or to the primary caregivers)
   b. Involve the patient directly in his or her own management
   c. Establish realistic time frames to achieve goals
   d. Reassess the patient's pain frequently
   e. Monitor for adverse side effects and treat in anticipation
6. DOCUMENT the pain assessment

skills is underscored by a survey of oncologists in which 75 percent identified clinical inadequacy in performing pain assessments as the leading barrier to effective pain management (Von Roenn et al, 1993).

COMPLETE HISTORY, PREFERABLY FROM THE PATIENT

Due to the fact that the perception of pain is so highly subjective, a detailed history is essential for a productive pain assessment. Remember that the focus of the pain assessment near the end of life is to reach a "pain diagnosis" rather than the "disease diagnosis" that is the usual goal of a patient–physician encounter. Thus, although the history of present illness is important to understanding the contextual basis of the complaint of pain, and the past history may identify causes for pain that may not be directly related to the terminal illness, the primary history of the pain itself is critical and sometimes overlooked. Questions about the characteristics of the patient's pain help to determine whether the pain is nociceptive, neuropathic, or mixed, and whether the pain is acute, chronic, or an exacerbation of acute pain superimposed on a chronic pain syndrome. Patients may have more than one site or cause for pain, with each pain having its own characteristics and therapeutic needs. As patients may be unaware of this complexity, the physician must maintain a high index of suspicion and take care to question the patient in sufficient detail to identify all painful areas.

HISTORY OF THE PAIN   The mnemonic device, PQRST, has proven to be a useful reminder of what questions need to be asked to complete an adequate pain history (Table 6–6). The "P" stands for both palliative and provocative: What conditions affect the perception of pain? Ask whether movement, rest, position, weight-bearing, or activities such as bathing, dressing, eating, or swallowing have a positive or negative effect. Determine what interventions, including current or past medications, make the pain better or worse.

The "Q" stands for quality: What are the properties and characteristics of the pain as perceived by the patient and how do they relate to the pathophysiology? Ask the patient to describe the pain in his or her own words. Because patients may have difficulty with this task, clinicians must become skilled at guiding the patient without being overly suggestive. Open-ended questions are preferable, but at times it may be necessary to ask directly whether the pain is sharp, dull, aching, or throbbing (think nociceptive pain), or shooting, piercing, burning, or tingling (think neuropathic pain).

The "R" stands for radiation. Attempt to localize the pain if possible. Determining patterns of radiation and whether the pain appears to be referred helps to differentiate somatic from visceral nociceptive pain and provides clues to the origins of visceral pain. In the case of neuropathic pain, pat-

Table 6–6

The PQRST of Pain Assessment

	MEANING	**EXAMPLE**
P	Palliative	What makes the pain better?
	Provocative	What makes the pain worse?
Q	Quality	How would you describe the pain?
R	Radiation	To where does the pain spread or travel?
S	Severity	On a scale of 0 to 10, how bad is the pain?
T	Temporal	Is the pain constant, or does it come and go?

Figure 6–1

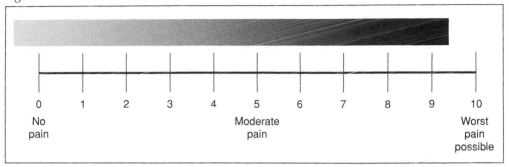

0–10 Numerical pain intensity scale. This is the gold standard for assessing pain severity. Patients should be asked about the severity of their pain with 0 representing no pain, 5 representing moderate pain, and 10 representing the worst pain possible.

SOURCE: Acute Pain Management Guideline Panel: *Acute Pain Management: Operative or Medical Procedures and Trauma. Clinical Practice Guideline.* AHCPR pub. no. 92-0032. Rockville, MD, Agency for Health Care Policy and Research, Public Health Service, U.S. Department of Health and Human Services, February 1992.

terns of radiation help distinguish peripheral from central nervous system lesions and identify specific nerve roots, plexi, and dermatomes.

The "S" stands for severity. Although pain is inherently subjective, for initial assessment, selection of treatment, and serial monitoring of response, it is useful to create a more objective and reproducible measurement system to quantify what the patient is experiencing. For this purpose, pain is rated by the patient according to its severity on a numerical 0 to 10 scale, with 0 representing no pain and 10 representing the worst pain imaginable. The utility of this method has been validated in a number of studies.

Figures 6–1 and 6–2 illustrate some of the tools that are helpful for assessing pain severity. The most common tool used is a linear scale (Fig. 6–1) consisting of a line 10 cm in length with or without marked gradations (0 to 10). The line may be augmented by a color chart with cool colors (blue) representing the lowest levels of pain and

Figure 6–2

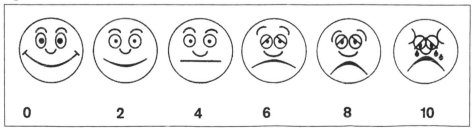

This measure uses faces to pictorially represent the severity of a patient's pain. This was originally developed for pediatric patients, and has also been found to be very useful in the elderly as well as patients who have difficulty reading. Numerical values (0–10) have been assigned to each face to allow for compatibility with the 0–10 numerical scale.

SOURCE: Wong D, Whaley L: *Clinical Handbook of Pediatric Nursing*, 2nd ed. St. Louis, Mosby, 1986. Printed with permission of the publisher and authors, who also give their permission for this scale to be duplicated and used in the care of children with pain.

hot colors (red) the highest pain levels. Patients who are able to write, mark the line at the point that corresponds to their perception of the severity of the pain. Alternatively, patients may verbally express their estimate of pain severity using the line scale to guide their response.

For children, or for patients with difficulty reading numbers or understanding numerical concepts, the Wong/Baker faces rating scale (Fig. 6–2) allows the patient to point to the face that best represents the severity of the pain. The clinician may then correlate the face with the 0 to 10 numerical scale.

When quantifying pain, the clinician should inquire not only about the immediate moment but also about the worst level of pain during the past 24 hours and during the past several days. Regardless of the method used to rate the severity of pain, it is mandatory that pain severity be measured as regularly as any other vital sign. All clinicians within an institution or practice should use the same scale and criteria to promote consistency and continuity of care.

The "T" stands for temporal. Understanding the pattern of pain expression over time helps differentiate acute from chronic pain and provides clues to the etiology and a framework for scheduling specific interventions. For example, a patient who complains of muscle stiffness and pain on awakening may require extra medication at bedtime and benefit from a new mattress or from a different sleeping position. Increased pain late in the afternoon, coincident with the return home of a spouse or caregiver, might suggest that the pain is intertwined with psychosocial issues that require exploration and counseling rather than an increase in analgesia.

PSYCHOSOCIAL, SPIRITUAL, AND FAMILY HISTORY A social history and a family history adapted to the special circumstances of terminal illness can add valuable information to the pain assessment. Knowledge about the patient's occupation or recreational interests might help the clinician better understand, for example, why a man with meticulous habits who loved opera, stopped attending performances after undergoing a colostomy, with the explanation that he now suffered from constant abdominal pain. A family history emphasizing

relationships can be instrumental in analyzing the difficult-to-control symptoms of a patient who, dying of advanced alcoholic cirrhosis, had not talked to his estranged daughter since her wedding, which he had missed due to a drinking binge.

The perception of pain can be influenced by a wide variety of psychosocial, familial, and spiritual issues that, if not detected and addressed, can sometimes blunt or even totally negate the efficacy of analgesics. There is ample evidence that anxiety, sleeplessness, anger, fear, fright, depression, discomfort, isolation, and loneliness can all lower the pain threshold and decrease the patient's ability to cope with discomfort that might be tolerable under other circumstances (Table 6–7).

MEDICATION HISTORY A complete medication history is crucial. Knowledge of all medications currently or previously in use, assessment of their efficacy and potential for drug interactions, and a determination as to whether treatment meets proper standards of care are critical for deciding the next steps in the patient's pharmacologic management. The medication history must include over-the-counter medications and information about recreational drug use and substance abuse.

PHYSICAL EXAMINATION

For the purposes of pain assessment, the physical examination should focus on painful areas and include a thorough neurologic evaluation. Assessment of pain in the neck or back requires a full motor, sensory, and reflex examination to identify spinal cord lesions and plexopathies. Patients with headaches or skull pain should be checked for possible cranial nerve defects that are characteristically found in certain well-defined cranial pain syndromes. Dermatologic inspection should be performed to look for herpes zoster or pressure sores. A complaint of oral pain should prompt a dental examination (dentures also) as well inspection of the oropharyngeal mucosa. The patient's environment should be inspected as well to identify uncomfortable furniture or other factors that might contribute to the patient's pain.

Table 6–7
Factors Affecting the Pain Threshold

EFFECT ON THRESHOLD	EFFECT ON PATIENT'S PERCEPTION OF PAIN	FACTORS
Lower	Increased severity	Poor pain control
		Depression
		Anxiety
		Sleeplessness
		Anger
		Fear
		Fright
		Isolation
		Loneliness
Raise	Decreased severity	Good pain control
		Treatment of depression
		Reduced anxiety
		Sleep
		Rest
		Diversion
		Empathy
		Sympathy

The physical examination is particularly important when evaluating pain in patients with cognitive impairment and in patients who are unwilling or unable to communicate verbally. Non-verbal phenomena such as gestures, facial expressions, guarding, restricted movement, and flinching that are observed in the course of physical contact with the patient can accurately signal the presence of pain even in confused and disoriented individuals.

ESTABLISH A PAIN DIAGNOSIS OR DIAGNOSES

Pain may be of single or multifocal origin, and may be attributable to the primary disease process itself or the result of previous treatment such as chemotherapy or radiotherapy. If the pain diagnosis is not evident from the history and physical examination, it is occasionally necessary to perform various diagnostic studies, even when patients are near the end of life. Indications for the use of diagnostic studies in end-of-life care are discussed in Chapter 17. A complete pain diagnosis also identifies those psychosocial, emotional, spiritual, financial, and any additional nonmedical factors that may modulate the patient's perception of pain.

INSTITUTE AN APPROPRIATE PLAN OF CARE BASED ON THE PAIN ASSESSMENT

The remainder of this chapter is devoted to treatment strategies for physical pain. However, there are also factors that affect a patient's perception of pain other than the physical causes. A number of pain management experts have redefined what is commonly referred to as pain with terms such as "total pain" or "suffering." These latter terms define the combination of physical, psychosocial, and spiritual components that all combine together to produce the sensation that the patient complains of as "pain."

Some components of "total pain" or "suffering" that influence a patient's perception of pain are listed in Table 6–8. Addressing these issues can help increase a patient's pain threshold, and render the physical pain more responsive to the pharmacologic and nonpharmacologic interventions in the plan of care.

In light of the complexity of the challenge, it is prudent to acknowledge that no single health care worker possesses the expertise and skills needed to manage all of the physical and nonphysical causes of pain. This fact is confirmed by the success of the hospice model of care. The structure of the hospice interdisciplinary team—which not only includes physicians, nurses, pharmacists, and home health aides (to address the physical symptoms and provide pharmacologic management) but also social workers, chaplains, and volunteers (to address the psychosocial and spiritual needs)—increases the likelihood the patient will benefit from "total pain" management. (See Chapter 4 for a discussion of how the interdisciplinary team functions to provide care to patients near the end of life.)

DIRECTLY INVOLVE THE PATIENT AND/OR PRIMARY CAREGIVERS

Regardless of the details of the treatment program, be careful to fully explain your findings and recommendations to the patient and/or to the primary caregivers. and involve the patient directly in the management effort. Instead of just telling the patient what to do, ask whether the proposed plan seems to make sense, and seek the patient's assent to be a partner in its implementation. By

Table 6–8

Factors That Affect a Patient's Perception of Total Pain and Suffering

An individual's basic psychological makeup
Loss of work
Physical disability
Change in social and familial roles and relationships
Fear of death
Cultural, ethnic, and religious background
Financial concerns

asking the patient for permission to treat, you are offering a degree of control—an action that may by itself be therapeutic.

Reach agreement with the patient on the goals of the treatment plan, and establish a realistic time frame for their accomplishment. For example, to avoid discouragement and premature abandonment of the course of treatment, patients should be aware that neuropathic pain usually responds less quickly to analgesic therapy than nociceptive pain. Establish an agreed-upon schedule for regular follow-up visits. Reassess the patient's pain frequently, anticipate incident pain (for example, increased pain associated with a particular activity), and monitor the patient for breakthrough pain, loss of pain control, or the development of new pain due to other causes. Be on the alert for side effects of therapy and initiate prophylactic treatment for expected adverse effects, such as opioid-related constipation.

DOCUMENT THE PAIN ASSESSMENT

Detailed and comprehensible documentation of the pain assessment is essential to ensure effective communication with all caregivers and to create a reference baseline for future assessments. Using a standard pain assessment tool (Fig. 6–3) is a good way to ensure uniform documentation. The body chart is an important component of the pain assessment tool because it clearly illustrates the loci of pain and allows for the depiction of pain radiation. Furthermore, by asking the patient to help complete or review the body chart, the clinician creates an opportunity to involve the patient in his or her own care.

Pharmacologic Treatment of Pain

Although nonpharmacologic interventions deserve careful consideration in a comprehensive treatment plan for pain (covered near the end of

Figure 6–3

PAIN

	LOCATION:	1._____ 2._____
P	PALLIATION:	1._____ 2._____
	PROVOCATON:	1._____ 2._____
Q	QUALITY:	1._____ 2._____
R	RADIATION:	1._____ 2._____
S	SEVERITY (0-10):	1._____ 2._____
T	TEMPORAL: ONSET	1._____ 2._____
	PATTERN	1._____ 2._____

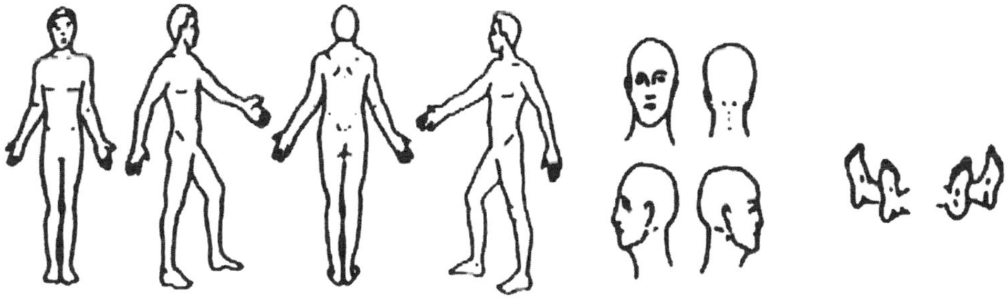

PATIENT'S PERCEPTION OF PAIN: _____

PRESENT MED.: _____ AMOUNT:___ SCHEDULE: _____ STARTED: _____ ADEQUATE: ☐ YES ☐ NO

PAST MED.: _____ AMOUNT:_____ SCHEDULE: _____ HOW LONG TRIED: _____

REASON FOR STOPPING: ☐ NAUSEA ☐ CONSTIPATION ☐ SEDATION ☐ ITCHING ☐ DIDN'T CONTROL PAIN

HISTORY OF DRUG OR ALCOHOL USE: ☐ YES ☐ NO

Pain assessment tool
SOURCE: Adapted with permission from Kinzbrunner BM. *Vitas Pain Management Guidelines*. Miami: Vitas Healthcare, 1995.

the chapter), in Western medicine these techniques are generally regarded as complementary to pharmacologic intervention, particularly in the context of end-of-life care. Expert knowledge in the use of analgesic drugs is essential for any clinician who cares for terminally ill patients, and alacrity in seeking appropriate consultation for difficult cases is highly recommended. Hospice medical directors, physicians who are certified by the American Board of Hospice and Palliative Care, and other trained pain specialists are available for consultation in most communities in the United States.

Guidelines for the pharmacologic treatment of pain are listed in Table 6–9 and are discussed in the next sections.

Table 6–9

Guidelines for the Pharmacologic Treatment of Pain

I. Develop a basic, generally applicable, drug armamentarium
II. Select the drug(s) best suited for the individual patient and type and degree of pain
   A. Patient considerations
      1. Prior experiences and drug history
         a. Prior response and adverse effects
         b. Allergies
         c. Substance abuse
      2. Physical condition and metabolic state
      3. Prognostic assessment
      4. Acceptability to patient and family
      5. Expense
   B. Drug-specific considerations
      1. Use specific type of drug for a specific type of pain
      2. Know the pharmacology of the drug(s) prescribed
         a. Achieve maximum benefit at lowest effective dose with fewest side effects
         b. Titrate to effect
         c. Choose the least invasive route of administration
         d. Select the most convenient schedule of administration
      3. Anticipate and treat complications and side effects
      4. Prevent acute withdrawal and the development of tolerance
      5. Use adjuvant drug combinations to provide additive analgesia and to reduce side effects
      6. Be aware of drug interactions
      7. Believe the patient:
         a. Working with the patient with a history of substance abuse
         b. Avoid pseudoaddiction

Develop a Medication Armamentarium

The pharmaceutical industry has responded to the increase in professional and public awareness about the problem of uncontrolled pain by rapidly developing new opioid and non-opioid analgesics and by adapting older agents for use as sustained-release products or via novel routes of administration. The proliferation of new and modified analgesic drugs provides the clinician with added flexibility, but may also be somewhat bewildering in terms of assessing claims of competing manufacturers and distinguishing agents with unique properties and advantages from drugs sometimes described as "me too." Effective pain management is best served by developing expert familiarity with two or three drugs within each class of analgesic agents and building on a base of personal clinical experience with this relatively restricted drug armamentarium.

Medication Selection: Patient-Specific Considerations

PRIOR EXPERIENCES AND MEDICATION HISTORY

The choice of an optimal analgesic regimen must be adapted to meet the needs and requirements of each individual patient. Information about the patient's prior experiences and a complete medication history should have been obtained during the process of pain assessment. Crucial information includes identification of agents that have been effective, as well as their dosages, routes, and schedules. The assessment should also identify allegedly ineffective agents, reasons for lack of efficacy, and a record of adverse reactions and side effects. A detailed investigation of "medication allergy" is important, as patients frequently attribute adverse side effects such as opioid-induced constipation and nausea, or morphine-associated, histamine-mediated pruritus to "allergy," although true immunologic hypersensitivity to opioids is quite rare. It is very important to properly educate patients and their families so that unfounded concern about allergic reactions does not become a barrier to optimal pain management.

Although the incidence of iatrogenic addiction in patients with no prior personal or family history of substance abuse is negligible, significant numbers of patients in need of pain management may be active or recovered substance abusers. (See "Pharmacologic Pain Management in the Patient with Previous or Current Substance Abuse" later in the chapter.)

PHYSICAL CONDITION AND METABOLIC IMPAIRMENT

The overall physical condition of the patient may restrict and limit pharmacologic options. The oral route, for example, may not be the best when patients have severe dysphagia, a high risk of aspiration, or suffer from esophageal, gastric, or small bowel obstruction. Transdermal fentanyl may be a poor choice in severely cachectic patients who lack subcutaneous fat depots. Renal impairment often precludes the adjuvant use of nonsteroidal anti-inflammatory drugs (NSAIDs) and may affect the dose and schedule of administration for opioids such as morphine and oxycodone whose active metabolites are renally excreted. For patients with severe renal insufficiency, hydromorphone, rather than morphine, may be the opioid of choice. On the other hand, morphine is preferable to other opioids for patients with hepatic impairment. Metha-

done, levorphanol, pentazocine, propxyphene, and meperidine can cause CNS depression that mimics hepatic encephalopathy in patients with poor liver function, and oxycodone must be used with caution when patients have severe liver impairment. Nonopioid analgesics or adjuvant drugs that should be avoided when patients have liver disease include acetaminophen and tricyclic antidepressants.

Pulmonary insufficiency should not be an insurmountable obstacle to effective pain management with opioid agonist agents, even for patients with severe chronic hypoxia whose ventilatory drive depends heavily on the response to CO_2. Clinical experience with COPD patients shows that when low starting doses of morphine are gradually titrated upward as needed to control pain, the risk of respiratory depression or arrest is negligible. In dying patients, the use of morphine for the palliation of terminal dyspnea is well documented in the literature (see Chapter 7).

PROGNOSTIC FACTORS

During the last few days of life, the principle that pain management should aim at maximal analgesia with minimal sedation may not necessarily be relevant. At this point in the patient's course, when pain and other symptoms may be particularly difficult to control, and may be accompanied with marked agitation, the concept of total sedation may be explored with the patient and/or family (see Chapter 12). As patients near death, and systemic organ dysfunction and metabolic failure ensue, dosage requirements for opioid medications may dramatically decrease, with a corresponding increase in opioid side effects. In these circumstances, opioids must not be abruptly and totally discontinued. Because of physiologic dependence, abrupt cessation of opioids will almost certainly provoke significant withdrawal symptoms that will compound terminal suffering.

ACCEPTABILITY TO PATIENT AND FAMILY

As previously discussed, patient resistance to the use of opioids is a significant barrier to optimal pain management. This behavior, known as opio-phobia, may sometimes be restricted to morphine, in which case substitution of other opioid agonists may win patient acceptance. However, some patients may refuse all pharmacologic analgesia because of fear of side effects, unrealistic denial, or due to a belief that pain is, in some way, either deserved or ennobling. These patients require intensive education and psychosocial interventions.

Input from primary caregivers and family members may also be critical to the choice of analgesic agents. Family members may sometimes minimize pain and other symptoms, even to the point of disbelieving the patient's complaints, withholding prescribed analgesics, decreasing the dosage, or prolonging the interval between doses. Patients and caregivers may object to short-acting analgesics as excessively burdensome in terms of remembering doses accurately, interfering with sleep, or otherwise disrupting the family schedule. In these circumstances, sustained-release analgesics may be selected to better advantage. Knowledge of suspicion of drug diversion by relatives or friends may also influence the choice and route of administration of analgesics, particularly those that are regulated as controlled substances.

EXPENSE

Although expense should generally not be the prime element in choosing either medication or other interventions in end-of-life care, neither should it be ignored, particularly when less expensive equipotent regimens are available. Prudent pharmacoeconomic management can conserve limited resources, expand the circle of patients receiving optimal end-of-life care, and alleviate a major source of anxiety for terminal patients and their families who are all too often under considerable financial pressure.

Medication Selection: Medication-Specific Considerations

USE A SPECIFIC TYPE OF DRUG FOR A SPECIFIC TYPE OF PAIN

The World Health Organization (WHO) recommends a three-step "ladder" guideline that provides for incremental analgesic therapy based on the severity of a patient's pain (Fig. 6-4). This approach was included in the Agency for Health Care Policy Research (AHCPR) 1994 gui

Figure 6-4

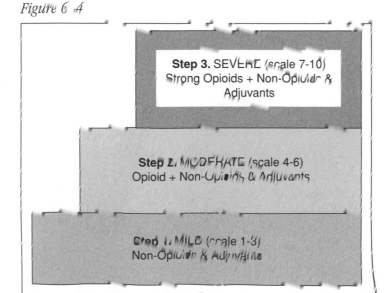

The World Health Organization (WHO) analgesic ladder

practice guidelines for the management of cancer pain, and is generally accepted as an appropriate guideline for patients with terminal nonmalignant diseases. Following a thorough pain assessment (described earlier), patients may rate their pain as mild (severity scale 1 to 3), moderate (severity scale 4 to 6), or severe (severity scale 7 to 10). Appropriate analgesic medication is selected based on this determination. Unlike a traditional "step ladder" (e.g., for hypertension), where treatment is usually started at the lowest rung and progressively intensified until the desired level of response is achieved, the WHO analgesic ladder is accessed at whatever level best represents the patient's pain on presentation. If a patient presents with a pain severity level of 9, treatment is initiated with a strong opioid per step 3 of the ladder, rather than with medications that are appropriate for step 1.

The WHO analgesic ladder favors the least invasive routes of administration and presupposes that appropriate nonopioid analgesics and adjuvant medications (e.g., acetaminophen, NSAIDs, corticosteroids, antidepressants, anticonvulsants) will be continued, if indicated, at all levels of the ladder. Should a patient advance from steps 1 to 3 because of progressive pain, nonopioid and adjuvant medications should not be discontinued (unless for reasons of toxicity) merely because a strong opioid is now prescribed. Step 2 is considered "weaker" than step 3 because it includes fixed combinations of an opioid and a nonopioid

(e.g., oxycodone and acetaminophen) that cannot be significantly escalated because of toxicity attributable to the nonopioid component. Its justification is questioned by many pain experts and criticized as pandering to the popular, irrational fear of the opioids, especially morphine.

STEP 1: MILD PAIN (SEVERITY SCALE 1 TO 3)   Nonopioid analgesics, recommended for the treatment of mild pain, include acetaminphen and the nonsteroidal anti-inflammatory drugs (NSAIDs), of which aspirin is the prototype. Some of the agents more commonly used to treat patients near the end of life are listed in Table 6–10.

Acetaminophen   Acetaminophen is currently the most widely recommended nonopioid analgesic for mild pain and is often used in combination with opioid analgesics such as codeine, oxycodone, and hydrocodone for patients with moderate pain. Acetaminophen has analgesic and antipyretic properties. However, it is not an anti-inflammatory agent, a point that should be remembered when selecting medication for patients whose pain is largely mediated by inflammatory cytokines (e.g., bone metastases). Acetaminophen is generally well tolerated and has a safety profile sufficient to allow government-authorized use as a nonprescription drug. It is frequently found in combination with other medications and packaged as a component of multiple over-the-counter preparations for colds, nasal congestion, cough, gastrointestinal upset, and

Table 6–10

Step 1 Analgesics

MEDICATION	ROUTES OF ADMINISTRATION	DOSAGE RANGE
Acetaminophen	PO, PR	325–650 mg q 4–6 h
Choline magnesium trisalicylate	PO	500–1500 mg 2–3 times/day
Ibuprofen	PO	200–800 mg q 4–6 h
Indomethacin	PO, PR	25–50 mg 2–4 times/day
Naproxen	PO	250 mg q 6–8 h
Piroxicam	PO	20 mg daily
Rofecoxib	PO	25–50 mg daily

insomnia. Because the public regards these wide-spread acetaminophen combination products as innocuous, patients may use multiple preparations simultaneously and in conjunction with prescribed medications. To avoid acetaminophen toxicity, it is important to have full knowledge of *all* medications taken by the patient.

Hepatotoxicity, including progressive, irreversible hepatic failure, is the major side effect associated with acetaminophen overdosage. For patients with normal liver function, it is usually recommended that the total daily acetaminophen dose should not exceed 4 grams. For patients with impaired liver function, a lower total daily allowance may be advisable, especially when prolonged chronic use is compounded by alcohol abuse. With prolonged use, acetaminophen may also cause phenacetin-like nephrotoxicity. Although this is unusual, particularly in the context of terminal illness, it is a point worth considering for patients with a relatively long prognosis and marginal renal function.

NSAIDs   Nonsteroidal anti-inflammatory drugs (NSAIDs) are the other major class of agents used to treat mild pain. As the name suggests, in addition to analgesic and antipyretic properties, NSAIDs have anti-inflammatory effects due to their inhibition of cyclooxygenase (COX) mediated prostaglandin synthesis. Among these agents, aspirin, like acetaminophen, is often combined with codeine or oxycodone to treat moderate pain. However, in terminally ill patients, aspirin and aspirin-containing preparations are usually avoided because of an enhanced likelihood of gastrointestinal toxicity and bleeding. A more generalized bleeding diathesis associated with aspirin treatment is attributed to impaired platelet function caused by irreversible acetylation of platelet surface glycoproteins. At analgesic doses, this effect supersedes aspirin-induced reversible inhibition of platelet COX-1, a phenomenon responsible for the vascular cardioprotective effects of low-dose aspirin therapy and one that is common to all NSAIDs. Because of the risk of clinically significant bleeding, aspirin is particularly to be avoided in patients with thrombocytopenia,

whether due to advanced disease or secondary to prior chemotherapy or radiotherapy.

The nonacetylated salicylates, including salsalate, choline magnesium trisalicylate, and diflunisal, have less gastrointestinal toxicity than aspirin and are less inhibitory to platelet function. Some of these products are inconvenient due to large tablet size and the need to ingest many tablets with each dose.

Other commonly used NSAIDs, some of which are available over-the-counter in doses usually lower than those restricted to prescription only, include ibuprofen, naproxen, and indomethacin. Although most of these short-acting NSAIDs exert analgesic effects within hours of initiating treatment, it may require 1 to 2 weeks of sustained therapy to achieve a maximal effect. Because of structural biochemical differences, one should not assume cross-resistance among different NSAID classes; and should the patient fail to respond positively to one NSAID, trial of another from a different category should not be precluded. However, combination therapy with more than one NSAID is not recommended due to likely additive adverse reactions.

Ibuprofen and naproxen are generally better tolerated than aspirin and are also available in fixed combinations with opioid analgesics. Indomethacin and naproxen are available as sustained-release preparations suitable for twice a day and three times a day dosing. Piroxicam is an NSAID in capsule form that is long acting and may be given in one daily dose. Ketorolac is often effective for managing acute inflammatory pain, especially when given parenterally. However, because of the high risk of gastrointestinal and renal toxicity, ketorolac is contraindicated for chronic use, and it should be administered for no more than 5 consecutive days or in no more than 20 doses. For patients who cannot swallow pills, there are liquid preparations of choline magnesium trisalicylate, ibuprofen, naproxen, and acetaminophen. Indomethacin, aspirin and acetaminophen may also be administered as rectal suppositories.

Although individuals may respond variably to different NSAIDs, there is little evidence that any one of the estimated 20 to 30 NSAID products available has greater analgesic efficacy than any other, when prescribed in equivalent dosage. However, there may be significant differences in toxicity profiles, presumably based on differential inhibition of the COX isoforms, COX-1 and COX-2. COX-1 is a ubiquitous, constitutive isoenzyme-producing prostaglandin necessary for homeostatic functions, such as maintenance of gastrointestinal mucosal integrity. COX-2 is believed to be largely induced and up-regulated by inflammatory cytokines, producing prostaglandins that mediate pain and inflammation. However, there is increasing evidence that COX-2 may also have significant constitutive, noninflammatory functions including ulcer healing, intravascular volume regulation, and regulation of bone remodeling. It is believed that the therapeutic effects of all conventional NSAIDs relate to inhibition of COX-2, whereas the adverse effects, particularly gastrointestinal toxicity, are caused by inhibition of COX-1 activity. This concept has led to a new classification of NSAIDs based on the degree of COX-2 specificity as well as the development of new COX-2 specific agents that, based on clinical trials, appear to have significantly decreased GI toxicity and platelet dysfunction.

The newer classification of NSAIDs identifies aspirin, ketorolac, ketoprofen, ibuprofen, naproxen, tolmetin, indomethacin, and fenoprofen as nonspecific COX inhibitors. Agents such as piroxicam, sulindac, and diclofenac are classified as preferential COX-2 inhibitors. However, this division is somewhat arbitrary as there is as yet no standard method for determining the ratio of COX-1 to COX-2 inhibition, and different assays give different results. Furthermore, in vitro results often do not correlate with clinical outcomes. These include the occurrence of relatively nonserious symptoms such as dyspepsia, heartburn, nausea, vomiting, epigastric pain, and diarrhea (found in 15 to 20 percent of NSAID users), as well as serious complications such as perforation, obstruction, ulcers, and bleeding (reported in 5 to 7 percent of NSAID users). Thus, agents such as nabumetone and etodolac, reported by some to be preferential inhibitors of COX-2, were not found to have a different spectrum of adverse events compared to other currently available NSAIDs.

In contrast, studies of the specific COX-2 inhibitor NSAIDs rofecoxib and celecoxib suggest a significant decrease in NSAID gastrointestinal and renal toxicity without loss of therapeutic efficacy. Both agents were recently approved by the FDA for symptomatic treatment of rheumatoid arthritis and osteoarthritis and are beginning to be offered to patients with terminal illnesses. In a recent study of 8000 patients, celecoxib, even at dosages greater than those clinically indicated, was associated with a lower incidence of symptomatic ulcers, bleeding, dyspepsia, abdominal pain, nausea, and constipation compared with other NSAIDs at standard doses. However, the favorable toxicity profile of celecoxib was adversely affected by concomitant low-dose aspirin therapy, and there have been sporadic case reports of fatal or life-threatening GI hemorrhage in a few patients using specific COX-2 inhibitors. Adverse renal events after celecoxib, such as peripheral edema (2 percent) and hypertension (0.8 percent), had a similar frequency as with other NSAIDs, but were not time or dose related, a phenomenon that may not be true for rofecoxib. There is no evidence of interactions between ACE inhibitors, beta-blockers, calcium channel blockers, or diuretics when used concomitantly with celecoxib.

As of this writing, there have been no trials published of the specific COX-2 inhibitors in terminally ill patients. It is assumed that the relative risk of NSAID toxicity is enhanced in these patients due to factors such as age, concomitant disease processes, and the concurrent use of multiple medications. However, in as much as endoscopically observed gastrointestinal ulceration may be detected within less than 3 months from initiation of NSAID therapy, the potential gain from specific COX-2 inhibitors in terms of equal efficacy and decreased toxicity may be relevant even for patients with a short life expectancy. It remains to be seen whether using these newer agents for end-of-life care is more efficacious and cost effective than the use of traditional NSAIDs with a gastroprotective agent such as misoprostol.

Regardless of toxicity profiles, NSAIDs, even those with COX-2 specificity, appear to have ceiling effects with regards to analgesic efficacy. Thus, as chronic pain becomes increasingly severe, acetaminophen and NSAIDs, which relieve pain primarily through peripheral mechanisms, are employed best when combined synergistically with opioid analgesics that have both central and peripheral activity.

STEP 2: MODERATE PAIN (SEVERITY SCALE 4 TO 6)

Most agents used to treat moderate pain are combinations of opioids and step 1 agents. The agents most commonly used to treat patients near the end of life are listed in Table 6–11, and are dominated by combinations of acetaminophen with codeine, oxycodone, or hydrocodone. The popularity of these agents stems from the fact that, unlike their plain opioid counterparts, the

Table 6–11

Step 2 Analgesics

MEDICATION	COMPONENTS	DOSAGE RANGE
Codeine with acetaminophen	Acetaminophen 300 mg (cap) or 325 mg (tab) with: #2 Codeine 15 mg #3 Codeine 30 mg #4 Codeine 60 mg	1–2 tablets or capsules every 4–6 hr
	Acetaminophen 500 or 600 mg with codeine 30 mg (tab)	1–2 tablets or capsules every 4–6 hr
	Acetaminophen 120 mg with codeine 12 mg per 5 mL	10–20 mL every 4-6 hr
Oxycodone with acetaminophen	Acetaminophen 325 mg with: Oxycodone 2.5 mg Oxycodone 5 mg Oxycodone 7.5 mg	1–2 tablets or capsules every 4–6 hr
	Acetaminophen 325 or 500 mg with oxycodone 5 mg	1–2 tablets or capsules every 4–6 hr
	Acetaminophen 325 mg with oxycodone 5 mg per 5 mL	5–10 mL every 4–6 hr
Hydrocodone with acetaminophen	Acetaminophen 500 mg with: Hydrocodone 2.5 mg Hydrocodone 5 mg Hydrocodone 7.5 mg Hydrocodone 10 mg	1–2 tablets or capsules every 4–6 hr
	Acetaminophen 650 mg with: Hydrocodone 7.5 mg Hydrocodone 10 mg	1–2 tablets or capsules every 4–6 hr
	Acetaminophen 167 mg with hydrocodone 2.5 mg per 5 mL	5–10 mL every 4–6 hr
Hydrocodone with ibuprofen	Ibuprofen 200 mg with hydrocodone 7.5 mg	1 tablet every 4–6 hr
Tramadol		50–100 mg every 4–6 hr, not to exceed 300 mg in the elderly

combination products are not Schedule II controlled substances, and therefore, are not subject to the same prescribing regulations as plain opioids are in states with triplicate prescription programs.

Along with the acetaminophen combinations, these opioids are available in combination with aspirin. However, the aspirin combination products are generally not prescribed to patients near the end of life due to the increased risk of gastrointestinal toxicity and bleeding from aspirin (discussed earlier). Recently, a combination of hydrocodone with the NSAID ibuprofen has been created to take advantage of the anti-inflammatory effects common to both aspirin and ibuprofen while avoiding the increased risk of bleeding associated with aspirin.

In view of the potential for acetaminophen toxicity (discussed earlier), dosing of the acetaminophen-containing agents should be limited to no more than two tablets every 4 to 6 hours. Patients should also be warned to avoid other acetaminophen-containing products (which are commonly available over the counter). Additionally, a ceiling effect further limits the use of codeine combination products. When codeine is administered in doses greater than 65 mg every 4 hours, side effects increase without any gain in analgesic efficacy. In addition to concerns about acetaminophen toxicity, these combination agents can cause typical opioid side effects including constipation, nausea, vomiting, drowsiness, and dysphoria, especially in opioid-naïve patients. (See "Anticipate and Treat Complications and Side Effects" later in the chapter.)

Propoxyphene is a synthetic analgesic, structurally related to methadone, and often prescribed, typically in combination with acetaminophen, for the treatment of mild to moderate pain. Propoxyphene binds to opioid receptors, but was originally believed to be free of potential for substance abuse. This has not proven to be the case. Furthermore, 65 mg of propoxyphene is at best equivalent in analgesic potency to 650 mg of acetaminophen, although there may be some synergy when used in combination. Propoxyphene crosses the blood–brain barrier, and is also metabolized by the liver to nor-propoxyphene, a highly neuroexcitatory, pro-

convulsant compound. Because there are ample equivalent or better alternatives with fewer side effects, propoxyphene combinations are not recommended for the management of pain in terminally ill patients, especially for elderly patients for whom propoxyphene may be particularly dangerous.

Tramadol is a synthetic, centrally acting, oral analgesic that possesses both opioid and nonopioid properties. It is a nonscheduled drug and available as a 50-mg tablet. For chronic pain, tramadol has analgesic potency roughly equivalent to codeine on a per-mg basis. There have been reports of seizures in patients receiving tramadol even within the recommended dosage range. The seizure risk is increased for patients who are simultaneously treated with selective serotonin reuptake inhibitors, tricyclic antidepressants, or other opioids. The usual doses are 50 to 100 mg every 4 to 6 hours. Daily doses of tramadol exceeding 300 mg are not recommended for patients over age 75. A parenteral preparation is currently being developed.

STEP 3: SEVERE PAIN (SEVERITY SCALE 7 TO 10) For treatment of severe pain, opioid agonist drugs such as morphine are the medications of choice. It is important to remember that to achieve pain control, adjunctive medications and other measures may be required in addition to opioid analgesics.

Mechanism of Opioid Action The mechanism of opioid action is related to the binding of opiate molecules to specific receptors in the brain, spinal cord, and peripheral nervous system. Opioid receptors are embedded within synaptic membranes. Formation of the opioid–receptor complex affects a number of events involving neurotransmitters including decreased levels of norepinephrine and dopamine.

The opioid receptors, classified as *mu* (μ), *kappa* (κ), *delta* (δ), and *sigma* (σ), are targets for the endogenous opioid peptides (enkephalins, dynorphins, β-endorphins) as well as the exogenous opioid analgesic drugs. Although analgesia is associated with *mu*, *kappa*, and *delta* receptors, only *mu* and *kappa* binding are currently relevant to analgesic drugs used in clinical practice. Responses to activation of the *kappa* receptor include spinal analgesia as well as sedation, dysphoria, and miosis. Activation of the *mu* receptor produces supraspinal analgesia as well as dysphoria, euphoria, respiratory depression, sedation, constipation, urinary retention, and drug dependence. In laboratory mice lacking a specific opioid receptor (gene "knockouts"), analgesia and all other effects associated with that receptor are not observed. Curiously, these knockout mice appear to develop and live normally despite their lack of opioid receptors, leading to the paradox that although opioid receptors may not be necessary for functional living (at least in mice), they are nonetheless essential for pain control in end-of-life care.

Table 6–12 lists many of the commonly available opioids based on their primary site of action. Opioids are classified as agonist, partial agonist, or mixed agonist–antagonist medications. An agonist drug, such as morphine, binds with its receptor(s) to activate and elicit a maximum response, whereas a partial agonist produces only a partial response. A mixed agonist–antagonist substance produces mixed effects; that is, it will activate one type of receptor but block a different receptor. Opioid agonist–antagonist drugs such as pentazocine have analgesic activity by virtue of binding the *kappa* receptor, but also have *sigma* receptor activity associated with undesirable psychotomimetic effects such as dysphoria, hallucinations, and confusion. Because of this dual agonist effect and coexistent antagonist activity, mixed agonist–antagonist drugs have a ceiling dose effect (as do the partial agonist drugs butorphanol, nalbuphine, and buprenorphine). Agonist–antagonist medications may also cause an acute withdrawal reaction and reverse opioid analgesia causing enhanced pain if administered to opioid-dependent patients or if given concurrently with an opioid agonist. For these reasons, partial agonist and agonist–antagonist opioid drugs are not recommended for managing chronic pain, particularly in terminally ill patients.

Table 6–12

Classification of Opioids Based on Receptor Interactions

RECEPTOR	CLASSIFICATION	MEDICATIONS	RESPONSES
Mu	Strong agonist	Fentanyl Hydromorphone Methadone Morphine	Supraspinal analgesia, constipation, urinary retention, dysphoria, euphoria, sedation, respiratory depression, drug dependence
	Partial agonist	Buprenorphine	
	Weak agonist	Meperidine	
	Antagonist	Naloxone Nalbuphine Pentazocine	Reverses opioid effects; withdrawal reaction in patients with physiologic opioid dependency
Kappa	Strong agonist	Oxycodone	Spinal analgesia, sedation, dysphoria, miosis
	Agonist	Morphine Nalbuphine Pentazocine	
	Weak agonist	Levorphanol Meperidine Methadone	
	Antagonist	Naloxone Buprenorphine	Reverses opioid effects; withdrawal reaction in patients with physiologic opioid dependency

Morphine Among the opioid agonists, morphine is the prototypical agent and the standard to which all others are compared. Morphine continues to be the drug of choice for the treatment of moderate to severe pain for most terminally ill patients because its pharmacology and pharmacokinetics are very well defined, and it may be administered by one of several routes. These include (1) orally as immediate-release liquid solution, tablets, and capsules, or as sustained-release tablets or capsules; (2) rectally as a suppository or in gelatin capsules; (3) subcutaneously or intravenously; or (4) via epidural, intrathecal, or intraventricular routes. (Morphine may also be administered in a nebulized form via inhalation for the treatment of dyspnea, as discussed in Chapter 7. However, due to poor systemic absorption—16 percent bioavailability—by this route, it is not an effective alternative route of administration for the treatment of pain.)

Morphine is rapidly absorbed via the gastrointestinal tract with peak plasma concentrations of free morphine occurring 15 to 30 minutes after oral administration of immediate-release products. The rapidity of absorption indicates that it is rarely necessary for patients with chronic pain to receive morphine intravenously solely for the purpose of accelerating the onset of analgesia. Due to first-pass metabolism by the liver and intestine following an oral dose, only approximately 40 percent of ingested morphine reaches the systemic circulation. As a result of differences in presystemic elimination, marked variations in bioavailablity occur from patient to patient, resulting in the need for individualized dosage titration to effect. Therefore, there is no standard effective dose for oral morphine. Some patients may achieve pain relief with milligram doses, whereas others may require tens, hundreds, or (rarely) even thousands of milligrams with each dose.

Morphine is metabolized by the liver into active and inactive metabolites that are excreted by the kidney. The main metabolite, morphine-3-glucuronide (M3G), is pharmacologically inert. However, a secondary metabolite, morphine-6-glucuronide (M6G), is pharmacologically active and is many times more potent than morphine itself. Unlike morphine, in which all analgesic and other side effects are dependent on binding to the *mu* receptor, M6G may cause additive analgesia via binding to a unique "heroin" receptor. Morphine blood levels are virtually undetectable 6 hours after a single oral dose, and the elimination of free morphine is unchanged in patients with impaired renal function. However, M3G and M6G blood levels remain elevated 12 hours after a single morphine dose, creating a risk of toxicity due to accumulation of M6G. The elimination of these metabolites is markedly prolonged with renal insufficiency. Another metabolite, nor-morphine, that is potentially neurotoxic and proconvulsant, is also renally excreted. However, it is not known whether accumulation of normorphine is a significant problem for patients with renal impairment.

Other Opioids As mentioned, morphine is the prototypical opioid agonist and the standard to which all others are compared. In addition to morphine, the clinician should be familiar with the pharmacology of several other commonly available opioid analgesics. This will allow for the effective pain management of patients who develop intolerable side effects (described later) or tolerance (described later) to morphine.

Table 6–13 lists some of these commonly used alternative opioids, and compares each to morphine. Included in this table are the bioequivalency ratios between oral and parenteral forms of the different medications (where applicable) as well the ratios between the oral form of each medication and oral morphine. The use of these ratios in titrating and managing the various opioid analgesics will be discussed.

Oxycodone is an excellent opioid for the treatment of moderate to severe pain. It is most familiar to clinicians when used in fixed combinations with either acetaminophen or aspirin (see "Step 2" earlier in the chapter). However, oxycodone in uncombined form is now available as immediate-release tablets and capsules, as a liquid solution, and as sustained-release tablets, making it an ideal step 3 agent as well. No parenteral forms of oxycodone are currently available. Since oxycodone is relatively unfamiliar to the lay public, it has not yet been subjected to the same stigma and fear as morphine. For this reason, pain-suffering patients who fear the use of morphine may sometimes accept oxycodone with equanimity.

Like morphine, oxycodone as a single agent has no ceiling effect, allowing upward titration to need. Unlike morphine, whose major effects are expressed via the *mu* opioid receptor, oxycodone has been reported to exhibit specificity for the

Table 6–13

Equianalgesic Conversion Table

Analgesic	Parenteral Oral Dose	Duration of Dose	Half-Life Action (hr)	Oral: Parenteral (hr)	Oral Morphine: Analgesic Ratio	Ratio
Agonists						
Morphine	30 mg[a]	10 mg	4–6	2–4	3:1[a]	1:1
Oxycodone	20 mg[b]	—	3–5	4–5	—	1.5:1[b]
Hydromorphone	7.5 mg	1.5 mg	3–4	2–3	5:1	4:1
Fentanyl	—	100 µg	1	3–12	—	See Table 6–18
Levorphanol	4 mg	2 mg	4–6	12–16	2:1	7.5:1
Methadone	Variable[c]	10 mg	4–6	15–50	2:1	Variable[c,d]
Codeine	200 mg[e]	130 mg	4–6	3	1.5:1	1:7
Hydrocodone	200 mg	—	3–6	3–4	—	1:7
Oxymorphone	6 mg[f]	1 mg	3–6	2–3	6:1	5:1
Meperidine[g]	300 mg	75 mg	2–4	2–3	4:1	1:10
Partial agonists						
Buprenorphine[h]	—	0.4 mg	4–8	2	—	25:1[i]
Agonist/ Antagonists						
Butorphanol[h]	—	2 mg	4–6	2–4	—	5:1[i]
Nalbuphine[h]	—	10 mg	4–6	5	—	1:1[i]
Pentazocine[h]	180 mg	60 mg	4–6	2–3	3:1	1:6

[a] This dose of morphine is based on chronic use. Older tables of this nature report the oral equivalent of 10 mg of parenteral morphine to be 60 mg. Practical experience has demonstrated that in the management of chronic pain, 30 mg of oral morphine is equivalent to 10 mg of parenteral morphine.

[b] There are some investigators who have reported that 30 mg of oxycodone is equivalent to 30 mg of morphine (ratio 1:1).

[c] The equivalent dose of methadone in chronic use has been shown to vary according to previously administered opioid doses.

[d] Recent studies indicate that methadone's potency increases as previous total daily morphine doses increase. Dose ratios from 8:1 to 14:1 have been reported when previous daily morphine doses exceeded 300 mg. Lower equivalent dose ratios of 3:1 to 6:1 have been demonstrated with lower morphine doses and individual titration at all doses is therefore recommended.

[e] Codeine has a ceiling dose of 360 mg/24 hr.

[f] Oxymorphone comes in suppository form only. There is no oral product available.

[g] Meperidine is not recommended for the treatment of patients with chronic pain and is included here for comparison purposes and so conversions to more appropriate analgesics can be made. With chronic usage, meperidine may cause significant toxicity, including seizures and myoclonus, due to accumulation of toxic metabolites such as normeperidine.

[h] Partial agonist and agonist/antagonist medications should not be used in the treatment of chronic pain and are included for comparison purposes only. They have dosage ceilings, and long-term use may increase risk of toxicity. Additionally, they should not be used in combination with opioid agonist medications, or given to patients who have been using opioid agonist medications on a chronic basis, as an opioid withdrawal syndrome could be precipitated.

[i] Parenteral morphine:analgesic ratio, because there is no oral form of the medication.

kappa opioid receptor, which may explain some reports that oxycodone causes less dysphoria and fewer nightmares and hallucinations than equipotent doses of morphine. However, not all investigators accept that oxycodone is *kappa* specific, especially since, as with morphine, oxycodone may cause side effects including euphoria, constipation, nausea, miosis, pruritus, orthostatic hypotension, suppression of the cough reflex, and respiratory depression.

The onset of action for immediate-release oxycodone is 30 to 60 minutes, and the recommended frequency of administration is every 4 hours. Oxycodone is extensively metabolized to noroxycodone, a considerably weaker analgesic than oxycodone, and one that is apparently not associated with neuroexcitatory effects such as occur with nor-morphine or nor-meperidine. Oxycodone should be dosed conservatively in patients with severe renal or hepatic impairment.

On a weight basis, oral oxycodone is generally considered more potent than oral morphine. For conversion purposes (Table 6–13), 1 mg of oral oxycodone is roughly equivalent to 1.5 mg of oral morphine, although potency ratios ranging from 1:1 to 1:2 have been reported. The variance in potency ratios may actually reflect the variable and unpredictable bioavailability of oral morphine.

Hydromorphone (Dilaudid) is another familiar opioid agonist analgesic that is available in multiple dosage forms: oral immediate-release tablets, oral liquid, rectal suppository, and parenteral. A sustained-release hydromorphone product, with the proposed name palladone, is in the late developmental phase at the time of writing.

The onset of action of oral hydromorphone is 30 minutes. Because of its short half-life, hydromorphone must be administered every 3 hours, limiting its use as an oral agent due to patient and caregiver inconvenience. Hydromorphone is 2 to 10 times more lipid soluble than morphine, and as an oral agent, has a potency ratio of 1:4 compared to oral morphine. Hydromorphone may cause fewer side effects and less sedation than morphine, especially in pediatric patients. Because of the lack of accumulation of toxic metabolites, hydromorphone may be preferable to morphine and oxycodone for patients with severe renal insufficiency. Because hydromorphone is approximately seven times more potent than morphine when administered parenterally and can be given in a small volume, hydromorphone is favored for use as a continuous subcutaneous infusion for patients who are unable to tolerate oral medications.

Methadone was developed as a synthetic opioid agonist more than 40 years ago and is available for oral use as tablets or liquid. In Europe, methadone is also available for use in subcutaneous infusions. Methadone is a broad-spectrum opioid that not only binds to *mu* and *delta* opioid receptors but also exerts analgesia through glutamate and serotonin receptor blockade. Therefore, methadone is more active for neuropathic pain than other opioid analgesics. Other features that make methadone an attractive alternative to morphine are its low cost and lower incidence of sedation and constipation.

Fentanyl is a lipid-soluble opioid analgesic whose use in chronic pain and in end-of-life care is significant because of its availability as a transdermal patch system and as an oral transmucosal preparation. Fentanyl solution is used intravenously for analgesia prior to surgery, as an adjunct for anesthesia, and in the immediate postoperative period, but has little relevance for chronic pain management. Fentanyl is metabolized in the liver and excreted in the urine. Drug interactions and adverse effects are similar to those of the other opioid agonists (described later).

Some opioid analgesics should be avoided. The disadvantages and hazards of the partial agonist and mixed agonist–antagonist opioids were previously discussed. Meperidine, which is widely prescribed for acute pain, should not be used to treat chronic pain. Meperidine has a very short half-life and must be dosed every 2 to 4 hours. It has poor and unpredictable oral bioavailability resulting in frequent underdosing, particularly after conversion from parenteral administration. Most important, meperidine is metabolized to normeperidine, which accumulates with repetitive dosing and may precipitate dangerous toxic effects including distressing mood changes, CNS stimulation, tremors, multifocal myoclonus, and seizures. Normeperidine accumulation is particularly marked when meperidine administration is prolonged, with high meperidine doses, and in patients with impaired renal or hepatic function. Information on the partial agonists, mixed agonist–antagonists, and meperidine has been included in Table 6–13 for comparison purposes only, and to facilitate switching patients already on these medications to bioequivalent doses of an appropriate agonist opioid.

USE OF ANALGESICS IN THE TREATMENT OF PAIN

AROUND-THE-CLOCK DOSING   As noted in "Acute and Chronic Pain" (and Table 6–4 earlier in the chapter), analgesia for the treatment of chronic pain should be provided on a regular, preventive schedule—in other words, around the clock. Figure 6–5 illustrates the pharmacokinetics associated with around-the-clock treatment versus "as needed" or prn dosing. Patients on a prn schedule (Fig. 6–5A) will receive medication only when they complain of and are experiencing pain. In con-

Figure 6–5

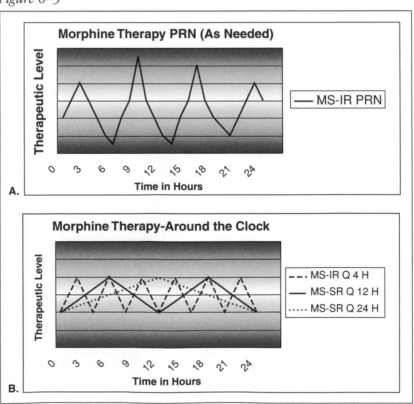

Morphine administered PRN (as needed) vs. ATC (around the clock). **A.** Morphine therapy provided PRN. Therapeutic levels are hectic, falling below pain threshold (lower red area), indicating that the patient is experiencing pain prior to next dose, and rising to toxic levels (upper red area). (MS-IR = immediate-release morphine.) **B.** Morphine therapy provided ATC. Therapeutic levels remain within the therapeutic range, and out of the red areas, indicating that the patient does not experience either pain or toxicity between doses. (MS-SR = sustained-release morphine.)

trast, when analgesic medication is provided on a regular basis, in anticipation of recurring pain, the establishment and maintenance of drug blood levels within a therapeutic range will effectively prevent the recurrence of pain (Fig. 6–5B). In addition, around-the-clock dosing avoids or minimizes the peaks and valleys in blood levels that result in uneven pain control punctuated by periods of drug toxicity.

ORAL ROUTE ADMINISTRATION   For patients with chronic pain who can take oral medicataion, oral administration of analgesics is the preferred route. Effective pain control may be accomplished using oral medications in 85 to 90 percent of patients. Orally administered analgesics are relatively safe, cost effective, and with the availability of sustained-release preparations, very convenient for patients and caregivers.

When patients who are opioid-naïve present with pain that is uncontrolled, it is generally recommended that patients be started on an immediate-release opioid, such as immediate-release morphine, immediate-release oxycodone, or hydromorphone. A typical starting dose of oral morphine is 10 to 20 mg every 4 hours, of oxycodone 7.5 to 15 mg every 4 hours, and of hydromorphone 2 to 4 mg every 3 hours, administered around the clock. Incremental increases in dose should be provided as necessary to achieve pain control. Additional doses at 50 percent of the basal dose every 2 hours should be provided on an as-needed basis to achieve adequate analgesia. Lower starting doses may be prudent in very elderly patients or when patients are known to have renal impairment. For a patient who has been managed on another opioid agonist or a step 2 opioid/nonopioid combination analgesic, the starting dose of morphine should be based on the equianalgesic dose of the prior medication. Keep in mind, however, that if the reason for switching the patient to morphine is uncontrolled pain, the starting dose should generally be higher than that calculated by the conversion formula (see Table 6–13).

Dosage adjustments are based on the patient's response, and the dose should be increased as necessary. Table 6–14 provides guidelines as to how to titrate opioid analgesic doses to achieve effective control of pain. Upward titration of the dose should continue until pain relief is achieved or until unacceptable side effects intervene.

Table 6–14

Titration of Immediate-Release Opioids for the Treatment of Uncontrolled Pain

1. Provide immediate-release analgesia around the clock. Recommended starting doses for opioid-naïve patients:
   Morphine 10–20 mg PO q4h around the clock
   Oxycodone 7.5–15 mg PO q4h around the clock
   Hydromorphone 2–4 mg PO q3h around the clock
2. Provide as-needed additional doses at 50% of starting dose every 2 hours.
3. If pain is almost controlled with the present regimen, but the patient still has some discomfort, the drug dose may be increased by 10–20%.
4. If pain is only partially controlled, increase the dosage by 25–50%.
5. If pain is severe, and little or no pain relief has been noted with the current dose, an increase of up to 100% may be appropriate.
6. Upward titration should continue until pain relief is achieved or until unacceptable side effects intervene.

Table 6–15

Oral Sustained-Release Opioid Products

1. MS Contin	Analgesic:	Morphine
	Frequency:	Every 12 hr
	Dosage form:	Tablet
	Dosage strengths:	15 mg, 30 mg, 60 mg, 100 mg, 200 mg
2. MS Extended Release	Analgesic:	Morphine
	Frequency:	Every 12 hr
	Dosage form:	Tablet
	Dosage strengths:	15 mg, 30 mg, 60 mg
3. Oramorph SR	Analgesic:	Morphine
	Frequency:	Every 12 hr
	Dosage form:	Tablet
	Dosage strengths:	30 mg, 60 mg, 100 mg
4. Kadian	Analgesic:	Morphine
	Frequency:	Every 24 hr
	Dosage forms:	Capsule
		Sprinkle (capsule may be broken open and sprinkled on applesauce or into water and flushed down a G-tube)
5. OxyContin	Dosage strengths:	20 mg, 50 mg, 100 mg
	Analgesic:	Oxycodone
	Frequency:	Every 12 hr
	Dosage form:	Tablet
	Dosage strengths:	10 mg, 20 mg, 40 mg, 80 mg, 160 mg

Sustained-Release Opioid Products   Around-the-clock dosing at 3 to 4 hour intervals is often burdensome for both patients and caregivers, and is particularly disruptive to needed sleep and rest. Therefore, with the exception of patients who are actively dying, once pain has been controlled with a stable dose of an immediate-release opioid, conversion to a sustained-release preparation should be accomplished.

Sustained-release opioid products that are currently available in the United States are listed in Table 6–15. They include the sustained-release morphine products MS Contin (q 12 hour schedule); its generic equivalent, "morphine extended-release tablets"; Oramorph SR (q 12 hour schedule; note that MS Contin and Oramorph SR are NOT considered generic equivalents); Kadian (q 24 hour schedule); and the sustained-release oxycodone product, Oxycontin.

To convert patients from immediate-release to sustained-release morphine products, the total amount of immediate-release morphine that is required in a 24-hour period is determined. The entire dose is then prescribed every 24 hours when Kadian is ordered; or the dose is divided in half, with 50 percent of the dose ordered every 12 hours for the other preparations.

It is important to remind the patient and caregivers that sustained-release tablets should not be broken or chewed, as this can result in a rapid and unintended release of a potentially toxic dose of morphine. However, a Kadian capsule may be opened and the contents sprinkled into food or administered via a feeding tube, provided that the morphine-containing pellets are themselves not chewed.

For patients taking Kadian, morphine blood levels peak at 8 to 12 hours. Some patients have reported somnolence during the period of peak blood levels at what is their therapeutic dose. A creative solution to this problem is to administer Kadian in the late afternoon so that peak blood levels will occur during regular sleeping hours when somnolence is of no consequence.

Some patients find that the sustained-release medication seems to lose its effectiveness 2 to 4 hours before the next dose of the product is due (20 to 22 hours for Kadian, 10 hours for the 12-hour products). This phenomenon, called "end-of-dose failure" can be resolved by either increasing the 12 or 24-hour dose of medication or by providing the same dose as before, or by increasing the interval of administration to every 12 hours for Kadian and every 8 hours for the other products. In no instance, however, should any sustained-release opioid be administered more frequently than at these intervals.

Unlike sustained-release morphine preparations, sustained-release oxycodone (OxyContin) exhibits a biphasic absorption pattern suggesting an initial immediate-release of oxycodone from the tablet followed by a prolonged phase of release. Whether this affords patients with an advantage is unclear, because, if one is following a proper dosage schedule, there should be no therapeutic need for immediate release of medication on a routine basis. Food has no significant effect on the absorption of oxycodone from Oxy-Contin, but does affect absorption of immediate release oxycodone, a point to remember when using the latter for breakthrough pain. As with sustained-release morphine, OxyContin tablets must be swallowed intact and may not be broken, chewed, or crushed without high risk of toxic effects. With reference to the commonly accepted oxycodone:morphine potency ratio of 1:1.5, at the time of this writing, OxyContin is somewhat more expensive than the sustained-release morphine preparations.

When patients first present with uncontrolled pain, some experts suggest that, rather than treating the patient with immediate-release morphine until control is achieved, the patient should be started on an empirical dose of a sustained-release product along with immediate-release "rescue" medication. The dose is then titrated upwards based on total 24-hour opioid consumption. Whether or not this method is as effective as using immediate-release opioids for initial pain control (which is the recommendation of these authors) remains to be determined, and is to some extent a function of clinician and patient preference.

Treatment of Breakthrough and Incident Pain Regardless of whether the patient is maintained on a short-acting opioid preparation or is converted to a sustained-release opioid, the availability of immediate release morphine for the treatment of breakthrough or incident pain is mandatory. Breakthrough pain refers to sporadic, self-limited episodes of acute pain due to the primary disease or to unrelated processes in a patient whose chronic pain is adequately controlled. Incident pain refers to an expected exacerbation of pain due to unusual physical activity, transfers, turning, or various diagnostic or therapeutic procedures.

For ease of titration of the sustained-release medication, it is recommended that whichever opioid is used in the sustained-release preparation should also be used in its immediate-release form for breakthrough or incident pain. In other words, immediate-release morphine should be used for any of the sustained release morphine products, and immediate-release oxycodone should be used for OxyContin. Recommended doses of immediate-release opioid for breakthrough or incident pain are calculated at 5 to 10 percent of the 24-hour total morphine dose given every 1 to 2 hours prn, or 25 percent of the doses of morphine administered over 12 hours given at intervals of 3 to 4 hours. Remember, whenever the dosage of the sustained-release product is increased, the dose of immediate-release medication for breakthrough or incident pain should be increased proportionately.

Should pain increase to the point that the patient is frequently requesting "rescue" medication for breakthrough pain, the patient requires new titration and adjustment of the dose of the sustained-release product at a higher level. It makes little sense to use a sustained-release preparation if the patient constantly requires medication every 2 to 4 hours. The use of oral, sustained-release products for chronic pain relief and prevention supplemented as needed by oral, immediate-release morphine is conceptually similar to the parenteral patient-controlled analgesia (PCA) that is typically used to manage acute postoperative pain.

Methadone Up until recently, oral methadone has been used primarily for drug detoxification rather than as an analgesic for chronic pain. This experience is largely the result of methadone's long blood half-life that extends well beyond its ability to sustain analgesia. To control pain, methadone must be dosed every 6 to 12 hours, but progressive drug accumulation to toxic levels is not uncommon, particularly in elderly and debilitated patients. Additionally, there are large individual variations in dose equivalency ratios and titration periods, and time to stabilization may sometimes be prolonged. In view of these issues, methadone has not been traditionally thought of as an opioid of choice in the treatment of chronic pain.

The view that methadone does not have a large role to play in the management of chronic pain near the end of life is changing. Methadone should be considered as a useful alternative to morphine in any of the situations listed in Table 6–16.

The unique characteristics associated with methadone are primarily related to a biphasic elimination process that allows methadone to be given less frequently than morphine. Methadone is initially dosed as often as every 3 hours, but once steady-state drug levels are achieved, methadone provides analgesia for 8 to 12 hours allowing for dosing every 8 to 12 hours. For patients who are opioid-naïve and who are starting methadone de novo, some experts recommend starting doses of 5 to 10 mg orally every 12 hours around the clock and every 3 hours prn for breakthrough pain. If necessary, the around-the-clock dose may be titrated upwards every 4 to 6 days.

For patients who are being converted from morphine, it is important to note that the potency of methadone appears to increase as previous total morphine doses increase. Counterintuitively, this places patients who are receiving higher morphine doses at greater risk for toxicity when they are converted from morphine to methadone. Methadone:morphine dose equivalency ratios varying from 1:8 to 1:14 have been reported when previous total daily morphine doses exceed 300 mg. Lower-dose potency ratios of 1:3 to 1:6 were reported with lower total daily morphine doses. For patients on relatively low-dose morphine (60 to 200 mg/24 hours), a dosing schema similar to that described for morphine-naïve patients is feasible. For patients on higher-dose morphine regimens, one widely accepted method for conversion to methadone is presented in Table 6–17.

Regardless of the dosing method or potency ratio used, individual titration and careful monitoring at all doses are essential. Most importantly,

Table 6–16

Clinical Indications for the Use of Methadone

1. Severe, persistent adverse effects with morphine at any dose such as heavy sedation, psychotomimetic manifestations, delerium, severe myoclonus, and allodynia
2. Increasing pain despite rapidly escalating doses of morphine compounded by increasing adverse effects
3. Neuropathic pain not responding to opioids plus adjuvant drugs
4. Renal failure, where, besides short-acting hydromorphone, methadone may be an opioid of choice because its metabolism and excretion are unchanged

Table 6-17

Protocol for Instituting Methadone for Patients Receiving Morphine or Other Strong Opioid Agonists (Morley–Makin Method)

1. Calculate total 24 hour PO morphine dose. (See Table 6–13 for conversion of other opioids to PO morphine equivalents.)
2. Discontinue morphine or other strong opioid.
3. Initial methadone dose depends on prior 24-hr PO morphine dose:
   A. <300 mg: Give a dose of methadone that equals 10% of 24-hr PO morphine dose.
   B. >300 mg: Regardless of the 24-hr morphine dose, the fixed dose of methadone is 30 mg.
4. During days 1–5, patients are titrated by adjusting the dosage frequency which should not be less than q3h or greater than q12h.
5. On day 6, the amount of methadone used during the previous 2 days is averaged as a daily dose and divided in half for q12h administration. The prior fixed dose is used for breakthrough pain at intervals not to exceed q3h.
6. If breakthrough medication continues to be needed frequently, increase the total daily methadone dose by 33–50% every 4–6 days until stable pain control is achieved.
7. It is unusual to require more than 40 mg q12h.

as a result of the secondary 36 to 60-hour component of the biphasic elimination, during which methadone metabolites persist but provide no analgesic effect, drug accumulation can cause toxicity that can unpredictably appear after days or even weeks of effective analgesia. Thus, careful monitoring for drug toxicity is mandatory.

Because of the considerable complexities associated with methadone usage, and the general lack of familiarity with methadone in hospice and palliative care in the United States, clinicians would be well advised to consult with experts and to review appropriate references before attempting to treat patients with methadone. One should also ascertain that there are no legal impediments to prescribing methadone for analgesia, as its use may still be restricted in some jurisdictions to drug detoxification programs.

NONINVASIVE ALTERNATIVE ROUTES OF ADMINISTRATION
Some patients cannot tolerate oral agents at some time during their illness due to disease-related nausea and vomiting, dysphagia due to oral or esophageal cancer or neurologic deficits, or depressed consciousness close to the end of life. In one retrospective study, 59 percent of patients with advanced cancer used more than one route of drug administration during the last 4 weeks of life (Coyle et al, 1990). Although it is all too commonplace in these circumstances to consider invasive, parenteral methods of drug delivery, a number of less invasive alternatives are available including buccal, sublingual, transdermal, and rectal routes of administration.

Buccal and Sublingual Routes   With the exception of fentanyl, all commonly used opioid analgesics that are available in the United States are hydrophilic, and as such are not absorbed across the lipid membranes, the buccal and sublingual mucosa. Nevertheless, it is fairly common practice in hospice and palliative medicine to medicate patients who are unable to swallow with high concentration (20 to 50 mg/mL) morphine liquid either buccally or sublingually. Although the medication is actually absorbed via the gastrointestinal tract by "trickle-down" swallowing, the method is widely accepted because of recognized efficacy and ease of administration.

Oral transmucosal fentanyl (Actiq) was designed to take advantage of the lipophilic nature of fentanyl, and its ability to be absorbed across mucous membranes. It is formulated as a solid drug matrix on an applicator handle (a lollypop-like device), and is designed to be dissolved slowly in the mouth. Dosage strengths range from 200 to 1600 μg. It is approved only for the management of breakthrough cancer pain for patients who are already receiving and who are tolerant to opioid therapy. The patient or caregiver places the Actiq unit in the mouth between the cheek and the lower gum, and the unit is occasionally moved from side to side. The unit must be sucked and not chewed. It requires at least 15 minutes for a full dose to be consumed. Unlike other opioids used for breakthrough pain, the dose of Actiq is not related to the dose of the around-the-clock maintenance opioid. Titration is empirical for each individual, beginning with the lowest 200-μg unit with advancement in 200-μg increments every 30 to 60 minutes until an effective dose is achieved.

Despite its being marketed as a transmucosal agent, only 25 percent of each dose is actually absorbed by the transbuccal route, with the remaining 75 percent being swallowed with the saliva and absorbed slowly from the gastrointestinal tract, the same mechanism of action by which morphine liquid administered sublingually is effective. It is not clear, therefore, that Actiq is more advantageous for breakthrough pain than concentrated morphine solutions (up to 50 mg/mL) administered sublingually.

Transdermal Route   Fentanyl transdermal (Duragesic) is particularly useful for managing chronic pain in patients with difficulty swallowing or complying with a schedule of oral medications. The latter problem includes situations in which either the patient or family members are unable or unwilling to administer oral doses reliably and on schedule. It also addresses problems with drug diversion, although it is now known that even fentanyl patches have a recognized "street value."

The transdermal patch releases fentanyl continuously by absorption through the skin into the subcutaneous tissue, where it accumulates and is then absorbed into the systemic circulation via capillary networks. The reservoir in the subcutaneous tissue is responsible for the 17 to 24-hour

half-life of this preparation and produces steady fentanyl blood levels over a period of approximately 72 hours. It is also responsible for the fact that following patch application, 17 to 24 hours must elapse before a significant medication effect is detected, thus rendering the fentanyl transdermal system inappropriate for the treatment of acute pain. The reservoir effect also explains the washout period of 17 to 24 hours after a patch is removed, such that toxic effects will not quickly dissipate after a patch is removed.

The fentanyl transdermal system is manufactured in four patch strengths: 25, 50, 75, and 100 μg/hr. In most instances, a patch will provide analgesia for 72 hours, although in some patients, "end-of-dose failure" similar to that with sustained-release oral opioids has been reported, with adequate pain relief lasting for only 48 to 60 hours. Because transdermal fentanyl is best begun after stable pain control has been established with immediate-release opioids, it is rarely started in opioid-naïve patients. For this reason, many hospice and palliative care specialists advocate a "fentanyl patch strength: 24- hour oral morphine" ratio of 1 μg/hr: 2 mg/day rather than the approximately 1:4 ratio recommended by the manufacturer in the product insert. Bioequivalent doses for transdermal fentanyl using the 1:2 ratio are shown in Table 6–18. When converting a patient to fentanyl transdermal from an opioid other than morphine, first calculate the 24- hour oral morphine dose equivalent using standard conversion tables (Table 6–13). Then, select the appropriate patch dose based on Table 6–18.

Table 6–18

Duragesic: Oral Morphine Equianalgesic Table

MORPHINE (MG IN 24 HR)	DURAGESIC (μG/HR)
50	25
100	50
150	75
200	100
Additional 50	Additional 25

Fentanyl patch doses in excess of 300 μg/hr (3 – 100-μg patches) are difficult to sustain because the amount of body surface area required to effectively place the patches, especially with the need for frequent site rotation, presents a formidable obstacle. After applying the patch or patches for the first time, the existing analgesic regimen should be maintained for 24 hours to allow fentanyl blood levels to reach the therapeutic range. As with any sustained-release opioid product, provision must be made for breakthrough pain by prescribing an immediate-release opioid for "rescue." Patch dosage adjustments are best made at 6-day intervals.

Should fentanyl patches have to be discontinued, begin treatment with the successor opioid 12 to 18 hours after removing the patches. Use 50 percent of the equivalent analgesic dose of the new opioid and then titrate the dose based on the patient's need and clinical response. Because of the half-life of 17 to 24 hours, any supportive care for adverse effects of transdermal fentanyl should be maintained for at least 24 hours after patch removal.

Fentanyl absorption is increased when the body temperature exceeds 102°F. Fentanyl patches should thus be avoided or used cautiously in patients with recurrent febrile episodes. Similar caution should be exercised in elderly, cachectic, or debilitated patients in whom the pharmacokinetics of transdermal fentany may be abnormal due to the lack of subcutaneous adipose tissue. CNS-depressant drugs can cause additive depressant effects, requiring one or both agents to be reduced by a minimum of 50 percent. Combination of transdermal fentanyl with other sustained-release opioids appears to lack clinical rationale and should be discouraged. Used fentanyl patches must be disposed of with care. They can pose a significant, even fatal, hazard for young children.

Rectal Route   Administration of opioids by rectal suppository is effective, although not necessarily perceived as noninvasive. Although rectal absorption of morphine is less than small intestinal absorption, because rectal blood flow bypasses the liver and first-pass metabolism, the actual blood levels after rectal administration are about the same as after oral ingestion. The efficacy of rectal morphine in terminally ill patients makes rectal morphine a viable alternative during the last several days of life. With the use of gelatin capsules and hydrophilic morphine tablets, virtually any dosage level of morphine can be achieved with the rectal route. Although not approved by the FDA, sustained-release morphine may be placed in a gelatin capsule and provide prolonged effects as long as the sustained-release morphine remains in contact with the rectal mucosa. This method reduces the frequency of suppository insertion.

Hydromorphone can also be administered by the rectal route; so can acetaminophen and several NSAIDs, including aspirin and indomethacin.

PARENTERAL ANALGESIA   Initiation of parenteral analgesia, which permits rapid attainment of analgesic blood levels, may be appropriate for patients with severe, uncontrolled acute pain. The intravenous route is preferable when venous access is present, with subcutaneous injections reserved for patients without venous access. Intramuscular injections should be avoided because of pain at the injection site and unreliable absorption of the medication. Continuous intravenous or subcutaneous infusion is preferable to intermittent boluses that provide only 45 to 60 minutes of analgesia and may rapidly cause the development of tolerance.

Continuous infusion provides patients with consistent blood levels and can be titrated to effect with ease. Some form of infusion control device, either mechanical (e.g., syringe driver or pump) or computerized, ensures proper drug delivery. Computerized delivery systems enable patient-controlled analgesia (PCA), with patients having the option of self-administering predetermined bolus doses for breakthrough or incident pain. Continuous subcutaneous infusion with PCA, using small-gauge Silastic needles that need to be replaced only infrequently and small computerized pumps, is particularly effective for ambulatory, terminally ill patients who are unable to tolerate oral analgesia and who require opioid doses that are too large for practical administration by the transdermal route. Adjunctive agents such as antiemetic and anxiolytic drugs that are compatible in solution with parenteral opioids can often be mixed together and administered with one syringe driver or pump.

When converting patients from oral to parenteral medication, and vice versa, remember that the relative potency of opioids is route dependent. Equianalgesic conversion doses for oral and parenteral opioids are depicted in Table 6–13. Except for opioid-naïve patients, in whom the ratio of oral to parenteral morphine is 6 mg:1 mg, most pain experts accept a conversion ratio of 3:1.

OTHER INVASIVE ROUTES OF ANALGESIA ADMINISTRATION
For end-of-life care, epidural, intrathecal, and intraventricular routes of analgesia should be reserved for the small percentage of patients whose pain cannot be controlled noninvasively or parenterally. For terminal patients with cancer, intraspinal therapy is most effective for patients with pelvic tumors or lumbosacral plexopathies. Although intraspinal opioid analgesia sometimes achieves effective pain relief with fewer side effects than with systemic routes of administration, respiratory depression and sedation may still occur. With disease progression, patients may also need to resume systemic therapy. Intraspinal analgesia is contraindicated for patients with musculoskeletal or spinal deformities, for patients with bleeding diatheses or coagulapathies, for patients with severe respiratory diseases, and in the presence of infections, increased intracranial pressure, or drug allergy. Rare cases of epidural hematomas associated with catheter placement have resulted in paraplegia. Infection associated with indwelling catheters is also a potential risk that may be minimized by total internalization of the catheter and pump. Comprehensive information about intraspinal analgesia may be found in review articles such as Bennett and associates (2000).

Anticipate and Treat Complications and Side Effects

Chronic opioid therapy predictably causes constipation. Nausea and vomiting occur in about 30 percent of patients starting opioid therapy, but unlike constipation, usually resolve within several days due to the development of tolerance. Transient sedation and confusion are also common. Less frequent side effects include dry mouth, myoclonus, urinary retention, pruritus, sleep disturbances, dysphoria, and inappropriate secretion of antidiuretic hormone. Respiratory depression, although a potential side effect in opioid-naïve patients who are being treated for acute pain, is generally not a factor in chronic pain management of terminally ill patients when proper titration guidelines are followed. The recommended treatments for the most common opioid-induced side effects, constipation, nausea, and sedation, are summarized in Table 6–19 and discussed next.

CONSTIPATION

Constipation occurs uniformly in nearly all patients receiving opioid analgesics. Therefore, any patient who is being treated for pain should be started on a bowel regimen with the objective of achieving a bowel movement at least every 2 to 3 days. Along with increased hydration, a bulk stool softener (psyllium) and a mild laxative (senna or bisacodyl) is usually adequate as primary therapy. In principle, patients should be encouraged to add fiber to the diet, avoid caffeinated beverages, and increase exercise. However, these recommendations may be impractical or irrelevant for many end-of-life patients who are often weak, bedbound, anorectic, or require fluid restriction. Patients who cannot increase fluids should not use bulk laxatives because of the risk of obstruction and bolus formation. The use of bisacodyl may sometimes be associated with fecal leakage due to excess colonic relaxation.

For resistant constipation, a strong laxative (lactulose, polyethylene glycol, citrate of magnesia) is required. Enemas may be indicated when stool is lodged in the rectum too proximal for digital disimpaction and the patient is unable to evacuate. For opioid-induced constipation that is refractory despite these interventions, oral administration of the opioid antagonist naloxone may be effective. The recommended dose is 3 mg three times a day,

Table 6–19

Opioid Side Effects

SIDE EFFECTS	TREATMENT	
Constipation (see Chapter 8)	1. Increased hydration 2. Bulk laxatives (psyllium) and stimulant (senna or bisacodyl) 3. Lactulose 4. The last option is to use castor oil or magnesium-containing products	
Nausea and vomiting (see Chapter 8)	Phenothiazines, such as:	
	Prochlorperazine	5–10 mg PO tid-qid 25 mg PR bid
	Promethazine	25 mg PO/PR q 4–6 hr
	Chlorpromazine	10 25 mg PO q 4–6 hr 50–100 mg PR q 6–8 hr
	Metaclopramide	5–10 mg four times daily
Sedation	Dextroamphetamine	2.5–5 mg bid
	Methylphenidate	2.5–5 mg bid

SOURCE: Information from: Levy, 1996; Jacox et al, 1994.

escalated daily in 3-mg increments as needed, up to 9 mg three times a day. With this regimen, many patients complain of abdominal cramps, and some patients—especially with the higher doses—experience sweating or shivering presumably due to an induced withdrawal reaction due to systemic absorption. A full discussion of constipation can be found in Chapter 8.

NAUSEA AND VOMITING

Opioids cause nausea and vomiting via a number of mechanisms including inhibition of gastric motility, stimulation of the chemoreceptor trigger zone (CTZ) in the brainstem, and stimulation of the vestibular nerve. Opioid-induced nausea and vomiting usually subside spontaneously within a few days. When nausea and vomiting persist, alternative etiologies unrelated to opioids should be considered such as electrolyte abnormalities, hypercalcemia, gastritis, obstruction, increased intracranial pressure, and other medications. Because nausea does not invariably occur in all

patients receiving opioids, prophylactic antiemetic treatment is not recommended except for patients with a prior history of opioid-induced nausea.

Nonpharmacologic interventions helpful to patients with opioid-related nausea and vomiting include elimination of provocative environmental stimuli (e.g., smells), providing adequate oral care, dietary consultation, and reassurance that the nausea will likely be transitory. Primary pharmacologic interventions include CTZ inhibitors (phenothiazines, haloperidol) and agents that promote gastric emptying (metoclopramide) rather than antihistamines, which are often tolerated less well. The newer 5HT3-receptor antagonists (odansetron, granisetron, and dolasetron) were developed primarily for treating acute nausea caused by cancer chemotherapy. Although these agents are generally not necessary for patients with opioid-induced nausea, they are sometimes effective for refractory cases. A sublingual odansetron preparation may be an effective alternative to parenteral antiemetics in patients with severe nausea and vomiting who are unable to tolerate or who fail to respond to an oral agent. For patients who do not respond to those measures, opioid rotation (discussed later) often results in effective relief. A full discussion of nausea and vomiting can be found in Chapter 8.

SEDATION

Opioid-related sedation, when it occurs, can be troublesome for patients and their loved ones, and may result in poor compliance with the prescribed pain control regimen, leading to therapeutic failure. It is thus very important to inform patients and caregivers that tolerance to sedation usually occurs within several days. They also need to be reminded that, due to the stimulant effect pain exerts, patients in pain often suffer from sleep deprivation. With initial pain relief, patients may be finally able to "catch up" on much needed sleep, creating the false impression that they are improperly and overly sedated. Careful observation and a review of the medication regimen, as well as inspection to determine what medications are actually given, and in what dosage, should allow one to distinguish between a patient in deep sleep and one experiencing medication-induced sedation. For those patients with sustained opioid-related sedation, small doses of methylphenidate (2.5 mg in the morning with dose escalation to effect) may be prescribed, often with good results.

Confusion, difficulty concentrating, mood changes, and hallucinations may occur with initiation of opioids or after dose escalation. These symptoms, especially hallucinations, can be extremely disturbing both for patients and for their families. Dysphoria is most common, whereas euphoria, absent the concomitant use of other medications such as corticosteroids, is uncommon when opioids are prescribed for pain control. Tolerance to these side effects occurs rapidly in most patients, but there is considerable individual variation. If confusion or dysphoria persist, the symptoms often remit with an opioid substitution. Oxycodone appears to cause hallucinations less frequently than morphine. When assessing persistent confusion near the end of life, it is also important to rule out causes other than opioids, especially terminal delirium associated with systemic and metabolic failure as the patient approaches death.

OTHER OPIOID-RELATED SIDE EFFECTS

Prutitus and flushing are primarily, but not exclusively, related to opioid-induced histamine release. Prutitus is most common in patients who are receiving intraspinal opioids although it may occur with any route of administration. Pruritus is usually treated with antihistamines. Should this prove ineffective, paroxetine and mirtazapine have antipruriutic properties. For severe cases, small doses of naloxone may offer relief.

Myoclonus and jerking movements may occur in conjunction with high doses of any opioid but are most commonly encountered in patients receiving high doses of meperidine or morphine, whose metabolites normeperidine and normorphine are particularly neuroexcitatory. Opioid-related myoclonus is more likely to occur when patients have concurrent renal or hepatic insufficiency. It usually responds to dosage reduction if possible, or to opioid substitution. Clonazepan (0.5 to 1 mg 2 or 3 times per day) is also often effective for controlling myoclonus when the existent opioid dose is necessary to maintain analgesic control. Myoclonus may sometimes be a prodrome to seizures. Should seizures occur, patients should be managed with dose reduction, opioid substitution, and benzodiazepine and/or nonbenzodiazepine anticonvulsants that should be continued for the several days usually necessary for clearance of the neuroexcitatory metabolites. Administration of naloxone should be avoided because this opioid antagonist can paradoxically aggravate CNS hyperactivity.

OPIOID WITHDRAWAL

In rare circumstances, terminally ill patients with chronic pain may improve sufficiently so that opioid analgesics are no longer required. An example might be a patient with lung cancer and advanced pulmonary and bone metastases whose bone pain has responded to palliative radiotherapy. Because chronic opioid treatment results in physical dependence, opioids must be tapered and never discontinued abruptly. There are two recommended methods for tapering opioid therapy:

1. Reduce the total daily dose by 10 percent per day over a 10-day period, or by 5 percent per day over 20 days.
2. Provide 25 percent of the previous daily opioid dose for 2 days, and continue to reduce the dose by 50 percent every 2 days until the patient is receiving 10 to 15 mg of morphine (or equivalent) per day. Administer this low dose for 2 days, and then discontinue.

The second method allows for rapid initial reduction of the opioid dose. With both methods, withdrawal symptoms such as chills, sweats, and generalized aches and pains tend to be mild and well tolerated.

When death is imminent, patients often exhibit evidence of multisystem failure, hypotension, poor tissue perfusion, decreasing renal function, and a depressed level of consciousness. At this stage, patients may appear to have a diminished sense of pain, and families (and even some physicians and other health care professionals) sometimes incorrectly attribute the patient's deterioration to opioid medication. In these circumstances, it may be appropriate to reduce opioid doses. However, precipitous discontinuation may provoke withdrawal symptoms even in actively dying patients. Therefore, the opioid dosage needs to be maintained at no less than 25 percent of the chronic daily dose in order to avoid additional discomfort for the patient, a goal with which most family members will readily identify after adequate explanation.

OPIOID TOLERANCE

The concept of opioid tolerance refers to the need to increase the dose of an analgesic medication to maintain the desired effect when there is no evidence that the loss of pain control is the result of disease progression or other pain-exacerbating cause. The development of tolerance appears to be dependent on a number of neurochemical adaptations to opioid administration including changes in neuronal concentrations of cyclic AMP, opioid effects on the calcium ion channel, and up-regulation of endogenous endorphins and competitive binding for opioid receptors. As a result of these multiple biochemical mechanisms, tolerance to the various opioid-induced physiologic effects develops differentially, and sometimes selectively. For this reason, most patients with chronic pain may be titrated to amounts of opioid medication sufficient to control pain without experiencing respiratory depression or sustained nausea or excessive sedation. In fact, the onset of analgesic tolerance in patients who are receiving opioids for chronic pain is unusual when the pain has an identifiable physical cause such as tumor growth and invasion or other sustained tissue injury. The increased need for opioid analgesics in patients with advanced cancer, for example, is most commonly due to disease progression rather than to the development of tolerance. Clinicians and patients should be aware of this observation, because the concept that strong opioids will become ineffective if started too early, and should be held in reserve until "really needed," continues to be one of the prevalent barriers to effective pain management.

Nevertheless, analgesic tolerance to a previously effective opioid may occur in some patients so that new pain relief is not achieved despite even rapid dosage escalation to high levels. In this circumstance, and after a thorough reassessment, it is advisable to switch to an alternate opioid. The justification for this approach, sometimes referred to as "opioid rotation," is that cross-tolerance among the various opioid agonist analgesics is frequently incomplete. Because of incomplete cross-tolerance, when converting such a patient to another opioid, the new analgesic should generally be started at no higher than 50 percent of the calculated bioequivalent dose (see Table 6–13) and at times, even lower doses may prove to be effective.

Although similar from a practical and conceptual viewpoint, opioid rotation, which addresses the issue of analgesic tolerance, should be distinguished from opioid substitution, which refers to the practice of changing patients with unacceptable, refractory adverse effects from one opioid to another member of the class. The purpose of this practice, which is based on the concept of individual, differential tolerance among opioids to various nonanalgesic effects, is to improve the adverse effect profile while maintaining equianalgesia. Perhaps only because its use is most prevalent, morphine is the opioid most often associated with uncontrolled adverse effects. In a recent study, substitution produced partial or complete relief from refractory opioid-related confusion in 18 of 25 cases, from refractory opioid-induced nausea and vomiting in 13 of 19 cases, and from drowsiness in 8 of 15 cases (Ashby et al, 1999). Unlike opioid rotation for analgesic tolerance, in which the effective analgesic dose of the new opioid is often less than that predicted from standard conversion tables, the effective analgesic dose of the new opioid when there is substitution for adverse effects is at least bioequivalent to the drug being replaced, or even higher than predicted.

Adjuvant Medications

Although opioid analgesics are the mainstay of effective pain management, other medications, used in conjunction with opioids, are frequently necessary to achieve effective pain control. Indications for these medications, termed coanalgesics or adjuvants, are determined according to the classification and etiology of the pain. The purpose of using drug combinations is to provide additive or synergistic analgesia and to reduce side effects. Failure to prescribe adjuvant medication, especially when patients have pain that responds incompletely to opioids, is one of the major causes for inadequate pain control.

BONE PAIN

Bone pain due to metastatic cancer is largely mediated by prostaglandins whose synthesis is catalyzed by cyclooxygenase. NSAIDs, which inhibit cyclooxygenase and decrease prostaglandin

production, are often effective, in conjunction with opioid analgesics, in reducing the pain and inflammation associated with bone pain (discussed earlier under type 1 pain).

Corticosteroids are also sometimes effective for skeletal pain. In terminally ill patients, especially those with a very short life expectancy, the adverse effects of chronic corticosteroid therapy are relatively inconsequential. Other than pain relief, patients treated with corticosteroids may realize an increased sense of well-being, or even euphoria. Another possible adjuvant treatment for bone pain is calcitonin. However, because calcitonin is expensive, and its effect appears to be totally mediated by increases in endogenous β-endorphins, it is not clear that adding calcitonin is more advantageous than merely increasing the exogenous opioid dose to achieve the necessary effect. Other adjunctive modalities for bone pain, including bisphosphonates, radiopharmaceuticals, and radiotherapy, may be selectively useful for end-of-life care, and are discussed in Chapter 17.

NEUROPATHIC PAIN

Neuropathic pain is sometimes described as being opioid resistant. This description is not entirely accurate because response rates up to 33 percent have been reported. Oxycodone appears to be useful for treating postherpetic neuralgia, tramadol is reported to ease the pain of diabetic neuropathy, and methadone has known activity for neuropathic pain. Additionally, patients often have mixed pain syndromes with nociceptive as well as neuropathic components. Therefore, it is reasonable to include opioids when treating neuropathic pain, but almost always in conjunction with other adjuvant medications.

Agents commonly used for the treatment of neuropathic pain are listed in Table 6–20. Unfortunately, no single agent or combination regimen is successful all of the time, and the treatment of neuropathic pain must be both empirical and individualized. A suggested stepwise schema, similar to the WHO stepladder, is illustrated in Figure 6–6 and discussed next.

Table 6–20
Neuropathic Pain Medications

CLASS OF MEDICATION	MEDICATION	DOSE
Steroids	Dexamethasone	16–96 mg PO daily in 2–4 divided doses
Tricyclic antidepressants	Amitriptyline	10–150 mg PO daily
	Nortriptyline	10–150 mg PO daily
Anticonvulsants	Gabapentin	300–1800 mg PO daily in 2–3 divided doses
	Carbamazepine	200–1600 mg PO daily in 3–4 divided doses
	Phenytoin	300–500 mg PO daily
	Clonazepam	0.5–1 mg PO 3–4 times a day
Others	Clonidine	0.1–0.3 mg PO or transdermally daily
	Baclofen	10–30 mg PO daily
	Mexiletine	300–1200 mg PO daily in divided doses

STEP 1: NEUROPATHIC PAIN   As the first step in the treatment of neuropathic pain, the clinician should combine an opioid with either corticosteroids or an NSAID.

Corticosteroids are especially effective in treating neuropathic symptoms accompanied by inflammation and edema. Headaches due to increased intracranial pressure and the pain and neurologic deficits of spinal cord compression are examples of neuropathic symptoms that may be alleviated with corticosteroids. Dexamethasone in high doses is generally the steroid medication of choice. Cor-

Figure 6–6

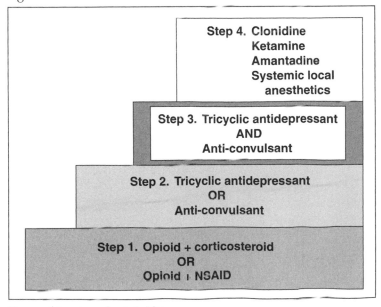

Neuropathic pain analgesic ladder

ticosteroids may also be helpful in treating other forms of neuropathic pain and plexopathy. They are especially effective when there is a significant component of inflammation and soft-tissue swelling. Corticosteroids may also be useful in the early management of herpes zoster and may possibly mitigate the later severity of postherpetic neuralgia.

Combinations of opioids and NSAIDs are also sometimes effective for cancer neuropathic pain. NSAIDs are discussed in detail earlier in the chapter.

Step 2: Neuropathic Pain   In the proposed schema for treating neuropathic pain (Fig. 6–6), either a tricyclic antidepressant or an anticonvulsant should be added as step 2.

Antidepressants   The tricyclic antidepressants (TCAs) address neuropathic pain by three different mechanisms: mood elevation, potentiation or enhancement of opioid analgesics, and direct analgesic effects. TCAs are particularly useful for dysesthetic neuropathy in which patients complain of burning, cold, or vise-like sensations. In general, TCAs are effective for 40 percent of patients with neuropathic pain.

Amitriptyline has been most extensively studied. Although some patients achieve analgesia with doses that are lower than those needed to treat depression, doses as high as 150 mg may sometimes be necessary. Analgesic effects may occur within 1 to 2 weeks, but the peak effect may not occur for 4 to 6 weeks. Patients need to be aware of this time response in order to avoid disappointment and frustration. The recommended starting dose, especially in elderly patients, is 10 mg at bedtime, with increases at similar increments every 3 to 4 days.

Other TCAs that are useful for neuropathic pain include nortriptyline, doxepin, and desipramine. These medications may have fewer adverse effects than those associated with amitriptyline; they include sedation, dry mouth, constipation, and urinary retention.

The selective serotonin reuptake inhibitors (SSRIs) have limited usefulness as analgesics for neuropathic pain due to their selectivity for the serotonin pathway. It has been reported that paroxetine has alleviated symptoms of diabetic neuropathy in approximately one third of patients treated, while fluoxetine, nefazodone, and sertraline have also been reported to be effective in treating symptoms of neuropathic pain for a small number of patients.

Venlafaxine, which shares properties of both SSRIs and TCAs, is reported to have enhanced activity against neuropathic pain. Mirtazapine has activity on both noradrenergic and serotonergic transmission and blocks 5HT2 and 5HT3 receptors. This biochemical profile reduces the likelihood of side effects related to nonselective serotonin activation, and decreases the risk of cardiotoxicity. Mirtazapine is relatively safe for elderly patients, has beneficial effects on sleep, and has anxiolytic and antipruritic properties. It is anecdotally reported to have analgesic properties beyond its antidepressant effects, but it has not yet been tested in a controlled clinical trial. Thus, although there may well be an emerging role for SSRIs and other new antidepressant medications for the treatment of neuropathic pain, at this point there is insufficient information to justify their routine substitution for TCAs.

Anticonvulsants   Older anticonvulsant medications, such as phenytoin, carbamazepine, valproic acid, and clonazepam, may be effective in treating episodic neuropathic pain that is lancinating or burning in nature. This type of pain is typically associated with nerve injury, trigeminal neuralgia, or postherpetic neuralgia.

Anticonvulsant drugs reduce or prevent pathologically altered neurons from excessive discharge and reduce the spread of excitation from abnormal foci to normal neurons. One of the major limiting factors in the use of the various anticonvulsants is the high incidence of side effects. Therefore, as with TCAs, the initial dose should be low and upward titration should be slow and cautious. For example, a starting dose of carbamazepine can be as low as 50 mg at bedtime in elderly patients or 100 mg in younger patients. Side effects may occur before any therapeutic benefit is realized.

Gabapentin, a new anticonvulsant, has a lower incidence of side effects than the other anticonvulsants and has been reported to effectively treat neuropathic pain in doses as low as 300 mg per day, up to the more commonly used doses of 600 to 1800 mg per day. (Doses as high as 3600 mg per day have been reported.) To achieve these doses, patients are titrated starting at 300 to 400 mg twice daily with increases over 4 to 5 days to 600 mg three times a day. These dosage levels may not always be attained due to excess sedation and onset of dysequilibrium. Gabapentin may be especially useful for patients with AIDS neuropathies because it does not interact with antiretroviral medications and, unlike carbamazepine, it does not cause bone marrow toxicity. Gabapentin may administered orally or rectally.

STEP 3: NEUROPATHIC PAIN   If there is an inadequate analgesic response to the addition of either a TCA or an anticonvulsant, concurrent use of both medications together is recommended as step 3. Anticonvulsants that work by different mechanisms (e.g. carbamazepine, phenytoin, valproic acid versus clonazepam, phenobarbital, gabapentin) may also be tried concurrently, although with increased risk of adverse side effects.

STEP 4: NEUROPATHIC PAIN

Clonidine and Local Anesthetics   Other agents with anecdotal success in the treatment of neuropathic pain include clonidine and systemically administered local anesthetic agents such as intravenous lidocaine and oral mexiletine and tocainide. Clonidine is a centrally acting α_2-adrenergic agonist that has been used successfully to treat phantom pain and pain associated with diabetic neuropathy, postherpetic neuralgia, and spinal cord injury. In larger studies, despite enthusiasm regarding the use of anesthetic agents, the responses reported overall have been disappointing, on the order of 10 percent of patients studied.

Baclofen and Tizanidine   Baclofen and tizanidine are best known as muscle relaxants, and have been found effective in the treatment of both neuropathic pain and the muscle spasm that so often accompanies neurologic injury. In cases of spinal cord compression or other CNS impairment that is associated with spastic paraparesis, for example, baclofen in gradually escalating doses from 10 to 30 mg per day, may be very effective, while tizanidine has been used to relieve severe muscle spasms for patients with multiple sclerosis.

NMDA Antagonists   While currently of limited clinical usefulness, most recent interest in the treatment of neuropathic pain has focused on agents that inhibit the N-methyl-D-aspartate (NMDA) receptor channel complex. The simplest NMDA receptor inhibitor is magnesium. Magnesium sulfate, 0.5 to 1.0 g intravenously, was effective in completely or partially alleviating pain for up to 4 hours in 10 of 12 cancer patients with neuropathic pain that was poorly responsive to opioids (Crosby et al, 2000). The practical clinical application of this finding is limited due to the short duration of response and the necessity for intravenous administration. However, it has also been postulated that hypomagnesemia may cause activation of the NMDA receptor, potentiate chronic pain, and blunt the response to opioids. For this reason, it may be worthwhile to identify and correct hypomagnesemia in terminal patients with intractable pain.

Primarily because of a high incidence of toxic effects, the use of NMDA receptor antagonists in humans has been restricted to a small number of clinical trials. These agents include methadone (discussed earlier), ketamine, dextromethorphan, and amantadine. Ketamine has been widely used as an anesthetic agent, but it produces analgesia in doses much lower than those required for anesthesia. Traditionally, it has been administered as a continuous intravenous infusion, and its utility for treating chronic pain was also limited by adverse side effects including excess sedation, psychotomimetic manifestations, and delirium. A number of recent studies indicate that ketamine, 10 mg tid to 20 mg qid, may be successfully used via the oral or sublingual route to treat postherpetic neuralgic pain as well as other neuropathic conditions including postlaminectomy radicular pain.

Dextromethorphan is an antitussive medication that is a component of many cough syrup formulations. It can be administered in a slow-release preparation, in doses of 15 to 500 mg bid. Its major side effect is sedation. In combination with morphine, dextromethorphan can potentiate pain relief and allow a reduction in the total daily morphine dose, although it is not clear that this effect alone is sufficient reason for the commercial development of morphine–dextromethorphan combination products.

Amantadine, used as an anti-influenza medication, is also an NMDA antagonist. In one report, three patients achieved complete and sustained relief of neuropathic pain after a single 200-mg intravenous infusion (Eisenberg & Pud, 1998). A follow-up, randomized trial in 13 patients confirmed that intravenous amantadine acutely relieves neuropathic pain, but that sustained long-term relief after a single dose is unusual (Pud et al, 1998). Oral amantadine may also have some activity and may be worth a try in patients with refractory neuropathic pain because it is less toxic, more easily available, and cheaper than oral ketamine.

ALIMENTARY TRACT PAIN SYNDROMES

A discussion on the treatment of pain related to mucositis and stomatitis can be found in Chapter 10 in the section "Disorders of the Mucous Membranes." A discussion of the etiologies and treatments of various forms of abdominal pain can be found in Chapter 8, in the section "Abdominal Pain and Dyspepsia."

Pharmacologic Pain Management in the Patient with Previous or Current Substance Abuse

It is particularly important to be aware of a history of previous or current substance abuse when patients present with chronic pain. Because of the complex neurophysiologic interplay between pain and addiction pathways, it may be necessary to modify pharmacologic interventions in these patients to achieve effective pain control and avoid toxicity. Characterizations of addictive behavior are listed in Table 6–21.

The complexities inherent in the management of pain in currently addicted patients and in recovered or recovering patients have led to the development of guidelines that are delineated in Tables 6–22 and 6–23. It should be noted that these guidelines are far from foolproof and require frequent adaptation and modification to meet the needs of individual patients.

PSEUDOADDICTION

A related concern of which clinicians must be aware is that of pseudoaddiction. This may occur in patients with or without a prior history of substance abuse. The natural history of this syndrome includes three characteristic phases:

1. Inadequate prescription of analgesics to meet the primary pain stimulus, resulting in persistent uncontrolled pain.
2. Escalation of analgesic demands by the patient associated with behavioral changes (similar to those listed in Table 6–21) to convince others of the pain's severity. Patients in this phase are often characterized as having a substance abuse problem, whether or not there was any prior history of substance abuse.

Table 6–21

Characteristics of Addictive Behavior

Overwhelming concerns about drug availability
Unsanctioned dose escalation
Continued use despite significant side effects
Manipulation of physicians to obtain additional drug supplies
Alterations of prescriptions
Drug acquisition from multiple medical or nonmedical sources
Drug hoarding or selling

Table 6–22

Guidelines for Treatment of Currently Addicted Patients

1. Encourage open communication with the patient.
2. Avoid charting comments about drug use behaviors unless you have discussed your concerns with the patient. (May be required under current Federal Privacy Protection rules.)
3. Remember that denial is a cardinal feature of addiction.
4. Within legal guidelines, obtain information about the patient's drug use from sources other than the patient.
5. Do not withhold opioids from patients with moderate or severe pain; doing so will only encourage craving and drug-seeking behavior.
6. Accept and respect the report of pain in spite of the possibility of being duped.
7. Assure patients that they will receive as much medication as needed to relieve pain.
8. Establish a written treatment plan or contract, negotiated with and agreed to by the patient to include:
   a. Allowable medications and doses
   b. Amounts of medication to be dispensed
   c. Policies regarding refills and "lost medications"
   d. Frequency of office or home care visits
   e. Consequences of failure to follow the plan
9. Arrange for all opioids and other adjunctive and psychotropic medications to be prescribed by the same physician.
10. Encourage participation of nurse addiction specialists and designate a nurse as coordinator for the management team, as traditionally done in hospice care.
11. These patients have often developed drug tolerance and may require much larger doses of opioids than the average patient. Therefore:
    a. Titrate to effect.
    b. Estimate the patient's usual daily intake and provide therapeutic dosing above this baseline dose to obtain effective analgesia.
12. Use regularly scheduled, long-acting opioids for baseline pain management. Avoid prn schedules except as indicated for intermittent or breakthrough pain.
13. Use adjunctive medications liberally, but appropriately. Do not use them as replacements for opioids.
14. Encourage the use of nonpharmacologic interventions.
15. Should the patient demand rapid or unexpected escalation in dosage requirements disproportional to the apparent extent or progression of the underlying disease, do not be too hasty to attribute this to the coexistent addictive disorder. Take the time to identify other potential areas of distress and suffering, including emotional, social, and spiritual pain.
16. Remember that relief of pain and maximization of quality of life are the common goals that should motivate the patient, family, caregivers, and health care team alike.

3. A crisis of mistrust between the patient and members of the health care team, resulting in the precipitation of a painful crisis.

Clinicians must always be alert to this problem. Awareness of the potential for pseudoaddiction and always remembering the operative definition, "Pain is whatever the patient says it is, existing whenever the patient says it does" are crucial to avoidance of this syndrome, and will result in improved pain management for patients near the end of life.

Table 6–23

Guidelines for Managing Pain in Recovered and Recovering Patients

1. Distinguish between abstinence and recovery.
    a. The abstinent person who is struggling with his or her abstinence is often still in denial, socially dysfunctional, and actively fighting drug craving.
    b. Pain in these patients is best managed similarly to actively addicted patients.
2. Believe the patient's complaint of pain.
3. Determine whether pain control techniques other than opioids are preferable.
4. Address patient and family concerns about dependence and relapse. Explain that physical dependency, which will occur, is not the same as addiction.
5. Reassure the patient and family that opioid use will be structured. Formulate and obtain patient agreement to a treatment plan contract.
6. One caretaker should be designated as responsible for pain management.
7. Use drugs in effective doses and titrate the doses to achieve adequate analgesia. Do not underdose, as this may lead to anxiety and drug craving.
8. Prescribe on a scheduled (around-the-clock) basis.
9. Limit quantities per prescription and do not allow refills.
10. Have spouse, friend, other caregiver, or pharmacist dispense each dose.
11. Maintain frequent contact with the patient and caregiver.
12. Remember that stress may increase the patient's request for analgesics.
13. Be alert for and address aberrant drug use behavior suggestive of true addiction, such as acquisition of drugs from multiple sources, repeated claims of lost medications, unsanctioned dose increases, and prescription fraud.

Nonpharmacologic Interventions for the Treatment of Pain

A total pain assessment that evaluates the physical, psychological, social, and spiritual causes of pain allows the clinician to formulate a holistic plan of care that targets each manifestation of a patient's overall perception of pain. This integrated approach to pain management extends treatment choices to include alternative therapies and nonpharmacologic interventions. Combining these techniques and treatment modalities with traditional analgesic medications will allow the patient, caregivers, and physician to select from the full range of pain management strategies that might be needed to adequately address pain's physical, mental and emotional components. Table 6–24 lists these interventions and categorizes them into four approaches.

Physical Invasive Approaches

Anesthetic and surgical procedures are used predominantly for managing cancer pain refractory to other less invasive modalities, and are discussed in Chapter 17. Realistic goals and expectations for these interventions should take into account not only the ability of the patient with advanced disease to tolerate the surgery or therapy but also patient preference. The guiding principle for all of these interventions should be that they have a high probability of success, they lack side effects that exact too high a price on the quality of life, and

Table 6–24

Nonpharmacologic Interventions for Pain Management

APPROACH	INTERVENTION/TECHNIQUE	ADVANTAGES	DISADVANTAGES
Physical—Invasive	**ANESTHETIC PROCEDURES** Nerve blocks (e.g., celiac plexus) Infusions: intraspinal clonidine CNS stimulation **SURGICAL PROCEDURES** Neurologic: rhizotomy Orthopedic: spinal decompression Oncologic: debulking **RADIATION THERAPY** Localized, wide-field Radiopharmaceuticals **CHEMOTHERAPY** Cytotoxic, hormonal	Can provide rapid pain relief Useful for pain that has not reponded to less invasive measures Effective for pain relief with certain diagnoses Can allow dosage reduction (and side effects) of systemic drugs Direct treatment of tumor	Possible infection at catheter site Requires special expertise, careful monitoring May require expensive expensive infusion pumps, specialized care and OR costs Procedures are irreversible
Physical—Noninvasive	**PHYSICAL REHABILITATION** Immobilization, movement, positioning Hydrotherapy **MASSAGE/MANIPULATION/STIMULATION** Superficial heat/cold applications TENS, ultrasound Acupuncture, acupressure, shiatsu Myofascial, craniosacral therapy Chiropractic, therapeutic massage Rolfing, Pruden, Feldenkrais, Trager Reflexology	May decrease pain and anxiety without drug-related side effects Can be used as adjuvant therapy with most other interventions Can be administered by patients or families	Heat and cold may sometimes be contraindicated Skilled therapist required for some interventions
Cognitive/Mind–Body	**INTERPERSONAL/SPIRITUAL** Therapeutic healing touch Prayer Bibliotherapy **ATTENTION/DIVERSION** Music, humor, art, pet therapy **IMAGERY** Guided, incompatible, transformative **EDUCATION** Information and instructions on care **PSYCHOLOGICAL–PHYSIOLOGIC** Self-talk, distraction Meditation, relaxation, yoga Guided imagery Biofeedback, hypnotherapy Autogenic training, cognitive restructuring	May decrease pain and anxiety for patients who have pain that is difficult to manage May increase patient's coping skills Gives patients sense of control over pain Can be used as adjuvant therapy with most other interventions Most are inexpensive, require no special equipment, and are easily administered	Patient must be motivated to use self-management strategies Some interventions require professional time to teach

(continued on next page)

Table 6–24 (continued)

Nonpharmacologic Interventions for Pain Management

APPROACH	INTERVENTION/TECHNIQUE	ADVANTAGES	DISADVANTAGES
Cognitive/ Mind–Body Alternative/ natural remedies	Rhythmic cognitive activity, problem-solving Herbal remedies Nutraceuticals Aromatherapy Homeopathy	Gives patient sense of control over pain Some interventions demonstrate analgesic efficacy	Some herbal remedies have the potential to cause drug interactions

that the benefit will be evident within the time frame of the patient's anticipated survival.

Physical Noninvasive Approaches

Physical medicine techniques include immobilization, range-of-motion exercises, hydrotherapy, massage, acupuncture, application of heat or cold, and transcutaneous electrical nerve stimulation (TENS). Incorporating traditional therapies delivered by physical therapists, nurses, and other rehabilitation therapists with alternative interventions that can be administered by the patient or caregivers will provide more opportunities and choices for the patient. These interventions achieve pain relief directly, by means of manipulation or stimulation of the musculoskeletal, nervous, and integumentary systems, or indirectly, by producing a generalized relaxation response.

Physical rehabilitation techniques may be used in limited settings for specific indications. Immobilization methods include use of a corset to help support the vertebral bodies and control back pain, a shoulder support to reduce pain secondary to brachial plexopathy, or splinting for a patient with a pathologic fracture in whom surgery is not contemplated or desired. Range-of-motion exercises may help reduce discomfort for patients with spastic paraparesis or prevent the development of contractures. The benefits of hydrotherapy are attributable to the buoyancy of water. They in-

clude increased strength and flexibility for patients whose joints are stiff and whose limbs are weak. TENS may occasionally benefit a small subset of patients, but it has generally not been successful for treating pain in terminal patients. The utility of superficial cold/heat treatments and ultrasound is restricted to localized somatic pain.

Acupuncture has been used for the treatment of pain for more than 2500 years, and its effectiveness for pain management has been documented in scientific studies. Acupuncture appears to elicit endorphin release at the level of the spinal cord and midbrain and may also lead to the release of anti-inflammatory cytokines. Its usefulness in managing patients near the end of life is uncertain, and should be evaluated on an individual patient basis. A detailed description of other alternative noninvasive physical techniques listed is beyond the scope of the chapter. Information about these techniques and the extent to which claims for efficacy have been validated scientifically is available from the Office of Alternative Medicine of the U.S. National Institutes of Health.

Cognitive/Mind–Body Approach

For terminally ill patients, the value for quality of life of achieving a perception of personal control over pain is evident when pain is defined as a multidimensional experience. This conceptual framework includes sensory, cognitive, affective, and behavioral parameters that are ultimately defined in terms of neurophysiology, as well as a spiritual dimension which, although metaphysical, appears to affect the processing of pain in people from widely disparate backgrounds and cultures. The cognitive/mind–body approach incorporates interventions such as prayer, therapeutic healing and touch, and music, art, humor, and pet therapy that help the patient cope with pain and provide a means by which a sense of personal control can be restored. These techniques are especially useful for patients who have strong psychosocial and spiritual issues that are influencing their perception and reaction to pain. Helping a patient understand that pain can exist both objectively (physical) and subjectively (emotional, mental, spiritual) will increase receptiveness to these interventions.

For the clinician, the cognitive/mind-body method requires a commitment to "total pain" management and the existence of a personalized therapeutic relationship with the patients and the caregivers and family. These techniques are very compatible with both primary care and with the hospice interdisciplinary model of care in which physicians, nurses, social workers, chaplains, home health aides, and lay volunteers work together with the patient and family and provide a therapeutic environment that encourages the concept of "total pain" control. Hospices are committed to the principle that even dying patients should be given every opportunity to experience the maximal fullness of living possible for them. The extent to which this goal may be enhanced with cognitive/mind–body interventions such as music therapy is apparent in the following quote: "At a time when I felt at the mercy of a situation and dependent on others for help, I was being offered a degree of self-determination. I was being challenged to take up with the tricky business of life again."

Alternative/Natural Remedies

Although herbal remedies contain physiologically active ingredients, the FDA classifies these products as dietary supplements rather than as controlled or regulated drugs. As dietary supplements, therapeutic efficacy cannot be attributed to herbal products and their use for treating pain is not yet based on substantiated research data. Based on anecdotal evidence, however, some of these products (e.g., feverfew, ginseng, green tea extract) have been promoted for the treatment of headaches and fibromyalgia. Clinicians need to be aware of this usage, not necessarily because of efficacy, but rather because of their growing popularity and the occurrence of documented herbal-related drug interactions (e.g., "serotonin syndrome" due to the combination of St. John's wort and meperidine).

Neutraceuticals, or foods that are used therapeutically, may have possible analgesic effects. Amino acid precursors to neurotransmitters such as serotonin and endogenous opioid peptides include tryptophan, phenylalanine, and leucine. Foods high in these amino acids such as protein, legumes, and certain nuts and vegetables have been reported to provide pain relief.

For aromatherapy and homeopathy, any benefits for treating pain are unproven and unsubstantiated at this time. Any analgesic effects from the oils used in aromatherapy would be due to their absorption and penetration of body tissues rather than due to their fragrance. Homeopathic preparations are based on the premise behind vaccines—"like cures like." These extremely diluted forms of substances might include products such as belladonna and chamolilla and have not yet been shown to be of important value in managing pain.

Conclusion

In end-of-life care, the key objectives in the treatment of pain include achieving relief of pain, preventing pain recurrences, optimizing the patient's sense of well-being, and restoring a modicum of hope and belief in the value of life, however chronologically limited. These goals are enhanced

Figure 6–7

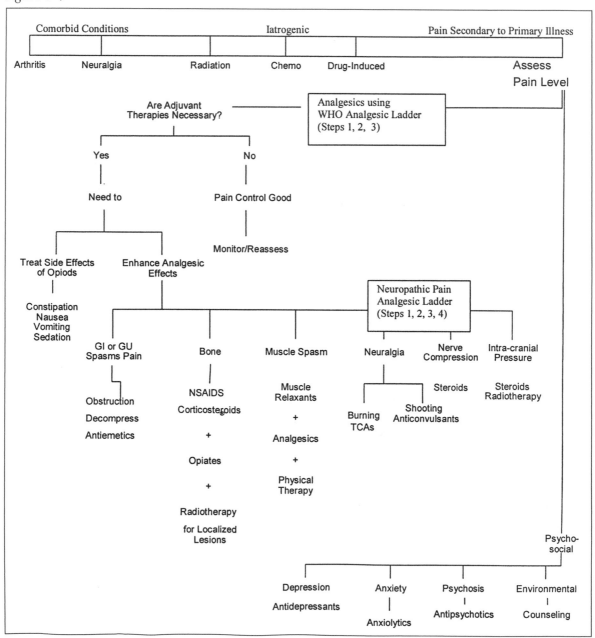

Pain management algorithm

Source: Reprinted with permission from Kinzbrunner BM: *Vitas Pain Management Guidelines*. Miami: Vitas Healthcare Corporation, 1995.

by comprehensive pain assessment and by choosing the least obtrusive, least sedating, and most effective analgesic techniques.

Pharmacologic intervention should incorporate the concepts of the analgesic ladder and appropriate use of adjuvant medications based on the pathophysiology of the patient's pain. Nonceiling-effect opioid agonist analgesics should be used in functionally effective doses, titrated according to individual need and response, and prescribed on a regular schedule with provision for additional "as-needed" doses for breakthrough and incident pain. Nonpharmacologic modalities and psychosocial and spiritual interventions should be integrated into the plan of care with the objective of addressing all dimensions of suffering. Parenteral and spinal analgesics and other aggressive "invasive" techniques should be offered to refractory patients with appropriate clinical and prognostic indications. Figure 6–7 presents the strategies for successful pain management in algorithmic fashion.

With the successful application of these concepts and principles, it may be theoretically possible to reduce the percentage of patients with truly intractable pain to less than 1 percent of the total population at risk. However, until data are available from further research and investigation—and more significantly, until the basic and well-founded principles of pain management described are widely disseminated and effectively applied—apparently intractable pain will continue to be a major source of suffering for patients and their loved ones. If physicians are willing to become better at managing pain both during and near the end of life, patients will be able to retain hope that they will not have to die in pain, and that dying does not have to be associated with unrelieved suffering.

References

Actiq (oral transmucosal fentanyl citrate). Reference 58-0645-R2, Abbott Laboratories, North Chicago, IL, 1999.

Acute Pain Management Guideline Panel: *Acute Pain Management: Operative or Medical Procedures and Trauma.* Clinical practice guideline. AHCPR Pub. No. 92-0032. Rockville, MD. Agency for Health Care Policy and Research, Public Health Service, U.S. Department of Health and Human Services. February, 1992.

American Pain Society: Principles of analgesic use in the treatment of acute pain and chronic cancer pain, 2nd ed. *Clin Pharm* 9:601, 1990.

Ashby M: The role of radiotherapy in palliative care. *J Pain Symptom Manage* 6:380, 1991.

Ashby MA, Martin P, Jackson KA: Opioid substitution to reduce adverse effects in cancer pain management. *Med J Aust* 170:68, 1999.

Bennett G, Burchiel K, Buchser E, et al: Clinical guidelines for intraspinal infusion: report of an expert panel. Polyanalgesic consensus conference 2000. *J Pain Symptom Manage* 20:S37, 2000.

Bennett G, Serafini M, Burchiel K, et al: Evidence-based review of the literature on intrathecal delivery of pain medication. *J Pain Symptom Manage* 2:S12, 2000.

Bolger J, Dearnly D, Kirk D, et al: Strontium-89 (metastron) versus external beam radiotherapy in patients with painful bony metastases secondary to prostate carcinoma. Preliminary report of a multicenter trial. *Semin Oncol* 20(suppl):32, 1993.

Bonica JJ: Cancer pain. In: Bonica JJ, ed. *The Management of Pain,* 2nd ed. Philadelphia, Lea & Febiger, 1990.

Borgeat A, Stirnemann HR: Odansetron is effective to treat spinal or epidural morphine-induced pruritus. *Anesthesiology* 90:432, 1999.

Brannon GE, Stone KD: The use of mirtazapine in a patient with chronic pain. *J Pain Symptom Manage* 18:382, 1999.

Brater DC: Effects of nonsteroidal anti-inflammatory drugs on renal function: Focus on cyclooxygenase-2-selective inhibition. *Am J Med* 107:65S; discussion 70S, 1999.

Bruera E, Breinneis C, Paterson AH, MacDonald RN: Use of methylphenidate as an adjuvant to narcotic analgesics in patients with advanced cancer. *J Pain Symptom Manage* 4:3, 1989.

Bruera E, MachEachern T, Ripamonti C, Hanson J: Subcutaneous morphine for dyspnea in cancer patients. *Ann Intern Med* 119:906, 1993.

Bruera E, Macmillan K, Pither J, MacDonald RN: Effects of morphine on the dyspnea of terminally ill cancer patients. *J Pain Symptom Manage* 5:341, 1993.

Bruera E, Neumann CN: Role of methadone in the management of pain in cancer patients. *Oncology* 13:1275, 1999.

Caraceni A, Zecca E, Martini C, Conno F: Gabapentin as an adjuvant to opioid analgesia for neuropathic cancer pain. *J Pain Symptom Manage* 17:441, 1999.

Carron AT, Lynn J, Keaneg P: End-of-life care in medical textbooks. *Ann Intern Med* 130:82, 1999.

Clarke S, Kitchen I: Opioid analgesia: New information from gene knockout studies. *Curr Opinion Anaesthiol* 12:609, 1999.

Cleeland CS, Gonin R, Hatfield AK, et al: Pain and its treatment in outpatients with metastatic cancer. *N Engl J Med* 330:592, 1994.

Cohen M: Post-surgical pain relief, patients' status and nurses' medication choices. *Pain* 9:265, 1980.

Cole L, Hanning CD: Review of the rectal use of opioids. *J Pain Symptom Manage* 5:118, 1990.

Courts NF: Nonpharmacologic approaches to pain. In: Salerno E, Willens JS, eds. *Pain Management Handbook, An Interdisciplinary Approach*. St. Louis, Mosby, pp. 137–178, 1996.

Cowcher K, Hanks GW: Long-term management of respiratory symptoms in advanced cancer. *J Pain Symptom Manage* 5:320, 1990.

Coyle N, Adelhardt J, Foley KM, Portenoy RK: Character of terminal illness in the advanced cancer patient: Pain and other symptoms during the last four weeks of life. *J Pain Symptom Manage* 5:83, 1990.

Crosby V, Wilcock A, Corcoran R: The safety and efficacy of a single dose (500 mg or 1 g) of intravenous magnesium sulfate in neuropathic pain poorly responsive to strong opioid analgesics in patients with cancer. *J Pain Symptom Manage* 19:35, 2000.

Dellemijn PL: Are opioids effective in relieving neuropathic pain? *Pain* 80:453, 1999.

Diemunsch P, Schoeffler P, Bryssine B, et al: Antiemetic activity of the NK1 receptor anatgonist GR205171 in the treatment of established postoperative nausea and vomiting after major gynaecological surgery. *Br J Anaesth* 82:274, 1999.

Edmundson EA, Simpson RK, Stubler DK, Beric A: Systemic lidocaine therapy for post-stroke pain. *Southern Med J* 86:1093, 1993.

Eisenberg E, Pud D: Can patients with chronic neuropathic pain be cured by acute administration of the NMDA receptor antagonist amantadine? *Pain* 74:337, 1998.

Enarson MC, Hays H, Woodroffe MA: Clinical experience with oral ketamine. *J Pain Symptom Manage* 17:384, 1999.

Enck RE: Understanding and managing bone metastases. *Am J Hospice Palliat Care* 3:3, 1991.

Enck RE: Adjuvant analgesic drugs. *Am J Hospice Care* 6:9, 1989.

Ettinger AB, Portenoy RK: The use of corticosteroids in the treatment of symptoms associated with cancer. *J Pain Symptom Manage* 3:99, 1988.

Farr WC: The use of corticosteroids for symptom management in terminally ill patients. *Am J Hospice Care* 5:41, 1990.

Felsby S, Nielson J, Arendt-Nielsen L, Jensen RS: NMDA receptor blockade in chronic neuropathic pain: a comparison of ketamine and magnesium chloride. *Pain* 64:283, 1995.

Ferrell BR, Grant MM, Rhiner M, Padilla GV: Home care: Maintaining quality of life for patient and family. *Oncology* 6(suppl):136, 1992.

Fine PG: Low-dose ketamine in the management of opioid nonresponsive terminal cancer pain. *J Pain Symptom Manage* 17:296, 1999.

Finlay I: Ketamine and its role in cancer pain. *Pain Rev* 6:303, 1999.

Foley K: The treatment of pain in the patient with cancer. *CA Cancer J Clin* 36:194, 1986.

Foley K: The treatment of cancer pain. *N Engl J Med* 313:89, 1985.

Galer BS, Harle J, Rowbotham MC: Response to intravenous lidocaine infusion predicts subsequent response to oral mexiletine: A prospective study. *J Pain Symptom Manage* 12:161, 1996.

Glare PA, Walsh TD: Dose-ranging study of oxycodone for chronic pain in advanced cancer. *J Clin Oncol* 11:973, 1993.

Grossman SA, Sheidler VR: Pain. In: Abeloff MD, Armitage JO, Lichter AS, Niederhuber JE, eds. *Clinical Oncology*. New York, Churchill Livingstone, 1995, p. 357.

Gurian B, Rosowsky E: Low dose methylphenidate in the very old. *J Geriatr Psychiatry Neurol* 3:152, 1990.

Hernon P: Hospice helps dull pain of dying patients (interview with Dr. C. Stratton Hill). *Montgomery Texas Advertiser,* March 17, 1992.

Herfindal ET, Gourley DR, Hart LL: *Clinical Pharmacy and Therapeutics,* 4th ed. Baltimore, Williams & Wilkins, 1988.

Jacox A, Carr DB, Payne R, et al: Management of cancer pain. Clinical practice guideline no. 9. AHCPR pub. no. 94-0592. Rockville, MD. Agency for Health Care Policy and Research, U.S. Department of Health and Human Services, Public Health Service, March 1994.

Jaffe JH, Martin WR: Opioid analgesics and antagonists. In: Gillman AG, Rall TW, Nies AS, Taylor P, eds.

Goodman and Gilman's The Pharmacological Basis of Therapeutics, 8th ed. Elmsford, NY, Pergamon, 1990, p. 502

Jones R, Hale E, Talomsin L, Phillips R: Kapanol Capsules. Pellet formulation provides alternative methods of administration of sustained release morphine sulfate. *Clin Drug Invest* 12:88, 1996.

Kaiko RF, Foley KM, Grabinski PY, et al: Central nervous system excitatory effects of meperidine in cancer patients. *Ann Neurol* 13:180, 1983.

Katz N: MorphiDex (MS:DM) double-blind, multiple-dose studies in chronic pain patients. *J Pain Symptom Manage* 19(suppl): S37, 2000.

Kaye P: *Symptom Control in Hospice and Palliative Care.* Essex, CT: Hospice Education Institute, 1989.

Kent JM. SnaRIs, NaSSAs, and NaRIs: New agents for the treatment of depression. *Lancet* 355:911, 2000.

Kinzbrunner BM: The terminally ill patient. In: Abeloff MD, Armitage JO, Lichter AS, Niederhuber JE, eds. *Clinical Oncology.* New York, Churchill Livingstone, 2000, p. 597.

Kinzbrunner BM, McGough JP: Cancer pain management. In: Salerno E, Willens JS, eds. *Pain Management Handbook, An Interdisciplinary Approach.* St. Louis, Mosby, 1996, pp. 293–341.

Kinzbrunner BM, Policzer, J, Miller B, Neiber L: Noninvasive pain control in the terminally ill patient. *Am J Hospice Palliat Care* 7:26, 1990.

Kreeger L, Hutton-Potts J: The use of calcitonin in the treatment of metastatic bone pain. *J Pain Symptom Manage* 17:2, 1999.

Kumar KS, Rajagopal MR, Naseema AM: Intravenous morphine for emergency treatment of cancer pain. *Palliat Med* 14:183, 2000.

Levy MH: Pharmacologic treatment of cancer pain. *N Engl J Med* 335:1124, 1996.

Levy MH: Pharmacologic management of cancer pain. *Semin Oncol* 21:718, 1994.

Levy MH: Pain management in advanced cancer. *Semin Oncol* 12:396, 1985.

Light RW, Muro JR, Sato IR, et al: Effects of oral morphine on breathlessness and exercise tolerance in patients with chronic obstructive pulmonary disease. *Am Rev Respir Dis* 139:126, 1989.

Lipman AG: Opioid analgesics in the management of cancer pain. *Am J Hospice Care* 6:13, 1989.

Lipsky LPE, Abramson SB, Crofford L, et al: The classification of cyclooxygenase inhibitors. *J Rheumatol* 25:2298, 1998.

Maloney CM, Kesner RK, et al: Rectal administration of MS Contin: Clinical implications of use in end-stage cancer. *Am J Hospice Care* 6:34, 1989.

Marks RM, Sachar EJ: Undertreatment of medical inpatients with narcotic analgesics. *Ann Intern Med* 78:173, 1973.

McCaffrey M, Beebe A: *Pain: Clinical Manual for Nursing Practice.* St. Louis, Mosby, 1989.

McCaffrey M, Ferrell BR: Does the gender gap affect your pain control decisions? *Nursing 92* 22:48, 1992.

McCracken AL, Gersden L: Sharing the legacy: Hospice care principles for terminally ill elders. *J Gerontol Nurs* 17:4, 1991.

McKenna F: COX-2: Separating myth from reality. *Scand J Rheumatol* 28(suppl):19, 1999.

McKenry L, Salerno E: *Mosby's Pharmacology in Nursing,* 18th ed. St. Louis, Mosby Yearbook, 1992.

Mercadante S, Casuccio A, Calderone L: Rapid switching from morphine to methadone in cancer patients with poor response to morphine. *J Clin Oncol* 17:3307, 1999.

Miser AW, Narang PK, Dothage JA, et al: Transdermal fentanyl for pain control in patients with cancer. *Pain* 37:15, 1989.

Morley JS, Makin MS: The use of methadone in cancer pain poorly responsive to other opioids. *Pain Rev* 5:51, 1998.

Mystakidou K, Befon S, Hondros K, et al: Continuous subcutaneous administration of high-dose salmon calcitonin in bone metastasis: Pain control and beta-endorphin plasma levels. *J Pain Symptom Manage* 18:323, 1999.

Nelson KA, Walsh TD: Metoclopromide in anorexia caused by cancer associated dyspepsia syndrome. *J Palliat Care* 9:14, 1993.

Patt RB, ed: *Cancer Pain.* Philadelphia, Lippincott, 1993.

Patt RB, Proper G, Reddy S: The neuroleptics as adjuvant analgesics. *J Pain Symptom Manage* 9:446, 1994.

Payne R: Cancer pain: Anatomy, physiology, and pharmacology. *Cancer* 63:2273, 1989.

Payne R: Novel routes of opioid administration in the management of cancer pain. *Oncology,* 1 (suppl): 10, 1987.

Perry S, Heidrich G: Management of pain during debridement: A survey of U.S. burn units. *Pain* 13: 267, 1982

Physician's Desk Reference (PDR), 51st ed. Montvale, NJ, Medical Economics, 1997.

Plezia PM, Kramer TH, Linford J, Hameroff SR: Transdermal fentanyl: Pharmacokinetics and preliminary clinical evaluation. *Pharmacotherapy* 9:2, 1989.

Portenoy RK: Drug therapy for cancer pain. *Am J Hospice Palliat Care* 7:10, 1990.

Portenoy RK: Practical aspects of pain control in the patient with cancer. CA *Cancer Clin* 38:331, 1988.

Portenoy RK, Coyle N: Controversies in the long-term management of analgesic therapy in patients with advanced cancer. *J Pain Symptom Manage* 5:307, 1990.

Portenoy RK, Hagen NA: Breakthrough pain: Definition, prevalence, and characteristics. *Pain* 41:273, 1990.

Porter J, Jick H: Addiction rare in patients treated with narcotics. *N Engl J Med* 302:123, 1980. Letter.

Pud D, Eisenberg E, Spitzer A, et al: The NMDA receptor antagonist amantidine reduces surgical neuropathic pain in cancer patients: A double-blind, randomized, placebo-controlled trial. *Pain* 75:349, 1998.

Ripamonti C, Groff L, Brunelli C, et al: Switiching from morphine to oral methadonen treating cancer pain: What is the equianalgesic dose ratio? *J Clin Oncol* 16:3216, 1998.

Robinson RG, Preston DF, Baxter KG, et al: Clinical experience with strontium-89 in prostatic and breast cancer patients. *Semin Oncol* 20:44, 1993.

Rosner H, Rubin L, Kestenbaum A: Gabapentin adjunctive therapy in neuropathic pain states. *Clin J Pain* 12:56, 1996.

Ross FB, Smith MT: The intrinsic antinociceptive effects of oxycodone appear to be kappa-receptor mediated. *Pain* 73:151, 1997.

Ross FB, Wallis SC, Smith MT: Co-administration of subnociceptive doses of oxycodone and morphine produces marked antinociceptive synergy with reduced CNS side-effects in rats. *Pain* 84:421, 2000.

Rupniak N, Kramer M: Discovery of the antidepressant and anti-emetic efficacy of substance P receptor (NK1) antagonists. *Trends Pharmacol Sci* 20:485, 1999.

Sindrup SH, Jensen TS: Efficacy of pharmacological treatments of neuropathic pain: An update and effect related to mechanism of drug action. *Pain* 83:389, 1999.

Smith H, Barton A: Tinazidine in the management of spasticity and musculoskeletal complaints in the palliative care population. *Am J Hospice Palliat Care* 17:50, 2000.

Storey P: Obstruction of the GI tract. *Am J Hospice Palliat Care* 8:5, 1991.

Storey P, Hill HH, St. Louis RH, Tarver EE: Subcutaneous infusions for control of cancer symptoms. *J Pain Symptom Manage* 5:33, 1990.

Tanelian DL, Brose WG: Neuropathic pain can be relieved by drugs that are use-dependent sodium channel blockers: Lidocaine, carbamazepine, and mexiletine. *Anesthesiology* 74:949, 1991.

Twycross RG: The management of pain in cancer. A guide to drugs and dosages. *Oncology* 2:35, 1988.

Twycross RG, Lack SA: *Oral Morphine in Advanced Cancer,* 2nd ed. Beaconsfield, England, Beaconsfield Publishers, 1991.

Twycross RG, Lack SA: *Control of Alimentary Symptoms in Far Advanced Cancer.* London, Churchill Livingstone, 1986.

USPDI: *Drug Information for the Health Care Professional,* vol. 1. Rockville, MD, U.S. Pharmacopeial Convention, 1994.

Vigano A, Fan D, Bruera E. Individualized use of methadone and opioid rotation in the comprehensive management of cancer pain associated with poor prognostic indicators. *Pain* 67:115, 1996.

Von Roenn JH, Cleeland CS, Gonin RS, et al: Physician attitudes and practice in cancer pain management. A survey from the Eastern cooperative oncology group. *Ann Intern Med* 119:121, 1993.

Watanabe S, Bruera E: Corticosteroids as adjuvant analgesics. *J Pain Symptom Manage* 9:442, 1994.

Warner TD, Giuliano F, Vojnovic I, et al: Nonsteroidal drug selectivities for cyclo-oxygenase-1 rather than cyclo-oxygenase-2 are associated with human gastrointestinal toxicity: A full in vitro analysis. *Proc Natl Acad Sci USA* 96:7563, 1999.

Watson CPN: Antidepressant drugs as adjuvant analgesics. *J Pain Symptom Manage* 9:392, 1994.

Watson CPN: Topical capsaicin as an adjuvant analgesic. *J Pain Symptom Manage* 9:423, 1994.

Watson CPN, Babul N: Efficacy of oxycodone in neuropathic pain: A randomized trial in postherpetic neuralgia. *Neurology* 50: 1837, 1998.

Weinreb NJ. Pain management in special situations. In: Salerno E, Willens JS, eds. *Pain Management Handbook: An Interdisciplinary Approach.* St. Louis: Mosby, 1996, pp. 465–523.

Weissman DE, Haddox JD: Opioid pseudoaddiction— An iatrogenic syndrome. *Pain* 36:363, 1989.

Welk T: An education model for explaining hospice services. *Am J Hospice Palliat Care* 8:14, 1991.

Whedon M, Ferrell BR: Professional and ethical considerations in the use of high-tech pain management. *Oncol Nurs Forum* 18:1135, 1991.

Wheeler WL, Dickerson ED: Pharmaceutical update: Clinical applications of methadone. *Am J Hosp Palliat Care* 17: 196, 2000.

Whelton A, Schulman G, Wallemark C, et al: Effects of celecoxib and naproxen on renal function in the elderly. *Arch Intern Med* 160:1465, 2000.

World Health Organization Expert Committee: *Cancer Pain Relief and Palliative Care*. Geneva, WHO, 1990.

Wilkinson TJ, Robinson BA, Begg E, et al: Pharmacokinetics and efficacy of rectal versus oral sustained release morphine in cancer patients. *Cancer Chemother Pharmacol* 31:251, 1992.

Wong D, Whaley L: *Clinical Handbook of Pediatric Nursing*, 2nd ed. St. Louis, Mosby, 1986.

Woodcock AA, Gross ER, Gellert A, et al: Effects of dihydrocodeine, alcohol, and caffeine on breath-lessness and exercise tolerance in patients with chronic obstructive lung disease and normal blood gases. *N Engl J Med* 305:1611, 1981.

Woods SW, Tesar GE, Murray GB, Cassem NH: Psychostimulant treatment of depressive disorders secondary to medical illness. *J Clin Psychiatry* 47:12, 1986.

Zhukovsky DS, Walsh D, Doona M. The relative potency between high dose oral oxycodone and intravenous morphine: A case illustration. *J Pain Symptom Manage* 18:53, 1999.

Zylicz Z, Smits C, Krajnik M: Paroxetine for prutitus in advanced cancer. *J Pain Symptom Manage* 16:121, 1998.

Elizabeth A. McKinnis

Chapter 7

Dyspnea and Other Respiratory Symptoms

Introduction

Irrespective of diagnosis, respiratory symptoms are common among patients at the end of life. The most common respiratory symptoms are dyspnea, cough, and hemoptysis. These symptoms can be very distressing for patients and families, and may have a profound effect on their quality of life. Therefore, it is vital for the practitioner to have an understanding of the definition, etiology, epidemiology, pathophysiology, clinical presentation, and appropriate palliative treatment for the most common respiratory symptoms near the end of life.

Dyspnea

Dyspnea is the uncomfortable awareness of breathing. Fifty-five to seventy percent of patients who are near the end of life experience this symptom and it can be distressing to both the patient and family. Breathlessness is often more distressing than pain but, like pain, dyspnea is most often multidimensional in its presentation. Nonetheless, the optimal treatment of dyspnea should be directed at a reversible cause; this may not be feasible in the terminal stages of disease. However, because dyspnea can lead to significant suffering, immediate palliation of the symptom should always be the primary goal.

Causes of Dyspnea Near the End of Life

There are many causes of dyspnea in the terminal patient, and these are outlined in Table 7–1. Primary pulmonary diseases responsible for dyspnea at the end of life include chronic obstructive pulmonary disease (COPD), pulmonary fibrosis, and lung cancer. Pneumonia, severe congestive heart

Table 7–1
Causes of Dyspnea

Pulmonary
    Chronic obstructive pulmonary disease
    Asthma
    Pulmonary fibrosis
    Pneumothorax
    Pneumonia
    Pulmonary embolism
Cardiac
    Congestive heart failure
    Pericardial effusion
    Myocardial infarction
    Cardiac arrhythmia
Cancer-related
    Superior vena cava syndrome
    Lymphangitis carcinomatosa
    Metastatic disease from any primary site
    Obstruction of bronchus
    Malignant ascites
    Pneumonectomy
    Anemia
Constitutional
    Generalized weakness
    Anorexia and/or cachexia
Psychological
    Hyperventilation
    Anxiety
    Uncontrolled pain
Neuromuscular
    Motor neuron disease
Metabolic
    Hyperthyroidism
    Metabolic acidosis
Miscellaneous
    Severe kyphoscoliosis
    Exogenous mechanical factors

failure, pulmonary embolism, superior vena cava syndrome, and metastatic cancer to the lung from other primary sites are common secondary causes of shortness of breath in patients near the end of life. Asthenia (see Chapter 11), anorexia and cachexia (see Chapter 16), and motor neuron disease may contribute to dyspnea due to weakness of muscles involved in the respiratory effort. Malignant ascites may cause dyspnea by diminishing movement of the diaphragm and decreasing lung capacity, while breathlessness from tachypnea may occur secondary to metabolic acidosis, hypoxia, anemia, or hypercapnia. The coexistence of pain can worsen dyspnea because of increased anxiety and guarded respiratory movements. In addition, the dyspneic patient with depression or anxiety will have increased sensitivity to pain.

Patients may have one or a combination of etiologies responsible for the symptom of breathlessness. The essential information needed to determine the causes of dyspnea in the hospice and palliative setting can usually be found by obtaining a thorough history and physical, with the occasional use of a few diagnostic tests.

Clinical Presentation

Dyspnea patients typically describe "shortness of breath," "tightness in the chest," "can't take a deep breath," or "smothering." The timing of dyspnea is often a clue to its cause. The terminal patient may present with sudden onset of dyspnea leading to consideration of an acute process such as pulmonary embolus, congestive heart failure, or cardiac arrhythmia. Dyspnea that occurs within hours or days may be related to the development of a pleural effusion (malignant or nonmalignant) or pulmonary infection. Gradual onset of dyspnea may be indicative of anemia, debilitated state, or growth of primary or metastatic tumor resulting in gradual obstruction of the airway. Chronic dyspnea is most likely related to the patient's primary illness.

Physical findings that may be important in assessing symptoms of breathlessness include the respiratory rate and pattern of respiration, presence of circumoral or nail bed cyanosis, the use of accessory muscles of respiration, and abnormal breath sounds, such as rales, rhonchi, and wheezes. Secondary physical findings that may help evaluate dyspnea near the end of life may include the presence of ascites; neck, facial, and upper body venous engorgement (suggestive of superior vena

cava syndrome); and lower extremity signs of deep venous thrombosis (suggestive of pulmonary embolism).

Laboratory and diagnostic tools used to assess dyspnea, such as pulse oximetry, pulmonary function tests, blood gases, x-rays, and scans, may be useful at times. However, the results of these tests frequently do not correlate with the patient's perception of distress, and therefore their utility near the end of life is limited, taking into consideration prognosis, goal of therapy, and risk versus benefit ratio.

Psychosocial factors can significantly affect the perceived severity of breathlessness. For example, the fear of suffocating or choking, or the implication that increasing dyspnea may be signaling disease progression or nearness to death, often leads to increased anxiety, which can further exacerbate the severity of the symptom.

Simple assessment tools are available to assist in measuring the level of distress the patient is experiencing. Verbal numeric (0 to 10) scales, verbal categorical scales such as none-mild-moderate-severe, and visual analogue scales can be used to allow the patient to self-report his or her level of shortness of breath. These scales have been validated and can be used to evaluate the effectiveness of the intervention.

Treatment

The primary therapeutic goal when confronted with a patient experiencing dyspnea is palliation of the breathlessness. The development of the treatment plan should involve the patient and family and reflect their goals and expectations. As previously mentioned, when it is feasible, an attempt may be made to assess and eliminate any reversible causes of the symptom.

Dyspnea, like pain, is a subjective experience and involves not only the physical aspect but also psychological and social aspects. Because dyspnea can be multicausal and multidimensional in nature, the optimal treatment combines measures to relieve symptoms, using pharmacologic and nonpharmacologic approaches, as well as specific treatments aimed at the underlying cause when possible and practical.

Table 7–2 summarizes treatments for dyspnea, categorized by the etiology of the symptom. The more common ones will be discussed next. As already stated, these treatments should be based upon the goals of therapy, prognosis, and the potential benefit and burden of those specific treatments.

TREATMENT OF DYSPNEA BASED ON ETIOLOGY

CHRONIC OBSTRUCTIVE PULMONARY DISEASE   Chronic obstructive pulmonary disease (COPD) may be a cause of dyspnea near the end of life, either as the primary terminal disease or as a comorbid condition in the terminal patient suffering from another life-limiting illness. Dyspnea may sometimes be chronic in nature, and often no longer responds well to bronchodilators, although the patient generally continues COPD maintenance medications. Exacerbation of COPD, often due to infection (discussed later), may require adjustment of bronchodilators, treatment with antibiotics, initiation or addition of corticosteroids, and adjustments in oxygen therapy. Opioids, whether oral or nebulized, play an important role in management of dyspnea, and will be discussed further below.

Similar therapeutic options exist for patients suffering from various forms of primary or secondary chronic asthma near the end of life. With the exception of there being less utility for bronchodilators, these same recommendations also apply to patients with primary or secondary pulmonary fibrosis.

CONGESTIVE HEART FAILURE   Congestive heart failure is another common cause of breathlessness in terminally ill patients. Fluid restriction, decreased sodium intake, diuretic therapy, oxygen, and morphine may all be initiated to relieve acute symptoms. If tolerated, left ventricular failure and volume overload may be treated more chronically with the addition of or adjustments in the patient's current diuretics, positive inotropic therapy, and/or angiotensin-converting enzyme inhibitors. The ongoing assessment of the clinical signs and symptoms such as jugular venous distention, peripheral edema, urinary output, and auscultation of the lung and heart will provide the clinician with sufficient information to properly manage the patient with congestive heart failure and ensure optimal comfort near the end of life.

RESPIRATORY INFECTIONS   Pulmonary infections including pneumonia, bronchitis, tuberculosis, or fungal infections occur in patients near the end of life who suffer from COPD, cancer, heart disease, HIV disease, dementia, and numerous other terminal illnesses. Decisions as to whether to use antibiotics near the end of life should be individualized, based on such factors as the type of infection, the patient's current condition and quality of life, the potential reversibility or irreversibility of the infection, and the desires of the patient and/or family. When a decision is made to treat a patient near the end of life with antimicrobial agents, the oral route of administration is preferable whenever possible. However, a parenteral route of administration may be considered appropriate on an individual patient basis.

SUPERIOR VENA CAVA SYNDROME   Superior vena cava syndrome is a clinical syndrome characterized by dyspnea; head, neck and facial edema; headache; cough; and upper extremity edema. It results from obstruction of the superior vena cava, usually by a cancer, with the most common cancers being bronchogenic carcinoma and non-Hodgkin's lymphoma. A variety of metastatic cancer may also be responsible for superior vena cava syndrome, as can fibrosis from prior chest radiation or the long-term presence of indwelling catheters.

Superior vena cava syndrome usually responds to a combination of high-dose corticosteroids and radiation therapy when the syndrome is of malignant origin. At the end of life, however, patient life expectancy and the ability of the patient to physically tolerate radiation therapy should be considered when determining therapeutic options.

PLEURAL EFFUSION   Pleural effusion is the excessive fluid collection in the pleural space. In the patient with a life-limiting illness, the etiology may

Table 7–2
Treatment of Dyspnea by Etiology

Chronic obstructive pulmonary disease	Bronchodilators
Asthma	Corticosteroids
Pulmonary fibrosis	Opioids
Congestive heart failure	Diuretics
with acute pulmonary edema	Opioids
Pneumonia	Antibiotics appropriate for pathogenic organism
Superior vena cava syndrome	High-dose corticosteroids
	Radiotherapy
	Chemotherapy
Pleural effusion	Thoracentesis
Pericardial effusion	Pericardiocentesis
	Pericardial window
Lymphangitic carcinomatosis	Corticosteroids
	Anxiolytics
Ascites	Paracentesis
	Diuretics
	Chemotherapy
Obstruction from primary tumor	Corticosteroids
or related	Radiotherapy
	Stent placement
	Cryotherapy
	Laser therapy
Pulmonary embolism	Anticoagulant
	Oxygen
	Benzodiazepines
Anemia	Transfusion of packed red blood cells

be related to malignancy, non-cancer illness, or a combination of both. Malignancies commonly presenting with a pleural effusion are lung cancer, breast cancer, and lymphoma. Congestive heart failure is a common nonmalignant cause for pleural effusion.

Patients with pleural effusions generally present with one or more of the following symptoms, depending upon the etiology and severity of the effusion: dyspnea, chest pain, cough, tachypnea, and/or hemoptysis. Physical findings may include dullness to percussion, a pleural friction rub, diminished breath sounds, and/or decreased tactile fremitus.

Pleural effusion may or may not need intervention depending upon degree of dyspnea, life expectancy, and the patient's desires regarding invasive therapy. Usually, by the time the patient has been referred to hospice, the options for disease-directed therapy to reduce the effusion, such as chemotherapy or radiotherapy, have been exhausted. Thoracentesis may provide symptomatic relief for patients with malignant pleural effusion, but relief may be brief (one month or sometimes only days). Patients with symptomatic persistent reaccumulation of pleural fluid may benefit from pleurodesis with or without chest tube drainage, with sclerosing agents to prevent the fluid from returning. (For further discussion of thoracentesis as a procedure near the end of life, see Chapter 17.)

ASCITES Ascites near the end of life is most often associated with end-stage liver disease, neoplasms that invade the abdominal cavity (ovary, endometrium, breast, stomach, colon, and pancreas), and in some cases, cor pulmonale due to chronic obstructive pulmonary disease or other causes of irreversible pulmonary hypertension. Ascites can cause breathlessness through decreased lung capacity related to restricted movement of the diaphragm and discomfort due to abdominal distension as well as due to the sympathetic development of a pleural effusion. Proper management of ascites can contribute to the alleviation of dyspnea.

Treatment of ascites at the end of life is primarily symptomatic, aimed at reducing the abdominal accumulation of fluid in sufficient quantities to provide comfort and relief from dyspnea. Diuretic therapy, using spironolactone combined with furosemide or another loop diuretic, is somewhat controversial, but is commonly employed and is shown to be effective in reducing ascites in some patients. Paracentesis, a minimally invasive procedure, can offer immediate albeit temporary symptom relief, even near the end of life. Fluid reaccumulation is common, sometimes forcing patients to undergo multiple repeat procedures. For such patients the placement of a catheter, either a temporary percutaneous or permanent indwelling catheter (the latter for patients with a sufficiently long life expectancy), may allow for more convenient maintenance of comfort without the burden of multiple invasive procedures. (For further discussion of paracentesis as a procedure near the end of life, see Chapters 8 and 17.)

LYMPHANGITIC CARCINOMATOSIS Lymphangitic carcinomatosis is caused by extensive lymphatic invasion of the lung by tumor cells, with surrounding fibrosis. It occurs most often in patients suffering from primary lung cancer or metastatic breast cancer to the lung. It is associated with severe dyspnea and is frequently undiagnosed or incorrectly diagnosed. In chemotherapy-sensitive neoplasms, symptoms may improve as a result of primary disease-directed therapy. For patients near the end of life, when chemotherapy is unlikely to be of benefit, some temporary symptomatic improvement may be obtained with the use of high-dose corticosteroids.

PHARMACOLOGIC INTERVENTIONS FOR THE TREATMENT OF DYSPNEA NEAR THE END OF LIFE

Pharmacologic interventions are the mainstay for providing symptomatic relief of dyspnea. As alluded to earlier, the use of these medications is dependent on the cause of the dyspnea. Commonly used medications for the treatment of dyspnea near the end of life include opioids, bronchodilators, corticosteroids, and anxiolytics (Table 7–3).

OPIOIDS Very near the end of life, especially when other commonly used medications such as bronchodilators and steroids in patients with end-stage COPD or diuretics in patients with congestive heart failure have limited benefit, opioids such as morphine are the medications of choice for rapid palliation of dyspnea. Opioids reduce breathlessness in several ways. They reduce breathlessness by decreasing the sensitivity to carbon dioxide in the medullary respiratory center, and they also reduce the response of the carotid body to hypoxia. Opioids have been shown to cause bradycardia and hypotension due to peripheral vasodilation and to reduce preload, which is also their mechanism of effect in the treatment of pulmonary edema. Finally, opioids also have anxiolytic effects.

Systemic Opioid-naive patients who require therapy with systemic opioids for dyspnea should be started on low doses of an immediate-release opioid, typically morphine 2.5 to 5 mg. For patients receiving a chronic opioid for pain, it is recommended that the patient receive a dose of an immediate-release opioid that is approximately 25 to 50 percent higher than the baseline dose they are receiving for pain to successfully palliate the breathlessness. This is due to the tolerance that patients develop to respiratory depression when receiving opioids on a chronic basis. The opioid

Table 7–3

Medication Table for Treatment of Dyspnea

MEDICATION	ROUTE	DOSAGE
Opioids		
Morphine	Oral, PR, IV, SC, IM	Starting oral or rectal dose 2.5–5 mg q4h
Nebulized morphine	Nebulized parenteral or oral solution	Starting dose morphine 2.5–10 mg q4h (May be administered alone or with dexamethasone 5 mg)
Bronchodilators		
Beta$_2$-Adrenergic		
Albuterol	Nebulized (0.083%)	2.5 mg q 4–6h
	MDI (90 µg/puff)	2–3 puffs q 4–6h
Lev albuterol	Nebulized (0.63 mg)	0.63–1.25 mg tid
Metaproterenol	Nebulized 5%	0.2–0.3 mL tid–qid
	MDI (650 µg/puff)	2 puffs q 3–4h
Terbutaline	MDI (200 µg/puff)	2 puffs q 4–6h
Pirbuterol	MDI (200 µg/puff)	2 puffs q 4–6h
Bitolterol mesylate	MDI (370 µg/puff)	2 puffs q 4–6h
Salmeterol	MDI (21 µg/puff)	2 puffs q 12h
Anti-cholinergic		
Atropine	Nebulized 1%	0.5–2.5 mg q 4–6h
Ipratropium	MDI (18 µg/puff)	2 puffs q 4–6h
Combination ipratropium and albuterol	MDI (120 µg and 21 µg/puff)	2 puffs q 4–6h
Methylxanthine		
Theophylline	Oral (sustained release)	Starting dose 10 mg/kg/day, titrate to effect and drug level
Aminophylline	IV	Loading dose 0.6 mg/kg, then 0.3 mg/kg/hr[a]
Anxiolytics		
Benzodiazepines		
Lorazepam	Oral, IV, IM	Initial oral dose 1–2 mg/day, 2 or 3 divided doses; adjust as needed[b]
Diazepam	Oral, IV, IM	Starting oral dose 2–2.5 mg qd or BID; titrate as needed[b]
Alprazolam	Oral	0.25mg bid - tid; adjust as needed[b]
Chlordiazepoxide	Oral, IV, IM	5 mg bid - qid
Miscellaneous		
Buspirone	Oral	75–150 mg/day divided doses

(continued on next page)

Table 7–3 (continued)

Medication Table for Treatment of Dyspnea

MEDICATION	ROUTE	DOSAGE
Oral Corticosteroids		
Prednisolone	Oral, IV, IM	Oral dose 5–60 mg/day
Dexamethasone	Oral, IV, IM	Oral dose 0.5–8 mg/day
Inhaled Corticosteroids		
Beclomethasone	MDI (42 µg/puff)	2 puffs tid - qid
Flunisolide	MDI (250 µg/puff)	2 puffs bid
Fluticasone	MDI (110 µg/puff)	1 or 2 puffs bid

MDI = metered-dose inhaler

[a] Dosages for older patient–need to consider all conditions that may effect the clearance and adjust dosage accordingly.

[b] Individual should be titrated to level of sedation desired—response is variable.

may be administered orally or, if the patient is unable to swallow, parenteral morphine may be given at one-third of the oral dose.

Although immediate-acting morphine is generally used to control acute breathlessness, some patients with chronic dyspnea have anecdotally benefited from the combination of a sustained-release opioid product to maintain baseline level of comfort, combined with an immediate-release opioid for acute exacerbations of dyspnea. For patients who do not tolerate morphine, other opioids such as oxycodone and hydromorphone may be used. (A complete discussion of how to use morphine and other opioids for the treatment of pain, which can be applied to the treatment of dyspnea as well, can be found in Chapter 6.)

Nebulized   Nebulization is another approach to the delivery of opioids to treat dyspnea near the end of life. Opioid receptors are located throughout the respiratory tract and are the likely target for nebulized opioids, although the exact mechanism of action by which nebulized opioids work is unclear.

Typically, nebulized morphine is used, with the starting dose being 2.5 to 10 mg, generally repeated at a 4-hour frequency as needed. Most reported studies have used injectable preservative-free morphine in 2 mL of normal saline, although anecdotal reports have also demonstrated efficacy

and safety with nebulization of preservative-containing injectable solutions and even oral morphine solution.

Morphine has been known to cause bronchospasm when nebulized due to histamine release in the airways; hence, professional observation during administration of the first dose is prudent. Some palliative care practitioners also add dexamethasone 5 mg to the nebulized morphine to reduce the risk of bronchospasm. It should be noted that in view of that fact that only 16 percent of inhaled morphine is absorbed systemically, the nebulized route of administration is recommended only for treatment of dyspnea, not for the treatment of pain.

Research evaluating the use of nebulized opioids is conflicting. Review of recent studies with small patient populations revealed effectiveness relieving breathlessness in approximately half of the studies, and the other half showed no difference between morphine and placebo. Although there is a need for large-scale randomized trials on nebulized opioids for treatment of dyspnea, its effectiveness in at least some patients warrants its use on a case-by-case basis for patients near the end of life.

BRONCHODILATORS

Inhaled   Inhaled bronchodilators are available in two classes: beta-adrenergics such as albuterol and metaproterenol, and anticholinergic such as ipratropium. Either class can be delivered via aerosol inhaler or nebulizer. These medications are primarily used for patients near the end of life who suffer from advanced chronic obstructive pulmonary disease. Occasionally, patients with malignant disease to the lung who experience bronchospasm may benefit from the broncho-dilatory effects of beta-adrenergic agents as well. Proper dosing of these medications can be found in Table 7–3.

Oral   Oral bronchodilators include the phospho-diesterase inhibitors, or methylxanthines, and oral beta-adrenergic agents. In addition to their broncho-dilatory effects, methylxanthines can affect dyspnea centrally through the medulla via stimulation of respiration, and peripherally by increasing the contractility of the diaphragm and other muscles involved in respiration, resulting in decreased sensation of breathlessness. Methylxanthines that are most commonly used are theophylline and amino-phylline. It should be noted, however, that due to significant cardiac side effects and the availability of safer drugs, such as the combination of inhaled beta-adrenergic agents and anticholinergic agents in patients with advanced COPD, the use of methyl-xanthines has fallen out of favor.

Oral bronchodilators in the beta-adrenergic class include albuterol, metaproterenol, and terbutaline. Unfortunately, systemic administration can cause undesirable side effects such as anxiety, restless-ness, tachycardia, insomnia, and tremors, which may adversely affect the quality of life of the patient. Therefore, the use of these oral broncho-dilators is not recommended because they are readily available for inhalation—a route that has fewer side effects and similar efficacy.

CORTICOSTEROIDS   Corticosteroids may be helpful as anti-inflammatory agents in patients with dyspnea due to exacerbation of chronic obstructive pulmon-ary disease, lymphangitic carcinomatosis, or with superior vena cava syndrome. By decreasing in-flammation, the obstruction, whether bronchial or vascular, may be diminished and breathlessness may be relieved.

Corticosteroids can also enhance well-being and improve appetite, thereby affecting dyspnea by reducing anxiety of the patient and family. Cortico-steroids may be administered orally, or for patients with chronic inflammation secondary to chronic obstructive pulmonary disease, inhaled cortico-steroids may be used. It is important to remember, however, that inhaled corticosteroids are not indi-cated for the treatment of acute dyspnea. Recom-mended corticosteroids that can be used for the treatment of dyspnea can be found in Table 7–3.

ANXIOLYTICS   Anxiolytics can be helpful in pa-tients with the concurrent presentation of anxiety with dyspnea. Like pain, anxiety increases the sensitivity to dyspnea. The dyspneic patient is often fearful of suffocating or smothering to death, thus precipitating anxiety. The resulting anxiety wors-ens the perception of dyspnea, which leads to a cyclical pattern of response.

The anxiety of the dyspneic patient responds well to treatment with benzodiazepines, with ben-zodiazepines such as lorazepam used to halt that cyclical pattern. Recommended anxiolytics to treat dyspnea can be found in Table 7–3.

OTHER PHARMACOLOGIC MEASURES   For patients with advanced congestive heart failure who develop acute dyspnea, the judicious use of diuretic agents such as furosemide, either orally or parenterally, may be of symptomatic benefit. Additionally, di-uretic therapy with the combination of furo-semide and Aldactone may be indicated for patients with ascites.

Another pharmacologic measure that may have benefit for patients with dyspnea is oxygen therapy, although its real efficacy is questionable. Correction in hypoxia has not been found to correlate with the amount of symptomatic benefit the patient experiences with oxygen therapy. A reason why oxygen therapy is able to palliate dyspnea, despite low oxygen saturation, may be airflow through the nasal cannula stimulating feedback to the respiratory center and thereby decreasing the sensation of breathlessness. Addi-tionally, oxygen therapy may have a psycho-logical benefit to patients and families as it is associated with active treatment, thus reducing the anxiety of patients and families.

NONPHARMACOLOGIC MEASURES USED TO TREAT DYSPNEA

Nonpharmacologic interventions are critically important in the treatment of dyspnea and can significantly improve a patient's quality of life. Many of these interventions are listed in Table 7–4, and include modification of the environment (for example, an exhaust fan for cooling and circulating the air), position changes, breathing techniques, diet, and physiotherapy. Meditation, relaxation techniques, and psychotherapy may also reduce dyspnea-associated anxiety. As mentioned earlier in the section on etiology-specific therapies, radiation therapy and procedures such as thoracentesis and paracentesis may also play a significant role in managing dyspnea. Careful consideration of these interventions, by collaboration between the clinician and the hospice interdisciplinary team, can support the goals and expectations of the patient and family, significantly improving the quality of life in the terminal stages.

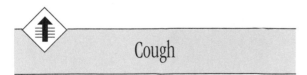

Cough

Introduction

Cough is defined as a sudden explosive forcing of air through the glottis, occurring immediately on opening the previously closed glottis. Cough is stimulated by mechanical or chemical irritation of the trachea or bronchi or by pressure from adjacent structures.

Cough occurs in 30 to 50 percent of all patients at the end of life, involving both cancer and noncancer diagnoses. Approximately 80 percent of lung cancer patients and patients prior to immediate death will have cough as a major symptom.

In the palliative care setting, cough requires aggressive management to prevent complications

Table 7–4

Nonpharmacologic Interventions for Dyspnea

Environment
   Cool air, low humidity
   Fan circulating air
   Quiet room
   Lightweight clothing and bedding
   Reduce pollen, dust, pet hair, etc.
Physical
   Positioning
      Sitting upright 45 degrees
   Breathing techniques
      Pursed-lip breathing
      Diaphragmatic breathing
   Energy conservation
      Plan activities
Relaxation techniques
   Progressive muscle relaxation
   Guided imagery
   Meditation
   Music therapy
   Massage therapy
   Therapeutic touch
Psychosocial support
   Active listening
   Reassurance
   Emotional support
   Education

that may adversely affect the quality of life. An inadequately treated cough may lead to laryngeal irritation, loss of sleep, thoracic muscular soreness, cough-induced fractures, syncope, and headaches. The persistent cough can also result in the development or exacerbation of anxiety involving both the patient and family. Therefore, the importance of prompt assessment and appropriate treatment is essential to the care of the patient in the terminal phase of disease.

Etiology

Similar to dyspnea, the common causes for cough in patients near the end of life are usually related to their terminal illnesses, lung cancer, chronic obstructive pulmonary disease, cardiac disease, or aspiration related to progressive weakness (Table 7–5). However, it must be remembered that patients near the end of life are also susceptible to the more common causes of cough such as postnasal drip syndrome, gastroesophageal reflux, and asthma. These other causes should be taken into consideration when evaluating terminally ill patients who are troubled by cough.

Clinical Presentation

The terminal patient may present with an acute cough related to an upper or lower respiratory tract infection, or may give a history of chronic cough associated with their terminal illness as mentioned. If the cough is exacerbated by supine position, this could be indicative of pulmonary edema, the presence of an endobronchial tumor,

Table 7–5
Causes of Cough

Neoplasms and related conditions	Primary bronchogenic carcinomas
	Metastatic lung tumors
	Mediastinal tumors
	Superior vena cava syndrome
	Lymphangitic carcinomatosis
	Pleural effusion
Cardiovascular disorders	Acute pulmonary edema
	Pulmonary infarction
	Aortic aneurysm
Respiratory infections and disease	Acute pharyngitis/laryngitis
	Acute tracheobronchitis
	Chronic bronchitis
	Lung abscess
	Pulmonary tuberculosis
	Fungal infections
	Bronchopneumonia
	Bronchiectasis
	Chronic obstructive pulmonary disease
Trauma and physical agents	Irritant gases
	Pneumoconioses
Allergic disorders	Bronchial asthma
	Seasonal allergies
	Allergic rhinitis
	Postnasal drip syndrome
Treatment-related	Chemotherapy-induced interstitial disease
	Radiation pneumonitis
Miscellaneous	Pulmonary aspiration
	Gastroesophageal reflux
	Diaphragmatic irritation
	Tracheoesophageal fistula
	Vocal cord paralysis
	Drug-induced (e.g., ACE inhibitor)
	Air quality
	Psychogenic

gastroesophageal reflux disease, or a postnasal drip syndrome. Chronic cough occurring at night might correlate with postnasal drip syndrome, congestive heart failure, or gastroesophageal reflux disease, while a predominantly daytime cough could represent a habitual or psychogenic cough.

Treatment

The optimal therapy for cough in patients near the end of life is to treat the underlying condition, if possible. Most often, however, as with dyspnea, the underlying condition is not identified, not easily treatable, or the patient does not wish to undergo aggressive treatment. For most patients, therefore, the treatment strategy will be to palliate the cough symptomatically.

PHARMACOLOGIC TREATMENT OF COUGH

Medications that may be effective in the management and control of cough near the end of life include cough suppressants, bronchodilators, inhaled lidocaine and corticosteroids.

COUGH SUPPRESSANTS   Cough suppressants are the mainstay of treatment for cough. They include soothing elixirs, dextromethorphan, local anesthetics, and opioids.

A soothing elixir provides first-line therapy and comfort without undesirable side effects. This first-line therapy works by forming a protective barrier over the pharyngeal sensory receptors, thus inhibiting the activation of the cough reflex. Caution is essential when administering such elixirs to patients with diabetes due to their high sugar content.

Dextromethorphan hydrobromide, available over the counter, is one of the most widely used cough suppressants worldwide. The drug acts centrally, raising the threshold for cough, and is almost equi-antitussive to codeine. Dextromethorphan is available in combination with antihistamines, decongestants, and expectorants, to meet the specific need of the patient.

Opioids are the most effective cough suppressants and appear to act centrally. Codeine and hydrocodone are the two most commonly prescribed antitussives, usually in the elixir formulation. They are often used in combination with a decongestant, antihistamine, or expectorant, depending upon the need of the patient. Recommended doses of these various elixirs are 5 to 10 mL by mouth every 4 hours. If the patient is already on an opioid, the current dosage should be increased, in lieu of adding a different opioid. The recommended dose increase in these patients should be an increase of approximately 25 percent over the routine dose to effectively suppress the cough. Remember, however, that cough suppressants, by causing mucus retention, can be problematic when patients are having difficulty with copious mucus production.

Anesthetic agents may be effective in the suppression of chronic cough. A commecially available product, benzonatate, is a peripheral anesthetic that affects the stretch receptors located in the respiratory passages, lungs, and pleura. This product is available in the form of "perles" and the standard dose is one 100-mg perle taken three times a day, with a maximum dose of 600 mg/day.

For more difficult to control chronic cough caused by an endobronchial malignancy, anecdotal reports suggest that inhaled lidocaine may be effective. The lidocaine inhibits the afferent nerve impulses from cough receptors in the pharynx that mediate the cough. The recommended dose is 5 mL of 2 percent lidocaine solution every 4 hours, nebulized and carefully titrated to effect, with the total dose not to exceed 300 mg of lidocaine per day. As there is a risk of bronchospasm when this treatment is initiated, close monitoring is imperative. Food and thick drinks should be avoided, to minimize the risk of aspiration, for approximately 1 hour after the treatment is provided, although small sips of water may be given. Patients should be made aware that injury to the oropharyngeal cavity may occur more easily when anesthesics are used.

OTHER PHARMACOLOGIC MEASURES   Other medications, including expectorants, antihistamines, decongestants, bronchodilators, and corticosteroids, may be useful in the treatment of cough. Guaifenesin is an expectorant found to be safe and mildly effective. Nebulized saline may assist in mobilizing thick secretions, especially for a patient with poor cough effort. Antihistamines/decongestants are effective for the patient with postnasal drip related to seasonal allergies or allergic rhinitis. Oral corticosteroids may be appropriate, when the cough is due to tumor compression of the bronchus; in such patients the steroids will decrease the edema from the tumor and thereby reduce the compression on the bronchus. Oral or inhaled corticosteroids are effective in asthma, bronchiectasis, chronic bronchitis, radiation pneumonitis, or any other cause for inflammation of the airways. In these situations, treatment should be initiated with oral corticosteroids, which can be tapered to the dose effective to control the cough, and/or switch to inhaled corticosteroids. Bronchodilators, such as albuterol or ipratropium, may be necessary for cough related to bronchospasm (refer to treatment of dyspnea, earlier).

For the patient with gastroesophageal reflux disease, treatment may include H_2 antagonists or proton-pump inhibitors with a prokinetic agent and elimination of any medications or foods that be contributing to an exacerbation of the symptoms (see Chapter 8).

Nonpharmacologic Measures to Treat Cough

Nonpharmacologic approaches to the treatment of cough include positioning, chest physiotherapy, changes in air quality, and oral suctioning. These can be used to keep the patient comfortable. Positioning can improve the patient's ability to cough up secretions. The optimal position for most patients is upright, whenever possible, to maximize mobilization of secretions. For the patient with pleural effusion, the best position is lying on the side of the effusion, thereby preventing mediastinal shift and tension on the bronchial tree. This position will avert the stimulation of cough.

Chest physiotherapy involving breathing exercises and postural drainage may be beneficial to some patients. Chest pounding and vibration, however, are not recommended in terminally ill patients, because of the propensity for pathologic fractures

related to osteoporosis or bone metastasis. Chest physiotherapy may also result in decreasing lung function by atelectasis or bronchoconstriction.

Consideration of air quality in the patient's environment can also assist in the palliation of the cough. Adjusting the environment can help if the air is either too hot or too cold. The air quality may be too dry, causing pharyngeal irritation that allows stimulation of the cough reflex. The use of a humidifier will aid in the alleviation of the stimulus for cough.

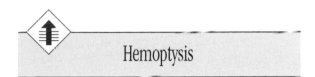

Hemoptysis

Hemoptysis is the expectoration of blood derived from the lungs or bronchial tubes as result of pulmonary or bronchial hemorrhage. It is one of the most frightening of all symptoms near the end of life. Hemoptysis can be extremely alarming both to terminally ill patients and their caregivers. True hemoptysis is defined as the expectoration of some quantity of blood, usually more than 2 mL. Massive hemoptysis is defined as blood loss of more than 200 mL/24 hours.

Incidence

Patients with primary lung cancers at diagnosis present with hemoptysis 30 to 50 percent of the time. The most common cause for massive hemoptysis is bronchogenic carcinoma, while nonmalignant conditions such as acute bronchitis and pulmonary embolus are most often associated with mild to moderate hemoptysis.

Etiology

The causes of hemoptysis are listed in Table 7–6. They include neoplasm, infection, cardiac or pulmonary disease, vascular or hematologic causes, trauma, or medication. Unfortunately, no cause can be determined in up to 40 percent of the cases.

Table 7–6

Causes of Hemoptysis

Neoplasm
　Bronchogenic carcinoma
　Metastatic carcinoma
　Tracheal tumors
Infection
　Bacterial pneumonia
　Fungal pneumonia
　Tuberculosis
　Parasitic
　Lung abscess
Cardiovascular
　Pulmonary edema
Pulmonary
　Pulmonary embolism
　Bronchiectasis
　Bronchitis
Vascular
　Arteriovenous fistula
　Pulmonary hypertension
Hematologic
　Thrombocytopenia
　Coagulopathy
　Disseminated intravascular coagulation
Trauma
　Bronchoscopy or lung biopsy related
　Lung contusion
Medication
　Anticoagulant therapy
　Aspirin
Miscellaneous
　Foreign body

It is important to differentiate true hemoptysis from blood coming from the nose, oropharyngeal cavity, or gastrointestinal tract. A thorough examination of those areas should therefore be performed, to rule out other causes for bleeding.

The patient's description of sputum may help to determine the etiology. Pink, frothy sputum may indicate pulmonary edema. Copious amounts of blood-streaked sputum may point to bronchiecta-

sis. Malodorous, purulent sputum may be consistent with a lung abscess.

Treatment

Once bleeding has been established as true hemoptysis, a treatment plan can be established (Table 7–7). The management of hemoptysis is dependent upon the cause, severity of bleeding, and life expectancy. Radiotherapy, laser therapy and bronchial artery embolization have all been found effective in controlling bleeding from endobronchial tumors. When respiratory infection is the cause, antimicrobial therapy should be considered.

MILD TO MODERATE HEMOPTYSIS

Mild hemoptysis usually warrants treatments with cough suppressants and the provision of psychosocial support in order to reassure the patient and family.

If a patient is experiencing moderate hemoptysis from an endobronchial lesion, visualization and therapy via bronchoscopy may be indicated if the patient's overall clinical condition and life expectancy warrant. Moderate hemoptysis due to endobronchial lesions is responsive to palliative radiotherapy in about 80 percent of cases. Alternative therapies to radiation may include bronchial artery embolization, laser coagulation, or cryotherapy.

Unfortunately, for most patients near the end of life, these interventions may not be realistic therapeutic options. Noninvasive therapeutic options for these patients include oral hemostatic agents such as tranexamic acid (1000 to 1500 mg PO 3 to 4 times a day), combined with psychosocial support and education of the patient and family as to the possibilities of massive hemoptysis.

MASSIVE HEMOPTYSIS

Massive hemoptysis is a rare condition occurring in about 1 to 4 percent of all patients presenting with hemoptysis. It is found more frequently with primary endobronchial tumors invading a bronchial artery, and is rare with lung metastases because metastatic lesions remain intrapulmonary.

Death from massive hemoptysis may occur very suddenly. Patients will classically cough up massive amounts of blood, leading to rapid and generally physically painless exsanguination. For the family, however, this event can be an exceedingly traumatic experience that will require all the skill of the hospice interdisciplinary team to support the family through a most difficult time.

When patients experience severe degrees of hemoptysis without rapid death, palliation is crucial to providing patients with comfort and to reduce awareness and anxiety related to fear. Opioids and benzodiazepines are available in the oral, rectal, or parenteral routes depending on the clinical situation. Patient positioning may be helpful, with the optimal position for patients with severe hemoptysis being to place the bleeding lung, if known, downward. Dark-colored towels are helpful at the bedside to reduce patient and caregiver anxiety.

Table 7–7
Treatment of Hemoptysis

Mild hemoptysis	Cough suppressant
	Reassurance
Moderate hemoptysis	Oral hemostatic agent
	Radiation therapy
	Laser therapy
Massive hemoptysis	Anxiolytics
	Opioids
	Proper positioning to minimize bleeding
	Family counseling and support

"Death Rattle"

Approximately 60 to 90 percent of patients who are within several days of death will develop noisy and moist breathing called the "death rattle." The patient usually appears unaffected by the noisy breathing, but family and staff may be distressed by its presence.

There are two types of death rattle. One type may be due to excessive oral secretions, and the other may be due to excessive bronchial secretions. Patients who receive artificial hydration or nutrition before death experience more excessive secretions than patients who are slightly dehydrated and are allowed a more comfortable, natural death.

Sometimes simply repositioning the patient from supine to lateral recumbent position may allow the patient to breath easier. Suctioning has been noted to be ineffective and unnecessarily invasive, and should be avoided in the dying patient. Anticholinergic medications are effective in most patients. Transdermal scopolamine patches are an effective, noninvasive method of administering a drying agent. Generally, one transdermal patch every 3 days suffices to control symptoms, but there are case reports of using as many as three patches at once. Lower doses of scopolamine have been found to be effective for oral secretions, while higher doses have been found to be beneficial for bronchial secretions.

Another effective agent for the treatment of "death rattle" is atropine. It may be administered via nebulizer in normal saline at a usual dose of 2 mg. (For patients with dyspnea in addition to death rattle, nebulized morphine with or without dexamethasone may be given with the atropine.) Another route of atropine administration is to utilize atropine ophthalmic drops sublingually.

Hyoscyamine 0.125 mg sublingual three to four times a day is another therapeutic alternative that may be used to decrease excessive secretions in actively dying patients. When using any of these medications, periodic moistening of the patient's oral cavity is important. The judicious palliation of excessive oral or bronchial secretions can help reduce the anxiety of the caregiver and family, and make the patient more comfortable.

References

Allard P, Lamontagne C, et al: How effective are supplementary doses of opioids for dyspnea in terminally ill cancer patients? A randomized continuous sequential clinical trial. *J Pain Symptom Manage* 17: 256, 1999.

Berger A, Portenoy RK, et al: *Principles and Practice of Supportive Oncology.* Philadelphia, Lippincott-Raven, 1998.

Booth S, Kelly MJ, et al: Does oxygen help dyspnea in patients with cancer? *Am J Respir Crit Care Med* 153: 1515, 1996.

Boyd KJ, Kelly M: Oral morphine as symptomatic treatment of dyspnoea in patients with advanced cancer. *Palliat Med* 11:277, 1997.

Chandler S: Nebulized opioids to treat dyspnea [see comments]. *Am J Hosp Palliat Care* 16:418, 1996.

Cooley ME: Symptoms in adults with lung cancer. A systematic research review. *J Pain Symptom Manage* 19:137, 2000.

Corr DM, Corr CA: *Hospice Care: Principles and Practice.* New York, Springer, 1983.

Doyle D: *Domiciliary Palliative Care: A Handbook for Family Doctors and Community Nurses.* Oxford, Oxford University Press, 1994.

Doyle D: *Palliative Care: The Management of Far-Advanced Illness.* London, Croom Helm, 1984.

Doyle D, Hanks GWC, et al: *Oxford Textbook of Palliative Medicine.* Oxford, Oxford University Press, 1998.

Dudgeon DJ, Lertzman M: Dyspnea in the advanced cancer patient [see comments]. *J Pain Symptom Manage* 16:212, 1998.

Dunlop R: *Cancer: Palliative Care.* London, Springer, 1998.

Duthie EH, Katz PR: *Practice of Geriatrics.* Philadelphia, Saunders, 1998.

Enck RE: The role of nebulized morphine in managing dyspnea. *Am J Hosp Palliat Care* 16:373, 1999. Editorial comment.

Enck RE: *The Medical Care of Terminally Ill Patients.* Baltimore, Johns Hopkins University Press, 1983.

Fallon M, O'Neill B: ABC of palliative care. BMJ 316:286, 1998.

Faull C, Carter Y, et al: *Handbook of Palliative Care.* Oxford, Blackwell Science, 1998.

Goroll AH, May LA, et al: *Primary Care Medicine: Office Evaluation and Management of the Adult Patient.* Philadelphia, Lippincott, 1995.

Hoegler D: Radiotherapy for palliation of symptoms in incurable cancer. *Curr Probl Cancer* 21:129, 1997.

Hoskin PJ, Makin W: *Oncology for Palliative Medicine.* Oxford, Oxford University Press, 1998.

Kaye P, Hospice Education Institute: *Notes on Symptom Control in Hospice and Palliative Care.* Essex, CT, Hospice Education Institute, 1990.

Kemp C: *Terminal Illness: A Guide to Nursing Care.* Philadelphia, Lippincott, 1999.

Kemp C: Palliative care for respiratory problems in terminal illness. *Am J Hosp Palliat Care* 14:26, 1997.

Kinzbrunner BM, Copeland J, Kinzbrunner E: Nebulized morphine using oral morphine solution. Poster presentation at the annual assembly of the American Academy of Hospice and Palliative Medicine.

Lalloo UG, Barnes PJ, et al: Pathophysiology and clinical presentations of cough. *J Allergy Clin Immunol* 98:S91, discussion S96, 1996.

Leung R, Hill P, et al: Effect of inhaled morphine on the development of breathlessness during exercise in patients with chronic lung disease. *Thorax* 51:596, 1996.

MacBryde CM, Blacklow RS: *MacBryde's Signs and Symptoms: Applied and Pathologic Physiology and Clinical Interpretation.* Philadelphia, Lippincott, 1983.

Manning HL, Schwartzstein RM: Pathophysiology of dyspnea. *N Engl J Med* 333:1547, 1995.

Patz EF Jr: Malignant pleural effusions: Recent advances and ambulatory sclerotherapy. *Chest* 113:74S, 1998.

Ripamonti C, Bruera E: Dyspnea: Pathophysiology and assessment. *J Pain Symptom Manage* 13:220, 1997.

Saunders CM: *The Management of Terminal Malignant Disease.* London, Edward Arnold, 1984.

Saunders CM, Sykes N: *The Management of Terminal Malignant Disease.* London, E. Arnold, 1993.

Stein WM, Min YK: Nebulized morphine for paroxysmal cough and dyspnea in a nursing home resident with metastatic cancer. *Am J Hosp Palliat Care* 14:52, 1997.

Twycross RG, Wilcock A, et al: *Palliative Care Formulary.* Oxford, Radcliffe Medical Press, 1998.

Vainio A, Auvinen A: Prevalence of symptoms among patients with advanced cancer: An international collaborative study. Symptom Prevalence Group. *J Pain Symptom Manage* 12:3, 1996.

Von Gunten CF, Twaddle ML: Terminal care for non-cancer patients. *Clin Geriatr Med* 12:349, 1996.

Waller A, Caroline NL: *Handbook of Palliative Care in Cancer.* Boston, Butterworth-Heinemann, 1996.

World Health Organization: *Symptom Relief in Terminal Illness.* Geneva, World Health Organization, 1998.

Zeppetella G: Nebulized morphine in the palliation of dyspnoea. *Palliat Med* 11:267, 1997.

Chapter 8

Elizabeth A. McKinnis

Gastrointestinal Symptoms

Introduction

The normal functioning of the gastrointestinal tract is something that occupies even healthy individuals. That is because the ingestion and digestion of food, as well as the excretion of its waste products, are central to the maintenance of a healthy life. The ingestion of food is an activity that pervades human existence, and serves a major social function in addition to its biological purpose. Therefore, it is no wonder that, when facing the end of life, symptoms related to dysfunction of the gastrointestinal tract can be extremely distressing to patients and families. For not only do the symptoms cause physical distress, but often cause psychological distress as well, by interfering with the patient's ability to socially interact with family members and others at a time when these interpersonal relationships are crucial.

This chapter will examine some of the more common symptoms that occur when patients are approaching the end of life. Nausea and vomiting will be discussed first, followed by perhaps the most troubling gastrointestinal symptom of all, constipation. Other symptoms, including diarrhea, dysphagia, dyspepsia and abdominal pain, bowel obstruction, and ascites will then be discussed. Anorexia and cachexia, two other common symptoms related to the gastrointestinal system, are reviewed separately in Chapter 16, with a discussion of the ethical issues involved with treatment of these symptoms. As with most other symptoms near the end of life, it is important to have knowledge of the etiology of these symptoms when possible, as the most appropriate treatment that leads to symptom relief is often dependent on the cause of the symptom.

Nausea and Vomiting

Introduction

Nausea is an unpleasant sensation in the region of the stomach, usually associated with an aversion to food, which may or may not be followed by vomiting. Vomiting, or emesis, is the sudden force-

Figure 8–1

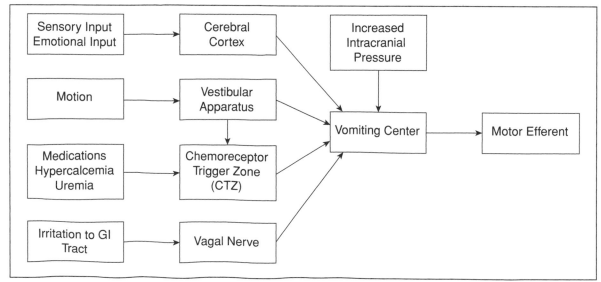

Pathophysiologic mechanisms of nausea and vomiting.

ful peroral expulsion of the contents of the stomach, often, but not always, preceded by nausea. Retching, or dry heaves, is to be differentiated from vomiting by the fact that although muscular contractions of the stomach and respiratory muscles occur with both, retching occurs without expulsion of gastric contents.

Nausea, with or without vomiting, occurs commonly near the end of life, being reported in more than half of all terminal cancer patients as well as in many terminal patients without cancer. That nausea and vomiting are troublesome symptoms goes almost without saying. It can prevent patients from not only taking in nutritional support, but perhaps more importantly, from ingesting the very medication that they need to prevent pain and other symptoms.

To manage nausea and vomiting effectively, it is important to identify the specific cause and to correct or remove it whenever possible. When it is not possible to remove or correct the cause, or while assessing the patient for the specific cause, various pharmacologic and nonpharmacologic treatments can be used to effectively control the symptoms.

The Vomiting Process

Understanding the mechanisms by which various stimuli cause nausea and vomiting is crucial to effectively treating these symptoms. To accomplish this, the vomiting process will be reviewed. As illustrated in Figure 8–1, the pathophysiologic process that results in nausea and vomiting is a complex one, involving the central nervous system, peripheral and central nerves, gastrointestinal tract, and motor efferent nerves that stimulate the diaphragm and abdominal muscles.

Central to the process is the vomiting center (VC), thought to be located in the lateral reticular formation of the medulla. The VC contains both histaminic and muscarinic cholinergic receptors. Vomiting occurs when the VC is stimulated by afferent impulses from one or more areas of the nervous system: the cerebral cortex, vestibular apparatus, chemoreceptor trigger zone (CTZ), and vagal and sympathetic afferent nerves from stim-

uli originating in the gastrointestinal tract. The many varied etiologic factors responsible for nausea and vomiting, as shown in Figure 8–1, will stimulate one (or sometimes more than one) of these areas, causing activation of the vomiting center and the symptom of nausea. If the stimulus to the vomiting center is sufficiently strong to stimulate motor efferents, actual vomiting will result.

With this basic outline of the process, some of the more common causes of nausea and vomiting seen in patients who are near the end of life can be examined in association with the specific sites of the nervous system that each one most directly affects (Table 8–1).

CEREBRAL CORTEX

Nausea and vomiting near the end of life that are caused by stimulation of the cerebral cortex often result from noxious inputs from the senses of smell, taste, or sight. Strong odors and strange or unusual tastes can sometimes invoke nausea and emesis even in healthy individuals, and they are more likely to cause symptoms in individuals who are terminally ill who often have a preexisting aversion to oral intake. Even the sight of food may be enough to invoke vomiting in these patients.

Anticipatory nausea and vomiting is an interesting form of sensory-mediated nausea and vomiting. Patients who have previously been exposed to a particularly noxious stimulus that resulted in severe symptoms of nausea and vomiting may develop recurrent symptoms by being exposed to something that reminds them of the primary stimulus, even in the absence of the stimulus itself. A well-described example of anticipatory nausea and vomiting is the cancer patient who has had particular difficulty with nausea and vomiting following chemotherapy. Such patients may experience recurrent nausea and/or emesis when, for example, they hear music similar to that played in the office when the chemotherapy was administered or when they merely drive by the office in which they received the chemotherapy.

Anxiety without other sensory input may lead to symptoms of nausea and vomiting under certain circumstances. Common examples of anxiety-

Table 8–1

Causes of Nausea and Vomiting in Patients Near the End of Life

PRIMARY SITE OF EFFECT	EXAMPLES
Cerebral cortex	Sensory inputs
	Anticipatory nausea and vomiting
	Anxiety
Vestibular apparatus	Motion sickness
	Vertigo
Chemoreceptor trigger zone (CTZ)	
Medications	Opioid analgesics
	NSAIDs
	Antibiotics
	Chemotherapeutic agents
	Theophylline
	Digoxin
Metabolic	Uremia
	Hypercalcemia
Gastrointestinal tract	Constipation
	Bowel obstruction
	Gastric outlet obstruction
	Gastroparesis
Direct effect on vomiting center	Increased intracranial pressure

related nausea might include the provocation of the symptom prior to the delivery of a major speech or before final exams.

VESTIBULAR APPARATUS

The vestibular apparatus, located in the inner ear, contains both histaminic and muscarinic cholinergic receptors. It causes nausea by signaling both the chemoreceptor trigger zone and the vomiting center (see Fig. 8–1). The role of the vestibular apparatus as a direct pathway to cause nausea and emesis near the end of life is somewhat limited. With the exception of patients suffering from advanced cerebrovascular disease with vertebrobasilar insufficiency, preexistent vertigo, or a malignancy affecting the vestibular apparatus, it is not that common for patients near the end of life to suffer from nausea primarily related to vestibular stimulation. Nevertheless, it is important to rule these

causes out when assessing terminally ill patients for symptoms of nausea and vomiting.

CHEMORECEPTOR TRIGGER ZONE

The chemoreceptor trigger zone (CTZ) is an important mediator of symptoms of nausea and vomiting in patients near the end of life. The CTZ is located in the area postrema at the ventral aspect of the fourth ventricle, and consists of dopamine receptors as well as 5-HT3 (serotonin) receptors. As the CTZ is outside the blood–brain barrier, it can be stimulated by various noxious substances that do not normally enter into the central nervous system.

The noxious substances that mediate nausea and vomiting by stimulation of the CTZ are many, with the majority being medications. For patients near the end of life, opioid analgesics are among the most common medications that cause nausea and vomiting through CTZ stimulation. However, one should consider other medications that patients are taking as well, such as nonsteroidal anti-inflammatory agents, antibiotics, and chronic medications such as digoxin and theophylline preparations. Chemotherapy agents also produce nausea primarily through stimulation of the CTZ, with cis platinum and related compounds more specifically stimulating the 5-HT3 receptors in the CTZ. This receptor specificity has led to the development of antiemetic therapy that effectively counteracts the emetogenic effects of these chemotherapy agents by specifically blocking the stimulation of the 5-HT3 receptor.

In addition to the effects of medications, metabolic abnormalities associated with nausea are mediated through stimulation of the CTZ. For example, uremia and hypercalcemia, two conditions commonly associated with patients who are near the end of life, cause nausea and emesis by this mechanism, and should be considered whenever patients near the end of life are symptomatic.

VAGAL AND SYMPATHETIC AFFERENT NERVE STIMULATION FROM THE GASTROINTESTINTAL TRACT

The main neural pathway from the gastrointestinal tract to the vomiting center in the central nervous system is via the vagus nerve. Nausea and vomiting mediated by the vagus nerve come by stimulation of chemoreceptors and mechanoreceptors located in the serosa and viscera of the gastrointestinal tract. Conditions commonly seen near the end life that may cause nausea and emesis mediated by vagal nerve stimulation include constipation, gastric outlet obstruction, gastroparesis, and bowel obstruction.

Assessment

As with most symptoms, a thorough assessment of the patient is key to determining the best therapeutic approaches to treat nausea and vomiting. Questions regarding the nature of the symptoms themselves are important. For example, projectile emesis with little or no nausea may be indicative of increased intracranial pressure, although increased intracranial pressure can also be associated with nausea and nonprojectile emesis. Gastric outlet obstruction often presents with vomiting after eating and the expelled material may include undigested food, while vomiting associated with intestinal obstruction may be associated with fecaloid emesis.

Querying the patient as to activities that occurred prior to the symptoms might provide additional clues to potential causes. This could be especially important in evaluating the potential for anticipatory nausea and vomiting, or symptoms associated with sensory input such as sight, smell, or taste.

Historical information may lead one towards the consideration of, for example, bowel obstruction from recurrent tumor or adhesions if the patient had prior abdominal surgery, or hypercalcemia if the patient is suffering from a progressive malignancy with bone metastases. Alternatively, it might lead to the uncovering of preexistent vertigo, unrelated to the patient's terminal illness, which would not have been suspected if specific inquiry were not made.

A key component to the assessment of the patient with nausea and vomiting near the end of life is a full medication review, searching for emetogenic medications, including opioid analgesics and antibiotics. Blood levels of medications that can cause nausea when toxicity is present, such as digoxin and theophylline, should be checked even if the patient has not had recent dosage changes, as changes in drug metabolism and clearance often occur as renal and liver function change during the dying process. Because patients are often on multiple emetogenic medications, looking for an association between the taking of the medication and the onset of nausea may be an important clue as to which medication may be responsible.

The physical assessment can provide additional information as to potential etiologies for symptoms of nausea and emesis. For example, abdominal distension with high-pitched, tinkling bowel sounds would be suggestive of intestinal obstruction, while the presence of a succussion splash in the gastric region would point toward gastric outlet obstruction. The presence of a fecal impaction might suggest constipation. Nystagmus or the reproduction of vertiginous symptoms when having the patient change positions would point to a vestibular problem, while the presence of papilledema could indicate the presence of increased intracranial pressure.

Treatment of Nausea and Vomiting

The majority of patients near the end of life have multiple coexistent causes of nausea and vomiting. Therefore, a combination of both nonpharmacologic and pharmacologic interventions is necessary for successful palliation. The following guidelines, which are summarized in Table 8–2, are designed to assist the clinician in deciding how to use the various interventions available to treat nausea and vomiting.

TREAT REVERSIBLE CAUSES WHEN INDICATED AND APPROPRIATE

The first step in the treatment of nausea and vomiting is to remove and/or avoid the cause, when possible. When removal or avoidance is impossible—for example, if the patient has a malodorous fungating skin lesion or cannot tolerate the taste of a necessary medication—masking the odor or the taste of the medication is an alternative way of addressing the patient's symptoms.

As noted, medications often cause nausea and vomiting, either as a primary side effect of the medication or when blood levels of the medication are at toxic levels. When possible, especially with chronic medications not directed at symptom

Table 8–2

Guidelines in the Treatment of Nausea and Vomiting in Patients Near the End of Life

1. Treat reversible causes when indicated and appropriate.
   a. Remove and/or avoid noxious stimuli.
   b. Discontinue unnecessary emetogenic medications.
   c. Reduce dose of medications at toxic levels or discontinue if unnecessary.
   d. Assess for and treat constipation if present.
   e. Decisions on whether to attempt to surgically correct bowel obstruction or to reverse metabolic abnormalities should be based upon patient's clinical condition, quality of life, and life expectancy.
2. Provide appropriate nonpharmacologic measures to ensure patient comfort (see Table 8–3)
3. Pharmacologic therapy should be used for irreversible causes and when emetogenic medications (e.g., opioid analgesics) must be continued.
   a. Choose an initial antiemetic based on potency and the primary site through which the nausea is being mediated (e.g., CTZ, vagal stimulation of GI tract).
   b. Avoid the oral route of administration when the patient is actively vomiting.
   c. If symptoms persist, do not start a second agent unless certain that use of the first agent has been optimal in dose, route of administration, and frequency.
   d. If symptoms persist after optimal use of a single agent, a second medication may be needed. Consider using an agent with site specificity that is synergistic with the first medication.
   e. If the addition of a second medication is not successful in ameliorating symptoms, the patient should be reevaluated. A third medication may be necessary to palliate symptoms while reassessing the patient.

management near the end of life, the offending medication should be discontinued. If the medication is essential for the management of symptoms, dosage adjustments should be considered if the blood levels are in or near the toxic range. A trial of an alternative medication with a similar action should be attempted, as patients may not have the same reactions to different medications in the same therapeutic class. Finally, if the medication is essential, and there is no other alternative, pharmacologic therapy with an antiemetic should be provided (discussed later).

A sometimes overlooked cause of nausea and emesis, especially in patients near the end of life, is constipation. By evaluating and treating for this common symptom, one can sometimes provide a simple solution to the patient's nausea and resolve the constipation as well. (Constipation is discussed later in the chapter.)

Finally, when patients are near the end of life, one must consider whether or not potentially reversible causes of nausea and vomiting can or should be reversed. For some patients, clinical condition, quality of life, or life expectancy might dictate whether or not a bowel obstruction can be surgically reversed, or whether or not it is feasible to reverse a metabolic abnormality such as uremia or hypercalcemia. These decisions are generally made on a patient-by-patient basis, and after discussion of the issues that the clinician needs to consider with the patient, family, and palliative care or hospice team to come to the appropriate conclusions (see Chapter 17 for further discussion).

NONPHARMACOLOGIC MEASURES

There are many nonpharmacologic interventions that can help ameliorate symptoms of nausea and vomiting in patients near the end of life. Some of the more common ones are listed in Table 8–3. As already mentioned, removal of noxious olfactory and visual stimuli, discontinuation of unnecessary medications, and avoidance of emotional or physical stressors are of great importance.

Table 8–3

Nonpharmacologic Interventions for Nausea and Vomiting

Create a comfortable environment
    Encourage patient to sit in fresh air
    Loosen clothing
    Apply a cool damp cloth to patient's forehead, neck, and wrists
    Discourage staff and family from wearing strong perfume, after-shave, and deodorants
Work with the patient
    Relaxation and visualization
    Practice deep breathing and voluntary swallowing to suppress vomiting reflex
    Avoid patient lying supine for two hours after eating
    Oral care after each episode
Modify the patient's diet
    Small, frequent meals encouraged
    Restrict fluids with meals
    Serve cold food (lessens the odor that may stimulate nausea)

Creating a comfortable environment for the patient is of great assistance. Such measures include encouraging the patient to sit in fresh air, loosening clothing, and applying cool compresses to the patient's forehead, neck, and wrists. Staff and family should be discouraged from wearing strong perfumes, after-shave lotions, and deodorants.

Patients should be taught relaxation and visualization techniques and should be encouraged to practice deep breathing and voluntary swallowing, each of which helps suppress the vomiting reflex. Patients should also be instructed to avoid lying in the supine position for at least 2 hours after eating. If emesis should occur, oral care should be provided after each episode.

The nature of food served to the patient may also have an ameliorating affect. If early satiety is a problem, small frequent meals should be encouraged and fluids should be restricted to avoid the sensation of bloating. Reducing food odor can be accomplished by serving food that is at room temperature or cooler.

PHARMACOLOGIC THERAPY

Despite application of many of the interventions outlined, the irreversible nature of the patient's clinical condition and/or the need to continue medications, such as opioids for pain, make continued nausea and vomiting irreversible. For such patients near the end of life, the appropriate and judicious use of antiemetic medications is critical to effective symptom management.

Table 8–4 lists many of the commonly used antiemetic agents, classified by the primary sites through which the nausea is being treated. By performing a good clinical assessment and having a good idea of the etiology or etiologies of the symptoms, the clinician can choose the best agent to use, based on the site through which the nausea and emesis are most likely being mediated. For example, patients who are experiencing nausea from a medication, such as morphine, which is primarily mediated via the CTZ, are best treated with a phenothiazine such as prochlorperazine, as these medications act on the CTZ. If olfactory or visual stimuli are causing nausea secondary to effects on the cerebral cortex, lorazepam might be a good primary agent because of its cortical effects. Nausea due to delayed gastric emptying without gastric outlet obstruction may respond best to metoclopramide, while that caused by increased intracranial pressure or a partial bowel obstruction with bowel wall edema generally will respond best to dexamethasone.

Table 8–4

Pharmacologic Interventions for Nausea and Vomiting for Patients Near the End of Life

MEDICATION	SITES OF ACTION	DOSAGE
Phenothiazines		
Prochlorperazine	CTZ, VC	5–10 mg PO tid-qid, or 25 mg pr bid
Promethazine	CTZ, VC	25 mg PO/PR q4–6 hr, or 12.5–25 mg IV/IM q4–6 h
Chlorpromazine	CTZ, VC	10–25 mg PO q4–6 hrs, or 50–100 mg PR q 6–8 h
Metoclopramide	GI, CTZ	5–10 mg PO/IV ac & hs
Dexamethasone	CC, GI	4–8 mg PO or IV qid
Haloperidol	CC, CTZ	1.5–5 mg PO tid
		2–5 mg SC or IM q4–8 h
Lorazepam	CC	0.5–2 mg PO or IV q4–6h
Diphenhydramine	VA, VC	25–50 mg PO, IM, or IV q4h
Scopolamine	VA, VC	Apply one patch transdermally
		to the postauricular area q 72 hr
Third-line agents (to be used in specific circumstances only)		
5–HT3 receptor antagonists[a]		
Dolasetron[a]	CTZ, GI	100 mg PO prior to chemotherapy
Granisetron[a]	CTZ, GI	1 mg PO prior to chemotherapy &
		1 mg 12 h after 1st dose
Ondansetron[a]	CTZ, GI	8 mg PO prior to chemotherapy &
		8 h after 1st dose
Dronabinol[a]	CC	2.5 mg–5mg PO q4–6 h & titrated

CC=cerebral cortex; CTZ=chemoreceptor trigger zone; GI=gastrointestinal; VA=vestibular apparatus; VC=vomiting center.
[a] These agents are indicated by the FDA for chemotherapy-induced nausea and vomiting, and not for primary treatment of nausea and vomiting from other causes.

When the primary symptom is nausea with little or no emesis, the oral route of administration is preferred. However, the clinician should be aware that when active vomiting occurs, an alternative route, which can be either rectal or parenteral, should be prescribed until the vomiting subsides, when oral medication can then be provided.

If symptoms persist, do not start a second agent unless certain that use of the first agent has been optimal in dose, route of administration, and frequency. If this has been assured, then choose a second agent that has a complementary primary site of action, based upon the cause of the patient's symptoms. If the addition of a second medication is not successful in ameliorating symptoms, the patient should be reassessed to ensure that no other potential cause of nausea and emesis has been overlooked, and that the medications prescribed are being taken appropriately. While the reassessment is being completed or if no new information is uncovered, a third medication, again with a complementary primary site of action, should be used to help palliate symptoms.

A word must be said here about the new medications, ondansetron, granisetron, and dolasetron. These agents specifically antagonize the 5-HT3 receptors in the CTZ, and to a lesser extent, the gastrointestinal tract. They were designed and have been approved primarily for treatment of nausea and vomiting secondary to severe emetogenic chemotherapy, such as cis-platinum and related compounds. Although they have found limited usefulness for nausea and vomiting due to other causes, their use should not be routine. However, they can be applied as third-line medications when primary and second-line anti-emetics have been ineffective.

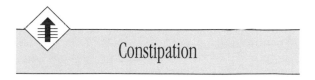

Constipation

Constipation is a subjective term describing the symptom of unsatisfactory defecation. Chronic constipation is a common complaint, with a prevalence of 4 to 30 percent among the elderly population, and a significantly higher prevalence for patients near the end of life.

Etiologies

The terminal patient is at increased risk for constipation for a number of reasons, many of which are listed in Table 8–5. Medications commonly used by patients near the end of life, especially opioid analgesics, are major causes of constipation, so much so that virtually all patients receiving analgesics should be preemptively treated for constipation at the time the analgesic is started. Other medications that may contribute to symptoms of constipation include aluminum-containing antacids, anticholinergic agents, calcium-channel blockers, and other calcium-containing supplements.

A number of advanced neurologic disorders commonly afflicting patients near the end of life, including Parkinson's disease, cerebral infarction, and multiple sclerosis, may have a high risk of constipation. Patients with spinal cord compression may suffer from constipation as well. Although they are more commonly perceived as having incontinence and loose stools due to loss of sphincter control, lack of peristalsis may actually lead to fecal impaction, with soft stool seeping around the impaction leaving the false impression that the patient has diarrhea rather than constipation. Therefore, patients with diarrhea and fecal incontinence should be routinely assessed for the presence of fecal impaction.

Bowel obstruction, due to various malignancies or adhesions in the patient with prior abdominal surgery, often presents with constipation as one of the initial complaints. Various metabolic disorders often associated with patients near the end of life, including uremia and hypercalcemia, may cause constipation, as can other metabolic abnormalities including hypokalemia and hypothyroidism. Patients suffering from advanced diabetes mellitus with autonomic neuropathy may suffer

Table 8–5
Causes of Constipation

ETIOLOGY	EXAMPLES
Medications	Opioid analgesics
	Aluminum-containing antacids
	Anticholinergic agents
	Calcium channel blockers
	Calcium-containing supplements
Neurologic disorders	Spinal cord compression
	Parkinson's disease
	Multiple sclerosis
	Cerebral infarction
Mechanical obstruction	Various malignancies
	Adhesions
Metabolic and endocrine disorders	Uremia
	Hypercalcemia
	Hypokalemia
	Hypothyroidism
	Diabetes mellitus with autonomic neuropathy
Changes in lifestyle	Dehydration due to lack of oral intake
	Lack of activity and exercise
	Low-fiber diet
	Inability to go to bathroom
	Unwillingness to use bedside commode or bedpan

from lack of bowel movements due to a decrease in the peristaltic activity of the colon.

Patients near the end of life experience changes in lifestyle that may adversely affect their ability to move their bowels on a regular basis. As a life-limiting illness progresses, patients often eat and drink less, leading to dehydration, which results in increased fluid absorption from the colon and harder stools. A decrease in dietary fiber is another contributing factor. Exercise has positive effects on the propulsion of bowel content, and the decreased activity that accompanies progressive illness near the end of life further complicates the situation. Finally, as patients lose their ability to ambulate to the bathroom, bowel function is inhibited by the lack of privacy and perceived lack of dignity often associated with a bedpan or a bedside commode, leading to a marked decrease in the frequency of bowel movements.

Clinical Presentation

Patients vary in their description of normal bowel movements, both as to the frequency and the degree of difficulty of defecation, which are the two basic parameters that define constipation. Studies suggest that most individuals have three or more bowel movements per week, while difficulty in defecation is almost entirely subjective. From this discussion it is clear that constipation may be perceived differently by different patients, highlighting once again the importance of an individual assessment as to the nature of the specific patient's symptoms.

Most patients will complain of a decrease in what they perceive to be their normal bowel movement frequency and/or complain of hard stools with or without pain on defecation. If constipation persists untreated over a prolonged period of time, patients may become confused, develop a decreased level of consciousness, complain of progressive abdominal pain, and even experience fever, severe abdominal distention, nausea and vomiting, and leukocytosis, depending upon the severity.

As noted already, the clinician must be alert to constipation presenting as loose stool or diarrhea as a result of fecal impaction. Although fecal impaction usually causes complaints of constipation, sometimes, especially after stool softeners are started, soft stool is able to pass around the fecal impaction, resulting in what the patient perceives as diarrhea, while in fact the constipation remains the major problem.

Treatment

The goal of treatment is evacuation of soft fecal material without straining and optimally, to have evacuation occur at least every 3 days. Non-pharmacologic measures that can be used to treat or prevent chronic constipation include increasing mobility and improving the state of hydration to the extent possible. Patients who are no longer able to ambulate to the bathroom should be provided with maximum privacy during defecation even when needing assistance with a bedside commode or a bedpan. Another nonpharmacologic intervention that is occasionally required is a manual disimpaction, if the patient is suffering from the complication of a fecal impaction.

Pharmacologic Treatment

The hallmark of the treatment of constipation is pharmacologic, and as alluded to earlier, therapy should be initiated prophylactically when patients are at high risk, such as when started on opioid analgesics. Table 8–6 lists commonly used medications for constipation.

The pharmacologic therapy of constipation has two major components, stool softeners and laxatives. Stool softeners, such as docusate sodium, are surfactants and act via detergent activity to facilitate the admixture of fat and water to soften stool. Laxatives promote fecal evacuation. Stool softeners and laxatives should be used together (either as two separate preparations or in a combination tablet) to allow softer stool to more easily be evacuated.

There are several different types of laxatives including saline laxatives, irritant or stimulant laxatives, bulk producing laxatives, lubricant laxatives, and hyperosmolar agents. An algorithm illustrating how these different medications may be used is presented in Figure 8–2.

Saline laxatives, such as magnesium hydroxide, attract and retain water in intestinal lumen, increasing intraluminal pressure and stimulating the release of cholecystokinin. The irritant and stimulant laxatives, such as senna and bisacodyl, have both motor and secretory effects on the colon, acting directly on intestinal mucosa to stimulate the myenteric plexus and altering water and electrolyte secretion.

Methylcellulose–psyllium is an example of a bulk-producing laxative, which acts by holding water in the stool and causing mechanical distention. The use of bulk-producing laxatives should be limited in palliative care due to the poor state of hydration experienced by most patients near the end of life, which when combined with a bulk-producing laxative, can place the patient at an increased risk for intestinal obstruction.

Lubricants, such as mineral oil, retard colonic absorption of fecal water and also soften stool. However, one must be aware of certain issues when using mineral oil. Chronic use of mineral oil can effect the absorption of lipid-soluble vitamins, though this is not often a concern near the end of life. On the other hand, aspiration of mineral oil can cause a lipoid pneumonitis, and this should be avoided when patients suffer from dysphagia. Use of docusate sodium in combination with mineral oil increases the absorption of the mineral oil, thus increasing the potential for mineral oil toxicity.

Hyperosmotic agents such as lactulose and sorbitol deliver osmotically active molecules to the colon to promote bowel function and also soften the stool. Glycerin suppositories cause local irritation and have hyperosmotic action resulting in rapid action after administration.

Finally, when oral stool softeners combined with oral or rectal laxatives are not achieving the desired results, enemas may be used. The most common type of enema provided to patients is hypertonic phosphate. When results are still not achieved, mineral oil or soapsuds enemas may need to be used. As already mentioned, one must be ever alert to and concerned about the problem of fecal impaction. Patients requiring enemas should be assessed for fecal impaction, and manually disimpacted, if necessary, prior to receiving an enema.

Table 8–6
Pharmacologic Treatment of Constipation[a]

MEDICATION	DOSAGE
Stool softeners	
Docusate sodium[a,b]	50–500 mg PO bid
Docusate calcium[b]	240 mg PO qd
Docusate potassium[b]	100–300 mg PO qd
Laxatives	
Saline	
Magnesium hydroxide	15–30 mL PO as needed
Citrate of magnesium	240 mL PO as needed
Stimulants	
Bisacodyl	5-mg tab PO or 10-mg suppository PR as needed
Senna	187-mg standardized concentrate or 33.3-mg/mL senna concentrate PO as needed
Cascara	325-mg tablets or 5 mL PO as needed
Castor oil	15–60 mL PO as needed
Bulk-producing	
Psyllium	1 rounded teaspoon or a 7-g packet of granules PO 3 times a day
Lubricant	
Mineral oil[c]	5–45 mL PO as needed
Hyperosmolar agents	
Lactulose	15–30 mL PO qd-tid
Sorbitol	15–30 mL PO qd-tid
Glycerin suppository	One suppository PR as needed
Combination laxative/stool softener	
Senna/docusate sodium	2 tabs PO at bedtime or bid
Enemas	
Fleet (hypertonic phosphate)	PR as needed
Mineral oil	PR as needed

[a] Preparations containing sodium should not be used by individuals on a sodium-restricted diet or in the presence of edema, congestive heart failure, or hypertension.
[b] Should not be used concurrently with mineral oil.
[c] May cause lipid pneumonitis in dysphagic patients and chronic use may interfere with absorption of lipid-soluble vitamins.

Figure 8–2

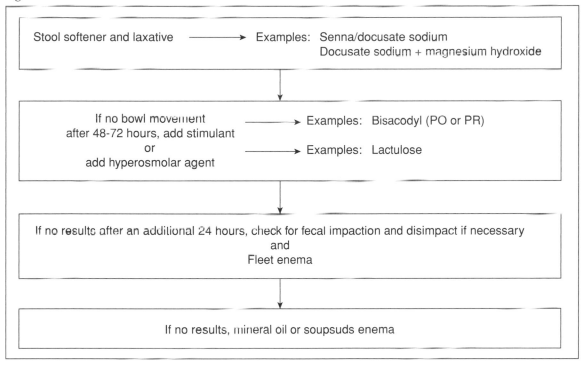

The treatment of constipation.

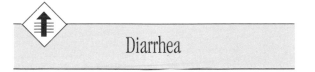

Diarrhea

Diarrhea is usually defined as the passage of more than three unformed stools within a 24-hour period. It can be a troubling symptom for patients near the end of life, and can lead to a number of associated problems, including fecal incontinence, skin breakdown, dehydration, electrolyte imbalance, and a painful rectum and perirectal skin. Caregivers of patients with diarrhea will have the additional burden of providing more frequent personal care to the patient as well as having to make frequent bedding changes, adding to patient distress because of the patient's awareness of the increased burden of care. Therefore, diarrhea should be resolved as quickly as possible by iden-

tifying the cause and initiating a plan to treat or palliate the symptom.

Etiology

The most frequent cause of diarrhea in patients near the end of life is the overuse of laxatives (Table 8–7). This problem should resolve within 24 to 48 hours of discontinuing the offending agent. The laxative can then be resumed if necessary, at a lower dose and titrated to the desired effect.

A thorough review of all other medications should be done and medications that may cause diarrhea, such as magnesium-containing antacids or antibiotics, should be discontinued or changed immediately. Certain chemotherapeutic agents that may occasionally be provided to patients near the end of life, such as the combination of 5-flurouracil and leucovorin and the single agent irinotecan, may also result in severe diarrhea. (See Chapter 17 for further discussion of the role of chemotherapy in the treatment of patients near the end of life.)

As discussed in the earlier section on constipation, fecal impaction may present with diarrhea and should not be overlooked. A complete history regarding bowel movements, including their frequency, consistency and amount, in addition to an examination of the rectal vault, will help to avoid missing this diagnosis.

Dietary habits that may contribute to diarrhea include excessive ingestion of fiber, fruits, and non-absorbable sugars. Radiotherapy can cause diarrhea 2 to 3 weeks after treatment is completed, due to damage to the intestinal mucosa, which releases prostaglandins that lead to increased bowel motility and also leads to malabsorption of bile salts. Malignancies of the pancreas and gastrointestinal tract, as well as other diseases of the small bowel,

may result in diarrhea secondary to malabsorption. Gastrointestinal infections that may occur in patients near the end of life, especially those suffering from AIDS, may be bacterial, viral, fungal, or protozoan in nature. (See Chapter 19 for further discussion of AIDS-related diarrhea.) Patients on chronic antibiotic therapy for other infections may also develop diarrhea secondary to antibiotic-related pseudo-membranous colitis.

Treatment

The initial step in the treatment of diarrhea should be to address any reversible causes of the symptom. Laxatives should be withheld and/or modified if necessary, and other potentially offending medications should be discontinued if possible. Fecal impaction should be considered and treated if found. Diet should be modified to avoid high-fiber content foods as well as fruits and other

Table 8–7

Causes of Diarrhea

ETIOLOGY	EXAMPLES
Constipation with fecal impaction	
Dietary intake	Supplemental drinks
	Increase in fruit, bran, hot spices, or alcohol
Medication and treatment	Laxatives
	Antacids
	Antibiotics
	NSAIDs
	Chemotherapy
	Radiation therapy
Disease related	Pancreatic insufficency
	Malignant bowel obstruction—partial
	Carcinoid
	AIDS related
	Infection
	Inflammatory bowel disease
	Irritable bowel disease
	Excess bile salts

Table 8–8

Treatment for Diarrhea

DISEASE STATE	MEDICATION	DOSAGE
Nonspecific diarrhea	Kaolin with pectin: 90 g kaolin and 2 g pectin/30 mL	60–120 mL PO q bowel movement
	Bismuth subsalicylate	2 tabs or 30 mL PO repeat dosage q 30 min–1 h, max 8 doses
	Loperamide	4 mg PO initial dose; 2 mg PO after each loose movement, not to exceed 16 mg/day
	Diphenoxylate with atropine	5 mg PO qid
Malabsorption due to pancreatic insufficiency	Pancrelipase	1–2 tabs PO with meals or snacks individualized to control steatorrhea
Malabsorption due to excessive bile salts	Cholestyramine	4 g PO tid before meals
Pseudomembranous colitis	Vancomycin	500 mg PO tid-qid for 7–10 days
AIDS-related, carcinoid tumors, tumors, bowel obstruction	Octreotide	100–500 µg SC or IV tid

offending agents, and foods low in fiber should be substituted.

Medications used to treat diarrhea are listed in Table 8–8. For some patients, specific agents should be chosen based upon the cause of the diarrhea. If an infectious cause of diarrhea is suspected, then appropriate antimicrobials should be prescribed. (See Chapter 19 for a discussion of appropriate antimicrobial agents used in the treatment of infectious diarrhea secondary to AIDS.) If pseudomembranous colitis from antibiotic therapy is suspected, then the offending antibiotic agent should be discontinued, and the patient should be treated with metronidazole or vancomycin. Diarrhea secondary to malabsorption, which may occur in patients with pancreatic and other gastrointestinal malignancies, may respond to pancreatic enzymes or cholestyramine. Secretory diarrhea, secondary to AIDS and carcinoid tumors, may require therapy with octreotide.

Patients near the end of life who do not have an identifiable or reversible cause of diarrhea should be treated symptomatically with antidiarrheal agents. Kaolin-pectin suspension or bismuth subsalicylate may be used if the diarrhea is mild to moderate. In more severe cases, or if there is no response to the kaolin-pectin suspension or bismuth, then medications that slow bowel motility, such as loperamide or diphenoxylate with atropine, should be prescribed.

Dysphagia

Dysphagia is technically defined as difficulty in transferring liquids or solids from the mouth to the stomach, but in more practical terms, the term is used to describe difficulties with swallowing. Dysphagia occurs in about 10 to 20 percent of patients with advanced cancer, and also occurs in patients near the end of life who suffer from advanced dementia and other advanced neurodegenerative disorders.

Common causes of dysphagia are listed in Table 8–9. Dysphagia in cancer patients is usually due to mechanical obstruction from direct tumor growth, inflammation caused by radiation therapy or chemotherapy, or infection such as candidiasis in the immunocompromised patient. Xerostomia secondary to medications, especially opioid analgesics, may also contribute to the patient's complaints of difficulty swallowing. (See Chapter 10 for a discussion of the treatment of xerostomia.)

Patients suffering from nonmalignant illness near the end of life who complain of or exhibit dysphagia may have abnormalities in the swallowing mechanism on a neuromuscular basis caused by their primary neurodegenerative disorder. Patients near the end of life, irrespective of diagnosis, may also have difficulty swallowing secondary to various commonly used medications, including anticholinergics, antihistamines, and phenothiazines.

Clinical Presentation

Patients with dysphagia may exhibit drooling, hesitancy in swallowing, holding food in the mouth, pain with swallowing, coughing, and/or choking or nasal regurgitation. Drooling is often associated with pain on swallowing or obstruction, while hesitancy in swallowing may be caused by a neurologic disorder. Coughing, especially after swallowing, may be a sign of a tracheoesophageal fistula. Patients with a mechanical obstruction, if they are alert, may be able to point to the location

Table 8–9
Causes of Dysphagia in Patients Near the End of Life

ETIOLOGY	EXAMPLES
Mechanical obstruction	Carcinomas of the head and neck
	Carcinoma of the esophagus
	Carcinoma of the upper stomach
	Thyroid carcinomas
Neurologic and neuromuscular disorders	Amyotrophic lateral sclerosis
	Alzheimer's disease
	Parkinson's disease
	Huntington's chorea
	Multiple sclerosis
	Cerebrovascular disease
	Head trauma
	Myasthenia gravis
Pain	Tumor related
	Candidiasis and other infections
	Radiation and/or chemotherapy-induced stomatitis
Pharmacologic agents	Anticholinergics
	Antihistamines
	Phenothiazines

Table 8–10

Pharmacologic Treatment of Dysphagia

ETIOLOGY	MEDICATION	DOSAGE AND ROUTE
Candidiasis	Nystatin suspension	400,000 U, 4–5 times per day via swish and swallow
	Clotrimazole lozenges	Dissolve in mouth 4–5 times per day
	Fluconazole	50–150 mg PO daily
Viral	Acyclovir	200 mg PO 5 times per day
Non-infectious inflammation or as an adjunct to antimicrobials	Liquid antacids	30 mL PO 3–4 times per day
	Sucralfate suspension	10 mL PO 4 times per day
	Cimetidine	400 mg PO bid or 800 mg PO hs
Mechanical obstruction	Prednisone	20–40 mg PO daily

of the blockage. Patients with dysphagia from either mechanical or neurologic causes may also present with aspiration pneumonia.

Treatment

Conservative treatment for dysphagia includes good oral hygiene and providing food of the type and consistency that the patient can swallow. Small meals served at room temperature may be of benefit. The head of the bed should be elevated during eating and for at least about 1 to 2 hours after eating, to facilitate food moving down the esophagus and reduce the risk of aspiration. Another physical maneuver that may help reduce aspiration risk is to keep the chin down toward the chest during swallowing, as this will close off the airway and decrease pressure in the throat.

Medications for the treatment of dysphagia (Table 8–10) may include topical or systemic antimicrobials for oropharyngeal or esophageal infection. Nystatin suspension 400,000 U via a swish and swallow technique, or clotrimazole lozenges 5 times a day, may be effective in mild cases of oropharyngeal candidiasis. However, if topical treatment is not effective, or when the infection extends into the esophagus, oral therapy with fluconazole 50 to 150 mg daily should be used. Viral

esophagitis caused by organisms such as cytomegalovirus may be treated with acyclovir, 1,000 mg a day in divided doses. For esophagitis secondary to noninfectious inflammation, agents that coat the mucosa, including liquid antacids and sucralfate suspension, are sometimes helpful. If swallowing problems are caused by gastroesophageal reflux, H_2-blockers such as cimetidine, or proton-pump inhibitors such as omeprazole, may be prescribed.

When there is a mechanical obstruction caused by tumor, corticosteroids may be helpful in improving symptoms by decreasing edema and hence tumor size, or reducing the size of mediastinal lymph nodes which may be interfering with swallowing. For patients near the end of life with appropriate prognoses and life expectancies, definitive treatment to alleviate the obstruction with radiation therapy, esophageal dilatation, stent placement, and/or laser therapy may be considered. (See Chapter 17 for a discussion of the utility of invasive therapies for patients near the end of life.) Finally, for patients with mechanical obstruction who are not candidates for more definitive treatment, and for patients with neurologic difficulties swallowing, placement of a gastrostomy tube may need to be considered under appropriate circumstances. (See Chapter 16 for further discussion of the indications and ethical considerations of gastrostomy tubes in patients near the end of life.)

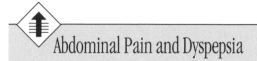
Abdominal Pain and Dyspepsia

Although the subject of pain is discussed elsewhere (Chapter 6), it is important to pay some specific attention to abdominal pain as a symptom, due to the multiplicity of causes and potential interventions other than analgesics that may be used to treat abdominal pain. Table 8–11 lists some of the more common causes of abdominal pain, as well as the various medications associated with treating those causes.

One of the more frequent abdominal complaints that patients experience near the end of life is, not surprisingly, dyspepsia, more commonly known as an "upset stomach." Dyspepsia is characterized by epigastric pain that is sometimes described as burning, nausea, or gaseous eructation.

There are two main types of dyspepsia, organic and functional. Organic dyspepsia is due to a specific lesion such as gastritis, peptic ulcer disease, gastroesophageal reflux disease, gastric carcinoma, or cholelithiasis. Signs of organic dyspepsia may include organomegaly, abdominal mass, ascites, fecal occult blood, dysphagia, weight loss, constant or severe pain, pain that radiates to the back, recurrent vomiting, hematemesis, melena, or jaundice. Functional dyspepsia is dyspepsia with no identifiable focal or structural cause, which accounts for approximately 40 percent of dyspepsia.

Table 8–11
Abdominal Pain: Etiologies and Pharmacologic Therapies

ETIOLOGY	MEDICATION	DOSE AND ROUTE
Dyspepsia	Liquid antacids	15–30 mL PO 3–4 times per day
	Cimetidine	200–300 mg PO qid, or 400 mg PO bid or 800 mg PO hs for up to 8 weeks
	Ranitidine	75–150 mg PO bid or 150–300 mg PO hs
	Lansoprazole	15–30 mg PO daily for 4–8 weeks
	Misoprostol	100–200 µg PO qid with food
Delayed gastric emptying without obstruction	Metoclopramide	5–10 mg PO/IV ac & hs
Gastric distention	Simethicone	40–125 mg PO qid
Abdominal cramping with or without partial bowel obstruction	Stool softeners and laxatives	See Table 8–6
	Antidiarrheals	See Table 8–8
	Hyoscyamine	0.125–0.25 mg PO q4h, max 12 tabs in 24 hours
	Dexamethasone	2–4 mg PO 2–4 times per day
Constipation	Stool softeners and laxatives	See Table 8–6
Bladder spasms	Belladonna/opium suppositories	1 every 4 hours as needed
	Hyoscyamine	0.125–0.25 mg PO q4h, max 12 tabs in 24 hours

Patients near the end of life may have abdominal pain for reasons other than dyspepsia. These include gaseous distention, diarrhea (with or without infection) associated with abdominal cramping, partial or complete bowel obstruction, and, perhaps, most commonly, constipation (discussed earlier). Hepatomegaly due to metastatic cancer may cause abdominal discomfort secondary to stretching of the liver capsule, which contains pain receptors. Finally, abdominal pain near the end of life is often due to bladder spasms or urinary retention.

Treatment

There are a number of nonpharmacologic interventions that should be attempted to address symptoms of abdominal pain, based upon the identified or suspected cause. Dyspepsia accompanied by reflux may respond to elevation of the head of the bed and avoiding foods such as mint, coffee, and fatty foods, which decrease the lower esophageal sphincter (LES) tone. Other foods that should be avoided include tomatoes, citrus fruits, and alcohol because of their direct irritating effect on the esophageal mucosa.

The patient's medication profile should be reviewed, and medications that may contribute to dyspepsia, such as NSAIDs and steroids, should be discontinued if possible. If the patient has symptoms of reflux, medications that decrease LES tone, such as calcium-channel blockers, anticholinergics, benzodiazepines, and theophylline, should be avoided.

Patients should always be assessed and treated for constipation, including manual disimpaction, if necessary, when a fecal impaction is identified. If urinary retention is suspected, placement of a catheter to drain the bladder might be a simple, nonpharmacologic way to resolve a troubling symptom.

Recommendations for the pharmacologic management of abdominal pain can be found in Table 8–11. For dyspepsia, antacids, H₂-blockers such as cimetidine, and the proton pump inhibitors

may be used. If a patient is complaining of early satiety suggestive of poor gastric emptying, and there is no evidence of gastric outlet obstruction, metoclopramide might be a good agent to try. Be aware, however, that if there is gastric outlet obstruction, metoclopramide will worsen rather than improve symptoms.

For gaseous distention, simethicone products, either alone or in combination with antacids if the gas is accompanied by dyspepsia, may be helpful; if there is constipation, stool softeners and laxatives should be prescribed (see Table 8–6). Patients with abdominal cramps and diarrhea who have an infectious or inflammatory diarrhea may require appropriate antibiotics and antidiarrheal agents (see Table 8–8). Antispasmodics, such as hyoscyamine either alone or in combination with phenobarbital, atropine, and scopolamine, may provide relief.

One must be aware of the possibility that the cramps and diarrhea are a sign of partial bowel obstruction, in which case the antidiarrheals and antispasmodic agents could aggravate rather than reduce symptoms. However, if the patient is suffering from an insoluble terminal bowel obstruction, these medications, combined with steroids, may be able to palliate specific symptoms by reducing cramps and keeping the bowels as open as possible. (Bowel obstruction is further discussed later in the chapter.) Antispasmodics, including belladonna/opium suppositories and hyoscyamine, have also been found useful in the palliation of bladder spasms.

Gastrointestinal Bleeding

Patients near the end of life are susceptible to gastrointestinal bleeding from many causes, with some of the more common ones listed in Table 8–12. Upper GI bleeding may be related to ulcer disease or gastritis, which near the end of life is often medication induced, with NSAIDs and

Table 8–12

Causes of Gastrointestinal Bleeding in Patients Near the End of Life

LOCATION	EXAMPLES
Upper GI bleeding	Gastritis
	Malignant gastric ulcer disease
	Benign peptic ulcer disease
	Esóphageal varices
	Erosive esophagitis
	Mallory–Weiss tear
	Esophageal carcinoma
Lower GI bleeding	Colorectal cancer
	Anal neoplasm
	Diverticulosis
	Hemorrhoids
	Angiodysplasia
	Inflammatory bowel disease
	Ischemic colitis
	Infectious colitis

steroids being the most common agents involved. Patients with esophageal or gastric malignancies may, of course, have bleeding directly from these lesions, while patients with end-stage liver disease and portal hypertension may develop bleeding esophageal varices.

In terminally ill patients, bleeding from colorectal and anal neoplasms is often obvious, but one must also be alert to common potential causes of lower GI bleeding seen in the general population, including hemorrhoids, diverticulosis, and arteriovenous malformations. Comorbid inflammatory bowel disease may also give rise to bleeding at times. Finally, patients near the end of life may bleed from ischemic or infectious lower bowel diseases.

The treatment of gastrointestinal bleeding near the end of life depends upon the cause, severity of the bleeding, and patient's overall clinical condition. If the bleeding is limited, symptomatic

therapy may be all that is warranted. Discontinuation of any potentially offending medications and the use of antacids and/or other antiulcer preparations (Table 8–11) may be effective in ameliorating upper gastrointestinal bleeding related to gastritis or ulcer disease. Patients with limited lower gastrointestinal blood loss may be observed, provided with iron replacement therapy, and if indicated based upon symptoms, receive periodic red blood cell transfusions. (See Chapter 17 for further discussion on the indications for transfusion therapy near the end of life.) If blood loss is not adequately controlled by these relatively conservative measures, then consideration for further evaluation, including the potential of upper or lower GI endoscopy with possible laser coagulation therapy, may be considered on a case-by-case basis. (See Chapter 17 for further discussion.)

Although acute bleeding may warrant replacement of blood products, fluids, and endoscopy, for some patients near the end of life, prognosis and clinical condition may dictate a more conservative approach, with comfort measures being provided, allowing the patient's life to end in a relatively painless way.

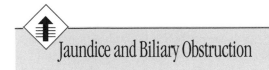

Jaundice and Biliary Obstruction

Jaundice and/or biliary obstruction occur in patients who are near the end of life suffering from primary and metastatic malignancies directly affecting the liver or gallbladder, from pancreatic carcinoma or lymphoma that obstruct the bile ducts, or from primary hepatic failure. Although jaundice itself is not necessarily dangerous, jaundice can cause severe pruritus. Pruritus can be treated symptomatically with antihistamines, such as diphenhydramine 25 mg or cyproheptadine 4 mg given every 4 to 6 hours. Cholestyramine 4 g given three times a day before meals may also reduce itching by binding and reducing the absorption of excess bile salts in the GI tract, which are responsible for the pruritus.

In some patients with obstructive jaundice, the placement of a biliary stent to relieve the obstruction may be indicated. This is discussed in more detail in Chapter 17.

Bowel Obstruction

Bowel obstruction is an unfortunate complication occurring in patients near the end of life, the majority of whom suffer from advanced abdominal or pelvic cancers. Some of the more common etiologies of bowel obstruction in patients near the end of life are listed in Table 8–13. Bowel obstruction near the end of life may be complete or partial, and its severity may fluctuate during the patient's clinical course.

Recurrent tumor is the most common reason for bowel obstruction, with the nature of the malignancy varying from a recurrent intraluminal mass to the more likely possibility of extraluminal metastatic implants. Nonmalignant causes of obstruction in patients with terminal neoplastic disease

Table 8–13

Causes of Bowel Obstruction Near the End of Life

Malignancy
  Intraluminal obstruction secondary to
    primary tumor or recurrence
  Peritoneal carcinomatosis
  Fibrosis secondary to prior radiation therapy
Adhesions secondary to prior surgery
Constipation with or without fecal impaction
Medications: anticholinergics, opioids, tricyclics,
  neuroleptics

may include radiation-related strictures and fibrosis. Terminally ill patients with or without malignant disease who have a prior history of abdominal surgery may develop obstruction from adhesions. And as already mentioned, constipation with or without fecal impaction, if allowed to become severe enough, may present with frank bowel obstruction. Medications that may contribute to symptoms of functional bowel obstruction include anticholinergics, opioids, tricyclic antidepressants, and neuroleptic agents.

Although the treatment of bowel obstruction is traditionally surgical, patients near the end of life are often not considered surgical candidates. A discussion of the indications for surgery to relieve bowel obstruction near the end of life can be found in Chapter 17. Patients with obstruction who are not surgical candidates generally suffer from symptoms of abdominal pain, intestinal colic, and nausea and vomiting. Obstructed patients may present with constipation; however, especially when the obstruction is partial, diarrhea may sometimes be a major complaint. When the obstruction is partial, interventions may include a liquid diet along with stool softeners to reduce complaints of constipation (see Table 8–6), antiemetics to reduce nausea (see Table 8–4), and antispasmodics to reduce abdominal pain and cramps (see Table 8–11). Stimulant laxatives should be avoided as they may worsen symptoms of intestinal colic. Steroids such as dexamethasone (see Table 8–11) may be useful as an adjunctive agent by reducing the edema or inflammation of bowel wall in the area of the obstruction, hopefully resulting in at least a partial opening of the intestinal lumen.

Despite these measures, emesis may be more difficult to control due to the natural secretion of fluids that accumulate in the obstructed gastrointestinal tract. For some patients, a once-a-day bout of emesis, with relative comfort the rest of the time, is acceptable. For others, the placement of a nasogastric tube (or a percutaneous gastrostomy tube) may need to be considered to provide periodic decompression without emesis. Patients who elect treatment with a a tube may still be permitted to take oral food and fluids by mouth to allow them to experience the pleasure of eating if they so desire. Another approach to reduce the incidence of emesis in these patients is with the use of the agent octreotide (see Table 8–8), which reduces gastric and intestinal secretions and hence the need for vomiting or tube decompression.

Ascites

Ascites is the pathologic accumulation of fluid in the peritoneal cavity that causes abdominal distention. Common causes of ascites that occur in patients near the end of life are listed in Table 8–14. Ascites occurs in 15 to 50 percent of patients with cancer, with the most common primary sites being the ovary, colon, stomach, endometrium, pancreas, breast, and lung. Ascites near the end of life may also occur in patients with nonmalignant conditions such as end-stage liver disease, cor pulmonale secondary to advanced chronic obstructive pulmonary disease or primary pulmonary hypertension, and end-stage congestive heart failure.

Peritoneal carcinomatosis produces ascites by obstructing of lymphatic flow and accounts for more than 50 percent of patients with malignant ascites. Primary and metastatic malignancies involving the liver cause ascites by obstructing the hepatic venous circulation. In cirrhosis with portal hypertension, abnormal renal function characterized by sodium and water retention is responsible for ascitic fluid accumulation.

Symptoms due to ascites are the result of increased abdominal pressure created by the accumulation of fluid. These symptoms include abdominal pressure or discomfort, anorexia, dyspepsia, dyspnea, and edema of the lower extremities. When the ascites is tense, the physical finding of shifting dullness to percussion may help differentiate ascites from abdominal distention due to obstruc-

Table 8–14

Common Causes of Ascites Near the End of Life

Peritoneal carcinomatosis
Gynecologic malignancies: ovary, endometrium
Gastrointestinal malignancies: colon, stomach, pancreas
Other malignancies: breast, lung
Liver metastases
Cor pulmonale
End-stage chronic obstructive pulmonary disease
Primary pulmonary hypertension
End-stage congestive heart failure
End-stage nonmalignant liver disease

tion. Measurement of the abdominal girth is an important way to assess the degree of fluid accumulation and the effectiveness of treatments.

Primary treatment of ascites includes a salt-restricted diet (<1000 mg/day) when possible, with fluid restriction (<1500 mL/day) if the patient becomes hyponatremic. Diuretic therapy is often attempted, with spironolactone 25 mg 4 times a day, either alone or in combination with furosemide 40 mg per day. It must be remembered that despite the large amount of fluid in the peritoneal space, many of these patients are intravascularly dehydrated, so both fluid restriction and diuretics should be used with care. With the aforementioned diuretic regimen, it has been found that approximately 70 percent of patients will have resolution of ascites in 2 to 4 weeks. If patients remain symptomatic despite treatment with diuretic therapy and salt and fluid restriction if necessary, then an abdominal paracentesis may be helpful. A full discussion of the indications for abdominal paracentesis for patients near the end of life, as well as the option of a peritovenous shunt for patients with chronic ascites who have a sufficiently long life expectancy, can be found in Chapter 17.

References

Baron TH, Dean PA, et al: Expandable metal stents for the treatment of colonic obstruction: Techniques and outcomes. *Gastrointest Endosc* 47:277, 1998.

Baumrucker SJ: Management of intestinal obstruction in hospice care. *Am J Hospice Palliat Care* 15(4):232, 1998. (Published erratum appears in *Am J Hospice Palliat Care* 15(5):137, 1998.)

Berger A, Portenoy RK, et al: *Principles and Practice of Supportive Oncology*. Philadelphia, Lippincott-Raven, 1998.

Conn HF, Rakel RE: *Conn's Current Therapy*. Philadelphia, Saunders, 1984.

Doyle D: *Domiciliary Palliative Care: A Handbook for Family Doctors and Community Nurses*. Oxford, Oxford University Press, 1994.

Doyle DG, Hanks WC, et al: *Oxford Textbook of Palliative Medicine*. Oxford, Oxford University Press, 1998.

Dunlop R: *Cancer: Palliative Care*. London, Springer, 1998.

Duthie EH, Katz PR: *Practice of Geriatrics*. Philadelphia, Saunders, 1998.

Enck RE: *The Medical Care of Terminally Ill Patients*. Baltimore, Johns Hopkins University Press, 1993.

Fainsinger R: Integrating medical and surgical treatments in gastrointestinal, genitourinary, and biliary obstruction in patients with cancer. *Hematol Oncol Clin North Am* 10:174, 1996.

Fallon BG: Nausea and vomiting unrelated to cancer treatment. In: *Principles and Practice of Supportive Oncology*. Berger, A, Portnoy RK, Weismann D, eds. Philadelphia, Lippincott-Raven, 1998.

Fallon M, O'Neill B: ABC of palliative care. Constipation and diarrhoea. *BMJ* 315:1293, 1997.

Fernandes JR, Seymour RJ, et al: Bowel obstruction in patients with ovarian cancer: A search for prognostic factors. *Am J Obstet Gynecol* 158:244, 1988.

Finlay I: End-of-life care in patients dying of gynecologic cancer. *Hematol Oncol Clin North Am* 13:77, 1999.

Fischer DS: Abdominal paracentesis for malignant ascites. *Arch Intern Med* 139:235, 1979.

Gilbar PJ: A guide to enteral drug administration in palliative care. *J Pain Symptom Manage* 17:197, 1999.

Gines P, Arroyo V, et al: Comparison of paracentesis and diuretics in the treatment of cirrhotics with tense ascites. Results of a randomized study. *Gastroenterology* 93:234, 1987.

Goroll AH, May LA, et al: *Primary Care Medicine: Office Evaluation and Management of the Adult Patient*. Philadelphia, Lippincott, 1995.

Hoegler D: Radiotherapy for palliation of symptoms in incurable cancer. *Curr Probl Cancer* 21:129, 1997.

Hurdon V, Viola R, et al: How useful is docusate in patients at risk for constipation? A systematic review of the evidence in the chronically ill. *J Pain Symptom Manage* 19:130, 2000.

Kaye P, Hospice Education Institute: *Notes on Symptom Control in Hospice and Palliative Care*. Essex, CT, Hospice Education Institute, 1990.

Kemp C: *Terminal Illness: A Guide to Nursing Care*. Philadelphia, Lippincott, 1999.

Kinzbrunner BM: *Vitas Pain Management Guidelines*. Miami, Vitas Healthcare, 1996.

Kinzbrunner BM, Coluzzi P, Gardner D, Geer-Pyron M: *Vitas Guidelines for Intensive Palliative Care*. Miami, Vitas Healthcare, 1996.

Kornblau S, Benson AB, et al: Management of cancer treatment-related diarrhea. Issues and therapeutic strategies. *J Pain Symptom Manage* 19:118, 2000.

Legg JJ, Balano KB: Symptom management in HIV-infected patients. *Prim Care* 24:597, 1997.

MacBryde CM, Blacklow RS: *MacBryde's Signs and Symptoms: Applied and Pathologic Physiology and Clinical Interpretation*. Philadelphia, Lippincott, 1983.

MacDonald N: *Palliative Medicine: A Case-Based Manual*. Oxford, Oxford University Press, 1998.

Maguire P, Faulkner A, et al: Eliciting the current problems of the patient with cancer—a flow diagram. *Palliat Med* 7:151, 1993.

McGann KP: *Griffith's 5-Minute Clinical Consult*. Philadelphia, Lippincott, 1999.

Morita T, Tsunoda J, et al: Contributing factors to physical symptoms in terminally-ill cancer patients. *J Pain Symptom Manage* 18:338, 1996.

Nevitt AW, Vida F, et al: Expandable metallic prostheses for malignant obstructions of gastric outlet and proximal small bowel. *Gastrointest Endosc* 47:271, 1998.

Ottery FD: Cancer cachexia: prevention, early diagnosis, and management. *Cancer Pract* 2:123, 1994. (Published erratum appears in *Cancer Pract* 2:263, 1994).

Philip J, Depczynski B: The role of total parenteral nutrition for patients with irreversible bowel obstruction secondary to gynecological malignancy. *J Pain Symptom Manage* 13:104, 1997.

Raijman I, Siddique I, et al: Palliation of malignant dysphagia and fistulae with coated expandable metal stents: Experience with 101 patients. *Gastrointest Endosc* 48:172, 1996.

Ripamonti C, Bruera E: Pain and symptom management in palliative care. *Cancer Control* 3:204, 2000.

Ripamonti C, Mercadante S, et al: Role of octreotide, scopolamine butylbromide, and hydration in symptom control of patients with inoperable bowel obstruction and nasogastric tubes: a prospective randomized trial. *J Pain Symptom Manage* 19:23, 2000.

Rossi RL, Traverso LW, et al: Malignant obstructive jaundice. Evaluation and management. *Surg Clin North Am* 76:63, 1996.

Saunders CM, Baines M, et al: *Living with Dying: A Guide for Palliative Carers.* Oxford, Oxford University Press, 1995.

Saunders CM, Sykes N: *The Management of Terminal Malignant Disease.* London, E. Arnold, 1993.

Sharma S, Walsh D: Management of symptomatic malignant ascites with diuretics: two case reports and a review of the literature. *J Pain Symptom Manage* 10:237, 1995.

Sleisenger MH, Fordtran JS, et al: *Sleisenger and Fordtran's Gastrointestinal and Liver Disease: Pathophysiology, Diagnosis, Management.* Philadelphia, Saunders, 1998.

Soetikno R: Palliation of malignant gastric outlet obstruction using an endoscopically placed Wallstent. *Gastrointest Endosc* 47:267, 1998.

Souter RG, Wells C, et al: Surgical and pathologic complications associated with peritoneovenous shunts in management of malignant ascites. *Cancer* 55: 1973, 1985.

Sykes NP: An investigation of the ability of oral naloxone to correct opioid-related constipation in patients with advanced cancer. *Palliat Med* 10:135, 1996.

Talmi YP, Bercovici M, et al: Home and inpatient hospice care of terminal head and neck cancer patients. *J Palliat Care* 13:9, 1997.

Twycross RG, Wilcock A, et al: *Palliative Care Formulary.* Oxford, Radcliffe Medical Press, 1998.

Vainio A, Auvinen A: Prevalence of symptoms among patients with advanced cancer: An international collaborative study. Symptom Prevalence Group. *J Pain Symptom Manage* 12:3, 1996.

Von Gunten CF, Twaddle ML: Terminal care for noncancer patients. *Clin Geriatr Med* 12:349, 1996.

Walsh D, Doona M, et al: Symptom control in advanced cancer: important drugs and routes of administration. *Semin Oncol* 27:69, 2000.

Watanabe S, Bruera E: Anorexia and cachexia, asthenia, and lethargy. *Hematol Oncol Clin North Am* 10:89, 1996.

World Health Organization: *Cancer Pain Relief and Palliative Care in Children.* Geneva, World Health Organization, 1998.

World Health Organization: *Symptom Relief in Terminal Illness.* Geneva, World Health Organization, 1998.

Wrede-Seaman L: Symptom management algorithms for palliative care. *Am J Hosp Palliat Care* 16:517, 1999.

Tina Maluso Bolton
Bruce Schlecter

Neurologic Symptoms

Introduction

Neurologic symptoms are extremely common near the end of life. Some of the most frequent neurologic syndromes are presented in Table 9–1. In terminal care, the complex nature of multisystem failure and extensive disease processes may render extensive, invasive, diagnostic workups inappropriate. Rather, the focus in palliative care is the management of neurologic symptoms, regardless of their cause. This chapter will discuss management of end-of-life neurologic symptoms, which frequently present challenging management issues for the patient, family, and palliative care clinicians.

Neurocognitive Disorders

Delirium and Terminal Agitation

DEFINITIONS

Delirium is a common occurrence in end-of-life care. The exact prevalence of delirium near the end of life is difficult to determine, partly because of the variety of terms used to refer to similar phenomena. For example, confusion, encephalopathy, cognitive failure, and impaired mental status are only a few of the terms used to describe what most experts refer to as delirium. Delirium is a disorder characterized by a fluctuating cognitive disturbance and change in mental status that develops over a short period of time and that can be associated with a known medical illness. Studies on delirium in cancer patients show this disorder to be experienced by 25 to 85 percent of patients. In dying patients, rates have been reported to be a high as 77 to 90 percent. However, a recent prospective study from an inpatient palliative care unit reported delirium in 42 percent of 44 patients on admission, with a total of 68 percent developing delirium at some time during their stay.

The occurrence of delirium is particularly disturbing to caregivers, both lay and professional, as difficult decisions must be confronted regarding informed consent and what constitutes appropriate treatment, without coherent input from the patient. Delirium is especially devastating to families and friends of the patient, as the onset of delirium frequently precludes hopes for a meaningful goodbye and emotional closure. Furthermore, delirium—particularly if accompanied by agitation—marks a situation in palliative care in which passive observation is no longer a viable option. Rather, intervention is essential because delirium may be easier to reverse in its earlier stages than in the final days of life, when rapid disease pro-

Table 9–1

Common Neurologic Symptoms Near the End of Life

Delirium or acute confusion	Neuropathic pain syndromes
Terminal agitation	Mononeuropathies
Dementias	Plexopathies
Seizures	Cervical
Headaches	Brachial
Primary brain tumors	Lumbosacral
Metastatic brain lesions	Radiculopathy
Meningeal carcinomatosis	Epidural spinal cord compression
Polyneuropathies	

gression and multisystem failure make reversal of delirium almost impossible. Once delirium is established, it frequently progresses to severe "terminal agitation."

Terminal agitation is a particularly distressing variant of delirium characterized by anguish, restlessness, agitation, and cognitive failure. Terminal agitation has a profound effect on the anguish and suffering experienced by families and caregivers, and therefore treatment of terminal agitation should be considered a palliative care emergency. As in delirium, terminal agitation is generally accepted to be multicausal and further complicated by coexisting multisystem failure, polypharmacy, and physical, emotional, spiritual, and psychological factors. If terminal agitation cannot be controlled, terminal sedation is often the only effective treatment alternative.

Given this background, it is clear that the implications of assessment and management of delirium have profound consequence. Assessment should rapidly identify and treat medical disorders that may be causing delirium. Treatment in turn should be based upon rational, evidence-based studies with careful consideration of the patient's life expectancy, comorbid conditions, goals of treatment, and patient/family desires. In addition, the treatment team should be guided by a commitment to the ethical principles of autonomy, beneficence, and nonmaleficence as well as the hospice principles to "neither hasten nor prolong death." Careful consideration must be given to quality of life and the burden of intervention and treatment. There is mounting clinical evidence that can guide decision making by exploration of the common reversible causes of delirium and terminal agitation.

CAUSES

Delirium and terminal agitation are generally accepted to be multicausal and often complicated by polypharmacy and multisystem failure in patients near the end of life. Some of the most common causes are presented in Table 9–2. Despite the reputation of delirium as being a potentially fatal disorder, studies have indicated that delirium and terminal agitation may be reversible in about 50 percent of patients without the extensive diagnostic interventions that would be incongruous with end-of-life treatment goals. Therefore, the focus of assessment should be on identifying the most common reversible causes of delirium and agitation.

One of the primary treatable causes of delirium and agitation in end-of-life care is prolonged or high-dose opioid administration. This is frequently seen with the use of morphine, which has active glucuronide metabolites that can cause neuro-excitation, myoclonus, hyperalgesia, allodynia (pain from a non-noxious stimulus to normal skin), and terminal agitation. Neurotoxic effects are thought to be caused when these metabolites accumulate in end-of-life patients because of diminished renal excretion due to multisystem failure, dehydration, and prolonged administration.

Medications other than opioids can also cause delirium and terminal agitation. Common offending agents include the psychoactive drugs, anticholinergics, and benzodiazepines. The anticholinergic drugs have been long associated with the risk of delirium in terminal care and should be used cautiously. Tricyclic antidepressants (TCAs) are known to increase plasma morphine levels as well as induce anticholinergic side effects. Fluoxetine, as well as other SSRIs, are known to be potent inhibitors of cytochrome P-450 hepatic enzymes, which may result in multiple drug interactions that may underlie delirium especially when used in conjunction with cisapride or the anticonvulsants. Fluoxetine can also cause plasma levels of TCAs to rise by three to five times, which may induce delirium as well as seizures.

Clearly, when reversal of delirium is the goal, the review of medications must take into account the most likely causative agents as well as the risk/benefit ratio of discontinuation. This challenges the palliative care professional to draw on a complex understanding of pharmacokinetics and pharmacodynamics in the midst of multisystem failure and unpredictable metabolite clearance. Table 9–2 provides a more complete list of the palliative care

Table 9–2

Potential Etiologies of Terminal Agitation

DRUG-RELATED CAUSES	NON-DRUG-RELATED CAUSES
Opioids	Dehydration
Hypnotics	Hypoxia/dyspnea
Antimuscarinic drugs	Anemia
Anticonvulsants	Infection
H_2 antagonists	Fever
Furosemide	Cerebral metastasis
NSAIDs	Increased intracranial pressure
Digoxin	Pain
Steroids	Urinary retention
Psychotropic drugs	Fecal impaction/constipation
Anticholinergic side effects	Fear, anxiety, spiritual turmoil
Neuroleptics	Environmental causes
Antihistamines	CA treatments (chemotherapy, radiation)
Antidepressants	Metabolic disturbances
Anti-parkinsonian agents	Hypercalcemia
Substance withdrawal	Renal failure
Alcohol	Hypoglycemia
Nicotine	Liver failure
Steroid	Hyponatremia
Anticonvulsants	
Benzodiazepines	
Opioids	

SOURCE: Reprinted with permission from Maluso-Bolton T: Terminal agitation. *J Hospice Palliat Nurs* 2:9, 2000.

drugs commonly implicated in delirium. Causes of delirium and terminal agitation not related to medications are also listed in Table 9–2.

TREATMENT

Table 9–3 provides strategies for the assessment of delirium and terminal agitation based upon the most likely treatable causes. It is important to exclude primary causes of agitation such as urinary retention, fecal impaction, unrelieved pain, urinary tract infection, and other environmental causes. The assessment must also include a thorough evaluation of all medications and substances ingested recently, as well as the current medication regimen, to evaluate the role of substance withdrawal or medication interactions in the evolution of delirium. After considering the relative risk/benefit ratio, potentially offending medications should be appropriately reduced, discontinued, or changed to an alternative agent whenever possible.

The development of delirium in the presence of high-dose or sustained opioid administration should be treated as opioid-induced neurotoxicity and opioid rotation should be undertaken. Opioid rotation is the process of switching from one opoid to another when tolerance or intolerable side effects develop. Research evidence supports opioid rotation as a sound, efficacious practice for alleviating side effects as well as for potentially improving analgesia (see Chapter 6 for further discussion).

Table 9–3

Checklist for Evaluation of Terminal Agitation

ASSESS FOR	INTERVENTION
Constipation	Medicate → disimpact → prevent with aggressive management of bowel regimen
Urinary retention	Catheterize and manage retention
Check hydration and urine output	Consider 1 liter of fluids/day[a]
Urosepsis	Urine dipstick → treat if symptomatic
High dose or prolonged opioid treatment	If pain is well managed, consider reduction of 25% of opioid delivered. If ineffective or in presence of pain, rotate opioid, consider fluids to excrete metabolites[a]
Dyspnea	Elevate head of bed. Remove environmental irritants. Use fan for comfort. Consider use of O_2 and/or morphine. Treat anxiety if present
Hypercalcemia	Consider hydration or treat according to patient/family wishes[a]
Drug side-effects or polypharmacy effects	Review medications and discontinue or taper offending medications if possible
Pain	If symptoms persist; rotate opioid with equianalgesic amount and monitor
Recent history drug/alcohol/nicotine addiction	Consider treating with benzodiazepines for drug/alcohol withdrawal or nicotine patch for nicotine withdrawal
Hypoglycemia	Consider glucose replacement
Liver/renal failure	Take this into account when ordering all medications
Metabolic abnormalities	Monitor for hypercalcemia and hyponatremia. Treat if desired by patient and/or family
Fever	Cooling measures and antipyretics
Anxiety/fear	Involve interdisciplinary team for intensive psychosocial, spiritual and emotional support. Treat cautiously with anxiolytics as needed. Music therapy, therapeutic touch, and nonmedicinal nursing interventions should be considered
Environmental causes	Reduce environmental stimulus; modify surroundings to provide orientation. Involve familiar social support system at bedside. Consider therapeutic use of aromatherapy to enhance soothing environment
If delirium or terminal agitation persists and patient is near death	Consider total sedation

[a] Consideration of fluids must always be weighed against the potential burden of fluid overload.

SOURCE: Reprinted with permission from Maluso-Bolton T: Terminal agitation. *J Hospice Palliat Nurs* 2:9, 2000.

Table 9–4

Medications for the Treatment of Delirium and Agitation Near the End of Life

DRUG	ROUTES OF ADMINISTRATION	USUAL ADULT DOSE	MAXIMUM DOSE
Lorazepam	Oral/ IV	0.5–1 mg bid to qid	12 mg/day
Haloperidol	Oral/IM	0.5–5 mg PO bid to tid	30–100 mg/day
		2–5 mg IM q 4–8 h prn	
Phenobarbital	Oral/IM/IV	90–180 mg tid in divided doses	320 mg/day
Chlorpromazine	Oral/rectal/IV	25–50 mg tid to qid	200 mg/day

Lawlor and colleagues (2000) demonstrated that delirium caused by opiate toxicity, psychoactive drugs, and dehydration was most often associated with reversible delirium; hypoxic and metabolic encephalopathy, on the other hand, were associated with irreversibility. Other studies have demonstrated similar results, with reversal of delirium associated with discontinuation of various medications, opioid rotation, and hydration to facilitate the excretion of toxic metabolites.

If measures to reverse potential primary causes of delirium or terminal agitation fail, or while waiting for metabolites to clear, appropriate pharmacologic interventions should be instituted (Table 9–4). Therapy may include administration of haloperidol, lorazepam, or phenobarbital. For severe, refractory cases of terminal agitation, however, recovery may be impossible. In these instances, sedation is widely accepted as an act of benevolence. More commonly known as total sedation, intractable suffering is relieved through the titration of medications such as midazolam, high-dose phenobarbital, or propofol to the desired level of sedation. The palliative care professional has an important role in differentiating between difficult symptoms and refractory symptoms thereby assuring that terminal sedation be accomplished with integrity. (See Chapter 12 for further discussion of total sedation.)

Dementia and Neurodegenerative Disorders

Dementia and neurodegenerative disorders include the clinical syndromes that cause a loss of cognitive and emotional abilities severe enough to interfere with daily functioning. More than 55 illnesses can cause dementia. While these disorders are, in reality, primary illnesses and not symptoms of patients near the end of life, many patients who are terminally ill have dementia as either a major or contributing component to their neuropsychiatric status. These disorders deserve mention, therefore, in view of the fact that many of symptoms that plague patients near the end of life—including uncontrolled pain, fever and sepsis, and dehydration—often exacerbate the degree of dementia suffered by the patient. Thus, worsening of dementia in patients near the end of life should trigger investigation for such reversible problems, and they should be treated when appropriate. A discussion of how to determine when patients with dementia and other neurodegenerative diseases should be receiving hospice and end-of-life care is found in Chapter 1.

Other CNS Symptoms

Seizures

CLASSIFICATION

Seizures differ in their characteristics and presentation according to the area of brain involved, behaviors elicited, level of consciousness, length of seizure, and postictal manifestation. The international classification of seizures is used most frequently to classify seizures according to whether they involve all or part of the brain from the beginning of the seizure (primary generalized seizure versus partial seizure). Further, there is a different distribution of seizure types according to age. With few exceptions, seizures in older individuals are of focal origin. Complex partial seizures are the most common type of seizure in persons 65 and older. Secondary generalized tonic clonic convulsions and simple partial seizures with motor manifestations may also occur.

CAUSES

The etiology of seizures varies with age. For older patients near the end of life, the causes are similar to those in other elderly persons. The most common causes are cerebrovascular disorders, brain tumors, metabolic disorders, and cerebral degeneration. Many physicians are not aware that seizures are a common complication of end-stage Alzheimer's disease progression, occurring in an estimated 20 percent of patients with advanced disease. Seizures can also be precipitated by medications, including tricyclic antidepressants and phenothiazines, which are commonly used at the end of life.

The differential diagnosis of seizures also includes disorders that may mimic seizures including, but not limited to, cardiovascular disease in the elderly, transient ischemic attacks including transient global amnesia, movement disorders, migraine, and psychological disorders. Despite the many known causes of seizures, it is important to note that epidemiologic studies suggest that seizures have an unknown cause in approximately 50 percent of older patients.

TREATMENT CONSIDERATIONS

Medications used to treat seizures are listed in Table 9–5, and some, such as gabapentin, phenytoin, and carbamazepine are also effective in treating neuropathic pain (discussed later in this chapter and in Chapter 6). While the preferred route of administration is typically oral, an individual with a seizure disorder who near the end of life can no longer swallow will still need seizure prophylaxis by some other route of administration. Thus, consideration should be given to using the medications that allow for the greatest number of routes of administration. The fewest daily doses and the least invasive route of administration will greatly enhance the comfort of a dying patient.

Because early aggressive treatment of prolonged seizures is thought to result in a higher percentage of termination of the seizure with smaller doses of medication and less risk to the patient, aggressive intervention to terminate the seizure should be instituted, even near the end of life. In an inpatient hospital setting, IV diazepam, 5 mg parenterally, has been the medication of choice to terminate seizure activity. The anticonvulsive effect for a single dose is brief, lasting about 20 minutes. In the home or hospice setting, reasonably good antiseizure effects have been achieved with the use of rectal diazepam. Lorazepam may be a good alternative agent in the acute treatment of seizure activity.

STATUS EPILEPTICUS

At some point during prolonged or repetitive seizures, the seizures are unlikely to end spontaneously. This point is the defining characteristic of status epilepticus. De facto criteria for the diagnosis of status epilepticus have been 30 minutes of continuous seizure activity or two or more discrete seizures without recovering consciousness in between. The focus of most discussions on treatment of status epilepticus has been generalized convulsive status epilepticus, but clearly other types exist (complex partial, epilepsia partialis continua).

MANAGEMENT ISSUES OF GENERALIZED STATUS EPILEPTICUS　Because prolonged seizures have a substantial risk of neurologic, cardiac, respiratory, renal, and orthopedic disorders, once the determination of status epilepticus is made, aggressive therapy should be instituted. Complex partial seizures should also be treated. It is recommended that sta-

Table 9–5
Anticonvulsant Drugs

Drug	Seizure Types	Usual Starting Adult Dosages	Usual Adult Dose (mg)	Therapeutic Range (mg/dL)	Usual Routes of Administration	Side Effects
Phenytoin	1. Generalized tonic clonic 2. Partial seizure	300 mg/day	300–400/day	10–20	Oral/ IV	Ataxia, gingival hypertrophy, acneiform rash, hirsutism, hepatic failure, lymphadenopathy
Carbamazepine	1. Partial seizures 2. Generalized tonic clonic	200 mg bid	800–1600/day	4–12	Oral	Drowsiness, blurred vision, diplopia, ataxia, leukopenia, hepatic failure
Valproate	1. Absence 2. Myoclonic 3. Partial seizure 4. Generalized tonic clonic	250 mg tid	1000–3000	50–100	Oral/IV	Weight gain, hair loss, tremor, thrombocytopenia, hepatic failure
Phenobarbital	1. Generalized seizures 2. Partial seizures	3 mg/kg/day	90–180	10–40	Oral/IM/IV	Sedation, hyperactivity, decreased concentration, depression
Gabapentin	Adjunct for partial seizures	300 mg tid	900–1800	Not established	Oral	lethargy, dizziness, ataxia, fatigue

tus epilepticus be treated with a single dose of lorazepam, 0.1 mg/kg, diluted with an equal volume of IV solution. The overall success rate in suppressing status epilepticus using lorazepam is approximately 65 percent. If the patient continues to have seizures, then a second agent, either phenytoin or phosphenytoin, 20 mg/kg, should be administered over 5 to 7 minutes. Other interventions include IV valproic acid, conventional as well as high-dose barbiturates, and high-dose benzodiazepines, but these are beyond the scope of this discussion.

Headaches

Headaches are among the most frequent of all pain disorders at the end of life. Headaches may result from progression of the patient's primary tumor. For example, growth of primary or metastatic brain tumors and meningeal carcinomatosis will cause headache because of increased intracranial pressure, while progressive skull metastases from multiple myeloma or breast cancer will result in headache from bone pain.

Patients with cervical radiculopathy, either from malignant or nonmalignant disease, may develop severe muscle spasm in the neck and head that will cause complaints of headache. Patients near the end of life are also susceptible to headache from causes not directly related to their terminal illness, such as migraine headaches, tension headaches, and headache due to fever.

Treatment of headache is directly dependent on the cause. For patients with suspected malignant disease of the brain or spinal cord with increased intracranial pressure, steroids may be an effective way of ameliorating symptoms. Such patients are commonly started on dexamethasone 4 mg orally or intravenously four times a day. Once symptomatic improvement occurs, the dexamethasone may be tapered slowly to the lowest dose that maintains the patient free of symptoms. For patients expected to live several months more, antineoplastic therapy, such as radiation therapy or intrathecal chemotherapy, may be considered in addition to the steroids. Nonsteroidal anti-inflammatory medications, opioid analgesics, and other measures that are effective against bone pain may be used for patients with headache caused by skull metastases (see Chapter 6). Other interventions may include antispasmodics for muscle spasms, and nonpharmacologic interventions such as heat, ice, or traction.

Peripheral Nervous System Disorders

The peripheral nervous system consists of the anterior horn cells, dorsal root ganglia, dorsal and ventral nerve roots, nerve plexi, peripheral nerves, and myoneural junctions. Damage to any part of the nervous system may result in neuropathic pain, which is widely accepted to be, at best, only partially responsive to opioid analgesia. Though the exact nature of neuropathic pain is unknown, its lack of sensitivity to opioid analgesics is thought to be due to a variety of factors including the mechanism of injury. Some commonly held theories to explain neuropathic pain include (1) inflammatory mediators at the injured nerve site, which lower nociceptive thresholds; (2) increased neuronal membrane excitability; (3) altered processing of neural impulses by the central spinal cord neurons resulting in activation of N-methyl-D-aspartate (NMDA) receptors; (4) stunted axonal regrowth, resulting in hypersensitive neuromas; and (5) a down-regulation of nociceptive inhibitory transmitters. Though knowledge of the exact pathway is unnecessary in the clinical setting, acquaintance with the variety of causal mechanisms will enhance the understanding of the need for serial trials of adjuvant medications to relieve neuropathic pain in individual patients.

A discussion of the general evaluation and treatment of neuropathic pain is presented in Chapter 6. In this chapter, the discussion will primarily focus on the different neuropathic pain syndromes that must often occur when patients are near the end of life. After reviewing the various causes of neuropathic pain, recommendations for treatment will be provided.

Focal Neuropathies

MONONEUROPATHIES

Mononeuropathies occur as a result of compression or infiltration of nerves by bony or soft tissues in the extremities. Common mononeuropathies include intercostal nerve injury from rib metastasis or local extension of chest tumors, and peroneal neuropathies at the fibular head, which are more common in cachectic, bedbound patients and patients with malignant lesions in the area of the popliteal fossa. Mononeuropathies of the cranial nerves can arise from tumors found at the base of the skull. Obturator and femoral neuropathies are seen when the tumor involves the soft tissues of the pelvis and thighs. Ulnar and radial neuropathies may result from bony lesions in the elbow or humerus.

Mononeuropathies can also result from nerve entrapment, which refers to peripheral nerve injuries that occur at specific locations where the nerve is constricted in a fibrous band or osseous tunnel. Some examples of entrapment neuropathies are carpal tunnel syndrome, ulnar neuropathy, thoracic outlet syndrome, femoral entrapment neuropathies from retroperitoneal or pelvic tumor masses, iliolingual neuropathy from tumors of the anterior superior spine, and sciatic entrapment neuropathy. Regardless of the exact mechanism or nerve involved, mononeuropathies frequently present with a combination of focal weakness, focal pain, and/or dysesthesia.

PLEXOPATHIES

Metastatic cancers can infiltrate peripheral nerves and plexi and result in severe pain and neuromuscular weakness. The most common plexopathies seen in cancer patients are cervical plexopathy, brachial plexopathy, and lumbosacral plexopathy. Low back pain is the most prevalent presenting symptom, followed by thoracic pain and cervical spine pain.

BRACHIAL PLEXOPATHY Metastatic brachial plexopathy is usually associated with spread from the supraclavicular lymph nodes, as in breast cancer or lymphoma, or from a superior sulcus (Pancoast's) tumor of the lungs. The most frequent presenting symptoms are pain located in the shoulder and axilla that radiates down the medial arm and forearm to the fourth and fifth fingers, and weakness. Pain is generally constant and severe and may be accompanied by areas of numbness and dysesthesias. Associated findings may include the presence of Horner's syndrome (ptosis, miosis, and anhidrosis due to tumor invasion of the cervical sympathetic plexus) or associated vertebral disk disease.

CERVICAL PLEXOPATHY Infiltration of the cervical plexus usually results from head and neck cancers, lymphoma, or metastasis from systemic tumors to the cervical lymph nodes or vertebrae. Pain frequently presents in the preauricular, postauricular, or anterior shoulder or neck area. Pain has been described as being both constant and intermittent with a lancinating component which may be exacerbated with swallowing or head movement. Associated findings may include an ipsilateral Horner's syndrome or hemidiaphragmatic paralysis if the phrenic nerve is involved.

LUMBOSACRAL PLEXOPATHY Invasion of the lumbosacral plexus usually results from direct extension of pelvic tumors, or from metastasis to the regional lymph nodes, sacrum, iliacus, or vertebrae. Lumbosacral plexopathies are most frequently associated with colorectal cancer, gynecologic malignancies, retroperitoneal sarcomas, lymphoma, or breast cancer. Pain is generally the presenting symptom and may be dull, aching, boring, or burning in nature and is generally unilateral, although bilateral plexopathies can occur. Pain may worsen following a bowel movement. Clinical symptoms will depend upon the level of nerve involvement. Upper lumbosacral plexopathies generally present with pain in the low back, flank, iliac crest, or anterior thigh and have associated L1-L4 dermatomal distribution deficits. Involvement of the lower plexopathies frequently presents with pain in the buttocks, perineum, and posterolateral leg and thigh with associated L4-S1 deficits including leg edema.

RADICULOPATHIES

A radiculopathy is characterized by pain or numbness in a dermatomal distribution in a region innervated by the spinal nerve roots. In cancer patients, radicular pain is most commonly caused by an epidural tumor mass, leptomeningeal carcinomatosis, or compression due to metastatic tumor arising from the vertebral body. Pain may be constant or intermittent, achy, dysesthetic, and may be localized or experienced anywhere throughout the dermatome. Radicular pain is frequently exacerbated by cough, sneezing, strain, or recumbent positioning. Herpes zoster and postherpetic neuralgias are common in cancer patients and frequently represent a classic, radicular pain pattern. Other implications of radicular pain include potential emergencies such as epidural spinal cord compression.

Epidural Spinal Cord Compression

Epidural metastasis is the most ominous complication of bony metastatic disease to the vertebral spine. It is a common complication in patients with cancer of the breast, prostate, and lung; multiple myeloma; melanoma; and renal cell carcinoma. Epidural spinal cord compression (ESCC) almost always presents with back or neck pain, either focally or in a radicular distribution, which then progresses over a period of several weeks until neurologic deficits appear. Pain is usually in the midline but sharp, shooting, radicular pain is frequently present in patients with nerve root involvement. Progressive back pain, which is aggravated by Valsalva maneuver, accompanied by a positive straight leg raise and/or positive Lhermitte's sign (shooting pain on neck flexion), and exacerbated by recumbency, should alert the clinician to the possibility of pending ESCC.

Neurologic symptoms usually begin in the lower extremities with motor weakness, paresthesias, sensory loss, and reduced or absent reflexes. The pain progressively travels proximally and patients eventually develop urinary retention and constipation. Once urinary or bowel problems appear, neurologic progression may be rapid and result in permanent dysfunction. Early recognition of symptoms and prompt initiation of treatment may reduce pain, minimize neurologic deficits, and preserve sphincter function, thereby improving the quality of life of terminally ill patients with epidural spinal cord compression.

Treatment of Neuropathic Pain

The treatment for neuropathic pain presenting as a plexopathy or mononeuropathy is primarily directed at decreasing the inflammation, preserving neurologic function, and aggressive management of pain. In patients with a reasonable life expectancy, diagnostic evaluation including a CT scan or MRI in conjunction with radiation therapy may be considered as part of primary palliative intervention. Nearer to end-of-life care, these invasive, costly, and energy-draining interventions may no longer be appropriate or desired.

The most appropriate therapeutic intervention will consist of oral steroids such as prednisone 20 mg two to three times a day or dexamethasone 4 mg four times a day. Steroids will reduce the edema that is at least partially responsible for the symptoms of cerebral and spinal cord compression, as well as manage pain due to perineural edema from infiltration or compression. An acute episode of very severe radicular pain related to a neuropathic lesion such as a plexopathy or spinal cord compression may respond dramatically to intravenous steroids followed by oral administration with dosage tapering over time. It is important to methodically reduce steroids to the lowest effective dosage to minimize the associated potential side effects such as steroid-induced myopathy, gastrointestinal distress, and neuropsychiatric manifestations including confusion, mental clouding, depression, and psychosis.

In addition to the use of steroids, most patients with neuropathic pain will require opioids and other adjuvant medications, listed in Table 9–6. See Chapter 6 for a full discussion of the treatment of neuropathic pain.

Phantom Pain

Phantom pain is manifested by symptoms of neuropathic pain in a limb that has been amputated. It may occur in patients who have amputation of a limb due to a malignancy or due to vascular disease. It has also been described in the chest wall area in women who have undergone mastectomy. Although it is thought to be of central nervous system origin, as is true of peripheral neuropathies it tends to respond to tricyclic antidepressants.

Conclusion

Neurologic symptoms present unusual challenges in end-of-life care. The manifestation of physical as well as cognitive symptoms may threaten quality of life, devastate caregivers, and tax physical, emotional, and financial resources. Furthermore, what constitutes "appropriate management" may be difficult to define as the neurologic symptoms are complicated by progressive disease and multisystem failure. Symptom control is frequently complex as self-care skills and activities of daily living are progressively compromised.

Management strategies must be based on a complete history, accurate physical assessment skills, prudent pharmacologic and interventional modalities, and comprehensive interdisciplinary support. Interventions should reflect the prognosis and life expectancy as well as the informed patient/family desires. In addition, management strategies should be guided by caring clinicians who, through conscientious application of ethical principles, acknowledge the limitations of our understanding, and support the patient and family through compassionate, individualized interventions.

Table 9–6
Medications for the Treatment of Neuropathic Pain

Drug	Routes of Administration	Usual Adult Dose	Maximum Dose
Amitriptyline	PO	10–150 mg/day	300 mg/day
Nortriptyline	PO	10–150 mg/day	150 mg/day
Dexamethasone	PO	16–96 mg/day	
Gabapentin	PO	300–1800 mg/day in 3 divided doses	1800 mg/day
Carbamazepine	PO	200–1600 mg/day in 3–4 divided doses	1600 mg/day
Clonidine	PO Topical	0.1 mg PO hs 0.1 mg/day	2.4 mg/day
Mexiletine	PO	300 mg/day in divided doses	1200 mg/day

References

Adams RD, Victor M, Ropper AH: Intracranial neoplasms and paraneoplastic disorders. *Principles of Neurology,* 6th ed. New York, McGraw-Hill, 1987, pp 642–690.

Allen RR: Neuropathic pain in the cancer patient. *Neurol Clin* 16:869, 1998.

American Pain Society: *Principles of Analgesic Use in the Treatment of Acute Pain and Cancer Pain,* 4th ed. Glenview, IL, American Pain Society, 1999.

American Psychiatric Association: *Diagnostic and Statistical Manual of Mental Disorders,* 4th ed. Washington, DC, American Psychiatric Association, 1994.

Argoff C, Wheeler A: Spinal and radicular disorders. *Neurol Clin* 16:833, 1998.

Ashby M, Fleming B, Wood M, Somogyi S: Plasma morphine and glucuronide (M3G and M6G) concentration on hospice patients. *J Pain Symptom Manage* 14:157, 1997.

Bennett G: Update on the neurophysiology of pain transmission and the modulation: Focus on NMDA-receptor. *J Pain Symptom Manage* 19:2, 2000.

Bergevin P, Bergevin RM: Recognizing delirium in terminal patients. *Amer J Hospice Palliat Care* 13:28, 1996.

Bleck TP: Management approaches to prolonged seizures and status epilepticus. *Epilepsia* 40:S49, 1999.

Bleck TP: Seizures in the critically ill. In: Parrillo JE, Bone RC, eds. *Critical Care Medicine: Principles of Diagnosis and Management.* Chicago, Mosby-Year Book, 1995, pp. 1217–1233.

Breitbart W, Bruera E, Chochinov H, Lynch M: Neuropsychiatric syndromes and psychological symptoms in patients with advanced cancer. *J Pain Symptom Manage* 10:131, 1995.

Bruera E, Franco J, Maltoni M, et al: 1995. Changing patterns of agitated impaired mental status in patients with advanced cancer: Association with cognitive monitoring, hydration, and opioid rotation. *J Pain Symptom Manage* 10:287, 1995.

Bruera E, Miller L, McCallion J, et al: Cognitive failure in patients with terminal cancer: A prospective study. *J Pain Symptom Manage,* 7:192, 1992.

Bruera E, Neumann CM: Cancer pain. In: Max M, ed. *Pain 1999; An Updated Review.* Seattle, IASP Press, 1999, pp. 25–35.

Bruera E, Neumann CM: Opioid toxicities: Assessment and management. In: Max M, ed. *Pain 1999; An Updated Review.* Seattle, IASP Press, 1999, pp. 443–457.

Burke A: Palliative care: An update on terminal restlessness. *Med Aust* 166:39, 1997.

Cairncross JG, Kim JH, Posner JB: Radiation therapy for brain metastases. *Ann Neurol* 7:529, 1980.

Cameron RB: *Practical Oncology.* Norwalk, CT, Appleton & Lange, 1994.

Caraceni A, Martini C: Neurological problems. In: Doyle D, Hanks G, MacDonald N, eds. *Oxford Textbook of Palliative Medicine,* 2nd ed. New York, Oxford University Press, 1998.

Chad D, Recht D: Neuromuscular complications of systemic cancer. *Neurol Clin* 9:901, 1991.

Chamberlain MC, Friedman H: Presentation, diagnosis, and management considerations of leptomeningeal metastases. In: Levin VA: *Cancer in the Nervous System.* New York, Churchill Livingstone, 1996, p. 281.

Cherny N, Foley K: Current approaches to the management of cancer pain: A review. *Ann Acad Med* 23:139, 1994.

Cherny N, Thaler HT, Friedlander-Klar H, et al: Opioid responsiveness of cancer pain syndromes caused by neuropathic or nociceptive mechanisms: A combined analysis of controlled, single-dose studies. *Neurology* 44:857, 1994.

Christrup L: Morphine metabolites. *Acta Anaesthesiol Scand* 41:116, 1997.

Commission on Classification and Terminology of the International League Against Epilepsy: *Epilepsia* 30:389, 1989.

Cummings JL: Current perspectives in Alzheimer's disease. *Neurology* 51 (suppl 1):S1, 1998.

Delattre JY, Krol G, Thaler HT, et al: Distribution of brain metastases. *Arch Neurol* 45:741, 1988.

Dreifuss FE, Rosman NP, Cloyd JC, et al: A comparison of rectal diazepam gel and placebo for acute repetitive seizures. *N Engl J Med* 338:1869, 1998.

England J: Entrapment neuropathies. *Curr Opin Neurol* 12:597, 1999.

Fabiszewski KJ, Volicer B, Volicer L: Effect of antibiotic treatment on outcome of fevers in institutionalized Alzheimer patients. *JAMA* 263:3168, 1990.

Fainsinger R: Use of sedation by a hospital palliative care support team. *J Palliat Care* 14:51, 1998.

Fainsinger R, Miller M, Bruera E, et al: Symptom control during the last week of life on a palliative care unit. *J Palliat Care* 7:5, 1996.

Fainsinger R, Tapper M, Bruera E: A perspective on the management of delirium in terminally ill patients on a palliative care unit. *J Palliat Care* 9:4, 1993.

Ferrante FM: Principles of opioid pharmacotherapy: Practical implications of basic mechanisms. *J Pain Symptom Manage* 11:265, 1996.

Fine P: Conflicts in medical care at the end of life. In: Slatkin N, chair, Rhoda G. and Bernard G. Sarnat symposium for supportive care of the patient with cancer and other life-threatening diseases. Conducted at City of Hope National Medical Center, Duarte, CA, October 1999.

Fitzgibbon D, Ready L: Intravenous high-dose methadone administered by patient controlled analgesia and continuous infusion for the treatment of cancer pain refractory to high-dose morphine. *Pain* 73:259, 1997.

Galer B: Neuropathic pain of peripheral origin: Advances in pharmacologic treatment. *Neurology* 45 (suppl 9):S17, 1995.

Galicich JH, Sundaresan N, Thaler HT: Surgical treatment of single brain metastases. Factors associated with survival. *Cancer* 45:381, 1980.

Geldmacher DS, Whitehouse PJ: Evaluation of dementia. *N Engl J Med* 335:330, 1996.

Greig NH, Ries LG, Yancik R, et al: Increasing annual incidence of primary malignant brain tumors in the elderly. *J Natl Cancer Inst* 82:1621, 1990.

Grond S, Radbruch L, Meuser T, et al: Assessment and treatment of neuropathic cancer pain following WHO guidelines. *Pain* 79:15, 1999.

Hanks G, Forbes K: Opioid responsiveness. *Acta Anaesthesiol Scand* 41:154, 1997.

Hauser WA: Epidemiology of seizures in the elderly. In: Rowan AJ, Ramsay RE, eds. *Seizures and Epilepsy in the Elderly.* New York, Butterworth-Heinemann, 1997, pp. 7–18.

Hewitt D, Portenoy R: Adjuvant drugs for neuropathic cancer pain. In: Bruera E, Portenoy R, eds. *Topics in Palliative Care,* vol 2. New York, Oxford University Press, 1998, pp. 41–62.

Iscoe N, Bruera E, Choo R: Prostate cancer: Palliative care. *CMAJ* 160:365, 1999.

Jacox A, Carr DB, Payne R, et al: *Management of Cancer Pain: Clinical Practice Guideline #9.* AHCPR pub. no. 94-0592. Rockville, MD, Public Health Service, 1994.

Jaeckle KA: Nerve plexus metastases. *Neurol Clin* 9:857, 1991.

Kelly JB, Payne R: Pain syndromes in cancer patients. *Neurol Clin* 9:937, 1991.

Kokkoris CP: Leptomeningeal carcinomatosis: How does cancer reach the pia-arachnoid? *Cancer* 51:154, 1983.

Lawlor P, Gagnon B, et al: Occurrence, causes, and outcome of delirium in patients with advanced cancer. *Arch Intern Med* 160:786, 2000.

Lipton RB, Stewart WF: Epidemiology and comorbidity of migraine. In: Goadsby PJ, Siberstein SD, eds. *Headache: Blue Books of Practical Neurology.* Boston, Butterworth-Heinemann, 1997, pp. 75–94.

Lloyd-Williams M: A survey of palliative care given to patients with end-stage dementia. *Palliat Med* 10:63, 1996. Abstract.

Lovejoy N, Matteis M: Pharmacokinetics and pharmacodynamics of mood-altering drugs in patients with cancer. *Cancer Nursing* 19:407, 1996.

MacDonald N, Der L, Allan S, Champion P: Opioid hyperexcitability: The application of alternate opioid therapy. *Pain* 53:353, 1993.

Mailis A, Bennett G: Painful neurological disorders: Clinical aspects. In: Aronoff GM, ed. *Evaluation and Treatment of Chronic Pain,* 3rd ed. Baltimore, Williams & Wilkins, 1999, pp. 93–114.

Maluso-Bolton T: Terminal agitation. *J Hospice Palliat Nurs* 2:9, 2000.

March PA: Terminal restlessness. *Am J Hospice Palliat Care* 15:51, 1998.

Martin LA, Hagen N: Neuropathic pain in cancer patients: Mechanisms, syndromes, and clinical controversies. *J Pain Symptom Manage* 14:99, 1997.

Massie MG, Holland J, Glass E: Delirium in terminally ill cancer patients. *Am J Psychiatry* 8:1048, 1983.

Mayeux R, Sano M: Treatment of Alzheimer's disease. *N Engl J Med* 341:1670, 1999.

Morita T, Inoue S, Chihara S: Sedation for symptom control in Japan: The importance of intermittent use and communication with family members. *J Pain Symptom Manage* 12:32, 1996.

O'Brien T, Kelly M, Saunders C: Motor neuron disease: a hospice perspective. *BMJ* 304:471, 1992.

Olsen AK, Sjogren P: Neurotoxic effects of opioids. *Eur J Palliat Care* 3:139, 1996.

Osborne R, Joel S, Slevin ML: Morphine intoxication in renal failure: The role of morphine-6-glucuronide. *BMJ* 292:1548, 1986.

Panerai A, Bianchi M, Sacerdote P, et al: Antidepressants in cancer pain. *J Palliat Care* 7:42, 1991.

Payne R, Gonzales G: Pathophysiology of pain in cancer and other terminal diseases. In: Doyle D, Hanks G, MacDonald N, eds. *Oxford Textbook of Palliative Medicine,* 2nd ed. New York, Oxford University Press, 1998, pp. 299–310.

Pereira J, Hanson J, Bruera E: The frequency and clinical course of cognitive impairment in patients with terminal cancer. *Cancer* 79:835, 1997.

Portenoy R: Current pharmacotherapy of chronic pain. *J Pain Symptom Manage* 19:16, 2000.

Portenoy R: Opioid and adjuvant analgesics. In: Max M, ed. *Pain 1999. An Updated Review.* Seattle, IASP Press, 1999, pp. 25–35.

Portenoy, R. (1998). Adjuvant analgesics in pain management. In Doyle D, Hanks M, MacDonald N, eds. *Oxford Textbook of Palliative Medicine,* 2nd ed. New York, Oxford University Press, 1998, pp. 361–390.

Portenoy R: *Contemporary Diagnosis and Management of Pain in Oncologic and AIDS Patients,* 2nd ed. Newtown, PA: Handbooks in Health Care, 1998.

Portenoy R: Neuropathic pain. In: Portenoy R, Kanner R, eds. *Pain management: Theory and Practice.* Philadelphia, F. A. Davis, 1996, pp. 83–125.

Posner JB: Management of brain metastases. *Rev Neurol* 148:477, 1992.

Posner JB. Clinical manifestations of brain metastasis. In: Weiss L, Gilbert HA, Posner JB, eds. *Brain Metastasis.* Boston, GK Hall, 1980, p. 207.

Rall TW, Schleifer LS: Drugs effective in the therapy of the epilepsies. In: Gilman AG, *The Pharmacological Basis of Therapeutics,* 8th ed. Maidstone, McGraw Hill, 1993.

Ray BS, Wolff HG: Experimental studies on headache: Pain sensitive structures of the head and their significance in headache. *Arch Surg* 41:813, 1940.

Rhiner MI, Coluzzi P: Managing breakthrough pain. *ADVANCE for Nurse Practitioners* Jan. 1998, pp. 41–68.

Ripamonti C, Zecca E, Bruera E: An update on the clinical use of methadone for cancer pain. *Pain* 70:109, 1997.

Rowan AJ: Reflections on the treatment of seizures in the elderly population. *Neurology* 51:3, 1998.

Sandyk R: Sodium valproate-induced analgesia: possible role of the GABA-ergic system in pain mechanism. *J Clin Psychopharmacol* 6:388, 1986.

Saper JR: Headache disorders. *Med Clin of North Am* 83:663, 1999.

Scheuer ML, Pedley TA: The evaluation and treatment of seizures. *N Engl J Med* 323:1468, 1990.

Shafer PO: Epilepsy and seizures. *Nurs Clin North Am* 34:3, 1999.

Sindrup S, Jensen T: Efficacy of pharmacological treatments of neuropathic pain: An update and effect related to mechanism of drug action. *Pain* 83:389, 1999.

Sjogren P, Thunedborg L, Christrup L, et al: Is the development of hyperalgesia, allodynia and myoclonus related to morphine metabolism during long-term administration? *Acta Anaesthesiol Scand* 42:1070, 1998.

Stiefel F, Fainsinger R, Bruera E: Acute confusional states in patients with advanced cancer. *J Pain Symptom Manage* 7:94, 1992.

Stone P, Phillips C, Spruit O, Waight C: A comparison of the use of sedatives in a hospital support team and in hospice. *Palliat Med* 11:140, 1997.

Teasell RW: Managing advanced multiple sclerosis. *Can Fam Physician* 39:1127, 1993.

Teener J, Farrar J: Neuromuscular dysfunction and supportive care. In: Berger A, Portenoy R, Weissman D, eds. *Principles and Practices of Supportive Oncology.* Philadelphia, Lippincott-Raven, 1998, pp. 465–476.

Thapar K, Laws ER: Tumors of the central nervous system: Diagnosis and therapy of brain tumors. In: Murphy GP, Lawrence W, Lenhard RE, eds. *Clinical Oncology,* 2nd ed. Atlanta, American Cancer Society, 1995, p. 382.

Thomas Z, Bruera E: Use of methadone in highly tolerant patients receiving parenteral hydromorphone. *J Pain Symptom Manage* 10:315, 1995.

Treiman DM, Meyers PD, Walton NY, et al: A comparison of four treatments for generalized convulsive status epilepticus. Veterans Affairs Status Epilepticus Cooperative Study Group. *N Engl J Med* 339:792, 1998.

Twycross R: Symptom control: The problem areas. *Palliat Med* 7 (suppl 1):1, 1993.

Ventafridda V, Ripamonti C, De Conno F, et al: Symptom prevalence and control during cancer patients' last days of life. *J Palliat Care* 6:7, 1990.

Vigano A, Fan D, Bruera E: Individualized use of methadone and opioid rotation in the comprehensive management of cancer pain associated with poor prognostic indicators. *Pain* 67:115, 1996.

Walker MD, Green SB, Byar DP, et al: Randomized comparisons of radiotherapy and nitrosoureas for the treatment of malignant glioma after surgery. *N Engl J Med* 303:1323, 1980.

Walton NY, Treiman DM: Rational polytherapy in the treatment of status epilepticus. *Epilepsy Res* 1996: 11(suppl):123, 1996.

Wasserstrom WR, Glass JP, Posner JB: Diagnosis and treatment of leptomeningeal metastasis from solid tumors: Experience with 90 patients. *Cancer* 49:759, 1982.

Watson CP, Babul N: Efficacy of oxycodone in neuropathic pain. *Neurology* 50:1837, 1998.

Weinberger J, Nicklas WJ, Berl S: Mechanism of action of anticonvulsants. *Neurology* 26:162, 1976.

Woodruff R: *Symptom Control in Advanced Cancer.* Melbourne, Australia, Asperula Pty, Ltd., 1997.

Woolf C, Decosterd I: Implications of recent advances in the understanding of pain pathophysiology for the assessment of pain in patients. *Pain* 6:141, 1999.

Woolf C, Mannion R: Neuropathic pain: Aetiology, symptoms, mechanisms, and management. *Lancet* 353:954, 1999.

Yaksh TL, Chaplan SR: Physiology and pharmacology of neuropathic pain. *Anesthesiol Clin North Am* 15:335, 1997.

Domingo Gomez
Joel S. Policzer

Dermatologic Problems

Introduction

Caring for the skin and mucous membranes of patients near the end of life can be challenging. The skin is in full sight of both the patient and the caregiver, and new lesions are usually noted immediately. Skin disorders can be very troubling to patients, causing interference with comfort, interpersonal interactions, eating, and voiding. Skin lesions can cause symptoms ranging from minor irritation to recurrent bleeding to intense, unremitting pain and itching. Lack of activity as the end of life approaches can lead to the development of skin breakdown, and foul-smelling drainage from secondarily infected wounds may keep both medical personnel and family at a distance.

Recognition of potential causes of skin and mucous membrane disorders is especially important because end-of-life patients do not have the luxury of waiting for diagnostic tests and biopsies to return from the laboratory before therapy is started. Thus, treatment planning is based on clinical identification of the most likely diagnosis, and therapy is instituted rapidly to effect palliation of discomfort as soon as is possible.

The goal of this chapter is to review common disorders of the skin and mucous membranes that occur in patients who are near the end of life. The all too common and challenging problems related to pressure ulcers will be examined first, followed by a review of the treatment of complications of neoplastic diseases such as fistula formation and the fungating tumor mass. Pruritis will be discussed next, and then the various skin lesions that can cause pruritis, including infections of the skin, drug reactions, and the dermatitides. Finally, there will be a discussion of the various lesions that can affect the mucous membranes of the mouth.

Paraneoplastic skin disorders (acanthosis nigricans, necrolytic migratory erythema) and other specific skin lesions (bullous pemphigus or pemphigoid) that occur uncommonly in terminally ill patients are not reviewed in this chapter. Rather,

the focus of this chapter is to examine skin disorders that occur across the spectrum of patients near the end of life, irrespective of diagnosis. Interested reader is referred to any good medical or dermatologic textbook for a review of uncommon disease-specific disorders.

Pressure Ulcers

Pressure ulcers are caused by unrelieved pressure to an area of skin over a prolonged period of time that results in damage of the underlying tissue. Pressure ulcers are staged based upon the depth of tissue damage (Table 10–1).

Pressure ulcers have a high prevalence among patients who are near the end of life. Some 14 to 19 percent of hospice patients cared for at home, and up to 28 percent of hospice patients cared for in long-term care facilities, have stage I pressure

Table 10–1

Staging of Pressure Ulcers

Stage I	Nonblanchable erythema of intact skin
Stage II	Partial-thickness skin loss involving epidermis, dermis, or both. This can appear as an abrasion, blister, or shallow crater
Stage III	Full-thickness skin loss involving damage to or necrosis of subcutaneous tissue; damage extends to, but not through, fascia
Stage IV	Full-thickness skin loss with extensive destruction or damage to muscle, bone, or supporting structures
Unstageable	Presence of eschar over the ulcer preventing assessment of depth

ulcers. Stage II pressure ulcers occur in approximately 8 percent of hospice home care patients and 11 percent of hospice patients living in nursing homes. Risk factors for pressure ulcers (Table 10–2) are well established and include many common conditions that are present when patients are near the end of life.

Pressure ulcers are associated with significant morbidity and mortality. Infection is the most serious complication. Infection may be localized; may spread subcutaneously, causing cellulitis; may spread to the underlying bone, causing osteomyelitis; or may result in septicemia. In fact, of patients who have pressure ulcers and bacteremia, the ulcer itself is the source of the organism in half the patients, and the mortality rate from sepsis associated with pressure ulcers is more than 50 percent. Pain is another major symptom associated with pressure ulcers, with about half of patients able to report pain indicating that there is pain in the affected area.

Prevention

Pressure ulcers result from exposure of the skin to high pressure over a short period of time, or to lower pressure for prolonged periods. In most patients, the exposure of the skin to such pressure is a result of decreasing activity from the immobility

Table 10–2

Risk Factors for Development of Pressure Sores

Increasing age
Male gender
History of cerebrovascular accident
Diabetes mellitus
Altered level of consciousness
Poor tissue perfusion and low blood pressure
Decrease in skinfold thickness
Contractures
Urinary and fecal incontinence
Decrease in serum protein and albumin

that is associated with progressive illness. Conditions responsible for this immobility may include primary conditions such as muscle weakness from deconditioning, paralysis, and fatigue. Decreased movement may also occur in patients who are still somewhat mobile but who have lost the motivation to change positions. For example, in situations where movement aggravates pain, patients will voluntarily decrease their activity. Depressed patients, as a symptom of the illness, also tend to remain in one position. Finally, conditions that block the perception of the pain that is evoked by pressure damage will prevent the pain stimulus from signaling the patient to move, thus allowing the pressure damage to continue. Examples of conditions in which this may occur, and which are common near the end of life, include damage to the central nervous system or peripheral nervous structures and the use of medications such as sedatives or analgesics that can cloud the sensorium.

Prevention measures are summarized in Table 10–3 and discussed in the next sections.

TURNING

Turning the patient is still believed to be the best preventive measure and it must be done frequently. The standard is to turn patients every 2 to 3 hours, based on the observation that patients turned on this schedule had fewer pressure ulcers than those turned less often. However, as with all facets of care near the end of life, this standard needs to be individualized for each patient. Some patients will require turning more often, while other patients may be at the phase of their life where they should be left alone and not moved at all.

SKIN CARE

A second key to the prevention of pressure ulcers is good skin care. The goal of such care is to maintain and improve tissue tolerance to pressure. The full skin surface, especially areas over bony prominences prone to pressure damage, must be inspected daily. The skin should be cleansed

Table 10–3
Prevention of Pressure Ulcers

ACTIVITY	INSTRUCTIONS
Turning	Frequently: Usually every 2 to 3 hours
Skin care	Wash with warm water, nondrying soaps
	Moisturizers
	Avoid hot water, drying soaps
	Avoid overhydration
Positioning	Heel: Lift leg to suspend foot
	Sacrum and coccyx: Side-position,
	less than 90 degrees
Lift patient without sliding	Undersheet
	Mechanical lift
Pressure-reducing surfaces	Air mattress or bed
	Water mattress or bed

with warm water, nondrying soaps, and moisturizers; hot water and drying soaps should be avoided. The skin should be cleansed as quickly as possible after soiling to prevent the added damage of prolonged contact with acidic body waste. Although the skin needs to be kept moist, overhydration will also compromise the skin's ability to serve as a barrier. Moist, damp skin is more permeable to irritants, and bacteria will colonize more readily. Therefore, moisture barriers should be used to prevent the accumulation of too much moisture.

POSITIONING

Positioning of various body areas susceptible to pressure ulcers is another important aspect of preventive care. The heels of the feet, which are the most common sites for pressure ulcers, should be protected by lifting the legs up onto a pillow to suspend the foot without pressure on the heels. The risk of sacral and coccygeal ulcers may be reduced by placing patients in a side-lying position, but this position should not place the body perpendicular to the bed, as placing the patient at a 90-degree angle places too much pressure over the greater trochanter of the hip, risking ulcer formation there.

Keeping frail and fragile skin from sliding and dragging across surfaces is another important preventative measure. Devices, ranging from a simple undersheet to full mechanical lifts, should be used whenever patients need to be lifted and moved.

MATTRESSES

Placing high-risk patients on pressure-reducing surfaces, such as air and water mattresses or full air or waterbeds, is another way to help prevent pressure ulcers. Studies do not seem to indicate that one system is superior to another; rather, any and all of these mattresess can produce benefit for some patients. In genereal, high-density foam mattresses are better than standard hospital mattresses and should be preferentially used. However, none of these surfaces is a substitute for frequent repositioning and proper care of the fragile skin, which must be provided to reduce the risk of pressure ulcers in patients near the end of life.

NUTRITION

Finally, improvement in nutritional status is believed to assist in the prevention and treatment of pressure ulcers, although in reality, the literature does not support this concept. It has been suggested that certain foods, such as citrus fruits, green leafy vegetables, grains, meat, fish, and eggs, may be helpful in the promotion of wound healing. However, for patients near the end of life, poor nutritional status is the norm, and it is unlikely that one will be able to reverse a patient from a state of poor nutrition. Therefore, aggressive nutritional support in this population in an effort to prevent or promote the healing of pressure ulcers is likely to be ineffective and may be more of a burden than a benefit.

Treatment of Pressure Ulcers

Although healing is the usual goal of pressure ulcer care, this goal may not be a realistic outcome for patients near the end of life. The potential for healing depends on the status of affected patients and their expected overall time of survival. For example, it may be possible to work toward the healing of a deep ulcer when a patient has a prognosis for survival of several months or more. On the other hand, if a patient has a life expectancy of days to a couple of weeks, the goal of care for even a shallow ulcer may be to simply keep the area clean and uninfected. The treatment strategy for pressure ulcers, based upon the stage of the ulcer, is summarized in Table 10–4 and discussed next.

STAGE I

Stage I pressure ulcers are defined by the presence of erythema without other signs of overt tissue injury. Despite the intactness of the skin, the patient is at increased risk for skin breakdown and

Table 10–4

Treatment of Pressure Ulcers

STAGE	GOALS OF TREATMENT	RECOMMENDED TREATMENT
I	Prevention	See Table 10–3
II	Keep area clean.	Gently cleanse area with saline and pat dry.
	Keep area infection free.	Cover with hydrocolloid or hydrogel dressing.
	Prevent further tissue damage.	Change dressing every 3–7 days or when drainage occurs.
	Freedom from pain.	
III	Keep area clean.	Gently cleanse area with saline and pat dry.
IV	Keep area infection free.	Minimal drainage:
	Prevent further tissue damage.	Apply thin coating of hydrogel.
	Freedom from pain.	Cover wound with saline-saturated gauze.
		Cover with dry gauze.
		Change once or twice a day.
		Large amount of drainage:
		Apply alginate pad or rope.
		Cover with gauze or transparent film dressing.
		Change daily.
		Eschar or necrotic tissue:
		Apply damp to dry normal saline dressings.
		Change every 8 hours.
		Debridement (mechanical, enzymatic, autolytic debridement).

the development of higher-stage lesions. Therefore, the treatment of choice is prevention, using the techniques described earlier and in Table 10–3. While some caregivers may consider the placement of dressings or other skin barriers as well, there has been no demonstrated benefit to these forms of intervention for stage I pressure ulcers.

STAGE II

Stage II pressure ulcers are shallow, have minimal necrotic tissue, and usually are not infected. They do not enter the subcutaneous tissue, muscle, or bone. The goal of treatment is to maintain a moist, physiologic environment by keeping the area clean and uninfected, and by preventing damage to surrounding normal tissue.

The wound should be gently cleansed with saline; scrubbing should be avoided. The area is then patted dry and covered with a dressing designed to keep the ulcer bed moist to keep the area clean and reduce pain. Optimal dressings include hydrocolloid or hydrogel preparations, semipermeable foams, and polyurethane films. The dressing should be changed every 3 to 7 days, or when drainage seeps out from under the dressing edge.

STAGES III AND IV

Stage III ulcers penetrate through the dermis and into the subcutaneous tissue, while stage IV lesions involve destruction through the subcutaneous tissue and involve fascia, muscle, joints, and/or bone. Healing of these ulcers is by secondary intent and can take many months, which is unrealistic for patients near the end of life. Therefore, the maintenance of a clean, uninfected wound with minimization of pain would be a much more achievable goal in this population.

All stage III and IV ulcers should be cleansed with saline and gently patted dry. Further treatment depends upon whether the wound has minimal drainage, large amounts of drainage, or an eschar or necrotic tissue present.

When there is minimal drainage, a thin layer of a hydrogel should be applied to the wound. The wound should then be loosely covered with gauze saturated in normal saline, and then covered with dry gauze. This dressing should be changed once or twice a day. Alternatively, a hydrogel or hydrocolloid wafer can be placed over the wound and covered with dry gauze. This only needs changing every 2 to 3 days.

For wounds with larger amounts of drainage, an absorptive dressing such as alginate, in the form of a pad or a rope, should be applied into the wound. The wound should then be covered with a gauze or transparent film dressing and changed daily or as needed. An alternative treatment would be to loosely pack the wound with gauze that is damp with normal saline and covered with dry gauze. This should also be changed daily.

When there is an eschar or necrotic tissue present, the wound should be covered with damp to dry normal saline dressings that are changed every 8 hours. It is important that necrotic tissue be removed to reduce the risk of infection, as necrotic tissue can support the growth of bacteria. Enzymatic debridement of necrotic tissue can be accomplished using topical enzyme creams such as collagenase or papain. Removal of this tissue could also be done by sharp debridement using forceps and blade, but this should be avoided, especially when patients are near the end of life.

Autolytic debridement is another method of removing necrotic tissue. This is accomplished by covering the ulcer with a dressing as outlined, and instead of changing the dressing as drainage increases, allowing the tissue fluid to accumulate. Macrophages and white cells in the fluid remove bacteria and necrotic debris via a natural process.

Fistulas

A fistula is defined as an abnormal communication between two hollow organs, or between a hollow organ and the skin. Patients who develop fistulas near the end of life are most often those suffering from complications of progressive and advanced malignant disease, although occasional patients will develop fistulas from nonmalignant causes. Fistulas can be extremely distressing to patients due to interference with normal bodily functions, alteration in self-image, and the uncontrolled leakage of fluid that is often malodorous and can damage surrounding skin. As with pressure ulcers, management of these fistulas near the end of life requires a systematic approach and the recognition that these patients often will not have healing as a goal.

Enterocutaneous Fistulas

Enterocutaneous fistulas occur between the gastrointestinal tract and the skin, usually as the result of progressive malignant disease affecting the gastrointestinal tract or as a complication of prior radiation therapy.

Due to the acidic nature of intestinal fluid, discharge of intestinal contents through the fistula will cause skin breakdown and concomitant pain. Proper skin protection needs to be planned so that irritated skin is soothed and further breakdown prevented. The affected area of the skin should be cleansed with warm water, avoiding soaps and irritant cleansers. An appliance, such as an ostomy bag, should then be placed to both capture the leaking fluid and to protect the surrounding skin. Application of the stoma adhesive as close as possible to the fistula borders is desirable to afford maximal protection to the skin. To make the best seal, the adhesive area of the appliance must be placed on as flat a surface as possible, which may be difficult when fistula sites are located on irregular anatomic areas. In such circumstances, anatomic creases may be filled with an ostomy sealing agent. The hole in the adhesive of the bag must be cut as closely as possible to the shape of the stoma. Once applied, the bag should be emptied and changed frequently to avoid the weight of the effluent from pulling on the adhesive and causing leakage.

If the fistula is very large or the skin is so excoriated that the appliance will not adhere, low-pressure suction may be applied to control the fistula output and allow the skin to heal. Carboxymethylcellulose or another barrier cream should be applied around the tube site.

A well-fitting appliance with a tight seal will prevent the other complication of fistulas—the malodorous nature of the discharge. These odors are embarrassing to the patient and often limit contact between the patient and family or other caregivers. Activitated charcoal, 4 to 8 grams per day, or cholorophyll tablets taken by mouth, may help to control the odor, though charcoal may also affect the absorption of other medication and, therefore, must be used with caution. In addition, use of scented candles and aromatherapy oil in the patient's room can serve to mask odor if necessary.

Urinary Fistulas

VESICOENTERIC FISTULAS

Formation of a fistula between the urinary bladder and the GI tract can occur at any level of the bowel. The problem almost always derives from pathology of the GI tract such as malignancy, inflammatory bowel disease, or diverticulitis. Rarely does the original problem come from the bladder. Symptoms can range from pneumaturia (passage of gas and froth in the urine), to urine with a foul smell, to passage of frank fecal material in the urine.

Management is dependent on the overall clinical status of the patient. If symptoms are severe enough, the patient's prognosis for survival is sufficiently long, and the patient's clinical condition warrants, surgical correction of the fistula may be attempted. If the fistula is large or not surgically correctable, diversion of the fecal stream with a simple loop colostomy (operative externalization of a loop of colon proximal to the fistula) can be considered. Patients near the end of life who are not surgical candidates require compassionate supportive care. Urine should be removed as quickly as possible after voiding. If odor is the main problem, bladder catheterization and collection of urine into a closed system may be effective palliation.

VESICOVAGINAL FISTULAS

Vesicovaginal fistulas are most often the result of gynecologic malignancy, surgery, or local trauma. Characteristically there is leakage of urine from the bladder into the vagina. If there is only a small leak, this may be managed by vaginal packing or by bladder catherization. In situations where there is extensive damage to the pelvic organs, urinary diversion from the upper renal tracts may be needed to avoid a situation where the patient is continually incontinent.

Cancers of the Skin

Malignant involvement of the skin can occur from a variety of neoplastic disorders. Primary cancers of the skin include basal cell carcinoma, squamous cell carcinoma, and malignant melanoma. Many solid tumors and hematologic malignancies will invade the skin secondarily, either through direct invasion or metastatic spread. As patients near the end of life, progressive malignant involvement of the skin, whether of primary or secondary origin, can be a troubling and distressing problem.

Treatment

Near the end of life, treatment of malignant skin lesions is usually symptomatic. Therefore, asymptomatic, slow-growing lesions can often be left alone. In patients with hematologic malignancies with skin involvement, small doses of oral antineoplastic agents such as hydroxyurea, or corticosteroids, may reduce tumor mass just enough to retard progression and keep the lesions from ulcerating and/or causing pain.

Rapidly enlarging, painful lesions, which often ulcerate or fungate over time, are much more difficult to treat. If the lesion is localized and the patient is a surgical candidate, then local excision may be indicated. If the malignancy is radiosensitive, then radiation therapy may be attempted. Occasionally, systemic chemotherapy may be effective as well. More often, however, the patient is not a surgical candidate, other antineoplastic therapy has been unsuccessful, and/or the size and location of the lesion prevents local excision with clear margins and a chance for healing. In such circumstances, local care of the lesion is the only treatment available. Treatment recommendations are listed in Table 10–5.

These lesions should be kept dry and uninfected if possible, and dressings must be changed frequently. As dressing changes may be painful, it is suggested that analgesics be given one-half to one hour prior. The lesion should be irrigated with warm saline. If bleeding is noted, gauze soaked in a solution containing 1:1000 epinephrine may be used for control. (Reports suggest that, depending on the extent of bleeding, undiluted solutions as well as solutions diluting the epinephrine to as little as 1:200,000 have been effective. There is minimal risk of side effects, as topically applied epinephrine solutions are poorly absorbed systemically.) If the lesions are red, inflamed, and malodorous, irrigation with metronidazole solution or application of sterile metronidazole gel may be useful. The gel is preferred because it soothes, stays on the skin, and helps reduce infection and any odors. Natural (i.e, unflavored) yogurt may also be used, as it is soothing and reduces anaerobic infection as well. Oral metronidazole, 500 mg three times a day, may be given to reduce any odor caused by bacterial overgrowth.

If the lesion is large or deep and there are signs of local infection, topical antimicrobial agents can be applied. If infection is more severe, then systemic antibiotics may be helpful, with the choice of antibiotics depending on the organism or organisms cultured. If the lesion is not infected, enzymatic debridement can be attempted, or if there is

Table 10–5
Treatment of Fungating Lesions

Administer analgesia one-half to one hour prior to dressing change.
Soak off prior dressing with warm water.
If bleeding noted, hold gauze soaked with 1:1000 epinephrine over bleeding points.
Irrigate lesion with normal saline.
If lesions are red, inflamed, and/or malodorous apply one of the following:
    metronidazole gel, metronidazole solution, natural yogurt.
If lesion appears infected, apply topical antibiotic. If infection appears severe, use
    systemic antibiotics as well.
If lesion is not infected, enzymatic debridement may be useful; if an exudate is
    present, pack loosely with an absorbent nonadherent hydrophilic dressing.
Apply a nonadherent dressing, made of absorbent material if an exudate is present.
Hold dressing in place with tubular elastic netting.
Place charcoal pads under the netting to absorb any odors.

sufficient exudate, absorbent nonadherent hydrophilic packing can be placed.

After the lesion has been cared for, it should be covered with a nonadherent dressing. If an exudate is present, the dressing should be of an absorbent material. The dressing should be held in place with tubular elastic netting; to help reduce odor, charcoal pads, which should be available from the pharmacy, may be placed under the netting.

Skin Lesions Caused by Physical Factors

Skin Tears

Due to the effects of long-standing chronic illness and poor nutrition, the skin of patients near the end of life often deteriorates into a state marked by poor elasticity and lack of lubrication. Use of steroids, as is common in many chronic illnesses, adds to deterioration of the supporting skin structures. As a result of these changes, any shear stress caused by moving the skin across sheets and bedclothes can cause a superficial tear.

The best treatment of skin tears is prevention. Because the main cause is loss of natural skin oils for lubrication, emollients that will trap moisture after bathing are very effective. Harsh cleansers that can dry the skin further are to be avoided. Attempts should be made to move patients as carefully as possible, with lifting rather than dragging movements.

Once a tear has occurred, it can be treated as a superficial burn with topical ointments and dressings (described in the next section). As these patients have compromised immune systems, tears are prone to infection and may require oral antibiotics if painful sequelae occur.

Thermal Burns

In an attempt to relieve the pain that can so often complicate the end of life, caregivers commonly use heating pads as a form of nonpharmacologic relief. Patients with altered mental status may not be able to complain of the heat, and therefore their frail skin may burn easily at settings that would be tolerated by otherwise healthy skin. These burns are usually first degree, involving the epidermis superficially and accompanied by tenderness and erythema, or second-degree, involving the epidermis and varying thicknesses of the dermis.

Treatment focuses on wound care, pain relief, and prevention of infection. For superficial burns, the affected area is soothed with cool compresses and then covered with an occlusive dressing. A hydrocolloid dressing is used if the burn is over a pressure site. Healing generally occurs within about one week. Analgesia can usually be provided by acetaminophen with or without a nonsteroidal anti-inflammatory agent. Infection is generally not a problem.

Burns that break the epithelium are exquisitely painful and usually require an opioid analgesic for management of the pain (see Chapter 6). Treatment involves cleansing the site with soap and sterile water to remove loose skin and debris, preventing these from becoming potential sources of infection. A topical antimicrobial agent is then applied. Silver sulfadiazine 1 percent is commonly used, but bacitracin or Polysporin can be used if the patient is sulfa allergic. Whereas bulky gauze dressings have classically been used, occlusive dressings are preferred, as they provide immediate pain relief, prevent drying of the wound, and speed healing. Dressings should be changed as necessary and once epithelialization begins, the lesions should be treated in a similar fashion to that recommended for first-degree burns.

Pruritis

Both pain and itch occur due to activation of the unmyelinated C-fibers in the peripheral nerves. The same chemicals—histamines, proteases, and prostaglandins—mediate both of these sensations. However, the two sensations are perceived differ-

Table 10–6
Causes of Pruritis

ETIOLOGY	EXAMPLES
Primary skin diseases	Xerosis (skin dryness)
	Many others
Metabolic	Hepatic dysfunction
	Renal impairment
	Hypo or hyperthyroidism
Hematologic	Iron deficiency
	Polycythemia vera
Cancer	Lymphoma (esp. Hodgkin's disease)
	Leukemia
	Cholestatic jaundice due to metasteses from many solid tumors
Drugs	Opioid analgesics
	Allergic drug reaction
Infestations	Scabies
Infections	Candidiasis
Allergic reactions, urticaria	Laundry detergents and soaps
Psychogenic	

ently by patients. Pain induces withdrawal, while pruritis induces scratching; opioids palliate pain, but can cause pruritis secondary to histamine release. Pain can occur anywhere, but pruritis is limited to the skin. Therefore, the transmission of the sensation of pruritis is likely via pathways distinct from pain.

Etiology and Treatment

As with any other physical symptom, the primary therapy of pruritis is dependent on first identifying the underlying cause or causes. Near the end of life, these causes (listed in Table 10–6) may be related to the patient's primary illness, comorbid conditions, allergies to medications and other substances, or infection or may be psychogenic in origin.

Once the etiology of pruritis is identified, treatment can be planned appropriately. When the cause of pruritis is due to skin infection or infestation, or is secondary to a medication allergy, the most effective strategy will be to treat the primary cause. Specific treatment recommendations for treating various causes of itching are found in other sections of this chapter.

In many situations near the end of life, one cannot influence the underlying disease sufficiently to relieve pruritis, and therefore effective palliation of the symptom is required. Skin dryness, which may be a primary cause of pruritis, is also present in most patients who have pruritis from another cause. Therefore moisturizers are an essential basic treatment for patients who experience itching. Wet wraps placed over a liberal application of a topical moisturizer are very effective.

Medications that can help counteract pruritis are listed in Table 10–7. A nonspecific topical agent such as menthol (0.5 to 2.0 percent) in aqueous cream may be beneficial as a soothing agent and it can also act as a mild anesthetic or counterirritant. Another approach is the use of topical steroids, especially when there is an inflammatory component to the skin that accompanies the itch. Providing the topical steroid as an ointment rather than as a cream has the added benefit of keeping the skin moist, palliating the dryness often present, and avoiding the stinging sensation that sometimes accompanies application of creams.

For most patients with pruritis, however, oral antihistamines such as diphenhydramine or hydroxyzine are the mainstay of empiric therapy. One needs to be concerned about the side effect of drowsiness, which can sometimes be exaggerated when patients are also on opioid analgesics. In patients with pruritis secondary to cholestasis, reduction in itching may be accomplished with cholestyramine.

Table 10–7

Medications to Treat Pruritis

MEDICATION	RECOMMENDED DOSE
Topical creams and ointments	
Menthol	Apply to affected areas 3–4 times per day as needed
Hydrocortisone	Apply to affected areas 2–4 times per day as needed
Oral medication (antihistamines)	
Hydroxyzine	25–50 mg 3–4 times per day
Diphenhydramine	25–50 mg every 4–8 hours as needed
Cyproheptidine	4 mg 3–4 times per day
For cholestatic jaundice	
Cholestyramine	4 g orally before meals and at bedtime

Cutaneous Infections

Due to the immunosuppression that is present in all patients near the end of life, susceptibility to infections, including cutaneous infections, is quite high. There is often an area of prior skin injury that permits the infection to begin, although this is not always the case. In terminally ill patients, common lesions from which cutaneous infection develops include pressure ulcers, malignant lesions, and stasis ulcers, although even areas of dry, cracked skin can serve as a focus from which a skin infection begins.

Infecting organisms may include bacteria, fungi, and viruses, and any of these organisms can either be indigenous or externally acquired. Although (as discussed in more depth in Chapter 17) treatment of infection with antibiotics near the end of life is often individualized, antibiotics are commonly prescribed for the treatment of cutaneous infections, because effective antibiotic therapy will significantly palliate pain and discomfort experienced from the inflammation and swelling that accompanies the infection.

Bacterial Cutaneous Infections

CELLULITIS

Cellulitis is an acute inflammation of the skin associated with pain and swelling of the affected area. It can be caused by indigenous skin flora (generally staphylococcus species) or by a wide range of exogenous flora. Bacteria gain access to the epidermis via cracks in the skin, abrasions, cuts, insect bites, and catheters.

Cellulitis due to *Staphylococcus aureus* spreads from a localized infection, such as an abscess or infected foreign body. Recurrent cellulitis of the lower extremities is commonly due to streptococcal organisms associated with chronic venous stasis, or chronic lymphedema

The treatment is with antibiotics. When patients are near the end of life, the choice of antibiotic therapy often needs to be empiric, based on the probably offending organism as culture diagnosis is possible in only a minimum of cases. Yield of tissue aspiration cultures is too low to be useful, and purulent drainage is not always present in sufficient quantity to permit obtaining cultures.

IMPETIGO

Impetigo is a more superficial bacterial infection than cellulitis and is usually due to either group A beta-hemolytic streptococcus or *Staphylococcus aureus*. The primary lesion is a pustule that ruptures to form a honey-colored crust. Impetigo occurs on normal skin or areas where other skin lesions are present

In view of the nature of the skin lesions, the treatment of impetigo includes topical therapy with soaks to debride the crusts together with topical antibiotics. Systemic antibiotics, usually oral, are often used as well.

ERYSIPELAS

Erysipelas is the abrupt onset of fiery-red swelling of the face and extremities, typically with well-demarcated indurated margins and the development of rapid progression and intense pain. The causative organism is group A beta-hemolytic streptococcus. As erysipelas is common in elderly, debilitated patients, it must be a consideration when patients develop a cutaneous infection near the end of life. Treatment with penicillin is effective, causing pain and other symptoms to rapidly resolve, followed by desquamation of the affected skin.

Cutaneous Fungal Infections

Fungal infections of the skin, hair, and nails can occur in the normal population, but as with other types of cutaneous infection they are more common in immuno-compromised patients, and, hence, in patients near the end of life. Common dermatophytoses—such as tinea pedis, cruris, capitis, corporis, and versicolor—are beyond the scope of this discussion, and although they can occur in patients near the end of life, the reader is referred to any medical or dermatologic textbook for further discussion of these common lesions.

CANDIDA ALBICANS

Candida albicans causes the most common and troublesome fungal infections occurring in patients near the end of life. *Candida* is a normal inhabitant of the gastrointestinal tract, but can cause infection due to overgrowth secondary to antibiotic treatment, diabetes, chronic intertrigo, and other immune deficiencies. The organism has an affinity for areas that are chronically wet and macerated, such as the intertriginous areas under the breasts or in the perineum. Cutaneous lesions caused by candidiasis are usually edematous, erythematous, and scaly with scattered "satellite pustules." In contrast to other dermatophyte infections in which inflammation is minimal, there is frequently a marked inflammatory response in *Candida* infections.

Therapy involves removing predisposing factors such as wetness, as well as applying topical antifungal agents such as nystatin or clotrimazole cream two or three times a day to the affected areas. If a marked inflammatory response is present, the skin can be treated with hydrocortisone cream or lotion, or with a combination antifungal/steroid cream. When cutaneous candidiasis is recurrent or refractory, systemic therapy with oral antifungal agents such as fluconazole 150 mg one time (combined with ketoconazole 2 percent cream twice a day for 2 weeks) or itraconazole 200 mg daily for 7 to 10 days may be used. Therapy of oral candidiasis is discussed later in this chapter.

Viral Infections

HERPES VARICELLA/ZOSTER

VARICELLA (CHICKENPOX) The herpes varicella-zoster virus causes two distinct clinical illnesses. First, infection with the virus causes varicella, commonly referred to as chickenpox, which is an acute illness highlighted by a prodromal febrile illness followed by the development of pruritic vesicular lesions, usually in a diffuse distribution. The lesions are often intensely pruritic, and if scratched off, may leave significant scarring. Varicella is typically a viral childhood illness that is well tolerated, although its course may be more virulent in previously unexposed adults, especially when the adult is immunocompromised. Therefore, although quite unusual, a patient near the end of life who has not been previously exposed to the varicella-zoster virus, is at risk of developing a severe case of chickenpox if exposed to, for example, a visiting child who is incubating or has active disease. In such a situation, treatment with varicella globulin could be provided at the time of exposure and before the development of active disease. If active disease occurs, treatment with acyclovir 4000 mg per day in divided doses for 5 days may be provided.

ZOSTER (SHINGLES) The more common problem with the varicella-zoster virus at the end of life is the reactivation of infection, as herpes zoster (shingles). Shingles presents as a very painful vesicular eruption classically in a dermatomal distribution. It most often occurs in the sixth to eighth decade of life. While the definitive mechanism for reactivation of the virus is unknown, it is clearly associated with immunosuppression, and hence can be a significant problem for patients who are near the end of life. Exposure of persons who were previously infected with the varicella virus to patients with active chickenpox has also been reported to be a risk factor for the development of shingles.

Pain of shingles may actually precede the skin eruption by several days to a week, and the duration of the skin lesions is usually 3 to 10 days, although it may sometimes take weeks for the skin to return to normal. The most distressing complication is post-herpetic neuralgia, which can occur in more than 50 percent of patients over the age of 50 and requires adjuvant medications that are effective for the treatment of neuropathic pain to provide the patient with adequate analgesia. (See

Chapter 6 for recommendations on how to treat neuropathic pain.) Treatment of the active infection consists of acyclovir 800 mg per day for 7 to 10 days. Although acyclovir therapy will speed healing of the skin lesions, it has no effect on the incidence of postherpetic pain.

HERPES SIMPLEX

Another virus that can be troublesome to some patients near the end of life is herpes simplex virus. There are two subtypes of the virus, HSV-1 and HSV-2. As with varicella-zoster, this virus is usually acquired early in life, and the major concern near the end of life is the reactivation of infection, usually in the oropharyngeal, perineal, and/or perirectal areas. In immunocompromised and terminally ill patients, the infection may be severe, extending into the mucosal and deep cutaneous layer, and the lesions appear clinically similar to mucosal lesions caused by chemotherapy, or fungal or bacterial infections. Systemic acyclovir can speed healing of the lesions and relief of symptoms.

Cutaneous Infestations: Scabies

Scabies is the most common cause of pruritic dermatosis worldwide. It is caused by infestation of the skin with the mite *Sarcoptes scabiei*. Person-to-person contact is the usual route of transmission and medical practitioners are at high risk of acquiring scabies. As outbreaks among patients living in nursing homes and hospitals are frequent, scabies can be a significant problem for patients who are near the end of life and hospitalized or living in a hospice or nursing home.

The itch and rash of scabies derive from a sensitization reaction. Thus, even through scratching destroys the mite, symptoms persist even in its absence. Patients report an intense pruritis, which is worse at night or after showering. Burrows may be difficult to find. They appear as wavy lines 2 to 15 mm in length that end in a pearly bleb. They are common on volar wrist surfaces, between fingers, on elbows, and on the penis. Papules, vesicles, pustules, and nodules are seen in these sites as well as under breasts, around the navel, in axillae, the belt line, buttocks, upper thighs, and scrotum. The face, palms, and soles are spared.

Treatment is topical, with 5 percent permethrin cream being recommended. Permethrin is much less toxic than the more commonly used 1 percent lindane cream. It is applied thinly behind ears and from the neck down, and washed off 8 hours later. While patients become noninfectious within one day of treatment, symptoms of pruritis and rash may persist for weeks to months. Pruritis may be symptomatically treated as outlined in Table 10–7.

Cutaneous Drug Reactions

Polypharmacy is common among patients near the end of life. Therefore, these patients are susceptible to adverse reactions to the myriad of medications used to help control symptoms. Whenever a patient who is near the end of life develops a new onset of pruritis associated with urticaria or maculopapular eruptions, a cutaneous drug reaction must be considered high on the list of possible causes, and a full review of all medication must be performed.

Urticarial drug eruptions are typically described as pruritic, red wheals that can vary from pinpoint to large in size, and usually last less than 24 hours. Involvement of the dermis and subcutaneous tissue can lead to more generalized swelling of skin, termed angioedema. Urticaria generally occurs early in the course of using a new medication. The urticaria may be allergic in origin. Or in the case of opioids, aspirin, and NSAIDs (medications commonly used in patients near the end of life), the reaction may be due to nonallergic release of histamine and other vasoactive mediators.

Maculopapular eruptions from medication tend to occur 1 to 2 weeks into therapy with a new medication. Erythematous macules and/or papules generally start on the trunk or on areas of pressure or prior trauma. They are frequently symmetrical and may become confluent.

The primary therapy for all cutaneous drug reactions is withdrawal of the offending medication. In the case of maculopapular eruptions, however, the eruptions may fade even if the offending agent is continued. In the absence of angioedema, primary treatment should include antihistamines (see Table 10–7), soothing baths, and emollients. If angioedema and/or anaphylaxis occurs, treatment must include epinephrine and/or corticosteroids, as needed, to halt the anaphylactic response.

Photosensitivity

A less typical cutaneous drug reaction may develop when the medication causes the skin to develop an increased sensitivity to light. Among the medications responsible for causing photosensitivity are sulfonamides, tetracyclines, thiazide diuretics, sulfonylurea, hypoglycemic agents, phenothiazines, and antihistamines. The skin reaction is very similar to the erythema of sunburn, but occasionally bullae may occur.

Primary treatment consists of breaking the connection between the medication and sun. Depending on the needs and goals of the patient, either the medication is stopped or sunlight is avoided. Treatment of the skin lesions is identical to that of first-degree or second-degree thermal burns (described earlier).

Dermatitis

Atopic Dermatitis

Atopic dermatitis is an extremely common skin disorder described as superficial, inflammatory, erythematous, pruritic, and eruptive. In adults, it is usually localized and chronic. It is in many ways a cyclic disorder, starting as a constant pruritis causing scratching, which in turns causes a rash that is pruritic, causing scratching, and so on. The causes of atopic dermatitis are unclear, although there is often intolerance to environmental irritants. Exacerbation of atopic dermatitis may be caused by conditions that are common to patients near the end of life, including emotional stress, temperature changes, and bacterial skin infections, and for this reason it is important to consider these factors as a potential etiology of dermatitis in these patients.

Therapy involves avoidance of rubbing on the skin, minimization of scratching, and decreasing exposure to triggering stimuli in the environment. The skin should be kept well lubricated. Medications that are useful in reducing symptoms are similar to those used for pruritis (see Table 10–7) and include hydroxyzine, diphenhydramine, and topical steroids. If lesions are resistant to this therapy then superimposed infection may be present. For such patients, antibiotic treatment directed against *S. aureus* may be of benefit.

Contact Dermatitis

Contact dermatitis is an inflammatory process caused by agents that injure the skin by direct contact. It is due to an antigen-specific immune response that can either be acute (edematous and wet) or chronic (dry, thickened, and scaly). Acute contact dermatitis can present as mild erythema or as a more pronounced skin eruption with the presence of vesicles and ulcers. Important clues that the skin reaction is due to contact dermatitis are that the area involved is strictly demarcated and may be unilateral. Patients near the end of life may develop contact dermatitis from contact with substances such as laundry detergents used to clean linens.

Treatment involves removing the offending agent, providing physical barriers to avoid contact, and high-potency fluorinated topical steroids. The dermatitis typically resolves in 2 to 3 weeks after treatment begins.

Stasis Dermatitis

Stasis dermatitis is a reaction that develops on the lower extremities due to vascular incompetence and chronic edema. Near the end of life it may be seen in patients who suffer from such illnesses as advanced congestive heart failure, advanced COPD with cor pulmonale, and advanced malignancies with obstruction of blood flow from the lower extremities due to tumor or radiation-induced fibrosis.

Early in the course of stasis dermatitis, one finds erythema and scaling with pruritis. Typically this starts over the medial aspect of the ankle at the site of an engorged vein. Eventually the area becomes pigmented due to hemosiderin deposition from extravasated red cells. The area can then become acutely inflamed with exudate and crusting. Chronic stasis dermatitis is associated with fibrosis, so-called brawny edema. Areas of brawny edema are highly susceptible to infection and superimposed contact dermatitis. In severe cases, ulceration can occur.

Treatment of early stasis changes is based on the use of emollients and mid-potency topical steroids for inflammation and decrease in chronic edema. Elevation of the affected limb and use of compression stockings of at least 30 to 40 mm Hg are effective.

Ulcers from stasis dermatitis are difficult to treat. The optimal goal near the end of life is to keep the ulcer clean and to avoid infection. This can involve gentle debridement of necrotic tissue with application of a semipermeable dressing under pressure. Antibiotics are used only for active infections.

Disorders of the Mucous Membranes

Xerostomia (Dry Mouth)

Xerostomia is an all too common complaint among patients near the end of life. The most common causes of xerostomia in this population are out-lined in Table 10–8. Patients with xerostomia usually complain of the need to continually do things to keep the mouth moist, the need to drink water at night, and difficulty with speech. If the dryness is severe, the patient may also complain of a burning sensation in the tongue or mouth. Other symptoms associated with xerostomia include halitosis, decreased taste acuity, and difficulty chewing and swallowing food. Difficulty chewing and swallowing is sometimes aggravated by ill-fitting dentures because of insufficient saliva to help seal dentures to the oral mucosa.

TREATMENT

Measures to reduce xerostomia include use of ice cubes, hard candy, or gum to maximally stimulate salivary flow. Frequent sips of cold liquids, frequent rinsing of the mouth with tapwater, and use of a saliva substitute are also helpful. If there is any evidence of oral infection (described next) appropriate therapy should be prescribed. The oral cavity should be kept as clean as possible by cleansing with a toothbrush, foam stick, or cotton bud soaked with water, as frequently as every 1 to 2 hours if needed. Mouthwashes that are alcohol based and astringent should be avoided, to prevent further drying of the tissues. Patients who have xerostomia due to prior radiation therapy may benefit from pilocarpine tablets 5 mg three times a day.

Oral Infections

The most common oral infections in terminally ill patients are fungal (oral candidiasis) and viral.

ORAL CANDIDIASIS

The presentation of oral candidiasis may vary. Patients can present with the typical white-yellow plaques that wipe off easily, generalized red lesions, or a diffuse red surface. Pain is present to a greater or lesser extent.

Treatment is available in both topical and systemic forms. Nystatin suspension is the classic

Table 10–8
Causes of Xerostomia

ETIOLOGY	EXAMPLE
Medication	Opioid analgesics
	Tricyclic antidepressants
	Antihistamines
	Phenothiazines
	Anticholinergics
Dehydration	Local: mouth breathing, oxygen use
	Systemic
Reduced salivary flow	Complication of local malignancy, radiation therapy, or surgery
Erosion of the buccal cavity	Infection (viral or fungal)
	Stomatitis
Depression	
Anxiety	

topical treatment with 400,000 U applied via a swish-and-swallow technique to the infected mucosa four times daily. Treatment is often disappointing because antifungal action is limited to the time the agent has contact with the fungus. Clotrimazole lozenges used five times daily are often effective, and may have the advantage of increased contact time with the infected mucosa. If topical treatment is not effective and systemic treatment is indicated, fluconazole 50 to 150 mg daily is effective with few side effects. Its long half-life allows once-daily dosing.

ORAL VIRAL INFECTIONS

Viral infections of the oral mucosa are primarily due to herpes simplex and zoster, cytomegalovirus, and Epstein–Barr virus, although the herpes species are most common. They generally present as yellow lesions that are easily wiped from the mucosa and are exquisitely painful. Pain may require systemic opioids for relief. Acyclovir, 1000 mg a day in divided doses, is the treatment of choice. Topical agents that may help soothe the mucosa include viscous lidocaine solution, often mixed with an equal part of liquid antacid to allow better and longer adherence of the anesthetic to the mucosa.

Stomatitis

Stomatitis is manifested in diffuse erythema, inflammation, and ulceration of the oral mucosa. It is most often a complication of chemotherapy and radiotherapy. The major risk factor is poor oral health and hygiene prior to initiation of these therapies. The inflammatory process most often affects the nonkeratinized oral mucosa, including the cheek, soft palate, lips, tongue, and floor of the mouth.

Treatment of stomatitis involves minimizing trauma to the mucosa and adequate pain management. Aggressive mouth care is needed to keep the mucosal surface clean, using soft brushes and hydrogen peroxide or chlorhexidine rinses. Lips should be kept moist with a petroleum-based jelly. The oral cavity can be cleansed with mouthwashes, but careful attention should be paid to avoiding alcohol-based preparations. Ice chips or popsicles can be very soothing, along with topical anesthetics.

An innovative technique is to make hard candy containing cayenne powder. Although the initial use of these candy lozenges may increase burning initially, the capsaicin in the pepper powder may well have an analgesic effect. Pain may be sufficiently severe to require systemic opioids.

References

Allman RM: Pressure ulcer prevalence, incidence, risk factors, and impact. In: Thomas DR, Allman RM, eds. *Clinics in Geriatric Medicine: Pressure Ulcers.* Philadelphia, Saunders, 1997.

Arnold HL Jr, Odom RB, James WD: *Andrews' Diseases of the Skin,* 8th ed. 1990.

Bergstrom NI: Strategies for preventing pressure ulcers. In: Thomas DR, Allman RM, eds. *Clinics in Geriatric Medicine: Pressure Ulcers.* Philadelphia, Saunders, 1997.

Bruera E: Skin disorders and their management. In: Portnoy RK, Bruera E, eds. *Topics in Palliative Care,* vol 3. New York, Oxford University Press, 1998.

Doyle D, Hanks GWC, MacDonald N: *Oxford Textbook of Palliative Medicine,* 2nd ed. Oxford, Oxford University Press, 1998.

Fauci AS, Braunwald E, Isselbacher KJ, et al: *Harrison's Principles of Internal Medicine,* 14th ed. New York, McGraw-Hill, 1998.

Goode PS, Thomas DR: Pressure ulcers: Local wound care. In: Thomas DR, Allman RM, eds. *Clinics in Geriatric Medicine: Pressure Ulcers.* Philadelphia, Saunders, 1997.

Jaffe R: Atopic dermatitis. In: Zuber TJ, ed. *Primary Care: Dermatology.* Philadelphia, Saunders, 2000.

Kinzbrunner BM, Pyron M, Coluzzi P, Gardner D: *Vitas Guidelines for Intensive Palliative Care.* Miami, Vitas Healthcare, 1996.

Mayer ME: The terminology of skin disorders. In: Zuber TJ, ed. *Primary Care: Dermatology.* Philadelphia, Saunders, 2000.

McEvoy GK, Litvak K, Welsh OH, et al, eds. *AHFS 98 Drug Information.* Bethesda, Maryland, American Society of Health-System Pharmacists, 1998.

Meyers D: *Client Teaching Guides for Home Health Care.* Rockville, MD, Aspen, 1989.

Pearson AS, Wolford RW: Management of skin trauma. In: Zuber TJ, ed. *Primary Care: Dermatology.* Philadelphia, Saunders, 2000.

Remsburg RE, Bennett RG: Pressure-relieving strategies for preventing and treating pressure sores. In: Thomas DR, Allman RM, eds. *Clinics in Geriatric Medicine: Pressure Ulcers.* Philadelphia, Saunders, 1997.

James B. Wright

Depression and Other Common Symptoms

Introduction

Previous chapters in this book have addressed major symptoms experienced by patients near the end of life. This chapter will discuss other symptoms commonly associated with terminal illness: depression, anxiety, delirium, asthenia, insomnia, urinary disorders, and hiccups.

Depression and Anxiety

According to the American Psychiatric Association *Diagnostic and Statistical Manual of Mental Disorders*, third edition (DSM–III), the prevalence rate of mental disorders among cancer patients is 47 percent. Of these, 68 percent suffer from reactive anxiety and depression, and 13 percent experience major depression. Extrapolating these data to all causes of terminal illness, depression and anxiety undoubtedly affect a significant number of patients near the end of life. These patients must be identified and offered appropriate medical and psychological treatment.

Depression and anxiety often have similar causes, although they may occur concurrently or separately in the same patient at varying intervals during the process of dying. Despite these simi-

larities, it is important to differentiate depression and anxiety, as well as to avoid confusing them with other mental disorders such as delirium and progressive dementia. Failure to appreciate the difference between each of these mental states may lead to inappropriate treatment and result in worsening symptoms. Table 11–1 compares and contrasts some of the common features of depression and anxiety, with delirium and dementia also included for comparative purposes. (For a full discussion of delirium and dementia, see Chapter 9.)

Depression

Causes

Depression near the end of life may be related to changes in a patient's life situation as the terminal illness progresses and/or to direct or indirect effects of the illness. In patients with a prior history of depression, these issues may cause an exacerbation of depressive symptoms that were previously controlled. Common causes of depression near the end of life are summarized in Table 11–2.

CHANGES IN LIFE SITUATION

LOSS OF CONTROL　Control entails managing oneself and one's environment in a self-satisfying manner. In an acute, reversible illness, loss of control

Table 11–1

Comparison of Depression, Anxiety, Delirium, and Dementia

	HALLUCINATION PRESENT	ONSET	SPEECH LOSS PRESENT	AWARENESS AFFECTED	LABILE EMOTIONAL RESPONSE PRESENT	AFFECT, MEMORY, JUDGEMENT, THINKING
Depression	—	Possible acute	—	—	Occasional	—
Anxiety	—	Possible acute	—	—	++	—
Delirium	+++	Acute	—	++	++	+
Dementia	—	Gradual	+	++	—	+

Table 11-3

Causes of Depression Near the End of Life

Changes in life situation
   Loss of control
   Loss of self-esteem or self-worth
   Loss of independence
   Alteration in environment
Direct or indirect effects of terminal illness
   Lack of knowledge concerning illness
   Unaddressed or uncontrolled symptoms of
     disease
   Medications
   Metabolic abnormalities
Exacerbation of preexisting condition

is generally viewed as a temporary impairment that will dissipate on return to normal health. Chronic illness, however—and particularly terminal illness—changes that outlook. As our society associates prestige and dignity with those who possess physical control and independence, progressive, irreversible disability due to illness or injury inevitably leads to a loss of independence and the sense of control. A loss of self-control often results in anger and frustration. Loss of independence also fosters feelings of low self-esteem, which may ultimately manifest as depression.

LOSS OF SELF-ESTEEM OR SELF-WORTH Most terminally ill people experience changes in body image and/or their place in society. The sense of loss that accompanies these changes usually causes a realistic and expected grief reaction. "Normal" grieving usually reflects not only the loss of physical prowess, but also the loss of time needed to take care of unfinished business, such as unresolved family problems and/or financial uncertainties. However, when grieving is disproportionate and accompanied by expressions of profound guilt or loss of self-worth, clinical depression should be suspected. Individuals most vulnerable are often those who provide the main financial support or otherwise serve as the titular head of the household, but no one is immune.

LOSS OF INDEPENDENCE Illness-induced dependency in activities of daily living is thought to contribute to the development of depression. However, its role in any given individual may be difficult to assess as it does not necessarily correlate with the physical state of the patient. Some physically dependent individuals can be very independent of mind, whereas individuals with apparently minimal physical problems can perceive themselves as being significantly dependent on others.

Patients who are unwilling to acknowledge the progression of their disease usually do not adjust well to progressive dependence. Using denial as an adaptive mechanism, patients sometimes readily discuss with the physician the signs and symptoms of their decline without focusing on the existential meaning of these changes indicative of impending death. This intellectualization of the process of decline may create a false impression that the patient is actually coping with his or her illness and its attendant dependency. However, input obtained from family, friends, or the hospice team may reveal that the patient appears to resent or even abuse the care providers, and this will clearly indicate the extent of the patient's maladjustment and discontent. The clinician should also suspect maladaptive behavior when patients begin to discuss their disease using medical jargon or scientific terminology rather than in personal terms. An attempt to divert such stilted conversation to a more personal and interactive level may be valuable.

ALTERATIONS IN ENVIRONMENT Patients with serious illnesses, especially those near the end of life, are rarely popular and may sometimes even be shunned by others. Isolation of a patient from family and friends often occurs, contributing to a patient's feelings of loneliness and loss of self-worth. Isolation may occur even in the home environment as families seek to protect or even hide the patient from others. Patients will often give in to such measures due to physical or mental decline. Due to infirmity, or out of desire not to be a burden, patients may passively accept social isolation as an inevitable outcome of their illness, withdraw further into themselves, and sink into despair.

DIRECT OR INDIRECT EFFECTS OF THE ILLNESS

LACK OF KNOWLEDGE CONCERNING ILLNESS   A patient's lack of knowledge concerning the nature of the illness, goals of therapy, or reason why definitive therapy is not offered, can lead to depression. Physicians must be aware that telling a patient about his or her disease or its treatment and prognosis may not ensure that he or she will understand or be able to recall that information at a later time. Unfortunately, many patients referred to hospice programs do not understand the implications of the referral and why the referral was made. In the absence of understanding the purpose and scope of hospice and palliative care services, patients and families may erroneously interpret a referral to hospice as synonymous with abandonment of all hope. In this circumstance, the patient cannot avoid feeling like a helpless victim of disease or of the medical system, and if the patient discloses this feeling at all, it may well be to nurses or a social worker rather than to the physician. Depression in such patients is often attributed directly to knowledge of the terminal illness (hence the common request: "Don't tell him he has cancer"). However, it is more likely that poor understanding of the disease process, fear of the unknown, fear of unrelieved physical and emotional suffering, and a conviction that there is no hope for continued useful and fulfilling life are really the causative factors. From a position of first blaming his or her condition on the system, the patient may well begin to blame himself or herself.

UNADDRESSED OR UNCONTROLLED SYMPTOMS OF DISEASE   Disease symptoms that are unaddressed or uncontrolled can promote depression. Although this is most commonly recognized when pain is poorly controlled, any symptom may lead to depression if not adequately treated. If the clinician fails to ask, listen, and act, symptoms may go unreported or inadequately treated. Forgetting to assess the response to a palliative intervention in a timely manner will increase the likelihood of therapeutic failure, and magnify the patient's sense of abandonment and hopelessness. Evasiveness and dishonesty about the limitations of treatment, whether curative or palliative, also often leads to disillusionment, anger, and despondency.

MEDICATIONS AND METABOLIC ABNORMALITIES   Signs and symptoms of depression may be evoked by medications prescribed for the patient, as well as by biologic or physiologic abnormalities associated with the terminal disease or other comorbid conditions. For patients with cancer, the rigors of radiation and chemotherapy treatments, especially when side effects are inadequately addressed, may provoke or potentiate a depressive reaction. Opioid analgesics, anxiolytic agents, corticosteroids, and antihypertensive medications are also known to produce depression. Altered biologic states, either incidental to or as a consequence of terminal disease, and including, but not limited to, fluid and electrolyte abnormalities, hypercalcemia, infections, brain tumors, cerebrovascular accidents, hypoglycemia, or progressive organ failure must be considered as potential causes of depression as a patient's illness progresses. However, it is important to remember that organic mental disorders such as delirium, which alter mood and mimic depression, should be distinguished, as they require a different treatment approach.

EXACERBATION OF PREEXISTING DEPRESSION

Patients with terminal disease may have a past history of significant depression or other psychiatric illness. In these patients, depression may recur or become more severe in the face of a terminal illness, even if all other predisposing or provocative factors are avoided or minimized.

Diagnosis

When assessing a terminally ill patient for depression, neurovegetative symptoms, such as fatigue, anorexia, weight loss and altered sleep patterns, which are often reliable indicators of depression in nonterminally ill patients, are nondiagnostic because these symptoms are often caused by the terminal disease itself. Therefore, psychological features will serve as more reliable indicators, and must be carefully evaluated. The depressed patient may exhibit loss of self-esteem, guilt, lack of interest in social interactions, suicidal ideation, sadness, crying, and mood disturbances. Although some of these phenomena are components of normal grieving that is part of the dying process, assessing the sum and/or depth of these various manifestations should help identify the patient with true depression. The single question "Are you depressed?" has been shown to be a reliable indicator of depression in terminally ill patients when answered in the affirmative. In any event, whether "normal" or "abnormal," psychological distress must be identified and should be treated aggressively with appropriate pharmacologic and nonpharmacologic interventions. When the diagnosis is questionable, a therapeutic trial of antidepressant medication is usually justified.

Treatment

PHARMACOLOGIC THERAPY

There are a number of different pharmacologic agents available for the treatment of depression in advanced illness (Table 11–3). With the exception of the psychostimulants, for which there are published, small, prospective trials, there have been no controlled studies of antidepressant medications in terminal patients near the end of life.

TRICYCLIC ANTIDEPRESSANTS Depression is associated with a relative decline in neuroactive chemical transmitters in the brain. Tricyclic antidepressants (TCAs), which were developed as derivatives of chlorpromazine, inhibit uptake of serotonin and norepinephrine at neural synaptic junctions, allowing for increased transmitter activity between nerves, thus enhancing neuronal activity. These agents, which include amitriptyline, imipramine, doxepin, and nortriptyline, have been standard antidepressant therapy for many years.

With specific reference to end-of-life care, depressed patients with terminal cancer often respond to lower TCA doses than those required in physically healthy patients with depression. Appetite and insomnia usually improve rapidly. TCAs are also frequently effective in treating neuropathic pain, which commonly coexists along with depression in patients with advanced or terminal cancer. Because the therapeutic dose for the treatment of neuropathic pain may be lower than for depression, patients on a TCA for neuropathic pain who develop depression may best be treated with an increased dose of the TCA rather than with addition of a new antidepressant from a different pharmacologic class. Other advantages include availability for oral, rectal, and parenteral routes; ability to monitor drug levels; and differential sedative effects and toxicity profiles.

Sedative TCAs, such as amitriptyline, are especially useful at bedtime for depressed patients with agitation and insomnia. Desipramine, which is less sedative, is more suitable for patients with apathetic depression and psychomotor slowing. Anticholinergic side effects such as dry mouth, blurred vision, constipation, urinary retention, and increased intraocular pressure can be particularly troublesome in elderly or debilitated patients, in whom there may be additional problems with drug interactions. In these patients, nortriptyline or desipramine may be preferred. TCAs can also cause postural hypotension, cardiac toxicity, seizures, extrapyramidal effects, and excess sedation. For this reason, many clinicians favor the use of newer, less toxic classes of antidepressant medications such as the selective serotonin uptake inhibitors.

SELECTIVE SEROTONIN REUPTAKE INHIBITORS The selective serotonin reuptake inhibitors, or SSRIs (fluoxetine, paroxetine, sertraline), are being used more often in the terminally ill, primarily for patients who have several weeks or months to live. Compared with TCAs, they cause fewer side effects and have a more rapid onset of action. Thirty to fifty percent of all patients with a poor response to TCAs will respond positively to a switch to SSRIs. Furthermore, due to differences in chemical structure, "cross-resistance" among the various SSRIs is less common than among TCAs, thus allowing intraclass switching for poorly responding patients. However, because SSRIs have relatively long half-lives, it may be necessary to allow a washout period before starting another SSRI. Paroxetine and ser-

Table 11–3
Antidepressants

MEDICATION	CATEGORY/DOSAGE	CLINICAL APPLICATIONS
TRICYCLIC ANTIDEPRESSANTS (TCAs)		

Amitriptyline
Nortriptyline
Desipramine
	75–150 mg PO daily in divided doses
	25–250 mg PO daily in divided doses
	10–150 mg PO daily
		Better for neuropathic pain
		Anticholinergic effects vary with
		  compound and dose
		Possibly more sedative and with slower
		  onset of action than SSRIs

SELECTIVE SEROTONIN REUPTAKE INHIBITORS (SSRIs)		
Fluoxetine Paroxetine Sertraline	10–80 mg PO daily 20–50 mg PO daily 50–200 mg PO daily	Fewer anticholinergic side effects and more rapid onset of action than TCAs
PSYCHOSTIMULANTS		

Methylphenidate	2.5–5 mg daily or in divided doses up to
	  20 mg per day. Up to 60 mg per day
	  has been used
		Rapid onset of action
		May be most effective for end-of-life
		  patients with short life expectancy
		Can cause anxiety and restlessness

traline, which have shorter half-lives and fewer metabolites than fluoxetine, also have fewer side effects such as nausea, headache, somnolence, insomnia, a brief period of increased anxiety, anorexia, and transient weight loss. Central nervous system stimulants may be more useful for patients in whom medication-related somnolence is a problem. Fluoxetine has an incompatibility with codeine and the two should not be used together.

PSYCHOSTIMULANTS Psychostimulants (methylphenidate, dextroamphetamine, pemoline) have generally been supplanted by MAO inhibitors, tricyclic antidepressants, and selective serotonin reuptake inhibitors for treatment of chronic depression. However, the rapid onset of action of psychostimulants makes them particularly valuable for end-of-life care. Methylphenidate is particularly appropriate in terminally ill patients with a very short life expectancy, except for those with advanced, unstable heart disease. It is generally well tolerated even in elderly, debilitated patients and can rapidly increase energy and appetite.

Methylphenidate counteracts opioid-induced fatigue and lethargy and has adjuvant analgesic effects. Psychostimulants may also be used to treat cognitive impairment in patients with AIDS. In the nonsustained-release form, a response can occur in 1 to 2 hours and continue for 3 to 6 hours. The sustained-release form may take 4 to 7 hours to begin to have effect, but activity persists for approximately 8 hours. Methylphenidate can initially be combined with a longer-acting antidepressant. When the longer-acting antidepressant begins to take effect, the psychostimulant can be discontinued.

MONOAMINE OXIDASE INHIBITORS AND ELECTROCONVULSIVE THERAPY Monoamine oxidase inhibitors and electroconvulsive therapy are not recommended for end-of-life care.

RECOMMENDED CLINICAL APPROACH

Patients who develop depressive symptoms should have a full medication review, as many medications can cause or exacerbate symptoms of depression. It may be possible to discontinue some medications, including beta-blockers and other antihypertensives, when patients are near the end of life. On the other hand, other medications, such as opioids, steroids, and anxiolytics, may need to be continued to address symptoms such as pain and anxiety. However, changing to an equianalgesic dose of an alternative opioid, reducing the dose of steroids to the minimum needed for symptom relief, and choosing an anxiolytic that does not contribute to depression may alleviate some depressive symptoms without further measures.

The clinician must also consider whether direct progression of the terminal illness or a secondary metabolic disorder could be contributing to symptoms of depression. If a reversible cause of depression is suspected, and the patient's overall clinical condition suggests that correcting the problem will improve quality of life, then even if the patient is on a hospice or palliative care program, appropriate diagnostic studies and therapeutic interventions should be undertaken. If the patient is close to death, or the problem is determined to be irreversible, then rapidly acting psychostimulant antidepressants and other symptomatic approaches should be provided. For severely depressed patients in whom the expected prognosis is several weeks or more, treatment should be started with a psychostimulant to achieve a rapid response. Thereafter, SSRIs or TCAs may be added and titrated upward to a therapeutic level, allowing a gradual withdrawal of the psychostimulant.

Other medications may be useful adjuncts in the treatment of depression. Trazodone, in low doses at bedtime, is useful for depressed patients with insomnia. Buspirone, an anxiolytic that does not possess antidepressant activity, has been found to augment the effect of antidepressants in doses of 2.5 mg twice a day. It is contraindicated for patients with known convulsive disorders or who are at high risk of having seizures. Pindolol is a postsynaptic antagonist that in doses of 2.5 to 7.5 mg per day for up to 6 weeks accelerates the onset of benefit of SSRIs. Because new antidepressants, including many not mentioned here, are frequently

introduced, hospice and palliative care specialists should be prepared to adapt these recommendations as evidence-based studies become available.

Exogenous thyroid hormones, both T_3 (Cytomel) and T_4 (levothyroxine), can augment the effectiveness of both tricyclic antidepressants and SSRIs when administered during the first 2 to 3 weeks of therapy. The exact mechanism of action is not known, but may relate to potentiation of noradrenergic activity. T_3 seems to be more effective than T_4.

NONPHARMACOLOGIC THERAPY

Regardless of the cause, treatment for depression in the terminally ill should not be restricted to pharmacotherapy (Table 11–4). Hospice patients are provided services from chaplains, social workers, and nursing personnel who are taught to offer psychosocial support for the patients and their families. This model is appropriate for all patients receiving end-of-life care.

A physician interview with the patient and his or her care providers can identify likely causes of the depression and help to relieve anxiety and stress. The most common nonmedical patient concerns involve personal or family problems and financial, social, and religious/spiritual distress.

Personal or family problems may be long standing and are often not resolvable prior to death. However, the physician and members of a hospice team should try to be aware of such problems. Careful thought must be given as to how such problems are to be discussed with the patient. Good intentions aside, increased stress can be

Table 11–4

Nonpharmacologic Therapy for Depression

Identify personal or family problems
Consider counseling
Address concerns about illness and therapy
Review level of care
Explore religious and spiritual concerns

experienced when personal relationships are explored. Professional counseling by chaplains, social workers, clinical psychologists, or psychiatric consultants should be recommended.

Financial concerns are nearly always present. Even well-to-do individuals can be stressed by the cost of medical care. The financial stability of the family is threatened when the patient is the main source of family income. The patient may feel guilty about the cost of care. Loss of income and dependency affects self-esteem and precipitates suicidal intentions as well as depression. The physician and allied health professionals can help to identify and marshal community resources and bolster the patient's self-image.

The focus of palliative care is different than acute care, but the layperson may find the distinction unclear and unsettling. Some patients perceive a hospice referral as "giving up," and may believe that no treatment will be provided. It is necessary to emphasize that although a cure seems to be out of reach, treatment will continue and symptoms will be controlled. An astute and caring clinician will realize that nonpharmacologic treatments such as listening, dialogue with the patient and family, careful exploration of the patient's concerns, and identification and reinforcement of adaptive mechanisms, although time intensive, are a vital part of the therapeutic armamentarium for combating both depression and anxiety.

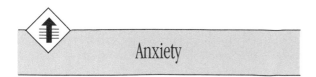

Anxiety

Causes

Anxiety shares many root causes with depression but may present acutely due to an exacerbation of symptoms such as pain or dyspnea (Table 11–5). In addition, chronic anxiety and depression often coexist. Therefore, when evaluating and treating an emotional reaction to terminal illness, it is best to anticipate the need to treat the other. Pain has

Table 11–5

Causes of Anxiety Near the End of Life

Changes in life situations
    Loss of control
    Loss of self-esteem
    Loss of independence
    Alteration in environment
Direct or indirect effects of terminal illness
    Lack of knowledge concerning illness
    Unaddressed or uncontrolled symptoms
    Drug interactions or medication effects
    Delirium/depression
    Hypoxemia
    Sepsis
    Impending cardiac or respiratory failure
Exacerbation of preexisting conditions
    Adjustment disorders
    Psychiatric conditions

been described as "being what the patient says that it is." To an extent, this dictum can be applied to anxiety and depression. Patients who complain of anxiety or depression need serious attention, and the physician must be alert to those patients who are suffering from anxiety and depression but who deny the presence of symptoms.

Anxiety may be viewed as denial or resistance to life changes resulting in physiologic and emotional stress, whereas depression reflects an attitude of resignation and hopelessness. Anxiety may be provoked by a lack of knowledge about the illness and its expected course and symptoms. There is some comfort in knowing that most people with the disease experience changes similar to those of the patient, and even more comfort in the knowledge that expert management will be offered. Listening to the patient's concerns may sometimes be the best form of therapy, but involvement of psychosocial specialists should be encouraged.

Acute anxiety commonly accompanies hypoxemia, sepsis, and cardiorespiratory and other systemic organ failure. In these circumstances, it may be associated with delirium. Exacerbation of preexisting conditions, including adjustment disorders or other psychiatric conditions, can be the cause of uncontrolled anxiety. The stress of a terminal illness can reactivate or accentuate latent pathologic mental states.

A delay in treating symptoms or inadequate treatment that results in poor symptom control will make patients anxious. Symptoms that particularly create anxiety are pain, dyspnea, and nausea and vomiting. Some drugs used to treat terminal illness such as neuroleptics, steroids, and psychotropic stimulators may cause anxiety as a side effect. Drug interactions may also play a role, especially when multiple medications are prescribed, dosages are varied frequently, or medications are rapidly withdrawn (especially those such as opioids, which cause physiologic dependence).

Diagnosis

Psychological expression of anxiety includes insomnia, irritability, poor coping skills, and poor concentration (Table 11–6). Poor concentration should be differentiated from disorientation, which is a feature of delirium. Poor concentration means distractibility and inability to focus. Anxious individuals do not lose awareness of self and their environment.

Table 11–6

Diagnosis of Anxiety

Psychological reactions
Insomnia
Irritability
Inability to concentrate
Poor coping skills
Symptoms and physical features
Anorexia
Nausea
Hyperventilation
Palpitations
Sweating

Physical features of anxiety include palpitations, sweating, hyperventilation, anorexia, and nausea. These physical symptoms represent reactions to psychological stress. As stresses build, a decline in the ability of the patient to perform usual levels of activities of daily living may result. Although functional disability usually is indicative of progression of the terminal illness, in some instances it may be attributable to undiagnosed anxiety.

Treatment

Because anxiety and depression often coexist, and because depression may be worsened by the use of antianxiety agents, it is advisable to first initiate antidepressive therapy for patients with mixed symptoms. If antidepressant therapy is not successful or depression is not present, benzodiazepines are usually first choice agents for treatment of anxiety (Table 11–7). They can be grouped into short acting (plasma half-lives of less than 5 hours), medium acting (plasma half-lives of 5 to 24 hours), and long acting (plasma half-lives of more than 24 hours). The short-acting benzodiazepines, such as triazolam and midazolam, are of little clinical value for treament of anxiety. The medium-acting agents like lorazepam, temazepam, and oxazepam are preferred. Temazepam has no active metabolites, and the World Health Organization and other organizations therefore find it preferable to the long-acting benzodiazepines. Low dosages in the range of 10 mg twice a day are recommended as the initial dosage level to decrease somnolence and sedation that often occur at "standard" doses. Lorazepam comes as a tablet or liquid, including a liquid with a highly concentrated formulation.

Long-acting benzodiazepines such as diazepam have accumulating active metabolites. As a consequence, blood levels may not reach a steady state for weeks. They are, therefore, not as useful as routine daily medication and side effects tend to persist after discontinuation of the drug. Diazepam is useful, however, for patients with anxiety and recurrent seizures.

Table 11–7

Pharmacologic Treatment of Anxiety

MEDICATION	DOSAGE	CLINICAL FACTORS
BENZODIAZEZPINES		
Lorazepam	PO 0.5–1 mg bid to qid IV 0.5–1mg bid to qid	Tablets, liquid concentrates, and IV 　forms available May be expensive
Temazepam	Initially given as 10 mg bid Titrate to effective dose Maximum daily dose 60 mg	No active metabolites that accumulate Causes somnolence and sedation, 　especially in the elderly
Oxazepam	10–30 mg PO tid to qid Titrate to effect Maximum daily dose 180 mg	Medium length of action Useful for alcohol withdrawal
Diazepam	2–4 mg PO bid to qid IV 2–10 mg Q 3–4 hours prn Maximum daily dose 40 mg	Long acting with accumulating active 　metabolites May be used for seizure control as well
Alprazolam	0.25–0.5 mg PO to TID	Long-term usage may cause dependence Useful as limited prn medication
BARBITURATES		
Pentobarbital	PO 50–100 mg bid to qid Maximum daily dose 400 mg Rectal 30 mg–200 mg bid or qid Higher dosage for terminal agitation only	Useful in terminal agitation and rectally 　for seizure control when PO dosage 　not appropriate
Thioridazine	25 mg tid	Useful in terminal agitation and rectally 　for seizure control when PO dosage 　not appropriate.

Because anxiety does not necessarily persist from day to day with the same intensity, it is a mistake to assume that the terminally ill *require* sedation as they advance in their disease. Clinicians should address the causes of anxiety, and only if the anxiety cannot be eliminated should extended sedation be considered.

Benzodiazepines have significant undesired effects such as sedation and confusion. Titration to effect is desirable. Sudden withdrawal should also be avoided as acute anxiety or an abstinence syndrome may result. Benzodiazepines should never be used with alcohol, because the effects are potentiated.

The literature suggests that alprazolam is not recommended in the terminally ill because of development of intense dependence and severe withdrawal reactions including seizures. However, with limited PRN usage, these reactions are less significant.

Barbiturates such as phenobarbital and pentobarbital can be useful if patients do not respond to benzodiazepines. Because benzodiazepines compete with endorphin binding sites, barbiturates—which do not compete—may be a better choice for patients with pain control problems. Pentobarbital is particularly useful for patients who can no longer swallow, as it is available as a suppository.

Phenothiazines also have a role in treating anxiety. Thioridazine is an older product, which is most effective when used to take advantage of its sedative side effects. In contrast, haloperidol can be given orally, intravenously, or subcutaneously, and it is not a sedative. In delirious patients with anxiety it is the drug of choice.

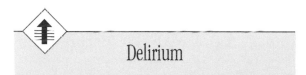

Delirium

This discussion concentrates on differentiating delirium from anxiety and depression. See Chapter 9 for a more in-depth discussion of delirium. Family and medical personnel frequently confuse delirium with anxiety, depression, or dementia. The earliest signs and symptoms may be subtle, and the most obvious reactions may be identified as the primary process. Consider the following case:

Mr. M is a 70-year-old retired Navy chief who has a primary brain tumor. Six months have elapsed since his last oncologic treatment. He is not having pain or any overt symptoms of disease except for a right hemiparesis. He was receiving sleep medication for insomnia, an H_2 blocker for reflux, and two anticonvulsants.

After many days of nocturnal wakefulness and daytime sleep, he began to refuse medications. He stated that he was fearful that the staff was trying to poison him. When pressed to take his medications, he became angry and belligerent. Antianxiety medications were ordered in large enough dosages to cause sedation and sleep. Unwilling but persuaded by family members, the patient took the new medication. After initially sleeping for several hours, Mr. M awoke and became even more agitated. He also began to experience visual hallucinations.

At this point, the hospice physician was consulted. All medications that had psychotropic effects were discontinued and the patient was started on haloperidol. Within 24 hours he returned to his prior mental status.

In this case, failure to recognize early evidence of drug-induced delirium resulted in interventions that exacerbated, rather than improved, the patient's delirium.

Because depression, anxiety, and dementia can occur in addition to delirium, these processes must be distinguished. Depression and anxiety do not significantly affect short-term memory, judgement, and ability to think, whereas delirium and dementia significantly affect cognitive skills. Dementia occurs gradually over months and years, whereas delirium is an acute process. Anxiety and depression can be chronic or acute. The course of dementia is progressive and follows a pattern of loss in activities of daily living and functional assessment staging. Delirium waxes and wanes with exacerbations often occurring at night. Dementia results in a limitation in speech content with progression to loss of vocabulary. Delirium is associated with occasional incoherent word usage but no actual verbal loss. There are no actual verbal deficits with depression or anxiety. Dementia patients progress slowly toward the unaware and unconcerned. Delirium is a state of hyperawareness and may be associated with increased emotional liability. In addition to anxiety, the patient may show apathy, fear, or rage.

Hallucinations are not associated with anxiety or depression, and are seldom seen in dementia. Hallucinations are common in delirium, however, because delirium is a state of altered wakefulness. The cerebral cortex is not fully aroused by the reticular activating system. Hence, the patient is rendered half-awake in a dream-like stupor. There are reversals of normal sleep patterns and inadequate rest when the patient does sleep.

To differentiate delirium from anxiety, depression, and dementia (see Table 11-1), a history should be taken to determine if the patient has or had hallucinations, speech loss, affected awareness, labile emotional responses, and problems with memory, judgement, or thinking. An acute onset suggests delirium.

The history should be obtained from people who know the patient best. Remember that a patient with delirium may not be blatantly abnormal at first appearance. For example, in midafternoon a delirious individual can appear quite normal. However, at night, usually when the physician is not present, the patient will exhibit diagnostic features. Thus, a careful recounting of the patient's behavior over 24 hours is necessary in order to avoid a missed diagnosis, the consequences of which might result in serious patient harm.

Treatment

When delirium is suspected, it is important to provide an orderly, calm environment free of stress or stimulation. Adherence to a routine daily schedule provides a coherent framework for the patient to hold onto. The presence of friends and familiar care providers is also beneficial. Hospice team members, particularly home health aides, who have established relationships with the patients, can be very supportive and provide a sense of comfort and stability. Pharmacologic interventions for delirium are discussed in Chapter 9.

Asthenia

Asthenia means a loss of energy or fatigue with an inability to maintain previous levels of performance or activities. The patient complains of a pervasive sense of generalized weakness.

Causes

Asthenia is usually caused by multiple interrelated factors (Table 11–8). To understand asthenia, it should be contextually related but also differentiated from anorexia and cachexia (Fig. 11–1). Anorexia is simply loss of appetite, whereas cachexia is severe muscle wasting with weight loss. Anorexia is sometimes reversible, but rarely so in the terminally ill. Cachexia is a cytokine-mediated inability to maintain muscle proteins, and it is not re-versed by increased food intake. Tumor products called cachectin are associated with cachexia, but no such markers have been found for asthenia. In asthenia, while decreased food intake contributes to weakness, correction of nutritional losses usually does not improve the debility. Inflammatory markers such as C-reactive proteins and ferritin may have some relationship to asthenia.

There are reversible forms of asthenia, such as occur with radiation and chemotherapy. Reversal is usually seen several weeks after treatments have ceased. On the other hand, progressive end-stage diseases with anorexia, cachexia, and asthenia most often are not reversible. Asthenia is also associated with specific end-organ failure like cardiac, renal, adrenal, and liver failure. Other related disease processes include anemia, hypocalcemia, hyponatremia, hypokalemia, Addison's disease, and Cushing's syndrome.

Because asthenia can occur with general inactivity, asthenia may be expressed through a muscle abnormality. Although loss of muscle and lean body mass and function can exist with normal calorie intake, and elevation of lactic acid is not necessarily noted in asthenic cancer patients, studies have shown atrophy of type II muscle fibers in

Table 11–8
Causes of Asthenia

End-organ failure
Comorbid and related disease process
Anemia
Hypocalcemia
Hyponatremia
Hypokalemia
Addison's disease
Polypharmacy
Chemotherapy
Radiation
Malnutrition
Anorexia–cachexia syndrome
Humoral tumor factors yet to be identified

Figure 11–1

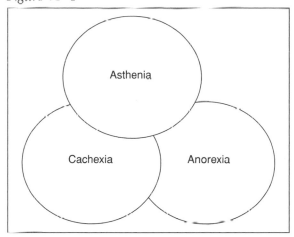

The intersection of asthenia, anorexia, and cachexia

are commonly used to control symptoms in terminally ill patients. Opioids exact a direct effect upon the reticular activating system, which in turn produces a sensation of fatigue.

Malnutrition or starvation causes asthenia, but as noted earlier, better nutrition does not reverse asthenia in the terminally ill. Anxiety, depression, and adjustment disorders have been reported to be associated with asthenia in 75 percent of terminally ill patients with noncancer diagnoses. Anorexia–cachexia syndrome, commonly found in patients with advanced AIDS, results in asthenia and eventual death. This syndrome is a disturbance of carbohydrate, fat, and protein metabolism with endocrine dysfunction and anemia. It is also common among patients with pancreas, lung, and colon cancer.

the adductor pollicis muscles in patients with advanced breast cancer, which seems to suggest that muscle dysfunction may be an underlying feature in asthenic cancer patients.

Medications may contribute to asthenia in the terminally ill. Polypharmacy may result in a general decline, but specific medications such as opioids, antidepressants, neuroleptics, benzodiazepines, diuretics, hypoglycemics, and antihypertensives are more specific contributors. Many of these drugs

Treatment

As the causes of asthenia are multiple, and not easily distinguished from the disease process, treatment is often more general than specific (Table 11–9). Future progress in treating asthenia may be dependent on a better understanding of cytokine interactions. Current treatment options are limited but could include steroids and progestogens that exert anticytokine effects, stimulate appetite, and increase the sense of well-being.

Table 11–9

Treatment for Asthenia

Medications	
Oral Steroids	
Prednisone	40–100 mg PO daily
Dexamethasone	16–96 mg PO daily in 2–4 divided doses
Progestogens	
Megestrol acetate	160–240 mg PO bid
Nonpharmacologic treatments	
Antidepressants when depression present	
Regular exercise	
Discontinuation of nonessential medications	
Psychostimulants	

Regular exercise limited to maintaining function and range of motion also helps, but it should not be overdone. Too strenuous a program could produce muscle fiber damage or exhaustion.

TCA and SSRI antidepressants and appetite stimulants do not have much of an impact on asthenia, unless there is coexistent depression. When possible, discontinue hypotensive agents, sedatives, and tranquilizers. Diabetes should be managed in a standard medical manner; oral hypoglycemics should be avoided whenever possible. Psychostimulants may cause arousal and lessen fatigue.

Insomnia

Insomnia is the subjective complaint of poor sleep. This problem includes insufficient sleep, difficulty initiating or maintaining sleep, interrupted sleep, or poor quality sleep. Causes of insomnia include pain, dyspnea, anxiety, depression, delirium, leg cramps, urinary frequency, and medication side effects from caffeine, steroids, diuretics, and sympathomimetics.

Treatment

Discontinue any suspected causative medications or agents that are not absolutely necessary. Identify, assess, and treat anxiety, depression, and delirium. Treat provocative symptoms effectively. Specific, problem-oriented interventions are much better than routinely prescribing sleep medication. For example, fear of dying is not relieved with temazepam. A psychosocial evaluation would be much more appropriate.

Even at home, daytime stimulation for a sedentary patient can be lacking. Such patients often doze throughout the day without even realizing how much sleeping they are doing. Daytime activities need to be enriched for such a person and naps, while often necessary, should be reduced in number and length.

For patients not able to sleep because of pain, stiffness, or night sweats, adding a nonsteroidal anti-inflammatory in the evening, 1 to 2 hours before bedtime, may be helpful. When using opioids, an increase of the daytime dose may be used at bedtime to extend the hours of sleep without pain. Try not to schedule routine medications during normal sleeping hours. Many drugs come in long-acting form that can be used prior to bedtime. Antidepressants are useful when depression is present. In particular, doxepin and amitryptyline have sedative properties.

Sedative/hypnotic medications are used only after the aforementioned treatments are tried, keeping in mind that terminal illness alone does not justify the need for sedation (Table 11–10). When used, barbiturates such as pentobarbital and phenobarbital should be prescribed in low initial dosages and titrated to effect. Benzodiazepines should be prescribed as single agents, using a higher nighttime dose of the regular daytime anxiety medication. The use of some benzodiazepines such as temazapam, flurazepam, and triazolam is controversial in that they have longer duration of effect, rebound effects, and increased anxiety or morning drowsiness. If these medications are used, watch for these side effects and consider using lorazepam or oxazepam instead.

Urinary Symptoms

Complications related to the urinary system commonly occur near the end of life. Early in the course of terminal illness, when a patient's overall functional abilities and performance score tend to be high, and life expectancy, although limited, is relatively long, most urinary tract problems are appropriately managed with conventional interventions such as would be offered to patients with nonterminal illnesses. In these circumstances, when failure to act will shorten life substantially, even invasive treatments such as surgical or radiologic intervention for upper or lower urinary tract ob-

Table 11–10

Pharmacologic Therapy for Insomnia

MEDICATION	DOSAGE	CLINICAL FACTORS
Oxazepam	15–30 mg PO HS Max dose 180 mg	
Lorazepam	0.5–4 mg PO HS Max dose 12 mg	May be given in large dose, at HS when used as routine daily antianxiety agent
Diphenhydramine	50 mg PO HS Max dose 200 mg	May be too sedating the following day in the elderly
Doxepin	75 mg PO HS Max dose 150 mg/day	
Amitriptyline	50–70 mg PO HS Max dose 300 mg	Also good for depression and pain control
Zolpidem	10 mg at HS Max dose 10 mg	Cannot titrate to response. Cost can be a limiting factor
NOT RECOMMENDED		
Temazepam: Slow onset of action Flurazepam: Accumulation of metabolites Triazolam: Withdrawal symptoms		

struction, or dialysis for renal failure, may properly be considered and discussed with patients and their families (see Chapter 17). Later in the course of terminal illness, when the patient weakens and functional capacity declines, urinary complications such as incontinence, retention, bladder spasms, infection, and hematuria often contribute to patient discomfort and detract from the quality of living. This section discusses aspects of the management of these problems that are specifically relevant to the patient with terminal illness in whom death appears to be quite near.

Urinary Incontinence

Urinary incontinence (oftentimes in conjunction with fecal incontinence) is one of the most common occurrences in end-of-life care and affects patients with both malignant and nonmalignant

terminal diagnoses. For patients who remain mentally alert, the problem is not only physically but also psychologically distressing, and is a tangible reminder of loss of control of bodily function and independence.

Urinary incontinence is caused by pathologic, anatomic, or physiologic factors that affect the pressure gradient from the bladder to the urethral sphincter (Table 11–11). Typically, patients experience uncontrolled detrusor contraction, poor sphincter function (stress incontinence), or inability to empty the bladder (overflow incontinence). In malignancy, these dysfunctions can be caused by direct tumor invasion that disrupts innervation and affects muscle function. Tumor invasion may also cause urinary leakage from external fistulas. Aging can lead to lax sphincter control, a phenomenon which is even more common in patients with debilitating, degenerative illnesses such as Alzheimer's disease or end-stage cerebrovascular or cardiovascular disease. A variety of medications may also cause urinary incontinence by several mechanisms, and a careful review of med-

Table 11–11

Causes of Urinary Incontinence

Pathologic factors
   Malignancy
Anatomic changes
   Aging
   Prostatic hypertrophy
   Bladder displacement
Physiologic factors
   Medications
   Trauma
   Irritation

ication history is mandatory for proper assessment of potential causes. Strong, involuntary detrusor muscle contractions (overactive bladder) may be idiopathic or caused by bladder irritation from internal bladder tumors, extrinsic compression, radiation or chemical cystitis, or bacterial or fungal infection. Prostatic enlargement may affect flow dynamics. Causes for overflow incontinence include neurogenic bladder, shrunken bladder due to radiation or chemical cystitis, medications such as anticholinergics, phenothiazines, antihistamines, and opioids, and bladder outlet or urethral obstruction.

An appropriate treatment care plan depends on the stage of terminal illness. For patients with a relatively long prognosis, diagnostic evaluations such as urinalysis, urine culture, or cystoscopy, ultrasonography, computed tomography, or cystometrics may be indicated in order to direct specific therapy. For patients closer to death, such a workup is more intrusive than helpful, and treatment should be empiric and symptom oriented. Discontinuing provocative medications may provide some relief. For patients with "overactive bladder" and bladder spasms, anticholinergics such as oxybutynin can be used but only to the point where troublesome side effects are not produced. Newer agents, such as tolterodine, have fewer systemic anticholinergic side effects, and may be preferable treatment for older, debilitated

patients. Nevertheless, one should be alert for problems such as dry mouth, constipation, and headache, especially when patients are receiving other palliative anticholinergic agents. For stress incontinence in alert mobile patients, agents that increase urethral sphincter tone such as pseudoephedrine and phenylpropanolamine can be tried, usually in conjunction with continence pads or adult diapers. For patients with overflow incontinence, catheterization is usually necessary, especially in immobilized, bed-bound patients who are actively dying. Even in such patients, a markedly distended bladder should not be emptied precipitously after catheterization in order to avoid hypotension and bradycardia. Proper catheter care including irrigation with normal saline, when necessary, and rigorous perineal care are extremely important in order to minimize unnecessary discomfort for the patient. Some patients, including those confused and disoriented, may find a catheter annoying or otherwise objectionable. When such patients are managed with diapers or incontinence pads, scrupulous perineal and skin care, including the use of a skin barrier, is essential. Hospice programs have learned that willing family members are capable of providing this care, provided they are properly instructed and supported.

Urinary Retention

Urinary retention is usually associated with a distended bladder that fails to empty completely. It can be detected with physical examination, ultrasonography, or postvoiding catheterization to detect and measure residual urine. Urinary retention is typically caused by denervation disorders leading to detrusor muscle failure or by bladder outlet obstruction at or distal to the bladder neck. Symptoms associated with detrusor muscle failure include hesitancy, impaired bladder sensation, longer time intervals to micturition, and decreased urgency. In contrast, patients with outlet obstruction usually complain of urinary frequency, urgency, nocturia, and a slow urinary stream. In the terminally ill, both mechanisms may sometimes coexist, and both may be exacerbated by exposure to various medications including opioids, antiemetics, antihistamines, antidepressants, and other anticholinergic agents that are commonly prescribed in hospice and palliative care.

Common causes of a neurogenic bladder in terminally ill patients include generally irreversible conditions such as spinal cord compression and sacral plexopathy associated with invasive tumor, radiation myelopathy, *Vinca* alkaloid neuropathy, nerve injury associated with abdominal–perineal resection, and diabetic neuropathy. Outlet obstruction in men is classically caused by benign prostatic hypertrophy (BPH) or prostatic cancer, but may also be caused by urethral stenosis or strictures associated with infections, including sexually transmitted diseases. In women, distal obstructive uropathy is associated with carcinoma of the cervix and vagina, meatal stenosis, urethral strictures, and tumors of the urethra.

From a pragmatic viewpoint, with the exception of urinary retention that may be reversed through adjustment of concurrent medications, for patients near the end of life, the treatment of urinary retention, whatever the etiology, is primarily via chronic transurethral or suprapubic catheterization. For some mobile patients with outlet obstruction who wish to remain free of catheters, metal, self-expanding urethral stents may prove to be a satisfactory alternative. Rarely, terminally ill patients with concurrent BPH and sufficient expected longevity may respond to conservative measures such as bladder rest for 1 to 2 weeks and institution of treatment with alpha$_1$-blockers such as terazosin or doxazosin. Usually, however, deconditioning and debility associated with terminal illness make recovery of micturition highly unlikely, and in the context of a short prognosis, also rule out, for all intents and purposes, surgical intervention. Patients terminally ill due to advanced prostate cancer are invariably refractory to hormonal therapy. However, androgen deprivation might reasonably be entertained for a patient with prostate cancer-related outlet obstruction and an unrelated terminal condition whose expected survival is thought to be measured in months rather than in weeks or days.

For a motivated, physically capable patient, clean intermittent catheterization is a preferable alternative to a chronic indwelling Foley catheter. Unfortunately, the majority of patients with advanced terminal illness do not fit this description, and the potential advantages in terms of decreased risk of infection, strictures, leakage, and bladder spasms are usually obviated by short life expectancy and other concurrent symptoms. Whether catheter use is intermittent or chronic, the risk of urosepsis relative to the risk of selecting progressively resistant microorganisms rarely justifies antibiotic prophylaxis or attempts to sterilize the urine in terminally ill patients.

Bladder Spasm

Bladder spasms are primarily caused by irritation of the bladder trigone. In the terminally ill, irritation can result from radiation, infection, blood or clots, stones, catheters, or tumor invasion. Spasm can originate in the bladder wall due to tumor invasion or radiation. Spinal cord injury from tumor invasion can also produce bladder wall irritability.

Treatment is directed at the cause. Catheters can be withdrawn or their balloons deflated. Urinary infection should be treated with antibiotics with the clear purpose of alleviating discomfort. If bleeding is present due to a reversible cause, invasive interventions may sometimes be indicated, depending on the patient's overall condition and prognosis. Otherwise, nonspecific measures discussed next can sometimes help in decreasing hematuria and clot formation. Increased fluids help to relieve irritation from infection, blood, or retained stones. If a stone will not pass, a palliative urology referral may be needed.

Nonspecific measures include anticholinergics such as flavoxate, oxybutynin, and tolterodine. In addition to the side effects described and the potential for drug interactions, these agents may cause drowsiness and blurred vision, and in noncatheterized patients may cause urinary retention. Nonsteroidal anti-inflammatory drugs may help to suppress spasms by inhibiting prostaglandin-related bladder irritation. However, NSAIDs may also increase the risk of hematuria and further compromise renal function. For actively dying patients, or for those unable to swallow oral medications, "B & O" suppositories can be useful; and in catheterized patients, irrigation with 0.25 percent acetic acid solution or bupivacaine 0.25 percent, 20 mL every 8 to 12 hours is sometimes effective.

Hematuria

The significance of hematuria in end-of-life care is often more psychological than physiologic. Gross hematuria, whether from the upper or lower urinary tract, may often be asymptomatic, and even urine that is very red in color may, in fact, contain only a small volume of red blood cells. Nevertheless, patients and families are often very disturbed, even agitated, at the site of blood even to the point of being convinced, against most probability, that the patient is bleeding to death. Therefore, controlling hematuria may be crucial for the relief of emotional suffering. Of course, hematuria may cause significant physical symptoms as well, especially clot colic due to upper urinary tract bleeding, and dysuria and bladder spasms due to lower urinary tract bleeding. Persistent gross hematuria may also cause symptomatic anemia in debilitated terminal patients, especially those dying with cancers that were previously treated with myelosuppressive chemotherapy or radiotherapy.

Near the end of life, hematuria is likely due to one or more of the following: urinary tract infections, tumors, radiation/chemotherapy cystitis, kidney stones, or acquired bleeding diatheses. Upper urinary tract hematuria results most often from renal cell carcinoma, transitional cell carcinoma of the renal pelvis and/or ureter, other metastatic cancers, or stone formation. In the lower urinary tract, hemorrhagic cystitis is usually due to infection, pre-

vious radiotherapy or chemotherapy, or neoplasia. Bleeding may also emanate from the prostate or bladder neck. Drug-induced hematuria (e.g., NSAIDs, coumadin) should also be considered if clinically relevant.

As has been repeatedly stressed throughout this book, the treatment plan is dictated by the patient's condition and prognosis, and ultimately by the patient's goals and wishes. Some diagnostic tests such as urinalysis and culture or coagulation screening are minimally invasive and may prompt relatively simple and rapidly effective palliative interventions such as antibiotics or reversal of anticoagulation. Hemorrhage due to tumors may respond to radiotherapy or cauterization. These interventions may be appropriate for select patients with longer prognoses. Aggressive palliative surgery including nephrectomy, cystectomy, and hypogastric artery ligation is rarely relevant for terminal hospice patients.

In end-of-life care, gross hematuria, especially when asymptomatic, may sometimes call for nothing beyond reassurance. When treating symptomatic hemorrhagic cystitis, patients should be encouraged to decrease physical activity and, if possible, to increase fluid intake. For persistent bleeding causing urinary clot retention, clots may be evacuated through a large diameter Foley catheter. Further bleeding and clotting can be minimized via bladder irrigation with saline chilled to 4°C at a rate of 3 L/24 hours. Empiric treatments to control bleeding from the bladder include ethamsylate 500 mg orally every 6 hours or epsilon-aminocaproic acid (Amicar) 5 g orally as an initial loading dose and 1g every 1 to 4 hours as needed. Amicar is contraindicated for patients with disseminated intravascular coagulation or with advanced liver disease. When hematuria comes from the upper urinary tract, Amicar can cause intrarenal obstruction due to clot formation and lead to severe pain from renal colic as well as to renal failure. Amicar may also be administered intravenously or intravesically, although these routes are generally not preferred for hospice patients. Another relatively innocuous treatment for hemorrhagic cystitis is 1 percent alum in sterile water given by continuous bladder irrigation. Formalin instillation, although highly effective, is also highly toxic, and requires general or regional anesthesia. It does not appear to have a place in palliative end-of life care. For terminal patients with symptomatic upper urinary tract bleeding and clot colic, treatment is best confined to fluid-induced diuresis and appropriate analgesics. Amicar may be excessively risky, as explained. For ethical reasons, the physician may be obligated to discuss the option of a palliative unilateral nephrectomy with the patient, but it is difficult to foresee the circumstance in which such a procedure would be recommended in end-of-life care.

Urinary Infections

Urinary infections in the terminally ill may be difficult to identify. Many elderly or debilitated patients may not be febrile despite significant infection. The basal body temperatures in such people may be lower than in a healthy person. A normal temperature reading in such a patient may actually represent a fever. The signs and symptoms of infection may be vague or attenuated. There may be some loss of appetite, a relative increase in fatigue or confusion, lower blood pressure, declining urine production, and tachycardia. Therefore, it is best to have a high index of suspicion for the presence of infection and sepsis.

Patients in long-term care facilities may have colonization of the urinary tract. Without signs or symptoms, a positive culture in such an individual may not warrant aggressive management that could cause selective growth of resistant strains of organisms. In the severely debilitated and/or demented patient, discussion of aggressive use of antibiotics needs to be done when formulating an overall plan of care. If the aim of treatment is primarily to relieve the symptoms of irritative voiding, acidification of the urine by drinking cranberry juice or the use of urinary analgesic drugs such as phenazopyridine (Pyridium) may be sufficient. The addition of anticholinergic drugs may also help to relieve symptoms.

If it is elected to prescribe antibiotics, treatment may be empirical pending culture results. Reasonably effective oral agents include amoxicillin, trimethoprim/sulfamethoxazole, and ciprofloxacin. Alternative, intravenous antibiotics may sometimes be indicated depending on the defined palliative goal.

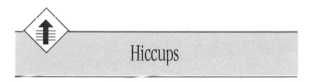

Hiccups

Hiccups are a pathologic respiratory reflex characterized by spasm of the diaphragm. This results in sudden inspiration (the "hic" portion) and then closure of the vocal cords (the "cup" portion).

Causes

The hiccup reflex is a result of irritation of the diaphragm, phrenic nerve, thoracic or upper lumbar spinal nerves, or the celiac plexus. In terminal patients, hiccups commonly occur with uremia, CNS lesions (CVAs and tumors), and tumors of the abdomen, esophagus, neck, chest, gall bladder, or pancreas. They may be associated with peptic ulcer disease, gall bladder disease, or pancreatitis, and with radiotherapy to the chest or neck.

Treatment

Treatment should focus on the underlying disease if possible. General principles include avoiding gastric loading, promoting gastric emptying, and avoiding foods and beverages that produce gas or irritation. Pharyngeal stimulation can disrupt spasms and suppress the reflex hiccups. This may be accomplished by drinking from the wrong side of the cup, rapid ingestion of granulated sugar or liquor, cold placed at the back of the neck, swallowing dry bread, and stimulation of the pharynx by an oral or nasal catheter. Breath

Table 11–12

Pharmacological Therapy of Hiccups

MEDICATION	DOSE	CLINICAL NOTES
Baclofen	5–10 mg PO tid	May cause excess sedation in elderly
Simethicone	40–120 mg PO after meals and HS prn Max dose 500 mg	Relieves gastric distention
Metoclopramide	10–20 mg PO bid to q 6 hours	Promotes gastric emptying
Chlorpromazine	10–20 mg PO bid to q 6 hours	Calms CNS response
Haloperidol	3–5 mg PO q 8 hours	Calms CNS response
Nifedipine	10 mg PO tid or XL 30 mg qd	If no cardiac contraindications
Phenytoin	300–500 mg PO daily in divided doses	Decreases nerve hyperstimulation
Carbamazepine	200–1600 mg PO daily in 3 or 4 divided doses	Decreases nerve hyperstimulation. In large dosages over time can cause bone marrow dysfunction
Prednisone	10 mg PO q 8 hours	Effective for inflammatory process from malignancies

holding or rebreathing to raise the levels of carbon dioxide in the lungs and blood may help as well. Medications that may be useful are listed in Table 11–12, and include baclofen, simethicone, metoclopramide, chlorpromazine, haloperidol, nifedipine, prednisone, phenytoin, and carbamazepine. Many experts in hospice and palliative care recommend baclofen as the agent of first choice. Prednisone is especially effective for inflammatory or destructive lesions in the thorax or abdomen.

References

Block SD: Assessing and managing depression in the terminally ill patient. *Ann Intern Med* 132:209, 2000.

Cadieux RS: Practical management of treatment—resistant depression. *Am Fam Physician* 58:2059, 1998.

Coluzzi P, et al: *Vitas Guidelines for Intensive Palliative Care.* Miami, Vitas Healthcare, 1996.

Doyle D, Hanks G, McDonald N: *The Oxford Textbook of Palliative Medicine.* New York, Oxford University Press, 1996.

Enck RE: *The Medical Care of Terminally Ill Patients.* London, Johns Hopkins, 1994.

Fallon MT, Hanks GW: Control of common symptoms in advance cancer. *Ann Acad Med* 23:2, 1994.

Hirshberg SJ, Greenberg RE: Urologic issues of palliative care. In: Berger A, Portenoy RK, Weissman DE, eds. *Principles and Practice of Supportive Oncology.* Philadelphia, Lippincott-Raven, 1998, pp. 371–383.

Johanson, GA: *Symptom Relief in Terminal Care.* Santa Rosa, Sonoma County Academic Foundation, 1994.

Rousseau P: Asthenia in terminally ill cancer patients. A brief review. *Am J Hosp Palliat Care* 14:258, 1997.

Storey P, Knight C: *Management of Selected Non-pain Symptoms in the Terminally Ill.* Gainsville, American Academy of Hospice and Palliative Medicine, 1996.

World Health Organization: *Symptom Relief in Terminal Illness.* Geneva, World Health Organization, 1998.

Vincent D. Nguyen
Jeanne Micklich Ash

Chapter
12

The Last Days:
The Actively Dying Patient

Introduction

"There is an appointed time for everything, and a time for every affair under the heavens. A time to be born and a time to die."

Ecclesiastes 3:1–2

Death is inevitable; dying is the concluding stage of life and death. For many, especially those who work in the hospice and palliative care arenas, death is seen as part of life's natural cycle and often as an accepted friend. Just as one feels joy when embracing a newborn as it leaves its mother's womb, hospice and palliative care providers feel a sense of satisfaction when having the privilege to care for a dying individual near the end of life.

While the satisfaction that one experiences in caring for the terminally ill occurs throughout the course of a patient's final illness, it is perhaps greatest during the final days of the patient's life, when attention is specifically focused on ensuring patient comfort and dignity as that life draws to its inevitable conclusion. During the final days of life, patients and families are often confronted with a multitude of shifting emotions, from hope to despair, from fear to courage, from relief to guilt. For some patients and families, it is the first time that the realities of the dying process are recognized and acknowledged. End-of-life caregivers are equally challenged, often torn between attending to the ever-changing needs of the patients in their charge, while trying to support the patients' family through the final dying process.

In view of the special nature of the final days of life, this chapter will focus on the signs of impending death. It will also offer contemporary palliative approaches to the most common chal-

Table 12–1

Characteristics of Phases of the Active Dying Process

Preactive (7–14 days prior to death)	Weakness and lethargy
	Increased dependence on caregivers
	Bedbound status in formerly active patient
	Increased sleep
	Progressive disorientation
	Limited attention span or withdrawal
	Restlessness
	Decreased interest in food and fluid
	Difficulty swallowing
	Loss of bladder and/or bowel control in previously continent patient
Active (2–3 days prior to death)	Clouding of consciousness
	Decreased responsiveness to external stimuli
	Eyes glassy, pupils unfocused
	No interest in food or fluid
	Abnormal respiratory patterns
	Blood pressure and pulse difficult to obtain
	Hypotension
	Progressive cooling and mottling of extremities
	Terminal congestion

lenging symptoms faced by the patients and families during the active dying process.

Clinical Signs of Approaching Death

Most patients die peacefully. The process is often described as a gentle withdrawing from the external stimuli and a slipping away into a very deep slumber. The multiple prominent cascading events that eventually occur before the patient's death will often include functional, cognitive, nutritional, and physical declines.

The active dying process is divided into two phases: the preactive phase, which begins around 7 to 14 days prior to death; and the active phase, which generally constitutes the last 2 to 3 days of life. The important clinical characteristics of each phase are outlined in Table 12–1, and described in detail next.

Preactive Phase

As patients enter the preactive phase of dying, they develop progressive weakness and lethargy, and become increasingly dependent on caregivers for the basic activities of daily living. Those patients who had previously been active are likely to become bedbound, and sleep occupies the majority of their time. Cognitively, patients may become progressively disoriented and their attention span is often limited. Some patients may withdraw from their surroundings while others may speak to external objects or persons not present. Restlessness is also common.

Nutritionally, the combination of lack of interest in food and fluid and difficulty swallowing result in severely diminished oral intake. Not surprisingly, urine output is reduced, and the loss of involuntary muscle control often leads to incontinence of bowel and bladder of patients who had previously retained these functions.

Active Phase

Patients are as unique in life as they are at the hours before their death. However, during the final phases of their dying process, patients will share similar clinical signs and symptoms. For example, patients generally remain in bed and lose any remaining interest in food or fluid. There is clouding of the consciousness as the body no longer responds to external stimuli. The eyes become glassy and the pupils appear to focus on unseen remote objects. The extremities, starting from the distal end, become progressively mottled, clammy, and cool to the touch. Blood pressure, heart sounds, and palpable pulses are often difficult to detect. Respiratory patterns can vary, from being slow, deep and regular to more rapid and irregular. Upper and lower airway congestion is often apparent. Periods of apnea occur, and over time may progressively lengthen until breathing finally ceases.

It is not easy to predict the exact time of death based on the development of any particular signs or symptoms, as this process often varies from several hours to many days. It is well known that on occasion, for inexplicable reasons, some patients may have a transient improvement in physical, cognitive, and/or functional abilities during the dying process. Hospice and palliative care workers characterize this phenomenon as a "surge of energy." When this surge occurs, the patient no longer appears to be imminently dying but instead, seems to have awakened from deep sleep with a new sense of vitality. This transitory episode can last from hours to days before the patient returns to the previous dying state. This surge of energy often makes families and caregivers confused and distraught as they go through an emotional roller-coaster of hope and despair. Sometimes, they will doubt that the patient is actually dying and may desire a shift to medical interventions in the hope of getting the patient back to normal. It is important for the professional caregivers to assist the family in characterizing the temporary nature of this "surge" as a precious memento from the dying person to them. It should be explained to the family that any medical intercessions made in an attempt to prolong this temporary phenomenon will not be beneficial, and may in fact be a painful and unnecessary intrusion on their loved one as life comes to an end.

As mentioned, however, most deaths are peaceful for the patient. The survivors often recall a nondramatic process. In a series of studies of dying patients, up to 98 percent of individuals died peacefully and 65 percent were peaceful 48 hours prior to death. However, in the final days, some patients may develop new symptoms or may experience a recurrence or an exacerbation of previously well-controlled symptoms. Pain, restlessness, confusion, agitation, hallucinations, myoclonic jerks, seizures, hemorrhage, nausea, vomiting, shortness of breath, and dyspnea are common symptoms from which dying patients can suffer. Oftentimes these symptoms can be terrifying for the witnessing friends and family members. The memories of the final moments will often linger in the mind and heart of the surviving members for many years to come. It is important, therefore, that health care professionals know how to recognize and treat these terminal symptoms.

Terminal Signs and Symptoms and Their Management

Pain Management as Life Concludes

The most important principle for pain management during the active-dying phase is that pain management practices employed in earlier stages do not change (see Chapter 6). Decreased levels of consciousness do not mean that earlier pain levels have lessened. Although there is some indication that metabolic changes induced by dehydration and diminished nutrition may have an analgesic effect, it cannot be assumed that pain abates as death approaches. In fact, pain during this stage of dying actually increases. Therefore, pain management protocols established earlier in the course of the disease should be maintained.

The issues related to pain management during this final phase of life revolve around assessment, route of medication administration, fear of hastening death through opioid use, and opiate withdrawal in the patient whose pain has been managed by opioids.

ASSESSMENT

Fundamental to pain management is the need to identify pain etiology and provide interventions that relieve the source of pain. Pain assessment in the mentally alert and verbally responsive patient does not change. In evaluating the nonalert and/or nonverbal patient, however, the clinician may have to rely on visual signs such as facial grimacing and motor restlessness, and auditory cues such as moaning that may imply physical discomfort.

As patients enter the actively dying phase of their illnesses, caregivers and health care professionals have often observed pain with movement of the patient. This pain has been variously described as "disturbance pain" and as "incident pain." This type of episodic pain is brief in duration and apparently occurs when the patient is moved or disturbed. The patient may cry out, moan, and/or grimace. It is probably attributable to the stiffness that occurs with immobility, although researchers have described it as an "alarm response" that is particularly evident in the blind, deaf, and confused.

This type of pain can be a source of distress for the family and/or caregiver, who may feel that they are agonizing the patient by touching them. It is therefore essential to teach the family and caregivers to expect this type of response and to ensure that they are comfortable with moving the patient. To this end, the patient caregivers must receive appropriate instruction in positioning techniques. Family communication with the patient should be encouraged even in the nonresponsive patient.

Management of disturbance pain includes explaining procedures and treatments carefully before performing them in addition to deliberate, careful, and planned movement of the patient. For prolonged manipulation of the patient or when performing certain treatments (e.g., wound care or Foley catheter insertion), the patient should be premedicated with a short-acting analgesic, such as liquid morphine, about half an hour prior to such activities.

Other common causes of physical discomfort during the final days of life may relate to the genitourinary and gastrointestinal tracts as well as the integument and musculoskeletal systems. Urinary retention leading to a distended bladder and/or promoting urinary tract infection can cause pain. Constipation can occur and be painful, complicated by the fact that many caregivers believe that with a lack of food intake, patients need not move their bowels. There is an increased incidence of pressure ulcers due to the immobility and incontinence associated with the last days of life. Although analgesics may be important in managing these symptoms, it is important to remember that interventions may also be nonpharmacologic in nature. Proper skin care, positioning, gentle range of motion, placement of a Foley catheter for bladder drainage, and maintenance of a bowel program are all examples of approaches that can increase comfort and decrease pain in the dying patient.

ROUTES OF MEDICATION ADMINISTRATION

ORAL ROUTE   In certain cases, the oral route remains the optimal choice for the administration of pain medication at this stage of life. A concentrated form of liquid morphine or oxycodone (20 mg/mL), administered every 4 hours (or more often if needed), can be used safely, noninvasively, and effectively. These medications are actually given by placing the liquid medication in the sublingual or buccal space, leading to the mistaken belief by many caregivers that these medications are actually being absorbed directly through the mucosa. However, our best understanding about the absorption of sublingually administered liquid morphine and oxycodone suggests that these two opioids are actually absorbed in the gastrointestinal and respiratory tracts after they trickle past the pharynx. Fentanyl is the only orally available narcotic analgesic that is truly absorbed sublingually and transmucosally (see the discussion on the oral transmucosal route later in the chapter). By anecdotal reports, these orally administered medications do not appear to contribute to symptomatic aspiration when given in small amounts. This is especially true for those patients requiring less than 120 mg/day of concentrated liquid oral morphine or oxycodone.

RECTAL ROUTE   In the patient with less than a few days left to live, the rectal route is an effective alternative route providing there is a willing caregiver who is comfortable medicating the patient via this route. Morphine and hydromorphone are the most common choices because they are readily available in suppository forms.

Absorption of rectally administered opioids can be affected by the presence of stool in the rectal vault, and defecation before complete absorption of the suppository can result in unreliable pain relief. Absorption and plasma levels of rectally administered opioids may differ from equivalent oral doses because the first-pass effect is diminished in rectal administration, although for most patients the ratio of oral to rectal opioid is 1:1. Careful assessment of level of consciousness, pain-related behaviors, and patient self-report of effectiveness, when possible, must be used to determine the efficacy of substituting the rectal for the oral route for pain medication delivery.

Continuous-release morphine and oxycodone preparations have been used as suppositories for rectal administration. Based an anecdotal reports, these are effective in sustaining patients' comfort, provided that the opioid suppositories are left in place. Theoretically, the vascular supply in the rectum is adequate for medication absorption, but there has been little research comparing the oral versus the rectal use of oral sustained-release compounds in terms of efficacy, plasma levels, and absorption.

The rectal route is especially useful for patients experiencing nausea and vomiting, and in those with partial or complete bowel obstructions. However, the rectal route cannot be used for long periods of time because it will cause discomfort from the irritation of rectal mucosa. In the presence of diarrhea, hemorrhoids, anal fissures, and neutropenia, the rectal route must be avoided or its use considered carefully. In these instances, other modes of administration may be more suitable.

ORAL TRANSMUCOSAL ROUTE   Fentanyl is lipophilic (lipid soluble), which makes it an ideal candidate for oral transmucosal use. The FDA recently approved an oral transmucosal fentanyl citrate delivery system. This system incorporates fentanyl citrate into a "lollypop" to be placed in or rubbed against the buccal area for 15 minutes, where it dissolves and is absorbed into the bloodstream. Fentanyl delivered transmucosally in this manner provides pain relief in 15 to 30 minutes. Dosages are often initiated at 200 µg and titrated to 1600 µg, stopping at the unit dose that provides adequate analgesia. Because of the newness and the much higher cost of this fentanyl delivery system compared to the oral and rectal medications described, its potential use in the actively dying patient remains extremely limited. See Chapter 6 for further discussion.

TRANSDERMAL ROUTE   Patients whose pain has been adequately managed by transdermal fentanyl should continue to use this medication during the last hours of life. However, transdermal fentanyl by itself is seldom the drug or route of choice to initiate in the actively dying patient. Transdermal fentanyl takes approximately 12 to 24 hours to reach peak plasma levels, so that the patient would have to use other additional means of pain management until peak blood levels are reached. The other drawback to using this method is that rapid titration is difficult. For further discussion of the use of transdermal fentanyl, see Chapter 6.

PARENTERAL ROUTES   Although noninvasive routes of administration are generally preferable, especially when the patient only has a short time to live, there may be times when it is necessary to provide analgesia via a parenteral route. For patients with an already existing venous access site the intravenous route would be most appropriate; while for the majority of patients, in whom no indwelling IV line is present, the subcutaneous route has been found to be an effective delivery system.

Subcutaneous Route   A continuous subcutaneous infusion with bolus doses for breakthrough pain has been shown to provide good pain relief during the final stages of life, with stable blood levels and the ability for rapid titration. The subcutaneous route compares favorably to the intravenous route in terms of efficacy and plasma levels without the complexities inherent in an intravenous delivery system.

Morphine is commonly used for subcutaneous pain management. Hydromorphone provides comparable pain relief and has the advantage of higher potency and concentration capabilities than morphine, and is thus useful in that it can be delivered in a lesser volume. This is especially valuable for those patients who require substantial amounts of opioids to adequately manage pain.

The biggest drawback to subcutaneous infusions for pain management is the limited volume that subcutaneous tissue can absorb without creating discomfort or side effects such as tissue damage. Subcutaneous tissue can absorb only about 2 to 3 mL/hour, though the use of hyaluronidase can significantly increase the capacity of the subcutaneous tissue to absorb fluid (see "Hydration During the Last Days of Life" later in the chapter).

Discomfort from needle placement is rarely an issue for this route. Butterfly needles are typically used, although there are also specialized needles designed specifically for subcutaneous infusion delivery. Typical subcutaneous infusion protocols call for needle and site changes every 72 hours to minimize the chance of infection and to promote fluid absorption.

For pain management by subcutaneous infusion to be effective, the patient must have adequate subcutaneous tissue. This means that cachetic patients are not ideal candidates for this method of pain management. Conversely, the grossly edematous patient is also not a good candidate for pain management via subcutaneous infusion. For immunosuppressed patients and those with coagulopathies, subcutaneous infusions must be carefully weighed against other choices because the possibility of side effects will increase.

Opioids used for subcutaneous infusions include morphine, hydromorphone, and also diamorphine, fentanyl, and methadone. Diamorphine, which is illegal in the United States, offers the advantage of high concentration per volume of fluid. Fentanyl has been used for subcutaneous pain management, but little research has been conducted on its pharmacokinetics during administration. The use of these referenced medications via this manner may cause site reactions in some patients.

Intravenous Route   Intravenous pain management is very effective in providing stable plasma levels, rapid titration, and bolus dosing for breakthrough pain. Medications used in subcutaneous infusion can likewise be used for the intravenous administration. For the patient with a functional central venous access device, this route is an ideal alternative. It is often the route of choice when large volumes of opioids are necessary to maintain pain control. In the absence of a central line or port, particularly during the last hours of life, venous access may often be difficult and often illogical. The use of the subcutaneous route is frequently the better alternative.

OPIOID WITHDRAWAL

Suspending the use of opioids in patients whose pain has been controlled will result in painful withdrawal symptoms (restlessness, agitation, tremors, and/or seizures). Withdrawal symptoms occur in patients taking oral medications who become less responsive as death approaches and, therefore, are unable to swallow large quantities of oral medications. For these patients, another route of opioid administration (rectal, subcutaneous, or intravenous) can be chosen to maintain controlled levels.

Alternatively (as described earlier) concentrated morphine or oxycodone preparations (20 mg/mL) can be administered into the sublingual or buccal space (where it is then swallowed) with good symptom control. To prevent withdrawal symptoms, it has been suggested that at least 25 percent of the original opioid dose must be maintained.

Dyspnea

Dyspnea is an uncomfortable awareness of breathlessness associated with shortness of breath. It is one of the most frequent and terrifying symptoms in the last days of a patient's life. Dyspnea may manifest as copious secretions, cough, fatigue, air hunger, anxiety, agitation, tachypnea, and chest pain. Some data suggest that dyspnea occurs in up to 70 percent of dying people, with the highest incidence in those with lung cancer, head and neck cancer, and degenerative neurologic diseases.

Terminal dyspnea is often multifactorial, and it is rarely possible to treat the underlying cause of dyspnea. Therefore, the treatment goal is aimed at relieving the perception of breathlessness and associated symptoms. Interventions that may be effective in the treatment of dyspnea in the last days of life are listed in Table 12–2.

Nonpharmacologic strategies include having the presence of a caregiver, a soothing calm voice, and added gentle touch to induce relaxation and relieve apprehension, especially when dyspnea is related to anxiety. In some circumstances, the use of a fan or opening of a window allows a cool draft of air to reach the cheek and nasal cavity, which can be useful in relieving dyspnea because perception of breathlessness is thought to be altered by stimulation of the areas innervated by the trigeminal nerve. A simple fan generally acts as well and provides as much relief as oxygen provided by nasal cannula. Oxygen may provide symptomatic relief for some patients, but is more beneficial for patients whose dyspnea is accompanied by cyanosis. Patients with cyanosis may benefit from the use of a noninvasive, positive-pressure facemask.

Pharmacologic strategies may also be required for the relief of dyspnea. Though bronchodilators (beta$_2$-agonists and xanthines) and steroids are effective treatments for those with airway obstruction and inflammation, respiratory sedatives such as the benzodiazepines, phenothiazines, and opioids are the mainstay of pharmacotherapy. (See Table 12–2 for appropriate dosing information.) They may be used alone or in conjunction with bronchodilators and steroids for added potency.

Opioids, in particular morphine sulfate, also have an established role in the treatment of dyspnea by suppressing respiratory awareness and at the same time improving the efficiency of breathing. In relatively "healthy" patients, morphine has been shown to improve exercise endurance. The precise mechanism for this is still unknown.

The overemphasized fear of potential for respiratory depression and hastening death has caused many health care professionals to withhold morphine for the treatment of dyspnea, especially for patients with lung pathology (COPD, lung cancer). This concern is not justified, and thus morphine should not be withheld. Rather, the dose should be titrated against the respiratory rate to achieve a rate of 12 to 20 per minute. For those patients already using opioids for pain control, a dose increase of 50 percent is needed to achieve adequate respiratory control. The route of delivery often recommended is oral; however, the subcutaneous, intravenous, and most recently the nebulized form (though with conflicting results in controlled studies) are routes of delivery used to treat dyspnea in the last days of life.

Table 12-2

Treatment of Dyspnea During the Last Days of Life

NONPHARMACOLOGIC
Presence of caregiver Soothing calm voice Gentle touch Relaxation techniques Circulation of air by the use of a fan or opening a window Oxygen
PHARMACOLOGIC

Benzodiazepines
    Lorazepam (oral, parenteral) 0.5–2 mg q4h prn
    Alprazolam (oral) 0.25–2 mg q4h prn
    Diazepam (oral, parenteral) 2–20 mg q4h prn
Phenothiazines
    Chlorpromazine (oral, rectal, parenteral) 30–100 mg q4h prn
    Thioridazine (oral, parenteral) 30–100 mg q4h prn
Opioids
    Morphine
        Oral[a], 5-10 mg q2-4h prn
        Parenteral[a], 2–5 mg q2–4h prn
        Already on opioids, increase dose 50% over baseline
        Nebulized, 5-20 mg q4h prn

[a]Opioid-naïve patient.

Table 12–3

Treatment of Terminal Congestion During the Last Days of Life

MEDICATION	ROUTE OF ADMINISTRATION	DOSE
Hyoscyamine	Oral	0.125–0.25 mg q4h prn
Atropine	Oral (ophthalmic solution)	1%, 2 drops q3h prn
	Parenteral	0.4 mg q1–2 h prn
Scopolamine	Transdermal	1 patch q3 days

The rationale for using nebulized morphine is based on the fact that opioid receptors have been found in the bronchial trees and along the sensory fibers of the vagus nerve. Nebulized morphine has a fast onset of 2 to 5 minutes, making this route of administration especially attractive. Morphine solution, prepared for either parenteral or oral use, diluted in 2 mL of normal saline (NS) solution, at the starting dose of 5 to 10 mg every 4 hours as needed, is recommended for administration via the nebulized route. The most common side effect is bronchospasm; thus the first treatment should be administered in a controlled setting.

In extremely rare cases, uncontrollable dyspnea can only be relieved by total sedation. This technique is discussed later.

Terminal Congestion (Death Rattle)

Terminal congestion, exhibited by noisy moist breathing or "rattling," is a common sign in patients nearing death. Though patients are not often troubled by it, the noise is often a source of distress to the family and caregivers.

This congestion, also known as death rattle, can simply be described as a collection of oscillating mucous secretion in the oropharynx and trachea during inspiration and expiration of the dying patient who is unable to clear the secretion. With empathetic explanation and assurance, positioning, and judicious usage of anticholinergic medication and occasional gentle aspiration of the secretion, this symptom can often be palliated. Hyoscyamine sulfate, atropine sulfate, and sco-

polamine have been recommended and are available in oral, subcutaneous, and transdermal forms. (See Table 12–3 for appropriate dosing information.) Suctioning should be avoided.

It is important to note that this moist respiration is different from congestion related to pulmonary edema. Anticholinergics will have minimal to no effect in reducing congestion related to cardiac failure. Morphine and gentle diuresis with furosemide or bumetanide in these cases are often required.

Xerostomia

It is believed by some that xerostomia (dry mouth) is a major cause of discomfort near the end of life, and is a primary reason for the desire to administer parenteral fluids to patients who have no fluid intake in the last days of life (see the next section). With fastidious oral care, however, discomfort from xerostomia can be relieved, obviating the need for fluids. Appropriate oral-care treatments include (1) cleansing and swabbing the oral cavity with peroxide and water or glycerin swabs, (2) lubricating the oral mucosa by offering sips of liquid or using a spray bottle, (3) using saliva substitutes, (4) application of moisturizer or petroleum jelly to the lips, and (5) administration of vitamin C, lemon drops, or pilocarpine to stimulate salivary flow. (See Chapter 10 for further discussion of xerostomia.)

Hydration During the Last Days of Life

Despite evidence that there is little benefit to artificial hydration near the end of life (see Chapter 16 for more discussion), families and medical professionals alike often feel compelled to provide fluids during the patient's last days. There are many reasons. For the families, it may seem to be the loving thing to do. For the clinicians, it is basic "standard" medical care; to withhold or discontinue fluids seem like a break in the sacred bond of patient–physician relationship. Also, the implications of allowing a person to die from dehydration and starvation may be perceived as acts of omission on the physician's part. Thus, for all parties involved, withholding the ever-so-available medical therapeutic interventions of IV fluids may lead to guilt, frustration, and "loss of control over death."

Another major reason why physicians and families want to give fluids to dying patients is the notion that death by dehydration will cause pain and suffering. This suffering has been hypothesized to be caused by thirst, dry mouth, fatigue, lethargy, nausea, vomiting, confusion, restlessness, as well as an increased risk of bedsores and constipation. In the presence of renal failure and accumulation of opioid metabolites, confusion, myoclonus, seizure, muscle cramping, and hastening of death may occur. Electrolyte imbalance, such as hypernatremia, may develop and cause confusion, weakness, lethargy, and eventually progression to obtundation, coma, and death.

However, several studies have examined the issue of pain and suffering and dehydration in the dying patient and have refuted some of the concern. Dehydration does not cause pain or discomfort because during dehydration, ketones are produced and serve as a natural anesthetic and euphorant. Ketones also cause a decreasing level of consciousness. Further, patients in end-state dehydration appear to experience less discomfort than do those receiving medical hydration.

Adverse effects of parenteral fluids are exhaustively long and include repetitive venipuncture from infiltration or self-removal, decreased patient mobility, congestion, increased respiratory secretions and pleural effusion that leads to coughing, and the common distressing signs of choking and drowning. Further adverse effects include fluid overload with resulting signs and symptoms of congestive heart failure; increased risk for intra-abdominal ascites; increased urinary output that can contribute to skin breakdown, which may lessen if an invasive urinary catheter is placed; increased GI fluid, which leads to an increased incidence of nausea and vomiting that may require a nasogastric tube to suction for relief; increased peripheral edema, which leads to an increased risk of pressure ulcers; increased tumor growth; and increased symptoms related to tumor size. Therefore, the many adverse effects of IV fluids and a lack of data suggesting that dehydration causes pain or discomfort for dying patients leads most experts in palliative care to not recommend IV fluids to prevent dehydration.

Hypodermoclysis

As noted, most patients die peacefully without the use of parenteral fluids. Nevertheless, there will be patients who will require some form of hydration because of symptoms (confusion, opioid toxicity) or, more often, for nonclinical reasons related to cultural or ethnic beliefs, or pressure from families. For most of these patients, provision of parenteral fluids by the intravenous route poses significant logistic challenges. Most patients do not have indwelling IV catheters and intravenous access can be difficult to obtain despite multiple attempts by the most skillful clinicians. Thus, hydration via the intravenous route can be cumbersome and discomforting for both the dying patient and the nursing staff.

Recently, there has been some resurgence of hypodermoclysis (HDC or clysis) usage within the palliative care community as a way to administer fluid and certain medications into the subcutaneous space for symptom control. HDC is a safe and simple technique of delivering fluid that can be used to provide short-term hydration. (Further discussion of HDC can be found in Chapter 16.)

In the last days of life, hydration by HDC may be provided via a continuous 24-hour infusion at 40 mL/hour, a 12-hour infusion at 80 mL/hour, or 3 times a day in 500-mL boluses over 1 hour each. The recommended solution used should contain electrolytes (normal saline or two-thirds 5 percent dextrose and one-third saline), because non-electrolyte solutions (D5W) tend to draw fluid into the interstitial space, which can lead to edema and swelling and cause tissue sloughing. Hyaluronidase, 150 U/liter of solution or prior to the first of the three 500-mL infusions, is added to facilitate fluid absorption.

In a study using HDC, researchers found the majority of patients receiving clysis tolerated the procedure well. If the needle was placed properly, patients did not have any discomfort, and some were not aware of the needle's presence. Needles used to administer fluids and medications are butterfly needles and Teflon cannula. The average duration of SQ sites using butterfly needles is 5.3 days versus 11.9 days using a Teflon cannula. The cost of the cannula, however, is reported to be ten times that of the butterfly needles.

Proctoclysis

The use of proctoclysis fluid administration via the rectal route has been described in the literature and appears as a reasonable and safe method for administering fluids. This mode of administration is based on the fact that fluid absorption occurs after enemas in normal volunteers. Though most patients would prefer the SQ route, the proctoclysis technique is an effective means of hydrating patients who are unable to receive fluid by any other route—provided there is no tumor involvement of the colon.

Proctoclysis requires the insertion of a 22-French NGT catheter 40 cm into the rectum. NS or tap water can be administered at 100 to 400 mL/hour 4 or 5 times a day. The two most common side effects are leakage and tenesmus (spasm of anal sphincter). Proctoclysis is more cost-effective than parenteral hydration, being 50 times less expensive than hypodermoclysis, and 30 times cheaper than IV hydration.

Confusion and Agitation

Confusion occurs in up to 10 percent of patients during the last hours of life. The spectrum of presentation can often be quite dramatic, ranging from disorientation to outright physical restlessness and agitation. The causes of confusion include environmental changes, anxiety, pain or generalized physical discomfort, constipation or distended bladder, dehydration, electrolyte imbalance, infection, and medications.

Treatment of confusion and agitation should begin by assessing and treating any correctable causes. Nonpharmacologic measures such as appropriate hygiene, positioning, calm reassurance, and keeping the room temperature at a comfortable setting should also be addressed. If there is no improvement in symptoms, medications are often required. Benzodiazepines and the phenothiazines are often used (Table 12–4). If symptoms are still not controlled, then total sedation may need to be considered.

Total Sedation

The cardinal goal of medicine in caring for the dying is the relief of distressing symptoms and phy-

Table 12–4

Treatment of Confusion and Agitation During the Last Days of Life

MEDICATION	ROUTE OF ADMINISTRATION	DOSE
Lorazepam	Oral, parenteral	1–2 mg q4h prn
Diazepam	Oral, parenteral	2.5–5 mg q4h prn
Haloperidol	Oral, parenteral	1–2 mg q4h prn
Chlorpromazine	Oral, parenteral	30–60 mg q4h prn

Table 12–5
Total Sedation during the Last Days of Life

CLASS OF MEDICATION	MEDICATION	ROUTE OF ADMINISTRATION	DOSE
Barbiturates	Phenobarbital	Rectal	30–60 mg q4h
	Pentobarbital	Rectal	2–6 mg/kg q4h
		Parenteral	2.5 mg/kg q15min
Benzodiazepines	Diazepam	Rectal (gel)	10–20 mg q4h
	Midazolam	Parenteral	0.02–0.1 mg/kg/hr
Anesthetics	Ketamine	Parenteral	0.1–0.5 mg/kg/hr
	Propofol	Parenteral	1 mg/kg bolus; 0.05–0.1 mg/kg/min

sical suffering. This obligation often brings about quandaries for physicians caring for those dying patients whose symptoms are recalcitrant to the aforementioned treatments. For fear of "robbing" patients of life in these situations, it is often more comfortable for clinicians to turn the other cheek and believe that there is less suffering than there really is. However, sedation is humanely acceptable and appropriate when suffering is presented.

The concept of total sedation is based on informed consent and the principle of double effect. The patient's family or the designated medical decision maker understands and acknowledges that the intention of the clinician is to mitigate symptoms rather than induce death purposefully, even though the treatment itself may result in the acceleration of the dying process.

Refractory symptoms that may require sedation include intractable pain, dyspnea, agitated delirium, multifocal myoclonus, hemorrhage, and intractable emesis. It is crucial, however, when considering patients for total sedation, that all appropriate and reasonable therapeutic options have been attempted prior to deciding to sedate the patient.

For patients already using opioids for pain and respiratory management, the dose of opioids can be titrated to the point of sedation. If the patient is not receiving opioids, is refractory to dosage escalation, or has developed neuroexcitatory side effects such as myoclonus or agitated

delirium (which may be contributing to the decision to totally sedate the patient) the addition and titration of anesthetics, barbiturates, benzodiazepines, or phenothiazines have been effectively used. (See Table 12–5 for appropriate dosing information.)

Caregiver Support

Death rarely occurs as it is depicted on television. The actual period immediately preceding death is in reality an evanescent phase: The dying individual gradually "fades" away. During this period, families and caregivers need information, emotional support, and concrete assistance with the physical as well as bureaucratic burdens that accompany death.

Information and Education

First and foremost, family members need to be told that death is approaching and given a general idea as to how soon it will occur. Time-frames can be given to families using "days versus weeks" or "hours versus days" types of terminology to give them an idea of when death is most likely to occur. While it is often difficult for health care providers to predict exactly when death will occur, the signs and symptoms that signal approaching death are easily identified. The need to identify impending death is important because most patients and family members need the emotional closure of being able to say "goodbye." Family members and caregivers should be advised that an unresponsive patient might still be able to hear and comprehend. Education as to what to expect during this phase should be given to the family at this time. Caregivers will require instruction in what to anticipate, physical care, interventions to control expected symptoms, and medication administration. Families may need assistance with physical care on an intermittent or full-time basis during this time of physical and emotional misery. This assistance can be provided via hospice and/or home care staff, hired caregivers, and additional help from friends and family.

Emotional Support

It goes without saying that patients, family members, and caregivers will require increased emotional support as death approaches. The hours before death will probably be intensely emotional for the family, and will be remembered long after the patient has died. Managing symptoms around the time of death will visibly reduce patient suffering, thereby providing families and caregivers with positive memories during bereavement. Patients, families, and caregivers should be reassured that events are proceeding as expected, that the patient is comfortable, and that they are "doing the right thing" by allowing the patient to die in their chosen environment. Positive reinforcement regarding their caregiving efforts should be given freely and often. Guilt at wishing for the patient's death, for example, needs to be supported by assuring the family that it is natural to wish for an end to the patient's suffering and family turmoil that often surrounds death. Survivors often take comfort in the fact that they have provided hands-on care to their loved ones in the last days.

Spirituality

Spirituality is an individual concept. Patients and families may or may not welcome spiritual support as their loved one enters the last phase of life. It should, however, be offered, with the emphasis that chaplain services are focused on spiritual issues and concerns of the patient and family, whatever those concerns and issues may be. The chaplain, in conjunction with the aid of a social worker, can also provide structured emotional support and concrete assistance with funeral, mortuary, cremation, and burial services. Planning for the necessary death services in advance will assist to decrease emotional turmoil at the time of death.

Time of Death

Families react in various ways at the time of death, often dictated by cultural or ethnic behavioral norms or expectations. These are so variable as to be beyond the scope of this discussion. What is important is for end-of-life care providers to be empathetic, understanding, and available to support the family through this period. Be sure that the body of the deceased is treated with the appropriate care and dignity, and that any cultural or religious customs are observed as requested by the family. Allow family members private time with the body, if desired, and reinforce the idea that the care they gave their loved one was appropriate and proper. If a family member gave a dose of sedating medication shortly before death, reassure the individual that the medication was not what ended the patient's life. Assist the family in calling the funeral home or other authorities if necessary.

Toward Death with Dignity

Death is an expected event that can be a positive experience for the survivors and a comfortable one for the dying person. By combining consistencies in the delivery of care to our patients and families, compassion balanced by rigorous scientific facts, knowledge and skill, we can ensure that our patients will die a dignified and peaceful death. The last days of life need not be terrible, painful, or lonely, but rather an opportunity for growth, remembrance, and closure.

References

AMA Council on Scientific Affairs: Good care of the dying patient [council report]. *JAMA* 275:474, 1996.

American Society of Clinical Oncology: Cancer care during the last phase of life. *J Clin Oncol* 16:1986, 1998.

Appleton M: Hospice medicine: A different perspective. *Am J Hospice Palliat Care* 13:7, 1996.

Baumrucker SJ: Management of intestinal obstruction in hospice care. *Am J Hospice Palliat Care* 15:232, 1998.

Bergevin P, Bergevin RM: Recognizing delirium in terminal patients. *Am J Hospice Palliat Care* 13:28, 1996.

Bernat JL, Gert B, Mogielnicki RP: Patient refusal of hydration and nutrition: An alternative to physician-assisted suicide or voluntary active euthanasia. *Arch Intern Med* 153:2723, 1993. Commentary.

Block SD, Billings JA: Patient requests to hasten death: Evaluation and management in terminal care. *Arch Intern Med* 154:2039, 1994.

Bottomley DM, Hanks GW: Subcutaneous midazolam infusion in palliative care. *J Pain Symptom Manage* 5:259, 1990.

Bozzetti F, et al: Guidelines on artificial nutrition versus hydration in terminal cancer patients. *Nutrition* 12:163, 1996.

Brant JM: The art of palliative care: Living with hope, dying with dignity. *Oncol Nurs Forum* 25:995, 1998.

Breitbart W, Jacobsen PB: Psychiatric symptom management in terminal care. *Clin Geriatr Med* 12:329, 1996.

Bruera E, Pruvost M, Schoeller T, et al: Proctoclysis for hydration of terminally ill cancer patients. *J Pain Symptom Manage* 15:216, 1998.

Burge FI: Dehydration symptoms of palliative care cancer patients. *J Pain Symptom Manage* 8:454, 1993.

Byock I: Patient refusal of nutrition and hydration: Walking the ever-finer line. *Am J Hospice Palliat Care* 12:8, 1995.

Caruso-Herman D: Concerns for the dying patient and family. *Semin Oncol Nurs* 5:120, 1989.

Chandler S: Nebulized opioids to treat dyspnea. *Am J Hospice Palliat Care* 16:418, 1999.

Cherny NI: The use of sedation in the management of refractory pain. *Principles and Practice of Supportive Oncology Updates* 3(4), 2000.

Cherny NI, Portenoy RK: Sedation in the management of refractory symptoms: Guidelines for evaluation and treatment. *J Palliat Care* 10:31, 1994.

Cleary JF: Pharmacokinetic and pharmacodynamic issues in the treatment of breakthrough pain. *Semin Oncol* 24:S16, 1997.

Coluzzi PH: Sublingual morphine: Efficacy reviewed. *J Pain Symptom Manage* 16:184, 1998.

Davis BD, Cowley SA, Ryland RK: The effects of terminal illness on patients and their carers. *J Adv Nurs* 23:512, 1996.

Doyle D, Hanks GW, MacDonald N, eds: *Oxford Textbook of Palliative Medicine*. New York, Oxford University Press, 1993.

Drickamer M, Lee MA, Ganzini L: Practical issues in physician-assisted suicide. *Ann Intern Med* 126:146, 1997.

Ellison NM, Lewis GO: Plasma concentrations following single doses of morphine sulfate in oral solution and rectal suppository. *Clin Pharmacy* 3:614, 1984.

Enck RE: The role of nebulized morphine in managing dyspnea. *Am J Hospice Palliat Care* 16:373, 1999. Editorial.

Erlen JA: Issues at the end of life. *Orthopaed Nurs* 15:37, 1996.

Faisinger RL, Bruera E: When to treat dehydration in a terminally ill patient? *Support Care Cancer* 5:205, 1997.

Faisinger R, Bruera E: The management of dehydration in terminally ill patients. *J Palliat Care* 10:55, 1994.

Faisinger R, MacEachern T, Miller MJ, et al: The use of hypodermoclysis for rehydration in terminally ill cancer patients. *J Pain Symptom Manage* 9:298, 1994.

Fine PG: Fentanyl in the treatment of cancer pain. *Semin Oncol* 104:694, 1997.

Gavrin J, Chapman R: Clinical management of dying patients. *West J Med* 163:268, 1995.

Gremaud G, Zulian GB: Indications and limitations of intravenous and subcutaneous midazolam in a palliative care center. *J Pain Symptom Manage* 15:331, 1998. Letter.

Hansen-Flaschen J: Advanced lung disease: Palliation and terminal care. *Clin Chest Med* 18:645, 1997.

Hanson LC, Danis M, Garrett J: What is wrong with end-of-life care? Opinions of bereaved family members. *JAGS* 45:1339, 1997.

Horn LW: Terminal dyspnea: A hospice approach. *Am J Hospice Palliat Care* 9:24, 1992.

Jecker NS: Medical futility and care of dying patients. *West J Med* 163:287, 1995.

Kemp C: Palliative care for respiratory problems in terminal illness. *Am J Hospice Palliat Care* 14:26, 1997.

Kinzbrunner BM, Copeland J, Kinzbrunner E: Nebulized morphine using oral morphine solution. Poster presentatation, annual assembly of the American Academy of Hospice and Palliative Medicine, June 2000.

Kinzel T: Managing lung disease in late life: A new approach. *Geriatrics* 46:53, 1991.

Levy MH: Pain management in advanced cancer. *Semin Oncol* 12:394, 1985.

Lichter I: Home care in the last days of terminal illness. *Home Health Care Consultant* 6:15, 1999.

Lichter I, Hunt E: The last 48 hours of life. *J Palliat Care* 6:7, 1990.

Lynn J, Teno JM, Phillips RS, et al: Perceptions by family members of the dying experience of older and seriously ill patients. *Ann Intern Med* 126:97, 1997.

MacDonald N: Suffering and dying in cancer patients: Research frontiers in controlling confusion, cachexia, and dyspnea. *West J Med* 163:278, 1995.

Macmillan K, Bruera E, Kuehn N, et al: A prospective comparison study between a butterfly needle and a Teflon cannula for subcutaneous narcotic administration. *J Pain Symptom Manage* 9:82, 1994.

Malone N: Hydration in the terminally ill patient. *Nurs Standard* 43:29, 1994.

March PA: Terminal restlessness. *Am J Hospice Palliat Care* 15:51, 1998.

McCaffrey-Boyle D, Abernathy G, Baker L, Conover-Wall A: End-of-life confusion in patients with cancer. *ONF* 25:1335, 1998.

McCann RM, Hall WJ, Groth-Juncker A: Comfort care for terminally ill patients: The appropriate use of nutrition and hydration. *JAMA* 272:1263, 1994.

McIver B, Walsh D, Nelson K: The use of chlorpromazine for symptom control in dying cancer patients. *J Pain Symptom Manage* 9:341, 1994.

Mercadante SG: When oral morphine fails in cancer pain: The role of alternative routes. *Am J Hospice Palliat Care* 15:333, 1998.

Mercadante S, DeConno F, Ripamonti C: Propofol in terminal care. *J Pain Symptom Manage* 10:639, 1995.

Miller FG, Meier DE: Voluntary death: A comparison of terminal hydration and physician-assisted suicide. *Ann Intern Med* 128:559, 1998.

Nuland SB: *How We Die.* New York, Vintage Books, 1995.

Oneschuk D: Subcutaneous midazolam for acute hemorrhage in patients with advanced cancer. *Can Fam Physician* 44:1461, 1998.

Pearlman RA: Forgoing medical nutrition and hydration: An area for fine-tuning clinical skills. *J Gen Intern Med* 8:225, 1993. Editorial.

Portenoy RK: Oral transmucosal fentanyl citrate (OTFC) for the treatment of breakthrough pain and cancer patients: A controlled dose titration study. *Pain* 79:303, 1999.

Portenoy RK: Treatment of temporal variations in chronic cancer pain. *Semin Oncol* 24:S16, 1997.

Ronan KP, Gallagher J, George B, Hamby B: Comparison of propofol and midazolam for sedation in intensive care unit patients. *Crit Care Med* 23:286, 1995.

Rousseau P: Terminal sedation in the care of dying patients. *Arch Intern Med* 156:1785, 1996. Commentary.

Simmonds MA: Pharmacotherapeutic management of cancer pain: Current practice. *Semin Oncol* 24:S16, 1997.

Spitalnic S, Blazes C, Anderson AC: Conscious sedation: A primer for outpatient procedures. *Hosp Physician* 5:22, 2000.

Stein WM, Min YK: Nebulized morphine for paroxysmal cough and dyspnea in a nursing home resident with metastatic cancer. *Am J Hospice Palliat Care* 14:52, 1997.

Steiner N, Bruera E: Methods of hydration in palliative care patients. *J Palliat Care* 14:6, 1998.

Storey P: *Primer of Palliative Care.* Gainesville, FL, Academy of Hospice Physicians, 1994.

Storey P, Hill HH, St. Louis RH, Tarver EE: Subcutaneous infusions for control of cancer symptoms. *J Pain Symptom Manage* 5:33, 1990.

Sullivan RJ: Accepting death without artificial nutrition or hydration. *J Gen Intern Med* 8:220,1993.

Taylor MA: Benefits of dehydration in terminally ill patients. *Geriatric Nurs* 16:271, 1995.

Thorns A, Sykes N: Opioid use in last week of life and implications for end-of-life decision making. *Lancet* 356:398, 2000.

Truog R, et al: Barbiturates in the care of the terminally ill. *N Engl J Med* 327:1678, 1992.

Ventafridda V, et al: Symptom prevalence and control during cancer patients' last days of life. *J Palliat Care* 6:7, 1990.

Zeppetella G: The palliation of dyspnea in terminal disease. *Am J Hospice Palliat Care* 15:322, 1998.

Sarah E. McKinnon
Bob Miller

Chapter
13

Psychosocial and
Spiritual Concerns

Introduction

In our death-denying society, the opus of those going through the dying process has been muted, only to be heard, if at all, among those living with and caring for the dying on a daily basis. Although there has been a significant increase in energy and focus on caring for pain and other physical symptoms near the end of life, less emphasis has been placed on psychosocial and spiritual issues including their influence on patient perceptions of pain and symptoms. In this chapter, therefore, the goal is to provide a basic overview of psychosocial and spiritual issues in end-of-life care while presenting a framework within which to discuss these subjects. The approach is intentionally non-clinical in nature. We will provide personal observations and share the opinions of dying persons and their families, as well as summarize literature that has been reviewed.

The understanding of psychosocial and spiritual issues that occur near the end of life is often of great importance to those who have received the least training about them, such as physicians and clinical nurses. In Buckman's book on *How to Break Bad News* (1992) he describes the paradox that occurs in health care. Those who have the most knowledge about psychosocial and spiritual issues (psychiatrists, psychologists, social workers, and chaplains) are those who "do not perform this task in daily practice." Rather, physicians do. Too often the stories patients and families share of their perceptions of their doctor delivering a terminal prognosis include words like "cold" or "insensitive," "in a hurry" or "just doesn't care."

> In a great majority of cases, those doctors were not cold or insensitive (most doctors aren't) but they were uncomfortable, edgy, and embarrassed. They may well have been aware that they did not know how to carry out the conversation effectively and supportively, and so may have backed off, attempting to end the interview quickly to reduce their own discomfort and sense of clumsiness. They may well have overused medical jargon to give an air of effi-

ciency and professionalism to the proceedings, and thus may have added to the perception that they were impersonal or indifferent (Buckman, 1992).

Much of this can be attributed to a physician's training. In the movie, *Patch Adams,* Dr. Hunter "Patch" Adams chronicles many of his real life experiences in medical school. In one scene, the dean of the school of medicine, in an opening lecture to all first-year medical students, tells them "It is our mission here to rigorously and ruthlessly train the humanity out of you in order to make you into something better. We are going to make doctors out of you." The objectivity necessary to deal with the realities of medical practice serves physicians well, as does the focus on the treatment of the symptoms and the disease process. However, to be overly emotionally involved with each and every patient might bring about an inability to effectively treat patients over a lifetime of practice. The challenge is to be able to include some subjectivity where and when it is truly "what is best for the patient." End-of-life care is just such a time.

Another piece of this puzzle is to attempt to fill the gap that exists between the professional role of the physician and the humanity of the individual who lives that role. In a recent gathering of community physicians the issue of bereavement for doctors was discussed. It should come as no surprise that these physicians, who deal repeatedly with death, identified their need to grieve the loss of their patients in some structured way. Too often we fall under the influence of the myth of the "doctor as God." For many years physicians have even contributed to that fable. Now it is not only the duty of doctors to move beyond this view, but the responsibility of the general public to remove physicians from the uncomfortable pedestal on which we have placed them.

Another challenge that physicians face in properly addressing the psychosocial and spiritual needs of their patients near the end of life relates to the evolving and changing nature of the health care industry.

> (Sarah) A patient I know who was dealing with cancer told a friend of his that "My doctor is my best friend for the 15 minutes a month I get to see him."

This was no reflection on the humanity of the physician, simply a comment on the reality of a medical practice and an ability to make a living (and pay off medical school loans) in this day and age.

(Sarah) Recently, a volunteer I work with mentioned that her own physician told her "Don't get me started" when she mentioned whether or not he referred to hospice. Further discussion unearthed the fact that he was under the mistaken assumption that he would have to turn over his patient to the hospice physician, who would then become his patient's primary physician. He is a doctor who is connected and involved in his patient's care to the point of making house calls when necessary. She educated him about a physician always being able to follow his or her patient on a hospice program and also his capability to continue to bill separately for his care of his patient. What resulted was a win-win: for the volunteer, the physician, and ultimately for his patients.

On the positive side, physicians are becoming increasingly aware of the psychosocial and spiritual issues that affect their patients near the end of life. What doctors seem to struggle with most, however, is what to do about these problems when they become manifest. More good news is that hospice care, which sets the standard in end-of-life care, addresses this struggle by including in its philosophy the need for psychosocial and spiritual components of care near the end of life. The hospice team includes trained social workers and chaplains to help the team address such issues. These team members can provide support for physicians in ensuring that patients receive appropriate psychosocial and spiritual care.

Although the title of this chapter differentiates spiritual aspects from the psychosocial, in truth, the range and depth of being human makes it impossible to know where one ends and the other begins. Therefore, psychosocial and spiritual concerns will be addressed as a continuum.

It is suggested that the first and most helpful resource for those traveling on the path toward the end of life is a new paradigm that reframes society's view of dying and brings to light the opportunities inherent in this end-of-life process. As stated by Dr. Ira Byock in his 1986 article on growth as the essence of hospice care:

Table 13–1

Psychosocial and Spiritual Opportunities Near the End of Life

The Opportunity to . . .
Reframe society's view of dying, grow on!
Expand our definition of quality of life
Focus on the individual, not the disease
Address as a whole physical pain,
    psychosocial issues, and spiritual concerns
Move through fear to peace
Move through confusion to meaning
Move through despair to hope
Move from isolation to community
Come to terms with your physical body
Move from loss to closure
Adjust to new roles
Get your affairs in order

Dying represents more than a set of problems to be solved. It represents an extraordinary opportunity. An opportunity for review, for restitution, for amends, for exploration, for development, for insight. In short it is an opportunity for growth.

Rather than looking at psychosocial and spiritual care near the end of life as problems to be solved, they should be viewed from the perspective of opportunities they provide to the patients, families, and caregivers, when the end of life is near. A list of these opportunities can be found in Table 13–1, and their discussion will constitute the content of the rest of this chapter. Therefore, a better title for this chapter might be "Psychosocial and Spiritual *Opportunities* Near the End of Life."

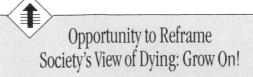

Opportunity to Reframe Society's View of Dying: Grow On!

One way to facilitate the shifting of one's view of dying from problem to opportunity is to redefine the end of life as an identifiable stage of human development. Instead of growing up, growing old, and dying, Dr. Byock suggests we grow up, grow old, and grow on:

> Growing on takes place for both the aged and ter-minally ill and their families. And although patients and families will universally find growth producing deaths as important and positive, it may not be easy. Indeed, there are typically many obstacles that must be overcome if the process of dying is to unfold in a productive manner.

In this light, the dying process may be seen as an established experience, attributed with specific tasks attached to the unfolding of the process itself. Fostering this understanding will be the challenge of established cultural and religious teachings that imply that death is the enemy, a sign of personal failure, betrayal by one's body, or a shortfall in the promise held out by medical science. Those of us who have journeyed alongside the dying know the other side of the story, that the dying process can be a time of great achievement.

Ironically, although illness and death come into each life, we tend to resist seeing these processes as "normal" or as opportunities to learn. Illustra-tive of this fact is that many quality of life instru-ments tend to "imply that a good quality of life is the result of an absence of problems rather than a reflection of favorable balance between positive and negative influences" (Cohen, et al, 1996). As with any new experience, there are aspects of what appear to be problems that, when you begin addressing them, become more comfortable and understandable due to the context created by the "problem" itself.

> (Sarah) I remember being in my sixth-grade math class when the "smartest" boy in the class com-plained to the teacher about how long it was tak-ing the rest of us to finish a problem. The teacher silently went to the board, wrote out a math prob-lem, and asked the boy to solve it. The look on his face was unforgettable. "But I don't know how to do that problem!" The teacher went to the board and within a minute, wrote out the answer. He then looked at the boy and said, "When you know how to do something, it is easy. The challenge is learning

something new. You understand how to do the problems the rest of the class is working on just as I know how to do calculus. Soon the rest of the class will know how to do what you have already learned just as someday you will learn to do what I know how to do now.

Unlike other experiences, the challenge in dying is that you don't really get any practice prior to doing it! However, seeing the process of dying as a stage of life development, which like every other life process is a balancing act of the good and the not so good, allows us a framework within which to comfortably explore this natural life event. Then and only then will we be able to see the psychosocial and spiritual experiences of dying as opportunities rather than concerns.

Opportunity to Expand Our Definition of Quality of Life

Early in adulthood, quality of life (QOL) is typi-cally thought of in terms of success in the world through work, family, friends, and personal activ-ities. Rarely do people include health in describ-ing their quality of life unless they have experienced the loss of it. Health has been defined by people with a life-threatening illness as a "sense of self-integrity encompassing physical, mental/emotional, and spiritual domains" (Cohen, et al, 1996). When one's health is compromised, a larger definition of quality of life must be devel-oped. Although many associate a lessening of functional status with a lessening of quality of life, it is not always the case, because the evaluation is subjective. "Patients' appraisal of QOL is thus dynamic and changeable across time and perhaps even across situations" (Cella, 1994).

When the first living will documents came into existence, they typically contained language that described the person's wish to be taken off life support when their "quality of life" was significantly diminished. Very soon, it was realized that more information was needed, specifically, what this unique individual meant by the phrase "quality of life." Each person's perception of quality will differ based on the importance and satisfaction the person gives each dimension or activity in life. For one person, that might mean the ability to get up every day and walk around the golf course; for another, it might mean the ability to interact and communicate with loved ones; for another, the feeling of still contributing something to society. It is the perception of the patient that defines quality of life for that individual. "For patients who are dying, appropriate care must respond to the patient's subjective and often changing quality of experience and needs" (Byock, Merriman, 1998).

Missoula-VITAS Quality of Life Index

The Missoula-VITAS Quality of Life Index has been an invaluable tool in exploring the patient's subjective experience of quality of life and the impact of illness on that perception. It also helps professional and family caregivers conceptualize broad concepts related to quality of life. The tool measures five dimensions of quality: symptom, interpersonal, functional, well-being, and transcendent. Each will be discussed here as it relates to psychosocial and spiritual care near the end of life. (For a more thorough discussion of the MVQOLI and quality of life in general, please refer to Chapter 5.)

The *symptom* section outlines the level of physical discomfort and distress experienced because of the progressive illness. For example, patients who have gone from having a few coughing fits throughout the day to one every time they speak are potentially going to have a lessened quality of life if they value social interaction and enjoy talking with others. This will not affect someone who prefers being alone to the same extent.

Function refers to the perceived ability to perform accustomed functions and activities of daily living (such as dressing, feeding, and bathing oneself) and the emotional response to this based on one's expectations.

(Sarah) My grandfather, as he grew more and more ill, had a terrible time with having others dress him and take him to the bathroom. He had been a vice-president of a major corporation and wore a suit and tie every day of his life, complete with an ironed cloth handkerchief. In direct contrast, I often kid with my friends that once a woman goes through childbirth any sense of privacy regarding her body is gone, and as far as mothers are concerned any type of help with anything is greatly appreciated, no matter how basic.

The *interpersonal* dimension deals with the degree of investment in personal relationships and the perceived quality of one's relations and interactions with family and friends. An illness may force, or provide an opportunity for, changes in one's significant relationships. These changes may be positive or negative in the eyes of the individual. The perception of satisfaction in this area may be dependent on the individual's ability to redefine and reframe important relationships, and the ability of the significant others in their life to do the same.

One's *well-being* is defined through a self-assessment of one's internal sense of wellness or disease, and weighed for importance related to a sense of contentment or lack of contentment with each identified area.

Finally, *transcendence* refers to the experienced degree of connection with an enduring construct and the resulting sense of meaning and purpose given to life. Spiritual issues are inherent in the measuring of quality of life in the patient near the end of life. "The data suggest that the existential domain is at least as important as the physical, psychological, and support domains in determining quality of life and therefore cannot be ignored" (Cohen, et al, 1996). Transcendence is about the connection to something beyond oneself, however one defines that something. For some this is God, for others it is simply a sense of meaning to the universe, and for still others it is the legacy they will leave behind as a result of having lived.

These dimensions are reviewed here because, near the end of life, there are specific opportunities available within each dimension. Although they will not form the outline of the remainder of this chapter, they underlie and inform much of the information that is to follow.

One disclaimer needs to be addressed at this point. Many professionals who care for patients near the end of life harbor the hope that the "perfect death" can happen for each patient and family. However, the reality is that many factors, both physical and psychological, are a part of whether this happens or not. As noted, in most cases individuals will die the same way they lived. This phenomenon is referred to as "remaining in character." As Cleary (1999) notes, "whether productive or maladaptive, the coping strategies one has utilized in the past will be called to the fore when faced with significant stress."

Typically, a kind, caring family man will be surrounded, supported, and loved by family members, and his dying process will reflect his way of being. If a woman was angry, hurtful, and resentful in her lifetime, unless there is an epiphany during the dying process, the chances are her dying experience will reflect the same. A patient's skill at adapting to changes during life prior to the terminal illness will play a large part in the capacity to make changes affecting quality of life as death nears. For many, the definition of what constitutes a true problem versus a minor inconvenience is redefined.

Opportunity to Focus on the Individual, Not the Disease

We all know that we are more than just our bodies. The mind–body connection, stress awareness, and caring for the "whole self" are becoming part and parcel of our understanding of ourselves rather than a fashionable part of the so-called new age movement. However, this holistic view continues to find a great deal of resistance within the traditional medical model. In the traditional model, our bodies and psyches are split. When someone has a physical problem, we address that problem with little regard for the rest of the person. Once

people are healed physically, and if they so are inclined, they can work toward emotional or spiritual healing of those areas affected by their illnesses. It is our experience that most individuals simply try to get back to "the way it was" prior to the illness. The problem with this approach is that it ignores the physical and psychosocial changes that have occurred as a result of the illness, leaving individuals wondering why things aren't the same or back to normal. The challenge is for them to embrace the fact that "normal" now has a new definition.

One of the results of emphasis on the traditional health care model, which tends to place importance only on the physical side of illness, is the reduction of the multidimensional nature of the individual into a single dimension, defined by the disease process. A patient loses his or her identity, and becomes "the lung cancer in room 203." There is a unique terror, known only to those diagnosed with serious or life-limiting illness, that their humanity will be somehow lessened by their relationship with the medical establishment. They fear that they will be known as, and perhaps become little more than, their disease in relationship to their doctors, the nurses providing care to them, and perhaps even to their families and friends.

Therefore, when caring for patients with terminal illnesses (and even with chronic longer-term diseases), physicians must be sure that their focus shifts away from a preoccupation with the disease back to paying primary attention to the patient. Inclusion of the family as part of the unit of care, as promulgated by hospice and palliative care programs, is also crucial. By viewing the patients and families that they care for from this perspective, physicians will be better able to recognize the importance of the psychosocial and spiritual needs of a person as essential elements of the treatment plan.

Of course, there is no reason to wait until someone has 6 months or less to live before addressing him or her as a whole person. For many people, however, the dying process represents the first time in their lives when they take the time to gain this awareness. There is much to be learned about life in general by examining this time when, outside of the need for controlled pain and other symptoms, the overwhelmingly urgent issues are psychosocial in nature.

Opportunity to Address as a Whole Physical Pain, Psychosocial Issues and Spiritual Concerns

Maslow's hierarchy of needs postulates that "higher" needs such as self-actualization cannot be met until more basic needs, such as food and shelter, are met. For example, a child who has not eaten will have a hard time studying ethics in school. Although life is rarely so neat or linear, this dynamic also applies to those dealing with a terminal illness. While a patient is in physical pain, it may be difficult to focus on psychosocial or spiritual concerns. As Cella (1994) states: "Patients in severe or excruciating pain often cannot relate to general questions about mood, social functioning, or even less severe symptoms." However, it would be a mistake to assume that psychosocial or spiritual concerns will wait until the physical concerns are resolved. While experiencing the pain, the person may be wondering "What did I do to deserve this?" or "Who can help me get through this?" or "Why is God punishing me so?" These concerns may or may not be spoken during the crisis, but as the physical pain is controlled, the opportunity to address psychosocial and spiritual issues increases.

Although patients may not focus on psychosocial and spiritual issues when physical pain is poorly controlled, it is equally important to remember the significant effect unresolved psychosocial and spiritual issues may have on the perception of physical pain.

(Sarah) I remember a patient in a nursing home who spent hours and hours moaning as though she was in physical pain. The nursing home staff had warned me about her and she had received plenty

of attention regarding medication to treat her pain, but she continued to engage in her behavior. As a clinical psychology student, she intrigued me. Everyday when I would visit Mrs. "Smith," I would hear her "complaining" down the hall and would gear myself up to see her. It would take about 10 minutes, but once she realized I was not going to come in and out and that I was going to stay with her for an extended period of time (1 hour), she quit her moaning. She simply wanted someone to be with her. Her "physical" complaints were psychosocial in origin. As our hospice care team worked with her, we were able to stop her groans completely.

Judy Szemplak (1997) writes in her article "The Effects of Physical and Emotional Pain on Quality of Life" about Mary Jo, a breast cancer survivor, who relates to her that the "emotional pain she experienced was worse than the physical pain." She described an "aloneness of the experience" and "despite the presence of a very supportive spouse and friends, her 'personal pain' was 'terrifying.'"

Sometimes it is the physical pain that leads to a psychosocial or spiritual symptom.

(Sarah) I remember a time when I dealt with an ongoing, undiagnosed medical condition. After more than 8 months with no relief, a friend said to me, "I think I know what the problem is: you're depressed." I remember telling her "Of course I'm depressed. I am in chronic pain."

In his article "An Educational Model for Explaining Hospice Services," Welk (1991) expounds on the interaction between physical pain and the psychosocial and spiritual challenges that occur at the end of life. He uses the word "suffering" to describe what many terminally ill patients experience, which should be distinguished from pain, even though the word "pain is frequently used interchangeably with suffering." Welk uses the word "pain" to describe physical pain only, and notes that someone may be in physical pain and may not be suffering. The corollary to that is true, too; someone may be free of physical pain but suffering none the less. Areas in which suffering needs to be addressed include emotional, social, and spiritual. Without emotional support, one may experience fear; without social support, there may be conflict and disconnection, without spiritual support, many lose their source of hope. Although one may address these areas separately, it is only by addressing all areas—the physical, emotional, social, and spiritual—that one may truly be successful in relieving suffering near the end of life.

Opportunity to Move Through Fear to Peace

During the dying process, we have the opportunity to look at the journey as one from fear to peace. Conversations with dying individuals show that there are a number of "unknowns" anticipated in this dying process that generate tremendous anxiety and fear, one of the greatest being the lack of knowledge as to what will happen physically as one nears death. In such circumstances providing a roadmap so that patients and caregivers know what to expect from the physical experience may be necessary. For example, end-of-life caregivers may be called upon to explain the reason for decreased appetite and thirst during the dying process, or the desire for a darker environment. Patients and families may need reassurance that fear of symptoms, such as increasing pain or the sensation of suffocating near the end of life, will be treated and controlled as the dying process continues. Family members' caregiving efforts may need to be directed away from cooking huge meals and toward providing simple mouth or skin care. Providing guidance to patients and families regarding these and other similar issues in a gentle and compassionate fashion, from the standpoint of experience with others who have been through similar disease processes, will reduce fear and provide patients and families with the support and peace they seek as life draws to a close.

Paul Tournier, in *Learn to Grow Old* (1972), discusses life as a task to be accomplished. Within

that task there is the paradox that one can never finish the task, and that the true task in the end becomes "acceptance of unfulfillment, acceptance of the unfulfilled." He goes on to say that it is hard to accept the unfulfilled and that it is one of the problems in dealing with death. He defines acceptance as an active choice, one which is decided upon rather than arrived at passively. "To accept is to choose the reality, choosing freely between the reality and the fiction . . . . You make the unity of your life by accepting the reality." For many, that unity can help to bring a sense of peace.

The only way one will know how to comfort an individual patient or family is to listen to their concerns and address them as directly and sincerely as possible. Often just having the information results in a greater level of comfort. Patients and families learn what is "normal" in the current situation. Remember, people don't get a chance to practice dying—it's a new experience for everyone.

Another aspect of the unknown is more existential in nature, and in this arena no one has ever "been there, done that." No one has been beyond death and come back to tell about it. No one can make the ultimate unknown known. Different people's faith systems will provide either comfort or create fear, depending on their orientation toward their faith. The crisis of facing death may cause some patients to be more open to the need for outside help, providing them with an opportunity to change a system of belief with which they are unhappy. It should be noted that there often needs to be a great deal of willingness and desire on the part of patients in order for this shift to occur.

The best that professional caregivers can offer in this circumstance is to be there and be present. To really listen to what is important to the patient, and if possible, build on the things that bring comfort. Even patients who reach what Elisabeth Kubler-Ross (1969) described as the "acceptance" stage outlined in her five stages of dying desire company as they make their transition.

(Bob) I had one patient, Fran, who didn't seem like she'd ever come to terms with her sense that God had abandoned her to her illness. She constantly said, "I've lost my faith." During the months I visited her, she found no comfort in anything I offered. Then, on her deathbed, she told me that she now understood that God had not abandoned her because I had not abandoned her. Sometimes just being there can make all the difference in the world, and you never know what patients will make of your relationship. In Fran's case, it wasn't anything I said; it was simply my presence with her.

Kathleen Dough Singh, in *The Grace in Dying* (1998), builds upon the Kubler-Ross model by addressing spirituality in the dying process. She describes three stages of dying: chaos, surrender, and transcendence. She offers "a different theoretical structure to the nature of the profound inner changes which are taking place as the personality restructures on a deep level in response to transpersonal forces." More and more people are coming to see themselves as spiritual beings living a human existence. Singh describes the process of letting go of one's "humanness" or one's ego connection to the world through the process of surrendering. The opportunity is then presented to acknowledge that part of oneself that is spiritual and eternal. This leads to a feeling of transcendence, a sense of unity with oneself and the world. The dying process takes on new meaning as the patient can see beyond the limits of the physical body and experience a sense of who one is beyond this singular life. These stages provide a framework within which to address the release of the struggle to hold on in the dying process and find tranquility.

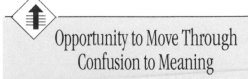

Opportunity to Move Through Confusion to Meaning

One critical factor in the capacity to "die well" is one's belief about the meaning of the illness. Is the illness seen as a punishment for past wrongdoing, invoked either by God or by some law of retribution? Exploring the source of that guilt may be helpful, especially if reconciliation is possible.

(Bob) One of the most difficult cases for me as a caregiver was a man who worked hard to develop a healthy form of detachment from his guilt regarding his illness. He tried to embrace the understanding that his disease was not a punishment from God. His last words to me were "I almost believed it." It took months for me to develop my own healthy form of detachment as a caregiver and to realize that although his journey didn't end up the way I wanted, it was his journey and my involvement was important just the same.

Perhaps the illness is seen as a fate, a random occurrence that is the result of an impersonal, uncaring universe. Exploring some sense of love and purpose may be helpful. Simply opening up the possibility that God may be grieved by the suffering of people, for example, may produce an unexpected insight, or at least produce a reaction worth exploring.

Is the illness seen as a sign of some personal failure, such as the case of a person whose smoking has resulted in emphysema, or a person who believes that anger has internalized in the form of a tumor? Exploring the cause and effect as well as the nature of the disease may be as helpful to a patient as taking responsibility to make amends with oneself and one's family where appropriate. The variations on these themes are many; the responses need to be equally diverse.

Walter Wangerin, in *Mourning into Dancing* (1992), makes an observation regarding the essence of tragedy and its meaning. He points to the time after an experience of despair, when there is awareness that "the griever had to suffer hopelessness in order to be astonished by her new life." Walter Brueggemann (1986), a biblical scholar, describes a similar dynamic as the basis of what we call pastoral care, which he describes as helping people enter into an experience of exile, to be in exile, and then to depart out of exile. He points out that, although the process is not as quick or easy as we would like it to be, "only grief permits newness."

Victor Frankl wrote about the meaning of suffering in *Man's Search for Meaning* (1959). He describes suffering as one way to discover meaning in life, and feels that "man's main concern is not to gain pleasure or avoid pain but rather to see a meaning in his life. That is why man is even ready to suffer, on the condition, to be sure, that his suffering has meaning." This is not to say that it is necessary to suffer; but that when suffering, there is an opportunity to transcend that suffering by attaching significance to it.

(Sarah) I will never forget a woman I'll call Anna. Anna was dying of cancer. The first time I met her, she told me that her cancer was the best thing that had ever happened to her. Now, I am a positive person, but this threw even me. Anna went on to share with me how she had never taken the time to "stop and smell the roses." Because of her diagnosis, she had learned to do many things— play with her grandchildren, have deep conversations with her daughter, garden, listen to opera, and take naps; things she was certain she would never had done had she not become ill. She had truly used her "suffering" to create new meaning in her life.

Opportunity to Move Through Despair to Hope

How a patient will find hope, and in what, is entirely a unique experience. For one patient, it may mean living until able to take part in some significant family event. For others it may be the sense of a life well lived, a sense that they have contributed something to the world or to someone important to them. For another it might be the hope that in the afterlife the wrongs of this world will be corrected. Whatever the source, our challenge is to support patients as they find, explore, redefine, or change the source of their hope, sometimes several times in the course of an illness (or in the course of a single day!).

Allowing the patient to take the lead in identifying his or her unique and preferred source of hope is not always easy, especially if we're inclined to

help by offering or suggesting our own values as an alternative to the patient's values.

(Bob) One of my patients, Otis, who was under the care of our local hospice for terminal cancer, was telling me about his brother who had previously died from cancer. He told me his brother had been increasingly weak and drowsy, developed a poor appetite, and shortly thereafter died. Otis asked me if I could tell him whether or not he had cancer, too. He said the doctor had told him he had a tumor. Evidently to Otis this didn't necessarily mean that he had cancer.

Then Otis proceeded to tell me that putting a "tube" down his throat had made the diagnosis. He scrunched up his nose. I said, "That must've been an uncomfortable procedure." He said, "They put me under for the procedure, but when I woke up, my throat was sure sore." Then he paused and a gleam came to his eye, "Come to think of it, my rectum was sore, too. I think they put the tube up there to get a look at the tumor from the other side." He fixed me in his gaze and said, with a straight face, "I sure hope they put it down my throat first!"

We laughed and together experienced what was a sacred moment. I say the moment was sacred because it was then that Otis began to tell me about feeling weak and sleepy much of the time, and that he was losing his appetite. He was letting me know that he knew he was dying of cancer as he was sharing with me the same symptoms he remembered about his brother's death. In this way he could communicate with me indirectly without having to acknowledge the "C word" or admit that he had cancer. We had an opportunity to laugh and let humor put some space between him and his tumor. My allowing him to do this, I believe, enhanced his sense of hope.

Opportunity to Move from Isolation to Community

The social conflict described by Welk (1991) refers to the changes that occur in our relationships with the onset of illness and terminality. In a perfect world, all individuals, upon death, would have full closure with all those whom they had connected with during their lifetime. Realistically, however, many come to this time of life with much left undone. Often there have been separations between family members. Many of these have gone on for years with no thought given to reconciliation until the onset of the terminal illness. Frequently, patients have been heard to say that they have forgotten what the argument was about in the first place. When a reconnection takes place, the internal conflict for the patient and family may be relieved.

The opposite also holds true.

(Sarah) I recently heard about a patient who had lost contact with his son. The hospice social worker tracked the son down only to hear from him a definite "no" in regards to visiting or even talking to his father on the telephone. This patient had been an alcoholic, was physically abusive to his wife, and had abandoned his family when they were very young.

Sometimes near the end of life the task is to come to terms with life's disappointments and what they mean. There may literally be no way to "fix" or make amends with what has happened. When there is no opportunity for reconciliation, caregivers may need to get creative in assisting a patient in their search for closure, maybe role-playing the hurt son, helping write a final letter, or making a tape recording of the father's "confession." Even if it doesn't lead to reconciliation, there may be some opportunity for healing in the simple act of confession, some absolution in the gentle listening presence offered, and maybe even some previously unrealized sense of a community established by the interaction.

As in the situation just described, sometimes one's community of choice does not have the capacity to remain constant and supportive of one who is ill. It is heartbreaking to listen to some of the those who have been shunned by friends or people in their condominium or neighborhood because of an illness, even one as noncommunicable as can-

cer. This forced isolation can cause the one who is ill to feel all the more abandoned. What is needed is someone who has the capacity to be close and not afraid: someone for whom the disease is not perceived as a threat; someone who can help patients understand that there is nothing wrong with them, that the distance their friends may establish says more about them than it does about the patient. It says that they are afraid of their own frailty, their own potential for loss or illness, or that they simply don't know what to say and because of that fear, they say and do nothing. That supportive "someone" is often a relative, or a best friend, or sometimes even a health care professional.

Opportunity to Come to Terms with Your Physical Body

As discussed earlier, physical changes associated with chronic or terminal illness often mean something in the subjective experience of the patient. If independence or control is central to an individual's ego, then the process of giving up roles in one's family can threaten one's sense of self. Or worse, a family system can be thrown off balance if cherished roles are reversed, such as when the breadwinner becomes the one in need, or the parent needs to be the one cared for. Often, how it will go depends on the family's or the individual's adaptability.

Body image concerns can be devastating, especially when illness is disfiguring. Our society, as part of its denial of death, celebrates youth and beauty. Women have a standard against which they are measured, one that is unattainable by most. Many are unable to come to terms with the changes that treatments such as surgery may bring, even if the surgery saves their life.

(Sarah) I know of a woman whose husband walked out on her the night before her mastectomy because he couldn't handle it.

Dealing with one's own responses to physical changes is difficult enough. This difficulty is doubled when others around you have trouble managing their reactions.

> (Sarah) Working in a cancer support community taught me about the ability to transcend this mindset. Through a gathering of people living with many of the same changes and challenges, a new model is created. I have seen women go into the bathroom together, five at a time, to look at a member's surgery results, to laugh and cheer and gather strength for themselves as a group. One member chose to have a tattoo of a smiley face put on her reconstructed breast rather than a nipple tattoo. She brought in cookies to her weekly support group decorated with, you guessed it, smiley faces.

There is also the issue of how an individual feels about his or her body.

> (Sarah) My grandmother was raised during a time when certain areas of the body were not discussed, described, or explored. She, at 77, was still referring to her pubic area as "down there," and it presented a challenge when her cancer necessitated treatment, dressing changes, and a catheter "down there."

Education and a nonjudgmental attitude will make a significant difference when dealing with these patients. Reminding them that they are more than just their bodies and approaching this new experience in a light-hearted and gentle manner will help. Depending on the relationship, humor can often cut through the worst embarrassment.

> (Sarah) My sister, who had cystic fibrosis, was a great teacher for me in this respect. She referred to her wheelchair and oxygen canister (which went everywhere with her towards the end of her life) by nickname. Once a woman on an elevator (who obviously had no idea she had this chronic and terminal illness) looked severely at her following one of her coughing spells. She proceeded to say to my mother "Gee, I guess it is about time I give up my two pack a day habit." Her responses to her realities paved the way for the rest of us.

Opportunity to Move from Loss to Closure

One's response to dying and the reactions of those around us are often tied to how openly we have or have not dealt with prior losses in life. A family member may shed a few tears and respond to bereavement follow-up with "I am doing great, fine, no problem," only to emotionally break down 3 months later when their dog dies. The pet's death opens the door for them to openly acknowledge their grief around both losses.

> (Sarah) I heard once of a woman who lived in a small house behind the larger, main house where her grandson and granddaughter-in-law lived. The grandson was on a hospice program and because of friction between the granddaughter-in-law and the grandmother, the older woman was not involved in her grandson's care. She would, however, talk with the hospice nurse when she came to care for him, and one day asked the nurse if she had any information on death and dying. At her next visit, the nurse brought some bereavement materials and the woman took them into her house to read them. Two days later when the nurse returned, the woman came running out of her house to greet her. She shared, in broken English, how grateful she was for the information the nurse had brought. It turned out that she had had a child who died over 50 years ago of sudden infant death syndrome. She had never taken the time to grieve this loss nor did she understand the importance of doing so. That hospice nurse is convinced to this day that had this woman been able to process that loss at that time, her role within her family and eventually in the life of her grandson, would have been different and better.

Attendant losses have been discussed as part of addressing the many changes that occur as one copes with the dying process. Already discussed earlier was the subject of prior losses and their potential effects on someone in the present. Another area of loss revolves around the loss of someone's future. In general, when the death of loved ones occurs, most will grieve the life they lived and the memories of the life that was shared between the deceased and those in mourning. Additionally, there is also the actual missing of that person in the present moment. An area of loss that is sometimes overlooked, however, is the loss of the future that one had hoped to experience with that person. The younger someone is when he or she dies, the greater the opportunity for this kind of loss. Dreams and aspirations for that loved one's future and one's future with the person may be more elaborate simply because there are potentially more lost years to grieve when someone dies at a younger age. There are all the "what ifs" and the "I wonder whats. . . ." This is especially challenging for the parents who lose a child, regardless of that child's age. "I wonder what she would have been had she had a chance to grow up." "I wonder if he would have gone to my alma mater if he had not gotten sick." "She'll never get to turn 16 or get her driver's license." So many parents, particularly those who lose young children, see themselves living a lifetime in the grief of "what might have been."

> (Bob) I remember talking with a woman whose grown son was on our hospice program. She said to me "A mother is not supposed to bury her child. It's just not right." In our minds the natural order of death is parent, then child.

Although one never completely recovers from the loss of a child, one can move on and continue with one's own life.

> (Sarah) One mother I know talks now about the "meaning" behind her experience in losing her 14-year-old daughter, which taught her to value life, love other people, and to stay connected to her faith. She remembers her child every day and then uses that memory to fuel her life.

Other parents use their experience to rally behind a cause, hoping to provide for other families that which they did not have, while honoring the life of their child at the same time.

"Anticipatory grieving," defined as grieving that occurs prior to death in anticipation of a coming loss, may affect terminally ill patients as well as families. For some, the diagnosis of a terminal illness results in an emotional withdrawal, interfering with the ability of the patient, family, or both to be present in the here and now. Many people feel that the knowledge of a terminal prognosis can be likened to an immediate death sentence, and revealing this information to patients may result in their withdrawal due to loss of hope and their no longer feeling a part of the "living" world. As previously mentioned, people generally have not prepared for the final stage of life or recognize the importance of "living until we die." Family members, trying to protect their dying loved ones, not only hide information but, assuming that the patients are too fragile to deal with the intense emotional reactions that may result from family members' feelings, hide them as well.

> (Sarah) I have heard many a family member say that they cannot cry in front of the patient because they do not want to upset them. Sometimes the patient is anxiously awaiting those tears as a symbol of the love and connection between them.

In these situations, the parties to a relationship prematurely treat each other as if the relationship were already over, and fail to see the importance of continuing to invest energy in this next, albeit probably final, stage of the relationship. When this occurs, tremendous opportunity for final closure is often lost.

Another aspect of loss is the "if only's." "If only we had caught it sooner." "If only he had stopped smoking 10 years earlier." "If only we had done this treatment instead of that treatment." "If only we had not tried that treatment at all." The best advice is that there is no advice. No matter what one might want to say in these instances, even if one has experienced similar situations, it is hard for the grieving individual to listen. For many, those are questions that they need to ask themselves as they make their way through their journey of grief. One can listen, support, and maybe even connect them with others who have had a similar experience.

An important understanding that most experienced end-of-life care providers carry with them is that one can never take away someone's denial or patterns of coping. One can simply join them in their model of the world and offer unconditional support. Caregivers must trust the patient's and family's process as they would their own.

Opportunity to Adjust to New Roles

So often, people define themselves and their relationships with others and to the world based on what they do and the roles in which they participate. Upon first meeting a new person, after asking them their name and where they are from, one most commonly asks, "What do you do?" Our society emphasizes "doing" more than "being," and our societal structure often places worth or lack thereof on individuals based on what they do. As discussed, when a patient is diagnosed with a terminal illness, he or she may ask, "Who am I, if physically I can no longer fulfill those roles?" Many of us fulfill many roles.

(Sarah) I am an employee, a mother, a daughter, a significant other, a friend, a volunteer, a spiritual student, an athlete, and an individual. Within each of these roles there are even more smaller, yet essential roles.

Illness may bring on changes in societal, familial, and sexual roles. As with all the areas discussed, each area is interconnected to the other areas. Physical changes may effect social roles. For those who were active in the community, it may be impossible to attend activities outside of the home. This could include church or synagogue, Kiwanis or Rotary, golf or tennis. Family roles change as well. For example, a man with a diagnosis of COPD will eventually become too ill to work and no longer be able to hold the position of breadwinner. He also may no longer be able to fulfill his other

roles such as driving the car, paying the bills, or even walking the dog. No longer is he the man his wife married. In long-term relationships, many of these roles have been assigned and fulfilled by only one of the partners for years. The wife may now need to take on several of her husband's roles, some of which she may be ill equipped to handle. Over time, resentment may build in the wife, which may, in turn, negatively affect their intimacy.

Although intimacy takes on many forms, sexual contact is an integral part of most adult relationships. Long-term illness brings about many changes in the way a couple interacts sexually. Many times there are concerns about possibly hurting the infirmed person—are they too fragile to engage in our usual form of lovemaking? Will it tire them out? There is sometimes the illogical yet strong fear of contracting the illness that the partner has even when it is noncommunicable. The simple truth is that few individuals will feel sexy or desirable when ill, and it takes energy to engage in sexual activity. Many couples have been living with the illness for years and have stopped connecting physically due to the distractions involved with the disease process and treatment. If this couple is from the "old school," in which one did not discuss sex and sexuality, then a further gap occurs. Bridging this gap means finding small ways in which to reestablish intimacy. The benefit of the terminal diagnosis and the choice to no longer pursue aggressive treatment also allows a couple to refocus on each other and turn their attention away from the disease. Although sexual intercourse may no longer be an option, there are many ways for couples to connect: talking, holding hands, back rubs, baths, and any sexual activity that makes allowances for the abilities of the patient.

Some of the best support we can offer families whose roles are rapidly changing is training in practical "survival skills." An 80-year-old man may have to learn to boil an egg or use a microwave. Another caregiver may need to learn, for the first time, how to balance the checkbook.

(Sarah) One caregiver I knew, upon his first trip to the grocery store alone, was uncertain which kind of margarine to buy because he wasn't sure why his wife had chosen the one they had been using. He left the store without any margarine.

In these cases concrete step-by-step instruction and participation during the first few trials can make all the difference.

It may also be very important to the one who is dying to know that we will continue to be there for the survivor with practical or emotional support. In this way, the dying person may be able to leave in confidence that the caretaking responsibilities that they would normally assume will be followed up by someone else. Not being the one to fulfill that role may still be a loss, but perhaps not an inconsolable one.

Many family members and friends need reassurance to understand how these changes will affect them and their relationship to the dying person. In this case, the opportunity is more for the healthy individual than it is for the dying one. Fear about the dying process is understandable, and it takes someone with courage to cross that threshold to visit within someone's home. Sometimes the challenge is due to the disconnection from the customary way of connecting. For instance, when you see someone at the mall in cutoff shorts and a T-shirt, someone who you have only seen in a suit at work, at first it seems strange and often it takes a moment before you can even identify them. Visiting a friend or family member who is now ill and homebound is similar in that it feels initially uncomfortable and strange because it is a similarly new and different experience. However, we can provide the reassurance that once the "comfort zone" is extended, it is likely that they will discover different ways to connect. Wouldn't you want someone to visit with you if the situation were reversed?

Imagine how much more intensely the spouse or significant other experiences these changes. For example, a wife might have cooked elaborate meals for her and her husband, and maybe they had long conversations together over dinner about politics and world events. Maybe the husband can no longer eat much or talk for long periods of time. The couple might connect now by eating a smaller dinner together while *listening* to the news.

If you are a family member living out of state and your loved one can no longer use the phone, a new link may need to be created. Perhaps e-mailing letters for the caregiver to read to your family member would keep the connection. As the dying process continues, it is important to continue to adapt the bonding experiences as much as possible. Ultimately, this may lead to the simplest, yet most enduring form of connection: the family member holding the hand of the patient as the patient takes the last breath.

There is also the dimension of one's relationships reflecting, in part, who we are as individuals. We make the assumption that if we have a compassionate, caring, committed support group who is with us throughout the dying process, then we must be all those things: compassionate, caring, committed, supportive. However, if we don't, what does that say about us? Many of us assume we will receive from others all that we have extended to them, especially in our time of need. Often, however, this is not the case. And often it is not because we weren't all those things to all those people. We have met many patients who simply outlived most of their families and friends and were at a time in their lives when creating new support relationships was a challenge. There are other patients who had wonderful friends and family but many lived out of state or were too ill themselves to visit or offer much support. In many cases these dying patients have been ill with their disease for years and have been unable to maintain a viable network of connections.

There may be no way to "make this better" in terms of adding new people to their lives, but one can spend time reminiscing about prior relationships and honoring the time, energy, and fun that went into them. It is a beautiful way to practice the art of storytelling while passing on interesting and historical information. It also allows the patient to relive wonderful memories and actually be with these people from the past in the present.

The practice of life review actually has a long tradition. In one sense, life review is part of the venerable old tradition of storytelling. In the Jewish faith, this process is recognized as a part of the person's legacy, called an "ethical will." In their book *So That Your Values Live On: Ethical Wills and How to Prepare Them* (1991), Jack Riemer and Nathaniel Stampfer give a wonderful overview of ethical wills, examples of historic and modern ethical wills, and guidelines for creating one. They point out that the ethical will does not have to be a written document—a cassette voice recording or videotape can be an amazing legacy to leave behind.

Opportunity to Get Your Affairs in Order

(Sarah) I spoke recently with a woman who was told by her oncologist to "get her affairs in order" as she had been diagnosed with stage three ovarian cancer. A year and a half later, she is here and cancer free.

This is one of those success stories that one loves to hear; but all too often, when the doctor tells a patient that it is time to get one's affairs in order, it is usually time to do so. "Affairs" in this context can include financial and medical matters, as well more practical matters such as funeral arrangements and issues surrounding those who will still be here after one is gone.

Sometimes the challenge is in addressing these practical matters while trying to cope with the overwhelming blow of being given a terminal prognosis. One might have to face up to the reality that efforts to combat the disease have been unsuccessful. It is hard enough to simply make it from minute to minute, hour to hour, much less decide who gets what and whether you want to be buried or cremated. Again, due to our death-denying society, few of us take the time to consider these matters when we are healthy and when these discussions would carry much less emotional trauma.

With the health care environment what it is today, many patients and families face a great deal of stress related to the cost of health care, as well as its bureaucracy, resulting in what can be termed "bureaucratic pain." Challenges related to payment for incredibly expensive treatments, which may not be as successful as first hoped; negotiating through the red tape of insurance companies, doctors' offices, and hospitals; together with the physical, social, and emotional challenges of being terminally ill, often contribute to what has been defined as "total or overwhelming pain" (Welk, 1991).

(Sarah) The best example of how to handle this came from a woman I knew who was dying of lung cancer. She talked about having worried about paying her bills during the years she was ill and all the companies calling her for payment and the anxiety it brought to her already strained life. She was laughing now about their inability to get "blood from a stone" because she was dying. This was a woman who had worked up until her illness, paid her bills on time and in full, and who had spent everything she had to pay to treat her illness. She taught me, through her experience, that each of us needs to do the best that we can, but there are times when our best must be "good enough."

One way to deal with bureaucratic pain is by doing what is referred to in psychology as "chunking it down." If a problem seems too big to handle, then chunk it down into manageable parts. Even financially, small payments over time add up to larger sums. Beyond that, there is only so much that it is in our control, and it is our job, as the "Prayer for Serenity" suggests, to accept what we cannot change, change what we can, and be clear on the difference between the two.

Conclusion

Each person's end-of-life experience is unique and individual. It can be as beautiful as a symphony, with numerous notes, instruments, and musicians coming together to create the exquisite final composition, or it can sound like a second-grader's first piano lesson. The difference between the two often rests with those of us working with people near the end of life. We must remember that in our lives, as in music, the finale is as important as the overture. As Tournier (1972) put it, "I live differently, but not less." For those caring for the terminally ill, psychosocial and spiritual issues that in the past had been seen as problems can, with information and compassion, become opportunities—opportunities that will allow each of us to live fully until we say goodbye.

In this chapter we have explored a number of psychosocial and spiritual issues affecting care of those near the end of life. These issues affect everyone from the physician to the patient's primary caregiver. With this knowledge, the physician's increased awareness of the psychosocial or spiritual issues might prompt earlier referrals and an interdisciplinary approach to pain management. A hospice nurse might recognize that a patient or caregiver's anger, so distracting in the past, is related to the dying process. This frees the nurse up to use professional skills to address the true problem and provide comfort while managing physical symptoms. The family member who is caring for a loved one might have new tools to understand and bridge the gap that the dying process sometimes creates.

In closing, the words of Henri J.M. Nouwen (1994) ring through.

Is death something so terrible and absurd that we are better off not thinking or talking about it? Is death such an undesirable part of our existence that we are better off acting as if it were not real? Is death such an absolute end of all our thoughts and actions that we simply cannot face it? Or is it possible to befriend our dying gradually and live open to it, trusting that we have nothing to fear? Is it possible to prepare for our death with the same attentiveness that our parents had in preparing for our birth? Can we wait for our death as for a friend who wants to welcome us home?

We think that the answer is yes! We hope the information in this chapter will help you to see that, too.

Bibliography

Becker E: *The Denial of Death*. New York, Free Press, 1973.

Brueggemann W: *Hopeful Imagination*. Philadephia, Fortress, 1986

Buckman R: *How to Break Bad News*. Baltimore, Johns Hopkins University Press, 1992.

Byock IR: Growth: The essence of hospice. *Am J Hospice Care* Nov/Dec 1986. 16–21.

Byock IR, Merriman MP: Measuring quality of life for patients with terminal illness: The Missoula-VITAS quality of life index. *Palliat Med* 12:231, 1998.

Cella DF: Quality of life: Concepts and definition. *J Pain Symptom Manage* 9:186, 1994.

Cleary E: Psychosocial palliation: Its role in cancer pain management. Ohio Cancer Pain Initiative (www.ocpi.orgla_psychosocial.html), 1999.

Cohen SR, Mount BM, Tomas JJN, et al: Existential well being is an important determinant of quality of life. *Cancer* 77:576, 1996.

Dough Singh K: *The Grace in Dying*. San Francisco, Harbor Books, 1998.

Frankl V: *Man's Search for Meaning*. New York, Touchstone, 1959.

International Work Group on Death, Dying and Bereavement. *Statements on Death, Dying and Bereavement*. Ontario, Kings College, 1994

Kaplan HI, Sadock BJ, Grebb JA: *Kaplan and Sadock's Synopsis of Psychiatry*. Baltimore, Williams & Williams, 1994.

Kubler-Ross E: *On Death and Dying*. New York, Free Press, 1969.

Nouwen HJM: *Our Greatest Gift: A Meditation on Dying and Caring*. San Francisco, Harper San Francisco, 1994.

Patch Adams (Dir: Tom Shadyac), Universal Studios, 1999.

Riemer J, Stampfer N: *So That Your Values Live On*. Woodstock, VT, Jewish Lights, 1991.

Sourkes BM: *The Deepening Shade*. Pittsburgh, University of Pittsburgh Press, 1982.

Szemplak J: The effects of physical and emotional pain on quality of life. Ohio Cancer Pain Initiative (www.ocpi.orgla_quality.html), 1997.

Tournier P: *Learn to Grow Old.* Louisville, Westminster/John Knox Press, 1972.

Wangerin W: *Mourning into Dancing.* Grand Rapids, Zondervan, 1992.

Welk TA: An educational model for explaining hospice services. *Am J Hospice Palliat Care* Sept/Oct 1991: 14–18.

Michael Bozeman

Bereavement

Introduction

The widely recognized principles of hospice and end-of-life care are effective symptom management, care of the patient and family, an interdisciplinary approach to the care of the patient, continuity of care, and bereavement follow-up care of the family. These principles serve to underscore the importance in end-of-life care of a comprehensive, integrative care approach to address the multiple and complex physical, psychological, spiritual, and socioeconomic concerns of the patient and family.

The involvement of physicians in all aspects of hospice and end-of-life care results in measurable improvement in the quality of care provided to terminally ill patients and their families. Additionally, hospice—with its principle of addressing the patient and family together as a unit of care, and with a built-in system for addressing the combined physical and psychosocial aspects of care—is consistent with the philosophy of primary care. Although most physicians feel comfortable in providing hospice care, most report receiving inadequate education about hospice care and associated death and dying issues, and they experience a heightened sense of their own mortality when dealing with these issues. This should not be surprising given our "death-denying" Western culture and an absence of a sufficient comfort level within it to openly discuss needs and fears associated with death, dying, and bereavement. The challenge, for physicians providing palliative care to patients dealing with these issues, goes well beyond simply acquiring knowledge about death and grief. Rather, physicians must be open to exploring their personal death awareness, feelings, and attitudes and be conscious of how these influence the physician–patient relationship.

With the shift of location of care from the hospital to the home, family caregivers play a primary role in caring for the patient while at the same time attending to and/or postponing their own physical and psychosocial needs. The physician providing palliative care has a rich opportunity and professional obligation to identify and address these needs. This obligation begins with assuming responsibility for appropriately breaking "bad news" to a patient about a terminal diagnosis (see Chapter 3), a step that is critical if the anticipatory grief process is to be as smooth as possible. When bad news is delivered indirectly, not only is the difficult work of grief obstructed for the patient and family, but the interdisciplinary team has the additional challenge of providing care to a patient who may not be ready to receive end-of-life services or even know what these services involve.

Bereavement care thus begins at the point of sharing the difficult news of a terminal diagnosis courageously and honestly. It must be shared in a relaxed setting that allows adequate time for the patient and family to express a plethora of painful emotions and reactions, some of which may be misdirected at the physician, who despite much discomfort, should realize that they are normal and necessary.

The physician continues to play an important role in care of the caregiver by remaining available during and following the patient's death and through being cognizant of when physical and psychological symptoms may be bereavement related. This is vital to determining appropriate treatment modalities, such as prescribing psychotropic medication, referring the bereaved caregiver for psychiatric assessment or bereavement counseling, or simply encouraging the expression of grief to decrease symptom severity. The physician needs at least a working knowledge of the use of pharmacotherapy for grief-related morbidity to provide appropriate medication when indicated, and to guard against prescribing medication when it may complicate the mourning process.

Studies examining the connection between patients' length of stay in hospice and spousal adjustment to loss are insufficient to draw any definitive conclusions regarding the importance of early enrollment in an end-of-life care program in reducing the risk of complicated bereavement. However, it is suggested that early referral allows palliative care providers more time to identify caregivers with risk factors for negative grief outcomes, as well as to initiate interventions both before and immediately following the loss when indicated. There is little disagreement that early enrollment helps the patient achieve the type of death that is regarded as preferred—that of dying in the home with the presence and support of loved ones. Recent studies indicate a relationship between caregiver health and level of caregiver satisfaction with a hospice experience and time of hospice enrollment, with spouses of patients who are moderately to severely sick being admitted to hospice later than those whose spouses are well. This demonstrates the need of all clinicians to not overlook the status of the caregiver and the demands that providing care places on them.

These demands continue after the patient's death. While bereavement care has historically been targeted at psychological adjustment, at least one third of survivors report financial problems due to postdeath economic sequelae of reduced income, disruption in their employment, and higher living expenses. An adjustment to loss occurs on a number of levels, and the socioeconomic and practical needs of survivors must receive much more attention if survivors are to adjust to both the emotional loss of a loved one and to the loss of a variety of roles the deceased assumed during the relationship.

Survivors have higher morbidity and mortality rates during the first year following the death of a loved one than do individuals in than the general population. Limited studies indicate that caregivers who participate in bereavement interventions following loss, such as bereavement counseling and support groups, may have lower health care costs and be healthier than survivors who receive minimal or no bereavement intervention. Hospices and other end-of-life care programs can be instrumental in assisting survivors to work through the mourning process by assessing and addressing caregiver bereavement needs beginning at the time of the patient's admission to the hospice and continuing to provide bereavement services for at least a year following the patient's death. It is for this reason that bereavement care is such a crucial part of end-of-life care, and is mandated by the Medicare Hospice Benefit for one year following the death of the patient.

Terminology

Bereavement

It may be helpful to provide a working definition of the various terms used when describing loss and bereavement. Bereavement is commonly understood as the objective situation or event in which an individual has suffered the loss of someone or something significant. "Bereavement" or "bereaved" are words that derive from the word "reave," which means "to despoil, rob, or forcibly deprive." A bereaved individual is someone who has been deprived or robbed of something valued. There is no bereavement or grief when there has not been attachment to a significant object. It is all too common in our society, in an effort to be helpful, to downplay one's experience of loss by dismissing or minimizing the importance of one's loss. Bereavement care, therefore, begins with an attempt to understand the importance of the loss to the bereaved person, and to communicate one's recognition of this significance.

Grief

Grief refers to the bereaved person's internal emotional response and subjective experience to the loss event. Grief has a number of components: somatic, behavioral, emotional, cognitive, social, and spiritual. The term appears to have arisen from the heavy weight experienced by an individual who is burdened by a loss. It is not uncommon for one who is experiencing grief to feel overwhelmed by a heaviness of something that cannot be easily thrown off.

An important element of grief often overlooked by health care professionals is that it affects all aspects of the self. Psychiatrist George Engel asked the question "Is grief a disease?" Horowitz sums up the response that is certainly the consensus of health care practitioners. "No, it is a normal human capacity for adapting to loss." He cautions against pathologizing grief unnecessarily and that no diagnosis is needed to warrant helping the bereaved with the mourning process. There are normal and abnormal responses to grief, which are defined in Table 14–1 and discussed next.

Normal Grief

Normal grief, also referred to as typical or uncomplicated grief, is the term used to describe the type of grief that is found in the vast majority of survivors. As will be mentioned later in this chapter, given adequate support and time both before and after a loss, most individudals are able to eventually readjust to their loss even though the loss may have produced dramatic changes in one's life. The word "recovery" is absent in most of the literature. One who suffers a loss does not recover in the sense of regaining or replacing what was lost. Neither does the bereaved individual return to a state in which one was the same person as before the loss. Survivors often talk about life after a loss

as "different" but never as the "same" as it once was. For some, loss changes virtually everything including the need of the survivor to search for identity, meaning, and purpose, especially when the sense of self had been dependent upon or inseparable from that of the deceased.

Abnormal Grief

Abnormal grief, also referred to as complicated, conflicted, or pathologic grief, describes grief disorders found in 3 to 25 percent of survivors (clinical studies vary, as do the rates with various types of losses). There are several types of abnormal grief reactions, and these are delineated in Table 14–1.

CHRONIC GRIEF

Chronic grief occurs when the person grieving cannot achieve closure or bring their grief to a satisfactory conclusion. Often an individual with chronic grief is unable to successfully integrate the loss into life and return to normal activities even over an extended period of time.

DELAYED GRIEF

Delayed grief refers to the intentional postponing of grief to a later date, usually precipitated

Table 14–1

Manifestations of Grief

TYPE OF GRIEF	DEFINITION
Normal (typical or uncomplicated)	Majority of survivors
	Eventual readjustment to loss
Abnormal (complicated, conflicted, pathological)	3%–25% of survivors
	Various subtypes depending on reaction
Chronic grief	No closure to grief
Delayed grief	Postponement of grief
Disenfranchised grief	Lack of acknowledgement of loss
Exaggerated grief	Intensification of normal grief reactions
Masked grief	Symptomatic repression of grief
Sudden grief	Unexpected loss resulting in lack of closure

by other events or losses. At least one study has shown that caregivers with prolonged caregiver roles may, out of exhaustion, not be able to have the emotional or mental energy to continue to work through the grief process.

DISENFRANCHISED GRIEF

Disenfranchised grief occurs when a person experiences a loss that "cannot be openly acknowledged, publicly mourned, or socially supported." Losses that may be associated with the risk of disenfranchised grief generally are those in which there is a discrepancy in how the mourner and society views its significance. Examples include losses related to AIDS, a miscarriage or stillborn child, infertility, or the loss of a homosexual lover that society does not accept as a real loss.

EXAGGERATED GRIEF

Exaggerated grief refers to the intensification of normal grief reactions with behaviors that may include nightmares, outbursts of fear, delinquent behavior, prolonged guilt, phobias, and suicidal ideation.

MASKED GRIEF

Masked grief, also referred to as the absence of grief, is a type of grief in which the grieving individual develops behavioral or psychiatric symptoms such as unexplained depression, usually through the repression of grief, which the griever is unable to associate with the loss.

SUDDEN GRIEF

Sudden grief is when a death takes place with little or no warning and does not allow for the grieving individual to accept the reality of the death or accomplish adequate closure with the deceased. When the circumstances of sudden death are of a traumatic nature (e.g., violent, random, or mutilating), bereavement reactions are more severe and complicated, sometimes resulting in posttraumatic stress disorder (PTSD) and other exaggerated grief reactions.

Mourning

Wolfelt defines mourning as "when you take the grief on the inside and express it outside of yourself," or "grief gone public" (Wolfelt, 1999). Mourning usually refers to the outward, public, cultural, and religious expressions of grieving such as the recognition of a special date through visiting the gravesite. It may also take on more private expressions, such as keeping a journal, leafing through a photo album, finding new ways to relate to or think about the deceased, or finding healthy ways to integrate the loss so as to move on with life. Some cultures have more dramatic expressions of loving that include intense wailing, the tearing of hair and clothes, and self-mutilation. Health care providers often mistake these more dramatic displays of grief as abnormal and believe that mourners who display these behaviors are in need of therapeutic intervention. The importance of culture in understanding grief and providing appropriate interventions will be addressed later in this chapter.

Grief Counseling and Therapy

Grief counseling is generally thought of as the process of helping facilitate normal, uncomplicated grief so that the mourner works through the various tasks of grieving within a reasonable time. As discussed later in the chapter, grief therapy involves the use of specialized techniques to help persons with abnormal or complicated grief reactions.

Reactions to Loss: The Grief Process

Although grief is a universal experience, every person responds differently to loss. There is no single blueprint by which all persons grieve, nor is there a set time frame in which one must adjust to a loss. Whereas in 1927, Emily Post mentioned that widows grieved for a period of 3 years following a loss, one newspaper article in the 1990s mentioned that it can be expected to last up to a week! Another newspaper article stated that, following the loss of his mother, the President of the United States would need at least "two full days" to grieve before he resumed his full duties. We now know that some adjust fairly quickly to a loss, usually within a year of the death, while others take several years. It has been shown that mothers who have lost a child and who are unwilling to relinquish their attachment to their child may still continue to grieve many years later.

Worden states that full resolution of grief usually takes 1 to 2 years, while Parkes' studies indicate that widows may take up to 4 years for grief to resolve. Davidson examined the intensity levels of separate reactions to grief (shock and numbness, searching and yearning, disorientation, reorganization) for 2 years following the loss. Instead of a gradual decrease in grief reactions, the findings were that survivors experienced "peaks and valleys" during the mourning period, with the most noticeable difficulties occurring between 4 and 6 months following the loss. After 24 months, most survivors were found to be readjusting adequately. Another study, which examined the course of spousal bereavement, supports the current thinking that survivors with either uncomplicated or complicated grief experience the most psychological distress at approximately 6 weeks following the loss, with a gradual decrease of distress and other symptoms over a 2-year period. This study also reinforced the common assumption that individuals with negative bereavement outcomes can be identified both before and following a loss using a standardized bereavement risk instrument or grief inventory instrument (see "Bereavement Risk Assessment" later in the chapter).

The novice health care professional who has just learned that persons progress through certain stages or phases of grief may mistakenly think that all grievers go through these phases in an orderly fashion. This type of linear thinking was popular after the publication of Elisabeth Kubler-Ross's sentinel work, *On Death and Dying,* on which she later commented that the stages of dying she elucidated were never meant to be taken in a literal,

predictable fashion. Clinicians report that some patients reach no level of "acceptance" in their resolution of grief, while others may stay angry or depressed, or "ping pong" between various stages. It is also common for grievers to "make one step backward for every two steps forward" and consciously or unconsciously take breaks from the mourning due to the amount of energy expended.

Thanatologist and clinical psychologist Alan Wolfelt discusses five "myths" about grief and mourning that the clinician should be aware of when managing bereaved family members. These myths are listed in Table 14–2 and are described below (Wolfelt, 1999).

Myth 1: *Grief and mourning are the same experiences.* Although these words are often used synonymously, an important distinction exists. Grief is the "composite of thoughts and feelings about a loss that you experience within yourself" while mourning is the process of moving toward healing by expressing one's grief outside of oneself.

Myth 2: *The experiences of grief and mourning progress in predictable and orderly stages.* Grief is unique and each person need not feel what they must experience in their grief journey.

Myth 3: *Move away from grief, not toward it.* Grief is often viewed as "something to be overcome, rather than something to be experienced." Grief must be experienced in order for the proper outcome to be achieved.

Table 14–2

Myths Related to Grief and Mourning

Grief and mourning are the same experiences.
The experiences of grief and mourning
   progress in predictable and orderly stages.
Move away from grief, not towards it.
The goal should be to get over your grief as
   soon as possible.
Tears expressing grief are only a sign of
   weakness.

Myth 4: *Following the death of someone loved, the goal should be to "get over" your grief as soon as possible.* The goal is not to get over one's grief but to "grow through it." The griever needs to mourn at his or her own pace.

Myth 5: *Tears expressing grief are only a sign of weakness.* While there are various theories regarding the causes and functions of crying, Wolfelt mentions that crying is nature's way of releasing tension and allows the individual to communicate a need to be comforted. One's capacity to express tears demonstrates one's willingness to work through grief.

The physician as well as other health care practitioners will come across a wide variety of reactions and behaviors in response to a loss. Although there are grief reactions, phases, and tasks that are common to most survivors, how and when the survivor completes these is very individual and determined by a great number of factors. Tables 14–3 through 14–8 detail many of the characteristics of normal, uncomplicated grief, divided into responses to loss that are physical (Table 14–3), behavioral (Table 14–4), emotional (Table 14–5), cognitive (Table 14–6), physiological (Table 14–7), and social (Table 14–8). These characteristics may also

Table 14–3
Physical Responses to Grief

An empty feeling in the stomach
Lack of energy
Muscle weakness, shaking, trembling
Fatigue
Extreme tension, irritability, oversensitivity
Diffuse aches
Headache
Dry mouth
Tightness in the throat, chest, jaw
Difficulty swallowing
Shortness of breath
Sweating, hot flashes, or chills

Table 14–4
Behavioral Responses to Grief

Changes in sleep patterns
Changes in appetite
Inability to concentrate, absent-minded behavior
Heavy and repeated sighing
Restlessness, overactivity, hypervigilance
Dramatic mood changes
Dreaming of the deceased
Crying
Calling out and searching for the loved one
Avoiding thinking of the deceased
Not wanting to go on living without the deceased
Repressing crying
Regression, feelings of insecurity
Apathy
Increase in psychoactive substances
Decreased productivity
Guarded or tangential in conversation
Attempting to embody the deceased by taking on his or her behavior
Treasuring or relinquishing objects belonging to the deceased
Visiting places or carrying objects of the deceased
Telling, retelling, and remembering aspects of the deceased

be present when individuals experience complicated grief, especially where they are present over a prolonged period of time.

Stages and Tasks of Grief

FOUR PHASES

There are several excellent models that describe the various stages and tasks of grief, listed in Table 14–9. Bowlby (1980) has divided the process of grief into four phases. The first phase is the period of numbness immediately following the loss. This is generally thought of as a healthy

Table 14–5
Emotional Responses to Grief

Sadness
Anger
Fear (death anxiety)
Guilt, shame, self-reproach
Loneliness
Fatigue
Shock
Yearning (pining)
Numbness (psychological distancing)
Relief
Helplessness
Anxiety

Table 14–6
Cognitive Reactions to Grief

Disbelief
Sensing the presence of or expecting the deceased to appear
Temporary visual and auditory hallucinations
Confusion, ambivalence about what to do
Preoccupation with thinking about the deceased
Feelings of inadequacy
Decrease in level of self-esteem
Increased spirituality, alienation, rejection
Search for meaning, identity

Table 14–7
Physiologic Responses to Grief

Hair loss
Diffuse somatic complaints
Gastrointestinal symptoms
Cardiopulmonary symptoms
Neurologic symptoms
Exacerbation of current complaints

Source: Adapted from Rando T: *Treatment of Complicated Mourning.* Champaign, IL, Research Press, 1993.

defense mechanism that allows the person in shock to disregard the death in order to survive emotionally. Following numbness is the second phase, searching and yearning (pining), characterized by yearning for the deceased to return. The grieving individual may experience weeping, anxiety, anger, self-reproach, confusion, and loss of security. It is in this stage that clinicians are often asked to provide assistance due to the perception that the mourner is acting pathologically, especially when the mourner is having panic attacks or hysteria. Statements by the mourner such as "I can't go on without him" are sometimes misinterpreted as suicidal gestures or threats. The third phase, disorganization and despair, is characterized by the desire to withdraw and disengage from others and from activities. Periods of apathy and despair become more intense while the severity and frequency of pining and yearning diminishes. The final phase is reorganization and recovery. Weight loss from the first couple of months of bereavement is regained, energy level increases, and the griever develops the desire to "engage in activities directed to the future rather than the past." While grief does not end, yearning for the loved one is diminished by recollection of positive memories of the deceased and the desire to make plans for

Table 14–8
Social Responses to Grief

Lack of or decreased interest
Withdrawal
Boredom
Misdirected anger, overly critical to others
Feeling alienated, detached, or estranged from others
Jealousy of others without loss
Dependency on others, avoidance of being alone
Self-destructive behaviors
Acting out, impulsive behaviors

Source: Adapted from Rando T: *Treatment of Complicated Mourning.* Champaign, IL, Research Press, 1993.

Table 14–9
Models of Stages and Tasks of Grief and Mourning

PROPOSER OF MODEL	TITLE OF MODEL	CHARACTERISTICS
Bowlby	Four phases of grieving	Numbness immediately following the loss
		Searching and yearning
		Disorganization and despair
		Reorganization and recovery
Stroebe and Schut	Dual-process model of coping with bereavement	Grieving is interrupted to attend to other issues
Sanders	Integrative theory of bereavement	Shock
		Awareness of loss
		Conversation-withdrawal
		Healing
		Renewal
Worden	Four tasks of mourning	To accept the reality of the loss
		To work through the pain of grief
		To adjust to an environment in which the deceased is missing
		To emotionally relocate the deceased and move on with life

SOURCE: Bowlby J: *Attachment and Loss: Loss, Sadness and Depression*, vol. 3. New York, Basic Books, 1980; Stroebe M, Schut H: The dual process model of coping with bereavement: Rationale and description. *Death Studies* 23:197, 1993; Sanders CM: Effects of sudden vs. chronic illness death in bereavement outcome. *Omega* 13:227, 1982–1983; Worden JW: *Grief Counseling and Grief Therapy: A Handbook for the Mental Health Practioner*, 2nd ed. New York, Springer, 1991.

the future. Most other descriptive models for the grief process build upon Bowlby's work.

DUAL PROCESS MODEL

Stroebe and Schut (1999) have developed a model to support their proposition that the grieving individual "at times confronts and at other times avoids the different tasks of grieving." This dual process model of coping with bereavement is based on the premise that those who grieve take respites from their grieving to attend to other stressors as well as to experience a "fluctuation of attention in the coping process." This concept is based on the notion that the bereaved is unable to maintain focus on the loss all of the time. This is compatible with other bereavement models that emphasize that grief is a process and not a state. Even though

grief theorists may have not have expressly detailed the respite that the bereaved take from grief, they are aware that the majority of grievers do not tackle their grief all at one time and that intervening variables in the grief continuum exist.

INTEGRATIVE THERAPY

Sanders (1982–1983) has developed an interesting model, referred to as the integrative theory of bereavement. The central element of this model is that "each of the psychological forces that operate during the process of grief also has a biological anlage that determines the physical well-being of the individual." She proposes five phases of bereavement: shock, awareness of loss, conversation-withdrawal, healing, and renewal, the first three based primarily on biological needs. This model also demonstrates how important the interactions of "external mediators" such as social support, concurrent crises, and "internal mediators" such as age, gender, and personality, can be for the survivor's grief outcome.

FOUR TASKS

The helpfulness of "the four tasks of mourning" in understanding the process of adaptation to loss cannot be underestimated. Worden (1991) states that following a loss, there are certain tasks of mourning that must be accomplished for equilibrium to be established and for mourning to be completed. Unlike "stages" or "phases," which imply that grief may go on at an unconscious level, the concept of tasks points out that effort is required to come to terms with the loss that occurred. The tasks, outlined in Table 14–9, are described next.

1. *To accept the reality of the loss.* "The first task of grieving is to come full face with the reality that the person is dead, that the person is gone and will not return." Without accepting that the loss has occurred, the bereaved cannot begin and continue through the mourning process.
2. *To work through the pain of grief.* It is important for the bereaved to acknowledge the pain and grief that has been caused by the loss. Avoiding or suppressing the pain only prolongs the mourning process.
3. *To adjust to an environment in which the deceased is missing.* The bereaved must adjust to the loss of roles played by the deceased. This includes, for example, searching and adjusting to one's sense of self and identity such as beginning to think of oneself as a widow or single person rather than as a "couple."
4. *To emotionally relocate the deceased and move on with life.* The bereaved is not compelled to totally give up the relationship with the deceased. Rather, the task is to "find an appropriate place for the dead in their emotional lives—a place that will enable them to go on living effectively in the world." There must be a letting go of the attachment so that new relationships can be formed. Worden shares a note from a teenage girl who was having a difficult time adjusting to the loss of her father. In this note to her mother, it is evident she was aware of the need for withdrawal and reinvestment: "There are other people to be loved," she wrote, "and it doesn't mean that I love Dad any less."

Determinants of Grief

A number of factors influence the grief process (Table 14–10). When assessing the bereaved individual using these categories to frame the discussion and keeping in mind risk factors for a poor grief outcome (Table 14–11), a fairly reliable picture can be painted as to some of the difficulties the mourner is likely to face in dealing with the loss.

Relationships

For example, a number of studies have shown that the loss of a spouse will be grieved differently in

Table 14–10

Determinants of Grief

The unique nature of the attachment to and relationship with the deceased
Characteristics of the deceased
Type and length of illness, mode of death
History of coping
Psychological history of functioning
Number and type of previous losses
Personality variables
Social, cultural, religious, spiritual factors, and expectations about grief and mourning
Concurrent crises
Level of support
Physiologic factors such as alcohol intake, use of sedatives, physical health

Table 14–11

Bereavement Risk Factors

CATEGORIES OF RISK	SPECIFIC RISK FACTORS
Related to current or prior losses	Sudden or unexpected death
	Death of a child
	Traumatic loss
	Multiple losses
	Unresolved losses
	Lack of acceptance of impending death
	Death from overly lengthy illness
	Death perceived as preventable
	Death results in financial hardship
	Death results in disruptions or multiple life-change events
Related to mental health	Low trust level in oneself or others
	History of poor mental health
	History of psychiatric illness
	Low tolerance of disturbing thought and feelings
	Clinging or pining
	Anxiety, depression, or suicidal ideation
	Substance use
	Concurrent crises or stressors
	Inhibition of feelings
	High levels of anger or self-reproach
Related to physical health	Poor physical health
	Prior pregnancy loss
Related to relationships	Ambivalence, anger, or dependence in the relationship
	Difficulty in relationship with parents
Related to age or social status	Young spouses
	Lower socioeconomic background
	Perceived low social support or isolation
	Children who lose a parent who had a low level of involvement
	Children who will experience a high level of change and/or disruption
	Children who lose a mother
	Female children who lose mother or sister
	Multiple children in the home
	Illness not socially acceptable
	Older adults with depression at time of death

terms of types of responses and intensity than the loss of a child. Bereaved parents have been shown to have more intense reactions than bereaved spouses, while bereaved spouses have been found to have more intense reactions than bereaved adult children. Male children appear to be affected more by the loss of a parent than by the loss of a sibling, whereas females seem to be more affected by sibling loss, especially the loss of a sister, than by the loss of a parent. One third of children who lose a parent show high levels of emotional difficulty in their readjustment, with complicated grief reactions often not being evidenced until the second year of bereavement. Interestingly, one study found that children who lost a parent did not have "any more significant school problems than those who hadn't lost a parent," suggesting that one must be cautious against assuming that all bereaved children need the same degree of intervention.

Cause of Death

The cause of death—whether natural, accidental, suicidal, or due to homicide—affects the grief response as well. It has been demonstrated that suvivors of sudden deaths have a more difficult adjustment than individuals who have had adequate time to prepare for the loss of a loved one. However, the sudden death of an elderly individual, whose death was not entirely unexpected due to advanced age, may not be grieved abnormally. Young survivors of loss by sudden death experience a more difficult time adjusting in the first or second years following the death than young survivors of losses that were expected, while family caregivers of patients who died following long-term illnesses were often too exhausted to complete the necessary grief work. In addition to the length of illness, the place of death influences grief.

Gender

There appear to be clear differences as to how males and females grieve, with most studies putting males at a disadvantage due to the greater ability of females to express emotion, accept temporary regression, and confide in others. As one male mourner said: "The only place I can cry is in my pickup truck where no one can see my pain." Male mourners are reported to be more reluctant to attend support groups, go for counseling, or in general, acknowledge problems associated with their grief. Caregivers working with grieving males quickly discover that expecting males to always cry or "open up" is counterproductive and that what is needed is to discover practices that are acceptable to the male mourner within his

upbringing and to present these practices as possible ways to process grief.

Cultural Issues

The first bereavement intervention when working with a person of another culture or religion is showing respect for and becoming willing to learn about the person's grief customs and practices and their potential for therapeutic value. Space does not permit adequate discussion of the social, religious, and cultural differences in grief as well as interventions and treatment approaches. Dealing with cultural differences is often viewed as a handicap to health care providers. This is unfortunate, because the opportunity exists to build upon cultural differences to facilitate provision of creative and effective cross-cultural care. This care begins by being grounded in cultural awareness sensitivity, and avoiding ethnocentrism and cultural stereotypes. The importance of this cultural awareness cannot be overstated as dramatic cultural shifts are occurring in the U.S. landscape, presenting enormous challenges in providing bereavement care to persons with vastly different ways of dealing with dying, death, and loss. Bereavement care has been misunderstood as a modern phenomenon in which medical interventions are offered before tapping into the mourner's cultural and religious resources, some of which have built-in therapeutic value. For example, in the Jewish religion, five major phases of mourning exist which are not just religious or social obligations but significant opportunities for healing that correlate with the changing experience of grief during the first year after a loss.

The Provision of Bereavement Care

It is the responsibility of all health care professionals to provide bereavement support to the families of all patients under their care. Support needs to be provided to families of patients, both before and following patient death, to facilitate the normal grief processes and attempt to short-circuit the development of abnormal grief responses. It is equally incumbent on end-of-life care providers to identify and provide the appropriate support to bereaved individuals who develop abnormal grief reactions, and assist them in coping with the loss in a fashion that will allow the grief responses to normalize.

Bereavement care may be accomplished in part by the clinician. It is best done in cooperation with an interdisciplinary team of caregivers (nurse, chaplain, social worker, aide, volunteer, hospice physicians, family clergy) so that each can provide their own unique perspective on the bereavement issues facing various family members. Hospice programs, in which interdisciplinary teams for end-of-life care are most readily available, are well suited to assist physicians in providing bereavement support to families who have suffered a recent loss. Hospices are required by federal law to complete a bereavement assessment and provide appropriate bereavement interventions, including counseling for up to a year following a patient's death. Generally, the psychosocial members of the team (chaplain and/or social worker) direct the bereavement care, drawing upon all that is known about the family and their needs to develop an individualized plan of bereavement care. However, any member of the team may provide bereavement support to the family, with the personnel involved often being chosen by the bereaved based upon relationships developed during the care of the patient.

Bereavement Assessment

BEREAVEMENT RISK ASSESSMENT

As with any clinical symptom, the first task of bereavement care is the assessment. In essence, assessment involves having the physician and end-of-life care interdisciplinary team determine the bereavement needs of the family and the risk for abnormal grief by the family members and significant others of the terminally ill patients under care. Any caregiver who has contact with the family (e.g., physician, nurse, chaplain, social worker, volunteer) may be able to contribute pertinent information to the assessment.

The bereavement assessment is performed prior to the death of the patient when possible, and it evaluates various factors that have proven useful in quickly identifying family members who may need additional support, as well as guiding clinicians as to the causes of problems encountered. A composite list of these factors can be found in Table 14–11. They are divided into five broad categories of (1) current or prior losses, (2) mental health, (3) physical health, (4) relationships, and (5) age or social status.

It should be noted that these factors cannot always be neatly inserted into a mathematical risk instrument to determine if an individual is at low, moderate, or high risk for a poor grief outcome and the problems likely to be encountered. Rather, most clinicians report a preference for making their own determination as to level of risk after examining all the variables presented, some of which may not neatly "fit" into a box associated with a particular risk factor. For example, an individual at high risk for abnormal grief based on having a history of psychiatric illness, might have that risk reduced somewhat if they have developed positive coping mechanisms during therapy and have a strong support system. Additionally, while an increased risk of abnormal grief is intuitively associated with recent negative life events, it has also been demonstrated that positive events may also increase the risk of an abnormal grief response, because any change, whether positive or negative, can produce stress by requiring individual adaptation and adjustment.

SYMPTOMS OF GRIEF

Physiologic, psychological, and spiritual reactions (see Tables 14–3 through 14–8) to the loss of a loved one are very broad and their connection with loss can easily be overlooked by the clinician. They can also be misinterpreted as an indication of complicated grief.

We now know that the primary difference between normal and complicated grief is not the types of reactions experienced but the intensity and the duration of these reactions. Manifestations such as sadness, anger, yearning, fatigue, helplessness, changes in eating and sleeping habits, and an inability to function may all occur in both normal and complicated grief. What differentiates the two is the intensity, degree of debility suffered by the bereaved, and duration of time the symptoms remain, all of which are exaggerated based on the type of loss experienced when the grief is complicated. For example, while it is common for grievers to go through brief periods of minor depression in their readjustment, Jacobs (1987) found that the majority of depressive episodes were transient and needed no professional attention. Therefore, intervention is needed only for those whose depression persists throughout the first year of bereavement.

Despite the fact that complicated grief is primarily differentiated from normal grief by differences in intensity and duration, there are also specific symptoms and conditions associated with complicated grief that can be easily recognized during the assessment process. These are listed in Table 14–12. Distilling this down, Horowitz and associates have proposed that bereaved individuals could be diagnosed as having complicated grief disorder if three of the seven symptoms listed in Table 14–13 were present 14 months after the loss, with a severity that interfered with daily functioning (Horowitz, 1997).

When assessing the bereaved for symptoms, it is important for the clinician to remember that while the bereaved may sometimes give a very detailed description of the problems being experienced, at other times the individual may only provide a "clue" as to what is transpiring. The clinician must be alert to this and must be able and willing to probe to determine if a grief component exists and what interventions, if any, are needed. Common complaints that are grief related may include symptoms of or caused by anxiety and/or depression. Probing questions will likely be necessary to determine the presence of emotional, social, or spiritual symptoms associated with a loss, and behavioral responses or symptoms.

Complaints that have a grief component can also be of a psychosomatic nature, as the mourner unconsciously takes a respite from overwhelming grief by redirecting energy from grief to a physical ailment. This redirection of grief into physical symptoms may serve as a purposeful temporary coping mechanism, allowing bereaved individuals to conserve at least some of their energy for continued grieving.

Following an assessment of presenting problems, including their duration, intensity, and how they affect the ability of the bereaved to function, the clinician must next determine if there is a connection between the presenting symptoms and the recent loss. Key factors to assist in determining this link are listed in Table 14–14.

PRACTICAL NEEDS OF THE BEREAVED

In addition to evaluating for the risk of an abnormal grief reaction, the bereavement assessment must include an examination of the socioeconomic and practical needs of the bereaved. Survivors, especially in the first first few months following a loss, often report that dealing with the loss of the deceased spouse's income, or taking over the practical roles assumed by the deceased (such as the payment of bills, cooking, cleaning, driving), are of significant concern. For many, the need to address these issues may be as important, or even more vital, than the psychological needs that are traditionally thought to be of primary concern.

Bereavement Therapy

The first step in providing appropriate bereavement therapy is to determine whether the grief reaction is normal or abnormal and whether or not the grief reaction is best left alone or whether it requires further investigation and possible therapy. Being familiar with risk factors for poor grief outcome (Table 14–11), and tasks of mourning that may be unfinished or in which the mourner is "stuck" (Table 14–9), will help determine the nature of additional interventions, if needed.

Table 14–12

Symptoms of Complicated Grief

CATEGORY OF SYMPTOM	SPECIFIC EXAMPLES
Intense preoccupation with the deceased	Reluctance to relinquish attachment to the deceased
	Manifestation of behaviors or illnesses of the deceased
	Prolonged yearning for the deceased
	Persistent intrusive thoughts regarding the deceased
	Searching for the loved one
	Idealization of the deceased
	Talking about the death as though it were recent
Anxiety and depression	Acute or prolonged
	Posttraumatic stress disorder
	Fear, panic, agoraphobia, feeling overwhelmed, confused
	Marked increase in death anxiety
	Despair, wish for death, frequent thoughts of suicide
	Adjustment disorders, inability to function or feeling out of control after a prolonged period
	Dissociative disorders, especially following traumatic deaths
Emotional or behavioral reactions	Excessive and/or chronic self-reproach, pronounced guilt, inappropriate guilt
	Extreme anger
	Continued withdrawal, alienation, feelings of isolation, antisocial behavior, social phobia
	"Stoic" affect, rationalizing rather than experiencing the loss
	Prolonged denial or delaying of emotion
	Obsessive compulsive behavior
	Continued avoidance of pain of loss
	Chronic feelings of desertion
Relationship with self and others	Finding others as unhelpful
	Neglect or changes in health practices
	Inability to form new relationships, reinvest in life
	Fear of intimacy, inability to engage in meaningful activities
	Lack of meaning and purpose, loss of identity
Physical symptoms	Persistent physical distress, shortness of breath, and/or choking
	Hypochondria and somatoform disorders
	Substance dependence or abuse

Guidelines for bereavement therapy are listed in Table 14–15. Once physical disease has been ruled out, and it has been determined that presenting symptoms are related to grief, the clinician needs to determine whether the bereaved individual is cognizant of the connection. Helping the individual become aware of the link between symptoms and the recent loss may sometimes be enough to effect a remedy. Provide grief counseling by making suggestions that universally apply to anyone suffering a loss, such as emphasizing that the emotional wound from the loss takes time

Table 14–13

Symptoms Predictive of Complicated Grief[a]

Unbidden memories or intrusive fantasies
  related to the lost relationship
Strong spells or pangs of severe emotion to the
  lost relationship
Distressingly strong yearnings or wishes that
  the deceased were there
Feelings of being far too much alone or
  personally empty
Excessively staying away from people, places,
  or activities that remind the subject of the
  deceased
Unusual levels of sleep interference
Loss of interest in work, social, care-taking, or
  recreational activities to a maladaptive degree

[a] Three of the 7 criteria must be present and sufficiently severe to
impair the bereaved's ability to function.
SOURCE: Horowitz and colleagues, 1997.

to heal, and the importance of moving toward
rather than away from the pain of grief. Medications can also be used (see later in the chapter),
but they should be used only when necessary,
and sparingly.

When appropriate, referrals should be made.
The clinician not experienced in these matters
should be comfortable seeking assistance from
those with the appropriate background, such as
from the members of an end-of-life care interdisciplinary team.

GRIEF COUNSELING

While grief counseling is often thought of as
something done formally through a referral process, it is important to realize that grief counseling
may take place in a variety of less formal settings,
such as during a brief phone call or an office visit.
Therefore, any clinicians who have contact with
the bereaved need to be aware of the principles
that govern grief counseling as well as when to
recommend such counseling on a formal level.

Worden (1991) has defined ten principles, listed in
Table 14–16, that provide guidance to the clinician or grief counselor in assisting the bereaved
through an acute grief situation and adjusting to
the loss.

While the clinician cannot provide the same
level of support as the professional grief counselor or therapist, the clinician can still participate
by reinforcing these principles whenever in contact with the bereaved. Emphasizing that grieving
requires time, normalizing the grief process, and
providing assurance to bereaved individuals that
the clinician will remain available throughout the
bereavement period, are all ways that the clinician can provide informal grief counseling that
supplements any formal support the bereaved may
be receiving.

One of the challenges to assisting patients with
grief counseling is its limited availability. For physi-

Table 14–14

Key Factors in Determining the Link Between Symptoms and Grieving

Date of the loss
Type of loss: (young or old, sudden or expected)
Relationship with the deceased
  Healthy or unhealthy
  Close or ambivalent
Personality
  Anxious or calm
  Stoic or expressive
Other crises or stressors
  Financial problems
  Dependents
  Other losses
  Poor health
Prior history of coping
  History of mental illness
  Is this a new problem?
Social or cultural components
  How is grief normally expressed in your family?
  How is grief normally expressed in your culture?

Table 14–15

Guidelines for Bereavement Therapy

Determine that presenting symptoms are related
   to grief.
 Rule out physical disease.
Assist the bereaved in becoming cognizant of
   the connection.
Provide grief counseling.
   Informal via phone or during visit.
   Formal through referral.
Use medication sparingly.
Make appropriate referrals.

cians and others in clinical practice, for example, grief counseling and therapy is time intensive and is only reimburseable in a limited way (i.e., based upon the diagnosis of a recognized clinical condition such as anxiety neurosis or sleep disorder). Insurance companies often do not pay for formal grief counseling with a licensed therapist. Fortunately, with the recognition that bereavement counseling reduces the time that the bereaved spend away from work due to illness and de-

creases overall use of the health care system, a small percentage of private insurance companies have begun to provide reimbursement for a limited number of bereavement counseling sessions.

As already noted, hospice programs may be an excellent source of grief counseling and bereavement care, provided at no cost to the bereaved whose loved one has died on the hospice program. Interdisciplinary hospice teams provide support in numerous ways, many of which are listed in Table 14–17. If grief counseling is indicated, the hospice chaplain and social worker can provide interventions within the scope of their discipline and training as well as help to make appropriate referrals to external grief counselors and therapists when indicated.

The last decade has witnessed a marked increase in the number of other grief resources available in the community. Most funeral homes offer support groups, with some even providing "aftercare" coordinators responsible for planning and conducting workshops, outings, and various social gatherings. Urban communites usually have a number of bereavement support groups offered by churches and temples, as well as grief centers or organizations such as the Dougy Center in Portland, the Warm Place in Ft. Worth, or the Center

Table 14–16

Principles for Grief Counseling

Help the survivor actualize the loss.
Help the survivor to identify and express feelings.
Assist living without the deceased.
Facilitate emotional relocation of the deceased.
Provide time to grieve.
Interpret "normal" behavior.
Allow for individual differences.
Provide continuing support.
Examine defenses and coping styles.
Identify pathology and refer.

SOURCE: Adapted from Worden W.: *Grief Counseling and Grief Therapy: A Handbook for the Mental Health Practitioner.* 2nd ed., New York, Springer, 1991.

Table 14–17

Bereavement Support Services Provided by Hospice Programs

Supportive telephone calls from employees and
   volunteers following the death
Closure visits at the home and or funeral service
Condolence cards and correspondence from the
   hospice describing its services and continuing
   availability
Memorial gatherings
Workshops and other educational offerings
Multimedia information on grief
Grief counseling and grief therapy
Pre- and postmortem grief support groups
Children's activities
Referrals to other professionals

for Sibling Loss in Chicago. Typing in the word "bereavement" or "grief" on the Internet will reveal a plethora of grief resources.

TREATMENT OF COMPLICATED GRIEF

Grief counseling and support groups are beneficial in facilitating the tasks of mourning for those who have recently experienced a loss. However, for the bereaved who exhibit the exagerrated symptoms consistent with complicated grief, other interventions, including grief therapy and medication, may be required.

GRIEF THERAPY　Grief therapy, which in some ways is an extension of grief counseling, is designed to "identify and resolve the conflicts of separation that preclude the completion of mourning tasks in persons whose grief is absent, delayed, excessive, or prolonged." Unlike grief counseling, grief therapy requires the intervention of specialists due to the complex psychotherapeutic process involved. In view of the exaggerated intensity of symptoms experienced by the patient, the time to successfully complete grief therapy is also prolonged when compared with uncomplicated grief counseling. Generally, at least 8 to 10 grief therapy visits are required to resolve whatever may be impeding the successful completion of tasks of mourning.

Psychiatric referral should be reserved for the small percentage of survivors who may be at suicidal risk or who exhibit frank manifestations of a psychiatric illness. Of this group, most will have a history of mental illness or history of poor coping/adjustment to loss.

MEDICATIONS　Much has been written concerning the use of medication and bereavement. With the bereaved often experiencing prolonged and intense anxiety and/or depression, the desire to prescribe anxiolytics and antidepressants can be quite strong. It is generally agreed, however, that such medications should be prescribed as an adjunct, and not as a replacement for other interventions. Additionally, these medications should be used sparingly both to avoid dependence and so as not to inhibit or circumvent the necessary process of mourning. The prescribing clinician needs to be aware of the potential for suicide in bereaved individuals receiving medication as well as the increase in use of other prescription and nonprescription drugs and alcohol in the bereaved.

If medications are used, anxiolytics can be helpful to persons experiencing acute distress including posttraumatic stress symptoms manifested in the early stage of a loss. (See Chapter 11, Table 11–7, for a list of recommended anxiolytics.) Antidepressants, on the other hand, are generally not indicated in persons with acute grief reactions. (See Chapter 11, Table 11–3, for a list of recommended antidepressants.) However, they are sometimes indicated in the presence of a major depressive episode. Reynolds and associates, in studying 80 subjects, aged 50 years and older with bereavement-related major depressive episodes, found that the use of the antidepressant nortriptyline was superior to placebo in achieving remission of these episodes. The combination of medication and psychotherapy, however, was associated with the highest rate of treatment completion, underscoring the importance of using grief therapy (or psychiatric therapy when indicated) and other supportive measures along with medications to properly manage complicated grief.

References

Bowlby J: *Attachment and Loss: Loss, Sadness and Depression,* vol. 3. New York, Basic Books, 1980.

Bowlby J: The making and breaking of affectional bonds, I and II. *Br J Psychiatry,* 130:201, 1977.

Bozeman M: Cultural aspects of pain management. In: Salerno E, Willens, J, eds. *Pain Management Handbook.* St. Louis, Mosby, 1996.

Brener A: *Mourning and Mitzvah.* Woodstock, VT, Jewish Lights Publishing, 1993.

Corr C, Corr D: *Hospice Care: Principles and Practice.* New York, Springer, 1983.

Corr C, Nabe CM, Corr DM: *Death and Dying, Life and Living,* 2nd ed. Pacific Grove, CA, Brooks/Cole, 1997.

Darwin C: *The Expression of Emotions in Man and Animals.* London, Murray, 1872.

Davidson G: Hospice Care for the Dying: Problems the Hospice is Designed to Correct, In *Dying: Facing the Facts*, e. Hannelore Wass, p. 169–181.

Derogatis LR, Spencer PM: *The Brief Symptom Inventory (BSI): Administration, Scoring and Procedures Manual*. Towson, MD, Clinical Research, 1982.

Doka KJ (ed): *Disenfranchised Grief: Recognizing Hidden Sorrow*. New York, Lexington Books, 1989.

Doka KJ, Davidson JD (eds): *Living with Grief: Who We are, How We Grieve*. Philadelphia, Brunner/Mazel, 1998.

Engel GL: Is grief a disease? A challenge for medical research. *Psychosomatic Med* 23:18, 1961.

Fenichel O: *The Psychoanalytic Theory of Neurosis*. New York, Norton, 1945.

Freud S: Mourning and melancholia. In: *A General Selection from the Works of Sigmund Freud*. New York, Doubleday Anchor, 1917.

Gorer GD: *Death, Grief, and Mourning*. New York, Doubleday, 1965.

Horowitz MJ: *Am J Psychiatry* 155:9, 1998. Letter.

Horowitz MJ: *Stress Response Syndromes: PSTD, Grief, and Adjustment Disorders*. Northvale, NJ, Jason Aronson, 1997.

Houts PS, Lipton A, Harvey HA, et al: Predictors of grief among spouses of deceased cancer patients. *J Psychosoc Oncol* 7:113–126, 1989.

Jacobs SC: Treating depression of bereavement with antidepressants: A pilot study. *Psychiatr Clin North Am* 10:501, 1987.

Kinzbrunner BM: The role of the physician in hospice. *Hospice J* 12:49, 1997.

Kubler-Ross E: *On Death and Dying*. New York, Simon and Schuster, 1997.

Lindemann E: Symptomatology and management of acute grief. *Am J Psychiatry* 137:45, 1944.

Lorenz K: *On Aggression*. London, Methuen, 1963.

Middleton W, Raphael B, Burnett P, Martinek N: A longitudinal study comparing bereavement phenomena in recently bereaved spouses, adult children and parents. *Aust NZ J Psychiatry* 32:235, 1998.

New Oxford Annotated Bible. Metzger B, Murphy R, eds. New York, Oxford University Press, 1991.

Owen G, Fulton R, Markusen E: Death at a distance: A study of family survivors. *Omega* 13:191, 1982.

Parkes CM: Risk factors in bereavement: Implications for the prevention and treatment of pathologic grief. *Psychiatr Ann* 20:6, 1990.

Parkes CM: *Bereavement Studies of Grief in Adult Life*. New York, International Universities Press, 1972.

Parkes CM, Weiss RS: *Recovery from Bereavement*. New York, Basic Books, 1983.

Prigerson HG, Frank E, Kasl SV, et al: Complicated grief and bereavement-related depression as distinct disorders: Preliminary emperical validation in elderly bereaved spouses. *Am J Psychiatry* 152:22, 1995.

Prigerson HG, Shear MK, Newsom JT, et al: Anxiety among widowed elders: Is it distinct from depression and grief? *Anxiety* 2:1, 1996.

Rando T: *Treatment of Complicated Mourning*. Champaign, IL, Research Press, 1993.

Rando T: An agenda for adaptive anticipation of bereavement. In: *Loss and Anticipatory Grief*. Lexington, MA: D.C. Health, 1986.

Rhymes J: Hospice care in America. *JAMA* 264:369, 1990.

Sanders CM: *Grief: The Mourning After. Dealing with Adult Bereavement*. New York, Wiley, 1989.

Sanders CM: Effects of sudden vs. chronic illness death in bereavement outcome. *Omega* 13:227, 1982–1983.

Sanders CM: A comparison of adult bereavement in the death of a spouse, child and parent. *Omega* 10:303, 1980.

Sanders CM, Manger PA, Strong PN. *A Manual for the Grief Experience Inventory*. Palo Alto, Consulting Psychologists Press, 1979.

Schuster SR, Zisook S: Treatment of spousal bereavement: A multidimensional approach. *Psychiatric Annals* 16:295, 1986.

Stroebe M, Schut H: The dual process model of coping with bereavement: Rationale and description. *Death Studies* 23:197, 1999.

Vachon MLS: Psychosocial needs of patients and families. *J Palliat Care* 14:49, 1998.

Videka-Sherman L: Coping with the death of a child: A study over time. *Am J Orthopsychiatry* 52:688, 1982.

Werner PT: Family medicine and hospice programs: A natural alliance. *J Fam Pract* 12:367, 1981.

Wolfelt AD: Dispelling 5 common myths about grief (www.mourning.com/5_common_myths.html), 1999.

Worden JW, Davies B, McCown D: Comparing parent loss with sibling loss. *Death Studies* 23:1, 1999.

Worden JW: *Grief Counseling and Grief Therapy: A Handbook for the Mental Health Practitioner*, 2nd ed. New York, Springer, 1991.

Wortman C, Silver R: The myths of coping with loss. *J Consult Clin Psychol* 57:349, 1989.

Wortman C, Silver R: Coping with irrevocable loss. In: VandenBos G, Bryant B, eds. *Cataclysms, Crises, and Catastrophes: Psychology in Action*. Washington, DC, American Psychological Association, 1987.

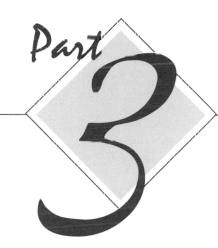

Ethical Issues and Controversies Near the End of Life

Domingo Gomez

Advance Directives and CPR

Introduction

Throughout history, decisions about how to care for people near the end of life have been made according to the cultural mores of the times. In primitive societies, the "medicine man" and the chief of the tribe would make these decisions based on their religious and political power, and their decisions went essentially unquestioned. As civilization evolved, various deities, the "oracles," and religious figures were often consulted as to life and death issues, although the ancient Greeks and Chinese also pioneered the use of physicians to provide expert advice on health and disease. Throughout most of the Middle Ages, religious groups remained the most important advisors to people who had to face serious or terminal illness. However, toward the end of the Middle Ages, Mediterranean Jewish and Arab physicians increasingly became the repositories of medical knowledge and providers of medical advice, to the point that even devout Christians called on them when faced with advanced illnesses. During the Renaissance, with medical knowledge advancing more slowly than the arts, religious leaders again took center stage away from physicians when it came to assisting patients and families in coping with serious illnesses and death.

The discovery of the nature of infectious diseases and isolation techniques during the latter half of the 19th and into the 20th centuries had a significant influence on prolongation of life, shifting public attention back to the physician as the chief health care advisor. The introduction of antibiotics in the 1940s made diseases like syphilis, tuberculosis, pneumonia, and cholera no longer dreaded as harbingers of certain death. New anesthesia techniques in the 1950s allowed patients to receive mechanical ventilatory assistance, supporting them during difficult surgical procedures and postoperative recovery, with a high likelihood of full recovery. Mechanical ventilatory support was eventually extended to trauma victims and, ultimately, to support vital functions in decompensated patients with acute and chronic medical illnesses. The addition of cardiac defibrillators further enhanced the ability to support and prolong the lives of patients who were victims of cardiac as well as respiratory arrest.

With the increased use of mechanical ventilatory support and other forms of advanced life support, medical facilities developed the intensive care unit (ICU) to ensure that patients received this care in the proper environment. During this same time period, improvement in nutritional support, both by enteral and parenteral methods, allowed physicians to provide nutritional support to patients who were unable to eat on their own. The refinement and widespread application of these techniques allowed physicians to effectively support and prolong the lives of patients who had previously succumbed to advanced and life-threatening illnesses.

As with all new modalities of treatment, the widespread use of advanced life support and artificial nutritional support has not only had benefits but adverse consequences as well. Although some patients who would otherwise have died have been given a new lease on life, other patients who had no realistic hope for recovery had their lives extended artificially for weeks and months. As patients and families became more aware of the futility of advanced life support in certain clinical circumstances, some began to assert their wishes not to have the dying process prolonged by artificial means. This philosophy of care began as a grassroots movement, with landmark legal cases, such as Quinlan, Cruzan, and Lane v. Candura, leading to legal precedents that gave patients the right to refuse life-prolonging treatment near the end of life. This ultimately led to the development of advance directives, documents that provide instructions to health care providers as to how individual patients choose to be treated near the end of life when they are unable to make independent health care decisions.

Efforts to encourage all patients to create advance directives while they are capable of making decisions about their care led to the passage of the Federal Patient Self-Determination Act (PSDA) in 1991. This legislation mandates that Medicare and Medicaid providers inform patients, in writing, of their rights to execute an advance directive and to assist them in executing such a directive if they choose to do so. The PSDA also mandates that Medicare and Medicaid providers may not deny patients access to health care services based upon their advance directive instructions.

It is the primary goal of this chapter to review the subject of advance directives, defining what they are, exploring the principles behind their development, and gaining an understanding of how they function. This chapter will then evaluate the historical driving force behind the development of advance directives, choices regarding cardiopulmonary resuscitation (CPR) at the end of life. A second major issue addressed by advance directives, choices regarding artificial nutritional support and hydration near the end of life, is covered in Chapter 16.

Advance Directives

Advance directives are specific instructions, prepared in advance of serious illness, that are intended to direct the medical care for specific individuals if they become unable to express their health care choices at a future date. This allows patients to participate in making their own decisions regarding the care they would prefer to receive if they contract a terminal illness. There are several different types of advance directives in use today in the United States, listed in Table 15–1 and discussed next.

Living Will

The living will is a legal document, written and signed by an individual in the presence of witnesses, that conveys the instructions of that individual regarding health care interventions, desired or not desired, in the event of terminal or irre-

Table 15–1

Types of Advance Directives

Living will
Verbal advanced directive
Durable (or special) medical power of attorney

versible illness and when the person is incapable of verbally communicating wishes regarding health care. This document should not be confused with a last will and testament, the purpose of which is to distribute assets after a person's death.

Although living wills have been traditionally thought of as addressing choices primarily limited to interventions such as CPR, nutrition, and hydration, they may in fact address a wide variety of other interventions (Table 15–2). State laws vary regarding living wills. Therefore, when advising patients on executing these documents, it is important to ensure that they meet the specifications of the state in which the patient resides. Information specific to individual states may be obtained from such organizations as the state medical association, the state nursing association, or the state bar association. Most hospitals, medical centers, and hospices will also be able to provide the appropriate information.

Table 15–2

Interventions Addressed by Living Wills

Cardiopulmonary resuscitation
Nutritional support by other than oral means
Hydration by other than oral means
Antibiotics
Transfusion of blood products
Invasive procedures and diagnostic studies including, but not limited to, blood tests, spinal taps, and x-rays and scans
Desire to be hospitalized or remain at home

Durable (or Special) Medical Power of Attorney

The durable (or special) medical power of attorney is a legal document that allows an individual to appoint a responsible person (usually called a health care surrogate or proxy) who is empowered to make health care decisions in the event the individual becomes unable to make and communicate such decisions personally. This document provides for power to make medically related decisions only, and does not give that individual the authority to make legal or financial decisions. Although health care proxies are usually family members, any individual—such as a close friend, clergy member, or even physician—may with the individual's permission be designated for this role. Unlike the living will, which provides specific instructions given directly by the individual concerned, the durable power of attorney allows the health care proxy to make decisions based upon his or her knowledge of the individual's wishes in the context of the specific circumstances under consideration at the time. The durable power of attorney also allows for the health care proxy to make decisions whenever a patient is incapable of making a choice, while living wills generally are only effective when the patient suffers from a terminal illness or is in a permanent vegetative state.

Verbal Advance Directives

Many individuals have, in the course of conversation with loved ones, expressed their desires concerning care near the end of life, but did not have the foresight to execute a written advance directive prior to becoming unable to make a health care decision. Alternatively, for psychological reasons, some individuals just cannot bring themselves to sign a document that addresses issues revolving around the end of life. For these people, the documentation of their verbal instructions by their physician and/or health care provider (hospice) may be sufficient to constitute a legitimate advance directive. In fact, nowadays these are the most common kind of advance care directives.

Verbal advance directives may be provided by patients or, in many states, by next of kin in the form of a health care proxy (akin to a verbal durable power of attorney). The ability of next of kin to make proxy decisions for patients varies from state to state, with most states defining a hierarchy of relatives who have precedence in health care decision making for incapacitated patients. In most states, there is also provision for a court-appointed guardian to make health care decisions for patients who have no relatives and have not left any written advance directive instructions. A small number of states still do not allow health care proxy decisions to be made for patients in the absence of written advance directives.

The key to the verbal advance directive is documentation. It is crucial that, whether the source of the information is the patient or the appropriate legal next of kin, the medical record should clearly document the nature of the conversation held regarding the patient's condition, offered options of care, and the decisions made around the various potential interventions discussed.

Do Not Resuscitate Order

A "do not resuscitate" (DNR) order is a physician's order that states that CPR is not to be initiated if a cardiac or respiratory arrest occurs. Technically, it is not an advance directive, but is the order given by a physician honoring the advance directive (written or verbal) of a patient or the patient's health care proxy that the patient does not desire CPR. Note that although a physician can theoretically give a DNR order on any patient for whom he or she deems it appropriate, it has become common practice (as well policy in many institutions and law in many states) for physicians not to give such an order in the absence of a verbal or written advance directive or the health care proxy's permission.

Advantages of Advance Directives

There are a number of potential advantages to the use of advanced directives (Table 15–3), the key advantage being the respect of patient autonomy. Autonomy derives from the deontological school of thought, which emphasizes duty and acting from the right intentions. One of those right intentions involves treating people with respect, which leads directly to the concept of autonomy, or respecting the capacity and the right of rational agents to self-determination. In a clinical setting, autonomy is defined as the right of patients to have self-determination when it comes to choosing between different therapeutic alternatives By choosing to execute an advance directive (an expression of autonomy unto itself), the patient provides family caregivers and professional health care providers with the information necessary to ensure that their choices regarding care near the end of life are respected and followed. In the form of a living will, autonomy is expressed in writing, while in the form of a durable power of attorney the assumption is made that the health care proxy is making health care choices for the patient based upon the knowledge of what the patient would have chosen.

Patients who execute advance directives may have the advantage of worrying less about the prospects of receiving therapy that they would otherwise not desire. Families are often appreciative of the fact that, especially when living wills are used, they do not have the anxiety and guilt associated with being forced to make life and death decisions for a loved one.

Advance directives may not only be advantageous to patients. Providers should also derive definable benefits from their use. By knowing what therapeutic interventions patients do and do not desire near the end of life, providers can care for patients in an appropriate, beneficial, and cost-effective manner, respecting patient autonomy and reducing the risk of medicolegal repercussions.

It must be emphasized that, as stated, many of the advantages discussed are potential at best. Studies have shown that although the majority of people believe having some form of advance directive is a good idea, only 7 to 8 percent of the population had actually developed any type of advance directive for themselves as of 1998. Many people state that they want their families to make health care decisions for them; however, fewer than half of these people have ever discussed the issue and their specific desires with family members. Studies also suggest that even when advance directives are executed, they are often not followed, usually due to perceived doubts and uncertainties about the patient's true wishes (even in the presence of the advance directive document) on the part of either the family or the physician caring for the patient.

Table 15–3

Potential Advantages of Advance Directives

PATIENT ADVANTAGES	HEALTH CARE PROVIDER ADVANTAGES
Expression of autonomy	Knowledge of patient's wishes
Decreased personal worry	Decrease in unnecessary therapeutic and diagnostic interventions
Decreased family anxiety and guilt	Decrease in health care costs
	Decrease in medicolegal concerns

How to Assist Patients in Executing Advance Directives

Physicians have a great deal of the responsibility to empower and encourage patients to execute advance directives. Physicians should have an advance directive discussion with all patients under their care. It is especially important for physicians to discuss these issues with patients who suffer from chronic illnesses that have a high risk of progressive mental and physical debility, and to do this before the patients become incapable of making health care decisions.

The timing of the discussion is important. Most often, physicians, as well as patients and families, tend to avoid advance directive conversations until the patient is nearing a time of crisis, when the need to make decisions about interventions such as CPR near the end of life are a virtual reality. As covered in depth in Chapter 3, many practitioners still have significant difficulty speaking with patients and families and "breaking the bad news" that the end of life is approaching. The additional burden of the discussion and decision making around advance directive issues is often too overwhelming for patients and families to comprehend and digest at the same time that the "bad news" is confronted. Therefore, it is recommended that advance directive conversations between physicians and patients be held at a time before bad news needs to be discussed. This will reduce the potential for overwhelming the patient and family during a time of great crisis and allow for more thoughtful decision making to occur.

The content of the discussion is of great importance. Table 15–4 lists some of issues that need to be reviewed by the physician. Patients should be offered the option of executing a living will, a durable power of attorney, or both, based upon individual and family preference. A thorough explanation of the structure and function of each of these documents should be provided to the patient and family. It is suggested that for many patients, it is desirable to execute both a living will and a durable power of attorney. As mentioned, living

Table 15–4

Content of Advance Directive Discussions

Types of Advance Directives
  Living Will
  Durable Power of Attorney
  Verbal instructions
State regulations regarding advance directives
Pros and cons of specific interventions (see Table 15–2)
Advance directives are not irrevocable

wills are only effective when a patient suffers from a terminal illness or is in a permanent vegetative state. If a patient's condition falls short of terminal or vegetative at a time when the capacity to make a health care decision is absent, the identification of the health care proxy will allow the necessary decisions to be made based upon the patient's expressed wishes.

Although it is better to have a written advance directive, verbal instructions remain important as supplements to written instructions as well as serving as advance directives on their own. Patients may be physically unable to execute an advance directive or may be unwilling to commit their wishes to paper for psychological reasons. In either event, in the absence of written advance directives, oral instructions that are reduced to writing by the patient's physician or another health care provider may adequately provide information on how a patient wants to be cared for near the end of life.

Specific state regulations regarding advance directives should be disclosed as well. Every state recognizes the living will, durable power of attorney, or both (Table 15–5). However, the laws of each state vary considerably regarding terminology, scope of decision-making, restrictions, and formalities required for executing an advance directive. Many states expressly recognize out-of-state advance directives if the directive meets either the legal requirements of the state where executed or the state where the treatment decision arises,

Table 15–5

Living Wills and Health Care Power of Attorney Statutes by State (as of 1998)

TYPE OF DOCUMENT	STATES
Living will only	Alaska
Health care power of attorney only	Massachusetts, Michigan, New York
Both	All other states and District of Columbia

while several states are silent on this question. However, even if an advance directive fails to meet technicalities of state law, health care providers are encouraged to value the directive as important, if not controlling, evidence of the patient's wishes. In the absence of written advance directives, many states have provisions that will allow documented verbal instructions to be followed. Most states also have provisions that allow various family members to serve as health care proxies for patients who are incapable of making health care decisions, although the order of precedence of the family members varies considerably from state to state. When all else fails, most states have provisions to provide court appointed guardianship to ensure that patients who have no instructions and no next of kin can have health care decisions made for them.

Therapeutic decisions that are commonly articulated in advance directives related to the interventions listed in Table 15–2 should be thoroughly discussed. The physician should present the potential benefits and potential harms of each intervention to the patient and family, so that informed decisions on each item can be made. It is urged that all patient decisions around specific therapeutic options be clearly spelled out both in the patient's medical record and in the advance directive documents.

It is very important for the physician to emphasize to patients and families that advance directives, once executed, are not irrevocable documents. Instead, they are evolving documents, reflective of the continuing conversations between physicians and their patients and families regarding patient wishes for care near the end of life.

Myths About Advance Directives

There are a number of misconceptions about advance directives that present barriers to their effective use. These are listed in Table 15–6 and discussed next. It is important for physicians to become familiar with these issues and be prepared to discuss or defuse them when they are raised as concerns by patients and families.

ADVANCE DIRECTIVES MEAN "DON'T TREAT"

There is a mistaken notion that when patients execute advance directives—especially when the directives include instructions not to provide CPR—that no treatment will be provided. Nothing could be further from the truth. The content of an advance directive is entirely dependent upon the

Table 15–6

Misconceptions about Advance Directives

Advance directives mean "don't treat"
Appointing a health care proxy means giving up control
Lawyers are necessary to execute advance directives
Doctors and health care providers do not have to honor advance directives
Families can make decisions in the absence of advance directives
Advance directives are only for old or sick people

patient's specific wishes and values. Questions regarding whether a patient chooses to receive any specific treatment modality can and should be clearly delineated in the advance directive discussion and document as discussed earlier. Even in the circumstance in which a patient has left advance directive instructions to not receive any form of life-sustaining treatment, standards of end-of-life care mandate appropriate interventions that provide pain and symptom control, comfort care, and respect for one's dignity.

APPOINTING A HEALTH CARE PROXY MEANS GIVING UP CONTROL

Another misperception about advance directives, specifically durable power of attorney documents, is that when individuals designate health care proxies, they relinquish their own authority to make health care decisions. In fact, as long as individuals remain able to make decisions, their consent must be obtained for medical treatment. The health care proxy only becomes directly responsible for decision making when the patient is incapacitated. Health care providers cannot legally ignore patients in favor of health care proxies when patients are competent and choose to make their own decisions. Indeed, in most states, advance directives have no legal effect unless and

until the patient lacks the capacity to make a health care decision. In a minority of states, immediately effective directives are permissible, allowing patients to defer to proxies when they could still make their own decisions—but patients always retains the right to override their proxies or revoke the directives.

LAWYERS ARE NECESSARY TO EXECUTE ADVANCE DIRECTIVES

An attorney is not necessary in order for an individual to complete an advance directive, although some persons may find a legal opinion helpful. To assist patients and families in executing advance directives in as easy a manner as possible, physicians' offices and other health care provider agencies should make the appropriate advance directive forms available. These can be obtained from several sources. In states that have advance directive statutes, "official" versions of living will and/or health care power of attorney documents should be readily available. In addition to the state forms, other organizations such as the American Bar Association, the National Hospice and Palliative Care Organization, Choices in Dying, and the Association of Death Education and Counseling have published advance directive documents. Table 15–7 provides information on

Table 15–7
Sources for Advance Directive Documents

NAME	ADDRESS	PHONE	INTERNET ACCESS
American Bar Association	740 15th St, NW Washington, DC 20005	202-662-8960	www.abanet.org
National Hospice and Palliative Care Organization	1700 Diagonal Rd Alexandria, VA 22314		www.nhpco.org
Choices in Dying	200 Varick St New York, NY 10014	800-989-WILL	www.choices.org
Association of Death Education and Counseling	638 Prospect Ave Hartford, CT 06105	860-586-7503	www.adec.org

how to obtain advance directive documents from these organizations.

DOCTORS AND HEALTH CARE PROVIDERS DO NOT HAVE TO HONOR ADVANCE DIRECTIVES

Doctors and health care providers must honor advance directives. The law is clear that medical providers cannot treat an individual against his or her wishes. If physicians act contrary to a patient's advance directive or contrary to the decision of the patient's authorized proxy, the physicians would risk the same liability as if they were to ignore the verbal instructions of a fully competent patient. Treatment could then be construed as constituting battery. However, there is a caveat that the written advance directive be clear regarding the specific circumstances being addressed. In the absence of a clear directive, physicians in many instances will use their best judgement, which could result in a patient receiving care contrary to his or her wishes expressed in advance directives.

Unfortunately, there are a number of circumstances in which, despite the existence of advance directives, patients receive care that they documented they did not want to receive. An example is when the doctor or health care facility is unaware of the existence of an advance directive. Whenever a patient is admitted to a hospital, nursing home, home health agency, or hospice, the Patient Self-Determination Act (PSDA) requires the facility or service to inquire whether or not the patient has an advance directive (as well as giving the patient the opportunity to execute one). If an advance directive exists, the facility or service has the responsibility to ensure that it is made part of the medical record. Unfortunately, this does not always happen. Therefore, the patient and/or health care proxy should make sure that any advance directives are available to the facility or service, and that copies of all appropriate documents are placed in the medical record.

Another important challenge to the proper execution of advance directives, as noted earlier, relates to the lack of detailed instructions in the documents. Simply using general language that rejects "heroic measures" or "treatment that only prolongs the dying process" does not give much guidance and leaves treatment decisions open to interpretation bias. Therefore, living wills should be detailed in defining what treatments a patient does and does not want. Likewise, when a patient designates a proxy via a health care power of attorney, the patient should have provided the health care proxy with specific instructions on how he or she desires to be cared for.

Conscientious objection to advance directive instructions is another important reason why these documents are not always followed. In most states, if a health care provider (whether a physician, facility, or service provider) objects to an advance directive based on reasons of conscience, state law permits the physician or the facility to refuse to honor it. However, providers are obligated to notify patients and/or families of their objections to advance directives at the time of admission or, in the case of the physician, when the issue arises. In circumstances where a provider cannot accept a patient's or health care proxy's advance directive choices, the patient's care should be transferred to another clinician who is willing to comply with the patient's and/or proxy's instructions.

Finally, people who are dying but living at home may receive unwanted efforts at cardiopulmonary resuscitation, despite having advance directives to the contrary, if a crisis occurs and emergency medical services (EMS) is called. EMS personnel are generally required to resuscitate and stabilize patients when they respond to a 911 call, irrespective of any advance directives that may exist. Many states are beginning to address this situation by creating procedures that allow EMS personnel to refrain from resuscitating terminally ill patients who are certified as having a "do not resuscitate order" via a state-approved document that identifies that the patient does not desire CPR. Most hospitals and hospices have these forms available. Physicians and other health care providers should ensure that patients complete this form when it is determined that the patient is near the end of life, and the patient has expressed, though an advance directive or via health care proxy, that CPR is not desired.

FAMILIES CAN MAKE DECISIONS IN THE ABSENCE OF ADVANCE DIRECTIVES

Many individuals believe that advance directives really are not necessary, relying instead on next of kin to make decisions for them when they become incapable themselves. Unfortunately, this is only partly true. In many states, if there is no advance directive, state law designates default "proxies," typically family members, who are permitted to make some health care decisions. The hierarchy of health care proxy among next of kin varies from state to state, which contributes to internal family conflicts at a time when family members need to be supportive of each other and their terminally ill family member. In the absence of family, a few states will allow a "close friend" to make proxy health care decisions, while in other states the lack of family forces a court-appointed guardian to be designated to make decisions. The end result in these circumstances is that individuals who have little or no contact with patients or knowledge of their wishes will be making health care decisions based on their own values, rather than on those of the patient.

ADVANCE DIRECTIVES ARE ONLY FOR OLD OR SICK PEOPLE

Advance directives are not only for the old and infirm. Although it may be natural to link death and dying issues with old age, younger patients and families may also be faced with making difficult decisions about end-of-life care. Consider that perhaps the most well-known landmark court cases addressing patient rights at the end of life (Nancy Cruzan and Karen Ann Quinlan) involved individuals in their 20s. The stakes are actually higher for younger persons in that, if tragedy strikes, their lives might be prolonged for years or even decades in an undesired vegetative condition. Therefore, advance directives are for all adults to execute

and make available to their next of kin as well as their physicians and other health care providers.

CPR Near the End of Life

As already noted, the Patient Self-Determination Act requires that all Medicare and Medicaid providers inform patients when the patient is admitted to the facility or service, in writing, of their rights to create an advance directive and to assist them in executing such a directive if they choose to do so. The PSDA also mandates that Medicare and Medicaid providers may not deny patients access to health care services based upon their advance directive instructions.

This latter statutory requirement raises major issues for patients receiving hospice care or other forms of end-of-life care when death is near. After all, it is generally assumed that a patient who elects hospice care has also agreed not to receive CPR when life comes to an end. However, the PSDA has been interpreted to require that a hospice provider (as well as any other provider of palliative care) must take a patient under care if he or she meets prognosis eligibility requirements, even in the face of an advance directive that states that the patient desires CPR. Needless to say, this interpretation of the PSDA has caused significant ethical dilemmas for end-of-life care providers regarding how to care for these patients in an appropriate and responsible fashion.

To more fully understand the scope of the ethical challenges confronted by end-of-life care providers when caring for patients who desire CPR near the end of life, the issue will be examined in the context of the four cardinal ethical values: autonomy, beneficence, nonmaleficence, and two forms of justice, distributive justice (availability of resources) and social justice (what is good for the society as a whole). (See the Preface for a definition of each of these ethical values.) In view of the fact that patient autonomy is currently the overriding ethical value, and the driving force behind the PSDA, it will be addressed last.

CPR and Beneficence

The basic procedure referred to as cardiopulmonary resuscitation was developed in the late 1950s and 1960s, primarily to revive patients who experienced cardiac and/or respiratory arrest (as with acute arrhythmia or drowning). As resuscitative techniques have been refined over the years, the use of CPR has been extended to patients with virtually any acute or chronic illnesses. In fact, CPR has become a "default" procedure, assumed to be desired by all individuals unless they specifically request that they do not want CPR performed.

Overall, survival rates for patients who require CPR is about 15 percent, but varies considerably depending upon the patient population studied. Table 15–8 lists reported survival rates, stratified by several key variables, for elderly patients (generally defined as 70 or older) receiving CPR. These variables include location, whether or not the arrest was witnessed, whether or not vital signs were detected at the onset of arrest, and the presence of chronic illness. Although 39 percent of a selected group of elderly cardiac patients have been reported to survive CPR, the outcome of CPR in all other reported studies is fairly dismal. Ambulatory elderly patients and patients who still had detectable vital signs are reported to have about a 10 percent survival rate, while those patients who arrest while in the hospital and/or have witnessed arrest survive about 5 to 7 percent of the time. Survival of patients following an unwitnessed cardiorespiratory arrest or an arrest outside the hospital, or who have no vital signs present when CPR is initiated, is 1 percent or less. Chronically ill elderly patients—including those with malignancies, neurologic disease, renal failure, respiratory disease, and sepsis (some of whom at least would potentially be receiving hospice or end-of-life care)—have a less than 5 percent probability of leaving the hospital alive. In many studies, survival of such patients approximates zero.

CPR and Nonmaleficence

The performance of CPR is not without the potential for harm, irrespective of whether the ultimate outcome is patient survival or death. Autopsy studies following CPR have demonstrated fractures of

Table 15–8

Survival to Hospital Discharge for Elderly Patients Requiring CPR for Cardiopulmonary Arrest

CHARACTERISTIC	SURVIVED TO DISCHARGE (%)
Out-of-hospital arrest	0.8
In-hospital arrest	6.5
Witnessed arrest	5.2
Unwitnessed arrest	0.9
Vital signs present	10.2
Vital signs absent	1.1
Ambulatory elderly	10
Selected cardiac patients, in hospital	39
Chronically ill elderly	< 5

ribs and sternum, bone marrow emboli, epicardial hemorrhage, mediastinal hematomas, aspiration pneumonia, and hemorrhage into various other cardiac and respiratory structures. Surviving patients may experience many of these same complications, as well as chest wall burns secondary to ventricular defibrillation. They also have the added risk of suffering from permanent neurologic sequelae including, but not limited to brain death, persistent vegetative state, seizures, and impairment of higher intellectual functions.

CPR and Justice

Examining distributive justice, one can intuitively conclude that performing CPR near the end of life is more costly than avoiding the procedure. Although hard data specific to CPR are lacking, it has been demonstrated that hospitalized patients who had advance directives in place prior to death spent less than one-third the resources of hospitalized patients who had no documented advance directive.

Social justice suggests that the society considers the ready availability of CPR to be in its best interest, based on the fact that, as already mentioned, CPR is considered a default condition. The question that needs to be asked, however, is whether having CPR as a default condition is in the best interest of society as a whole. This is a far more complex question than one might surmise, especially in view of the facts related to beneficence and nonmaleficence already presented. While it is beyond the scope of this chapter to answer the question as it affects society as a whole, one must seriously question whether the societal good is met by having CPR be the default situation in patients who are near the end of life.

CPR and Autonomy

That autonomy is the preeminent value regarding the question of CPR near the end of life has been made abundantly clear by the passage of the PSDA. Autonomy in this area is further emphasized by the fact that hospice and end-of-life care providers must serve eligible patients who request

CPR. Hospice and end-of-life care providers are respectful of patient autonomy in this area, and most hospice providers, in compliance with the PSDA, will admit patients who are eligible for care and have requested CPR. Physicians are generally supportive of allowing patient preference to dictate whether or not CPR is performed near the end of life, although it is suggested that patient autonomy is more often respected when CPR is desired than when it is not.

For autonomy to properly function in this setting, however, there needs to be a caveat that patients possess the necessary information that allows them to make appropriate choices. Herein lies a major challenge, for the literature suggests that, at least to date, patients as a whole are not well informed when making decisions about matters such as CPR near the end of life.

There is a great deal of public misperception about the nature of CPR. Although 94 percent of people who participated in a study evaluating their knowledge of CPR knew that CPR included chest compressions, only 43 percent recognized that CPR might entail needing "paddles on the chest" and only 36 percent knew that it could include placing a "tube in the windpipe." The mass media have seriously affected the public's perception of the successfulness of CPR, with television shows and movies often depicting a much higher degree of successful resuscitation than has been demonstrated in the medical literature. That proper information is vital to helping patients express autonomy in this area is underscored by a study evaluating the influence of patient knowledge regarding the probability of survival following CPR and patient preferences. When patients were questioned about CPR preferences during an acute or chronic illness, the percentage of patients desiring CPR significantly decreased (acute, 41 to 22 percent; chronic, 11 to 5 percent) after they were informed of the probability of survival following the procedure. By demonstrating that most patients do not want to undergo CPR when they are informed of the probability of survival after the procedure, this study affirms the importance of physicians providing their patients with the information necessary to help them express their autonomy in this area (Murphy, et al, 1994).

Unfortunately, despite the fact that patients are capable of synthesizing the information necessary to make informed and autonomous decisions about CPR near the end of life, only about 25 percent of patients are having such discussions with their physicians. (A full discussion on the subject of physician–patient communications near the end of life can be found in Chapter 3.) More importantly, over 50 percent of patients who have not had a discussion with their physicians about CPR near the end of life do not want to have the discussion in the first place. This serious lack of communication between patients and physicians has led, not surprisingly, to many patients receiving CPR in support of their autonomy, where if they had been properly informed, their expressions of autonomy might have been very different.

CPR Near the End of Life: Synthesis of Ethical Values and Final Thoughts

Table 15–9 summarizes the salient issues regarding CPR in relationship to each of the cardinal ethical values. Analysis of this information suggests that, with little if any medical benefit and the potential for significant medical harm, the ethical values of beneficence and nonmaleficence would clearly be violated if one were to provide CPR to patients near the end of life. Distributive justice would also dictate that CPR near the end of life be avoided. The ethical position of social justice in relationship to CPR is less clear and remains the subject of continued debate. Finally, autonomy clearly dictates that if desired, CPR should be provided to patients who request this procedure.

Weighing this all together, with three of the four major ethical values suggesting CPR should be avoided at the end of life, one could certainly make the ethical case, autonomy notwithstanding, that to provide CPR to patients near the end of life would be in violation of the principles of medical ethics. Reality is quite different, however. Autonomy is clearly the dominant ethical value in our society today, to the point that on the issue

of CPR, it actually supercedes all the other values. Therefore—and reinforced by federal law—patients who desire CPR near the end of life are entitled to receive it, despite the medical evidence that it is ineffective near the end of life and despite the violation of most other medical ethical values.

While awaiting shifts in societal values or changes in legislation, how is the provider of end-of-life care to proceed? Clearly, good autonomous decision making needs to be accompanied by information. Physicians need to meet with patients and families and discuss their CPR preferences with them, disclosing to them all the medical facts related to the benefits, risks, and outcomes of CPR near the end of life. Likewise, hospice providers and other providers of end-of-life care should discuss these issues carefully and thoroughly with patients and families when patients are referred and admitted for palliative care. If these conversations are held thoughtfully, it is likely that most patients and families will choose, either verbally, or with a written advance directive, to avoid CPR near the end of life.

The dilemma is how to properly care for patients who continues to express the desire to receive CPR near the end of life. Physicians will usually address this issue by simply acquiescing to the patient or family wishes while keeping the lines of communication open. Hospices and other end-of-life care providers confronted with patients who desire CPR, recognize a challenge and an opportunity. Being respectful of both patient autonomy and the PSDA, hospice providers will admit these patients. Integral to the hospice plan of care for these patients and families is appropriate and continual patient/family education, with the goal being to convince these patients and/or health care surrogates to alter their decisions and no longer desire CPR. For the rare patient or family where such education does not result in the choice that the patient forego CPR, the patient or health care proxy always has the option to leave the hospice program at any time to receive the care that they desire.

When dealing with human beings, especially as life is drawing to an end, there are no circumstances that are perfect or ideal. There will always

Table 15–9

Ethical Issues Related to CPR Near the End of Life

ETHICAL VALUE	PROS	CONS
Autonomy	1. Legislated by the PSDA	Lack of patient information to make an informed autonomous decision, as indicated by:
	2. Respected by hospices and other end-of life-care providers	1. Public misperception of nature of CPR
		2. Public misperception of successfulness of CPR
	3. Physicians supportive—more so when choice is for CPR	3. Only 25% of patients speak with physicians about CPR preferences
	4. Patients would make appropriate CPR choices if properly informed	4. More than 50% of patients do not want to speak with physicians about CPR preferences
Beneficence	None in patients with chronic or terminal illness	1. Overall survival rate about 15%
		2. Arrest unwitnessed, out of hospital, or no vital signs survival 1% or less
		3. Chronically ill elderly survival rate < 5%
Nonmaleficence	None reported	1. Autopsy studies indicate risk of fractures, hematomas, and aspiration
		2. Survivors also risk chest wall burns and permanent neurologic sequelae
Justice		
Distributive	None reported	Threefold increased in average cost of final hospitalization in patients without advance directive versus patients with advance directives
Social	CPR is default situation	No clear evidence that providing CPR to patients near the end of life is in the best interests of the society

be specific situations where, despite the best efforts of all concerned, individual patients and/or families will opt to receive CPR when it will be clearly be ineffective. Physicians, hospices, and other providers of end-of-life care can all be instrumental in reducing these situations to a minimum by better understanding how to help their patients provide advance directive instructions that are legal and binding, by properly documenting these instructions, and most importantly, by educating their patients and families about the medical facts of procedures such as cardiopulmonary resuscitation near the end of life.

Bibliography

Bedell SE, Delbanco TL, Cook EF, Epstein FH: Survival after cardiopulmonary resuscitation in the hospital. *N Engl J Med* 309:569, 1983.

Chambers CV, Diamond JJ, Perkel RL, Lasch LA: Relationship of advance directives to hospital charges in a Medicare population. *Arch Intern Med* 154:541, 1994.

Curtin, LL: DNR in the OR: Ethical concerns and hospital policies. *Nursing Management,* February 1994.

Curtis JR, Park DR, Krone MR, Pearlman RA: Use of the medical futility rationale in do-not-attempt-resuscitation orders. *JAMA* 273:124, 1995.

Gordon M, Cheung M: Poor outcome of on-site CPR in a multi-level geriatric facility. Three and a half years experience at the Baycrest Centre for Geriatric Care. *J Am Geriatr Soc* 41:163, 1993.

Hoffmann JC, Wenger NS, et al: Patient preferences for communication with physicians about end-of-life decisions. *Ann Intern Med* 127:1, 1997.

Members of 1991 NHO Ethics Committee: *Do-Not-Resuscitate (DNR) Decisions in the Context of Hospice Care.* Arlington, National Hospice Organization, 1992.

Moss, AH: Informing the patient about cardiopulmonary resuscitation. *J Gen Intern Med* 4:349, 1989.

Murphy DJ, Burrows D, Santilli S, et al: The influence of the probability of survival on patient preferences regarding cardiopulmonary resuscitation. *N Engl J Med* 330:545, 1994.

Murphy DJ, Murray AM, Robinson BE, Campion EW: Outcomes of cardiopulmonary resuscitation in the elderly. *Ann Intern Med* 111:199, 1989

Schonwetter RS, Teasdale TA, Taffet G, et al: Educating the elderly: Cardiopulmonary resuscitation deci-sions before and after intervention. *J Am Geriatr Soc* 39:372, 1991.

Scofield GR: Is consent useful when resuscitation isn't? *Hastings Cent Rep* December 1991:28–36.

Singer GR: Do-not-resuscitate orders. *J Florida Med Assoc* 8:30, 1994.

State in End-of-Life Care. Focus: Oregon's POLST Program. A publication of the National Program Office for Community–State Partnerships to Improve End-of-Life Care. Midwest Bioethics Center, 1021–1025 Jefferson Street, Kansas City, MO 64105-1329. April 1999, issue 3.

Teno JM, Lynn J, Phillips RS, et al: Do formal advance directives affect resuscitation decisions and the use of resources for seriously ill patients? *J Clin Ethics* 5:23, 1994.

Internet Sources

Health Answers Medical Reference Library, advance care directives: http://www:healthanswers.com/adam/top/view.asp?filename=001908.htm

Hospice Net Advance Directives: http://www.hospicenet.org

Legal Developments: http://www.choices.org/legal.htm//MAP

Resources Advance directives: http://wouncare.org/newsvol3n3/fy10:htm

Barry M. Kinzbrunner

Chapter

16

Nutritional Support and Parenteral Hydration

Introduction

Among the major challenges facing physicians who care for patients near the end of life are issues related to the continuation or withdrawal of nutritional support and/or hydration. Multiple court decisions have affirmed that patients or their surrogates have a right, drawn from the ethical principle of autonomy, to decline forced nutrition and hydration. The importance of patient autonomy (defined as the patient's right to choose what he or she believes to be best for him or her) in these decisions has been further emphasized by the passage of the federal Patient Self-Determination Act (PSDA) in 1991. This legislation mandates that Medicare and Medicaid providers inform patients of their rights to execute a living will or other advance directive, documents that may include instructions regarding the acceptance or refusal of hydration or nutritional support in the event of a terminal illness. (For a further discussion of advance directives, see Chapter 15.) Unfortunately, the PSDA, designed to foster patient–physician interaction on end-of-life issues, has not yet had its intended effect, with recent studies showing that only about 25 to 30 percent of hospitalized patients have documented advance directive conversations with their physicians within 48 hours of admission. When advance directives concerning nutrition and hydration are discussed, the ethical principles of beneficence and nonmaleficence, providing benefit and avoiding harm, are often overshadowed by cultural and social beliefs that food and fluids are essential to sustain life and provide for increased well-being and recovery in illness, even in the face of a terminal prognosis. In many instances, therefore, patients, families, surrogates, or health care providers find it difficult to come to fully informed, thoughtful, and objective decisions on these most important issues.

It is the responsibility of the physician, therefore, to assist the patient and loved ones in wrestling with the intellectual, philosophical, and emotional conflicts that present themselves whenever decisions involving nutritional support and hydration near the end of life need to made. To facilitate this process, this chapter will review the medical literature on the subject of nutritional support and hydration near the end of life.

Nutrition Near the End of Life

Factors that interfere with the ability of patients to receive adequate nutrition near the end of life can be directly caused by the terminal illness, secondary to treatment of the illness, or due to indirect or unrelated causes. It is, therefore, incumbent upon the physician to understand the various causes of anorexia and weight loss in order to be able to provide appropriate remedies and set appropriate expectations for patients and families. The most common causes are listed in Table 16–1. Patients with nutritional impairment will most often experience symptoms of anorexia and weight loss.

Cancer Anorexia–Cachexia Syndrome

Anorexia and weight loss are common symptoms in patients with end-stage cancer, reported to occur in from 30 percent to over 70 percent of terminally ill cancer patients. The pathophysiologic and etiologic factors that contribute to these symptoms are quite complex, and include metabolic abnormalities, possible circulating humoral substances, and direct and indirect physical and psychological effects of the malignancy and/or its treatment. Increased understanding of these factors has led to coining the term cancer anorexia–cachexia syndrome (CACS) to describe these abnormalities.

The metabolic alterations caused by the CACS are primarily related to glucose metabolism with secondary effects on protein and lipid metabolism. In simplified summary, glucose, the major source of calories for malignant tumor cells, is

Table 16–1

Causes of Anorexia and Weight Loss in Patients
Near the End of Life

Cancer Anorexia–Cachexia Syndrome
  Abnormalities in carbohydrate, lipid, and
    protein metabolism
  Humoral mediators
    Tumor necrosis factor/cachectin
    Interleukins
    Gamma interferon
Direct effects of tumors and antineoplastic therapy
  Abdominal fullness
  Taste change
  Dry mouth
  Constipation
  Uncontrolled nausea and emesis
  Dysphagia
  Mechanical obstruction
  Uncontrolled pain
Impaired mobility
Impaired cognition
Modified consistency diets
Upper extremity dysfunction
Abnormal oral and pharyngeal function
Impaired dentition, ill-fitting dentures

rendered less available to the abnormal cells as well as to the rest of the body during the early phases of the neoplastic process, due at least in part to development of insulin resistance and glucose intolerance. This results in the increased conversion of lactate to glucose by induction of the Cori cycle, and induction of gluconeogenesis from sources that include proteins and amino acids from lean muscle mass and lipids from adipose tissue stores.

One would expect that the increased requirement of malignant cells for glucose and other nutrients would be accompanied by the physiologic host response of increasing food intake to meet the increased energy needs of both the host and the disease. However, the opposite, a reduction in appetite and food intake, is what actually occurs.

This has led to speculation that anorexia in patients with the CACS may be independently mediated by circulating humoral factors, secreted either by the tumor or the host. Certain endogenously produced cytokines that have been isolated and appear to play a role in this process include tumor necrosis factor (TNF or cachectin), interleukin-1, interleukin-6, and gamma interferon.

Symptoms of malignant diseases that may directly contribute to anorexia and weight loss include abdominal fullness and early satiety, taste change, nausea, emesis, and mouth dryness. Uncontrolled pain is often associated with decreased oral intake, as are changes in smell, mucositis secondary to opportunistic infection, and a learned aversion to specific foods. In patients with head and neck or gastrointestinal malignancies, mechanical obstruction may contribute to malnutrition, especially late in the course of the illness. Malabsorption is only rarely implicated in the CACS, occurring in some patients with gastrointestinal or hepatobiliary carcinomas, and in other patients, already severely anorectic and cachectic, secondary to enzymatic deficiencies from atrophy of small intestinal villi. Various therapeutic interventions aimed at the malignant disease—surgery and its accompanying postoperative period, and chemotherapy and radiotherapy, with side effects including gastrointestinal mucositis and ulceration, nausea, and emesis—may also contribute to poor nutritional status.

Anorexia in the Debilitated Elderly

Elderly, debilitated patients who suffer from a non-malignant terminal illness will generally experience anorexia and weight loss primarily due to the functional loss of the ability to independently eat, rather than due to metabolic or humoral factors. (It should be noted that patients with terminal malignant disease may experience anorexia and weight loss from this as well, compounding the changes that occur secondary to the CACS.) The loss of functional independence in eating has been associated with impaired mobility, impaired cognition, modified-consistency diets, upper extremity dysfunction, abnormal oral–motor examinations, absence of teeth and dentures, and behavioral indicators suggestive of abnormalities in the oral and pharyngeal stages of swallowing. Consistent with these problems, the vast majority of elderly patients who require nutritional support suffer from various forms of chronic neurologic debilitation, including severe cerebrovascular disease, Parkinson's disease, Alzheimer's disease, and other forms of dementia. A small but significant number of patients will be malnourished secondary to severe chronic obstructive pulmonary disease or congestive heart failure, and a few patients will experience dysphagia secondary to a nonmalignant obstructive process, such as presbyesophagus.

 ## Treatment of Malnutrition

With a better understanding of some of the underlying mechanisms responsible for anorexia and weight loss in patients suffering from advanced terminal illnesses, strategies can theoretically be designed to reverse the abnormalities and restore patients to a more positive nutritional state. The importance of attempting to remedy this situation for physicians as well as for patients and families cannot be understated.

The desire of clinicians to improve the nutritional status of terminally ill patients is driven by evidence that for both patients with cancer as well as patients with nonmalignant advanced illnesses, weight loss and nutritional status have a negative effect on prognosis. This, of course, suggests that an improvement in a patient's nutritional parameters could result in a prolongation of survival.

For the patients themselves, and for their families, effective nutritional support is also an essential component of the care they desire to receive. There are strong ethnic and cultural beliefs that food is essential for maintaining life and a sense of well-being. Additionally, weight loss in many patients emphasizes significant physical changes that take place during the course of their terminal illness, and these alterations in appearance may create significant anxiety for the patient and family by serving as a constant reminder of deteriorating health.

The delivery of nutritional supplementation may generally be accomplished parenterally or enterally (Table 16–2). For example, a study comparing the metabolic effects of enteral and parenteral nutritional support in a group of patients with localized squamous cell carcinoma of the distal esophagus demonstrated no major differences, suggesting that equivalent levels of nutritional supplementation can be provided by either means. Decisions regarding the use of parenteral or enteral supplementation, therefore, should be based on whether or not the patient has a functional gastrointestinal system, as well as other potential benefits and risks to the patient.

Total Parenteral Nutrition

The development of intravenous hyperalimentation (IVH), also known as total parenteral nutrition (TPN), was viewed with great excitement as having the potential to reverse the negative effects of the anorexia and cachexia associated with malignant dis-

Table 16–2
Methods of Delivering Nutritional Supplementation

Parenteral nutritional support
    Total parenteral nutrition (TPN)
Enteral nutritional support
    Oral supplementation
    Gastrointestinal intubation
        Nasogastric tube
        Percutaneous endoscopic gastrostromy
            (PEG)
        Operative gastrostomy

eases. The hope was that TPN would have a positive effect on prognosis by improving nutritional status and by improving patient tolerance to aggressive surgery, chemotherapy, and radiotherapy. Once principles and guidelines for using TPN to treat patients with malignant diseases were established, early studies suggested that TPN had some beneficial effects on the nutritional status of at least some patients. Subsequently, however, studies have shown that—with the exception of patients undergoing bone marrow transplantation—cancer patients being treated with chemotherapy or radiotherapy have obtained no significant benefits in terms of survival, treatment tolerance, treatment toxicity, or tumor response with the addition of TPN. Additionally, patients treated with TPN were observed to have an increased risk of infectious, metabolic, and mechanical complications that, in at least one analysis, resulted in decreased patient survival (Klein, 1993). Similarly, enhancement of quality of life, perhaps the most important factor in determining the efficacy of any treatment recommended for patients with terminal illness, has not been demonstrated in the majority of studies involving TPN.

Based on the demonstrated lack of efficacy of TPN, the American College of Physicians (1989) published a position paper stating that "(t)he evidence suggests that parenteral nutritional support was associated with *net harm,* and no conditions could be identified in which such treatement appeared to be of benefit. Thus the routine use of parenteral nutrition for patients undergoing chemotherapy should be strongly discouraged." One could certainly draw the logical conclusion that TPN would play even less of a role in providing nutritional support for patients with even more advanced cancer who are no longer candidates for chemotherapy.

Enteral Nutritional Support

Oral Nutritional Support

Interest in providing oral nutritional support to patients with malignant diseases dates back at least

to 1956, when nine patients with progressive cancer were force fed on a metabolic ward, in an attempt to document any alterations in nutritional status (Terepka & Waterhouse, 1956). While positive findings included weight gain and nitrogen retention for some patients early in the course of treatment, the weight gain was primarily due to intracellular fluid accumulation, and nitrogen balance reequilibrated from positive to the baseline negative state in short order. More importantly, in about half the patients there was clinical evidence to suggest that the supplemental feedings caused the malignant process to accelerate.

More recent randomized controlled studies on oral nutritional support have suggested that neither aggressive dietary counseling nor specific dietary instructions significantly improved patient response to chemotherapy, quality of life, or survival. Additionally, there is no scientific evidence to support benefits from other popular dietary interventions, such as macrobiotic diets, hypervitamin therapy, or shark cartilage.

Gastrointestinal Intubation

For patients who are unable to swallow—whether due to obstructing malignant lesions in the oropharynx or esophagus or chronic neurologic disorders—enteral nutrition via intubation of the gastrointestinal tract has been the method of choice for providing nutritional support. The nasogastric tube is the least complex way to provide nourishment to these patients, although there is a high incidence of pulmonary aspiration and self-extubation, the later resulting in subsequent trauma to patient, family, and health care staff when replacing the tube. This has led to the development of alternative methods to provide more reliable access to the GI tract, which include surgical and percutaneous–endoscopic techniques for placing a feeding tube directly into the stomach. Studies comparing nasogastric tube placement with gastrostomy via percutaneous endoscopy have suggested that the latter is associated with a lower risk of self-extubation. In addition, the gastrostomy patients generally received a greater proportion of their prescribed feedings than patients receiving nutritional support by nasogastric feedings. A separate study comparing operative gastrostomy with percutaneous–endoscopic placement of a feeding tube demonstrated no difference in morbidity, mortality, tube functionality, or overall cost (Stiegman, et al, 1990).

As with TPN and forced oral nutrition, however, data concerning the effectiveness of enteral nutrition for patients with advanced illness is equivocal at best. In a prospective analysis of 70 patients receiving enteral nutrition, it was observed that while most patients were able to maintain weight for the first 2 to 6 months following intervention, beyond 6 months, about 33 percent of patients experienced recurrent weight loss (Ciocon, et al, 1988). During the entire 11 month study period, only 6 percent of patients were observed to experience any appreciable increase in weight. Metabolic parameters, including hemoglobin measurement and serum albumin, were essentially stable for all patients during the study period. Two studies examining the effect of enteral feedings on nutritional parameters of patients with head and neck carcinomas demonstrated that weight and serum albumin levels could, at best, be stabilized (Heber, et al, 1986; Campos, et al, 1990). A retrospective analysis of 31 patients with severe dysphagia from motor neuron disease compared the outcomes of 13 patients who were provided nourishment by nasogastric tube with 18 patients managed conservatively and without gastrointestinal intubation (Scott, 1992). (Conservative management included such techniques as assistance in oral feeding; modifications in the form, consistency, and nutritional content of the food; and proper positioning.) Results of the study showed no difference in survival between the two groups of patients, with intubated patients having significantly more complications related to increased oropharyngeal secretions.

In other reports, enteral nutritional support by either nasogastric tube or gastrostomy is demonstrably associated with significant morbidity and mortality. Almost paradoxically, patients who are at the highest risk for complications—those with advanced neurologic impairment, who are non-communicative, recumbent, and have a history of aspiration when fed orally—are the most likely to be considered candidates for gastrointestinal intubation. In a study of severely neurologically impaired patients who underwent surgical gastrostomy, mortality was reported as 48 percent within 1 month of the procedure (Wasiljew, et al, 1982). Another study, examining patients with a variety of debilitating conditions who had either percutaneous–endoscopic or surgically placed gastrostomy tubes, demonstrated a 38 percent mortality rate within 1 month of tube placement, with disease-specific mortality rates of 28 percent (19/67) in patients with neurologic disease, 37 percent (3/8) in patients with metastatic cachexia, 90 percent (9/10) in patients with pulmonary cachexia, and 12 percent (2/16) in patients with obstruction secondary to head and neck carcinoma (Stuart, et al, 1993).

Self-extubation and aspiration pneumonia are the most common causes of morbidity reported in patients who are fed with a nasogastric or gastric tube. In one study comparing the complications of nasogastric feeding with gastrostomy, 67 percent (36/54) of patients with NG tubes extubated themselves within 2 weeks of tube placement, while 43 percent (23/54) had aspiration pneumonia (Ciocon, et al, 1988). Gastrostomy patients had a somewhat lower incidence of self-extubation at 44 percent (7/16), with a slightly higher risk of aspiration pneumonia at 56 percent (9/16).

In summary, it would appear that with exception of selected patients who are unable to swallow due to tumor obstruction of the oropharynx or esophagus, enteral nutritional supplementation is not of significant benefit to patients with the cancer anorexia–cachexia syndrome. For patients with advanced neurologic illnesses or other non-malignant terminal conditions, enteral feeding may provide transient nutritional stability, but this advantage is lost over time. For all patients who require nutritional support, there are significant increases in morbidity and mortality associated with gastrointestinal intubation. Thus, these interventions are generally not appropriate for patients in a palliative care setting near the end of life.

Pharmacologic Interventions

Despite the fact that, as of today, there is no single medication that will provide appetite stimulation and weight gain for all patients treated, several agents have been studied and some have shown at least modest success. A list of these agents can be found in Table 16–3 and will be discussed next.

STEROIDS

Steroids have been widely used to treat various symptoms for patients with advanced cancer, including pain, weakness, nausea, and anorexia. These agents also provide an increased sense of well-being. These agents are commonly used in the hospice setting, with one British hospice reporting that 58 percent of patients evaluated over a 16-month period received some form of steroid.

Various forms of steroid medication, including dexamethasone, methylprednisolone, and prednisone, have been shown to improve appetite in 50 to 75 percent of patients with advanced cancer. The improvement generally occurred within several days of initiation of the medication. Maximum appetite stimulation was achieved within 4 weeks and anorexia tended to recur over the next several weeks. Reported toxicity to steroids includes oral candidiasis in about one-third of patients and the development of edema and cushingoid features in fewer than 20 percent, while 5 to 10 percent of patients develop dyspepsia, weight gain, psychic changes, or ecchymoses. Other gastrointestinal complications, occurring in less than 10 percent of treated patients, include esophagitis, gastrointestinal bleeding, and perforation. Thus, although steroids may have some efficacy as an appetite stimulant in the terminally ill, the lack of durability of this effect and concerns over toxicity have tended to limit the use of this class of agents.

MEGESTROL ACETATE

The observation that megestrol acetate induced undesirable weight gain in women being treated for breast cancer, led to studies concerning the use of this agent as an appetite stimulant for patients with cancer anorexia–cachexia syndrome. Controlled trials comparing megestrol acetate to placebo in patients with advanced cancer have shown positive drug effect on appetite and food intake, although weight gain has not been demonstrated in many patients. Doses between 160 mg and 1280 mg/day have been assessed, with improvements in appetite and food intake seeming to peak at a dose of 800 mg/day.

Improvement in quality of life has also been reported for some patients, suggesting that megestrol acetate may have a role to play in the treatment of the cancer anorexia–cachexia syndrome. The goals of therapy, consistent with palliative care, should be focused on improvement in appetite, which is much more clearly demonstrable and correlates well with quality of life, rather than weight gain, which seems to be a much less consistent observation. The maximum beneficial dose appears to be 800 mg/day, although the lower, more traditional dose of 160 mg/day is still recommended as the starting dose, with upward titration if symptomatic benefit is not achieved. As it takes some time for megestrol to be effective, it is recommended that megestrol be started early in the course of the disease to derive maximal benefit.

Table 16–3

Pharmacologic Treatments of Anorexia

MEDICATION	RECOMMENDED DOSAGE RANGE
Steroids	
Dexamethasone	1.5–4 mg qd to qid
Methylprednisolone	20 mg qd to tid
Prednisone	20 mg qd to tid
Megestrol acetate	160–400 mg bid
Metoclopramide	10 mg tid ac and hs
Tetrohydrocannabinol (THC)	2.5 mg tid
Cyproheptadine	4 mg tid

METOCLOPRAMIDE

As mentioned earlier, one of the causes of anorexia may be early satiety, often due to delayed gastric emptying. Metoclopramide, an agent that increases lower esophageal sphincter pressure and increases gastric emptying, has been demonstrated to be effective in the treatment of anorexia, as well as for symptoms of bloating, belching, and nausea, in patients who suffer from what has been described as the cancer-associated dyspepsia syndrome (CADS). Improvement in similar symptoms in diabetics with gastroparesis suggests that in some patients who would otherwise require gastrointestinal intubation, metoclopramide may be beneficial in improving symptoms without resorting to mechanical intervention.

TETRAHYDROCANNABINOL

Studies with tetrahydrocannabinol (THC), the active chemical in marijuana, have been limited. In patients with HIV disease, preliminary results have suggested that there is some stimulation of appetite and mood, without concomitant weight gain. In patients with cancer, a dose of 2.5 mg of THC three times a day showed varying degrees of appetite and weight gain, but nausea was common. Significantly, THC causes fluid retention and has significant untoward central nervous system side effects including dizziness, somnolence, and dissociation. These symptoms limit the usefulness of THC in the elderly and in patients with already impaired cognitive abilities.

CYPROHEPTADINE

Cyproheptadine is an antihistamine that has been demonstrated to cause weight gain in a number of clinical conditions including childhood asthma, anorexia nervosa, and with patients with tuberculosis, prompting its use as a potential appetite stimulant. A controlled clinical trial comparing cyproheptadine with placebo in patients with advanced cancer showed that patients treated with cyproheptadine had significantly less nausea, less emesis, more sedation, and more dizziness than patients receiving placebo. Appetite enhancement was of borderline significance and there was no demonstrable weight gain. Therefore, use of this agent in terminally ill patients has been relatively limited.

NONPHARMACOLOGIC MEASURES

There are many other simple and often overlooked treatments that can be recommended to patients in dealing with anorexia (Table 16–4). It is important to recognize that stomatitis, mouth ulcers, or other oral lesions may present a significant impediment to food consumption, and can generally be treated with topical antimicrobials if there is an infectious etiology, topical anesthetics, and meticulous mouth care. Patients who complain of chronic nausea and other gastrointestinal symptoms need to be promptly assessed and aggressively treated.

Be creative in suggesting modification of eating habits. Patients with early satiety can be given more frequent smaller meals rather than insisting that they follow the traditional pattern of three meals per day. Serving the smaller meals on smaller plates may provide patients with a psychological boost, the sense of accomplishment by being able to finish a meal. Most importantly, allow patients to eat what they want, when they want. Many patients are on dietary restrictions for other chronic medical conditions and would like nothing better than to eat what has been in the past a forbidden food. In the palliative care setting, encourage this, and compensate by adding an additional dose of a medication if needed. These maneuvers are relatively simple and may add significantly to the quality of a patient's remaining life.

Hydration Near the End of Life

A majority of hospitalized patients receive intravenous fluids in the period just prior to death, despite evidence that hydration is of negligible

Table 16–4
Nonpharmacologic Treatments for Anorexia

Assess for treatable causes	Oral thrush
	Nausea, emesis, constipation
	Metabolic disturbances
Dietary counseling to help patient adjust eating habits	Increase attractiveness of meals
	Smaller portions
	Smaller plates
	Allow patient to eat whenever desired
	Lift dietary restrictions (low salt, ADA)
	Allow favorite foods
	Avoid strong smells, spices
	Avoid hot foods
Dietary counseling to explain changing dietary needs to patient and family	Need for less food
	Lifting of dietary restrictions

benefit to these patients and in fact may be accompanied by significant adverse effects. As already noted, there are emotional and cultural imperatives that often compel patients and families to insist that parenteral hydration is provided, regardless of whether it is beneficial or harmful to the patient. In addition, physicians and other health care professionals are concerned about patient discomfort caused by symptoms of dehydration near the end of life.

Symptoms of Dehydration Near the End of Life

Symptoms of dehydration and potential interventions to treat these symptoms are listed in Table 16–5. They include thirst, dry mouth, nausea, headaches, cramps, postural hypotension, and central nervous system effects including lethargy, drowsiness, and fatigue. Thirst is believed to be the symptom of overriding concern to families and physicians, although for some patients the loss of the pleasure in drinking may be more important.

In fact, thirst may be less of a problem then most perceive, as it has been shown that healthy elderly males who were deprived of fluid for 24 hours experienced a reduction in thirst and fluid intake as compared to normal younger male adults treated in the same fashion. Furthermore, it may even be that dehydration at this last stage of life is beneficial for most patients because it results in the development of starvation ketosis, which reduces sensations of thirst and hunger and may additionally provide some relief from pain due to its possible anesthetic effects.

Metabolic abnormalities resulting from dehydration that are of concern to clinicians include azotemia, hyperosmolality, hypernatremia, hyperkalemia, and hypercalcemia. While these conditions should be appropriately treated with parenteral fluids and other measures when the patient still has significant quality time remaining, concerns that these abnormalities cause discomfort in the last days of life are greatly exaggerated. Studies have demonstrated that, despite lack of parenteral hydration, patients near the end of life do not experience significant changes in serum sodium, osmolality, or blood urea nitrogen. Alteration in level of consciousness is somewhat more controversial with some reports showing no correlation between level of consciousness and the use or nonuse of intravenous fluids, while other investigators have suggested that providing small amounts of parenteral fluid to patients may have beneficial effects on sensorium.

Negative consequences of parenteral hydration, however, are often overlooked by physicians and family members caring for terminally ill patients who are actively approaching death. Near the end of life, fluid needs decrease, and it is more difficult for the body to properly mobilize and incorporate fluids that are provided. Significant third-spacing of fluid can often be the result, leading to increased edema as well as increased pulmonary and gastrointestinal secretions. An increase in urine output, either due to the fluid itself or due to diuretics admininstered to reduce third-spacing, brings with it a number of untoward complications. For patients with impaired mobility, the increased need for toileting required might result in physical discomfort or the potential stresses associated with a bedside commode or bedpan. For bedbound and incontinent patients, increased urine output brings with it either the risk of skin breakdown or the discomfort and potential of infection secondary to a Foley catheter.

Treatment of Dehydration Near the End of Life

Interventions to treat symptoms of dehydration near the end of life are listed in Table 16–5. Most symptoms can be treated without resorting to parenteral fluids. Thirst—the symptom about which families worry most—may be managed in the majority of patients by providing them with small amounts of oral fluid and/or ice chips. While clearly insufficient to alter any of the metabolic abnormalities associated with decreased fluid intake (which are of minimal concern, as noted), the small amount of oral intake provided will usually satisfy the patient's desire to drink fluids as well ameliorate any thirst the patient may be experiencing. Dry mouth may be successfully managed with meticulous mouth care. Symptoms of lethargy, drowsiness, and fatigue are not uncommon, but in most cases are not believed to be harmful, especially when patients are close to death. Symptoms of nausea, cramping, and headaches are not as commonly reported as generally thought.

If parenteral fluids are used to treat any of these symptoms, small amounts, generally less than 1 L/day, should suffice, which avoids the negative consequences of fluid overload. For patients with symptoms of postural hypotension, short-term parenteral hydration of sufficient quantity and duration to allow the patient to resume his or her prior level of activity may be very appropriate and should be considered.

Table 16–5
Symptoms of Dehydration of Patients Near the End of Life

SYMPTOM	OCCURRENCE	TREATMENT
Thirst	Common	Small amount of oral fluid or ice chips
Dry mouth	Common	Meticulous mouth care
		Small amounts of artificial saliva
Nausea and emesis	Rarely reported	Symptomatic medications
Headache		Parenteral hydration may be indicated
Cramps		in selected patients
Postural hypotension	Occasional in ambulatory patients	Parenteral hydration may be indicated
Lethargy	Common but w/o distress in	May protect against pain and other
Drowsiness	bedbound patients	discomforting symptoms in
Fatigue		bedbound patients

Subcutaneous Infusion: Hypodermoclysis

Parenteral hydration has traditionally been provided to patients via the intravenous route. For patients near the end of life who require parenteral fluid support and have an indwelling intravenous access site or who have peripheral veins that can accept an intravenous catheter, this route of fluid administration may still be used. However, the majority of terminally ill patients do not have intravenous access devices in place, and the condition of their peripheral venous system makes use of an intravenous catheter difficult, creating the need for an alternative method of providing parenteral fluid when indicated near the end of life.

The development of improved techniques for subcutaneous infusion of fluids and medications, also known as hypodermoclysis, appears to have met this need. Use of this technique near the end of life to provide both fluids and medications has increased substantially over the last decade.

Hypodermoclysis is performed by placing a 23–25 gauge Teflon cannula or butterfly needle into the subcutaneous tissue of the medial thigh, abdominal wall, or upper chest wall. Studies suggest that a little more than 1 L/day can be safely and effectively delivered by this technique, with the usual fluid infused being either normal saline or 5 percent dextrose and one-third normal saline. The enzyme hyaluronidase, 150 U/L, is added to the infusate to break down the interstitial barriers in the subcutaneous space and promote fluid absorption. Multiple medications can be delivered by hypodermoclysis, making it a viable alternative route of medication administration when a patient cannot be medicated orally and no intravenous site is available. A partial list of medications that may be provided via subcutaneous infusion is in Table 16–6.

With increased refinement in the technique of hypodermoclysis, some experts suggest that subcutaneous infusion might be indicated for all patients receiving palliative care, much as intravenous infusion has traditionally been viewed in the acute

Table 16–6

Medications That May Be Administered by Hypodermoclysis

SYMPTOM	MEDICATION
Pain	Morphine
	Hydromorphone
Sedation and other CNS symptoms	Midazolam
	Haloperidol
	Phenobarbital
	Dexamethasone
Gastrointestinal	Metoclopramide
Respiratory secretions	Atropine
	Scopolamine

care setting. One has to wonder, however, whether the motivation for this is based upon sound clinical indications, or whether, as has been the case with intravenous hydration in the past, it is mostly due to the overwhelming desire among physicians and families to provide the patient with "something" near the end of life. The decision to provide parenteral fluid support, whether by the intravenous or subcutaneous route, should be made in the same fashion as is any other decision to provide a therapeutic intervention in palliative medicine. It should be based upon evidence that the intervention is the most appropriate therapy to provide relief of a specific symptom for the individual patient being treated. Such evidence is severely limited.

No controlled clinical trials have been performed addressing the potential benefits and risks of parenteral hydration of patients near the end of life. Based upon the physiologic evidence discussed earlier, it would appear that routine parenteral hydration in this population should be avoided. Use of parenteral fluids, either by the intravenous route or by hypodermoclysis, should be reserved for symptomatic patients who have a distressing symptom that will improve with fluid administration, or when medication cannot be administered by a noninvasive route. For the overwhelming majority of patients who are near the end of life, symptoms of decreased fluid intake will respond just as effectively to palliative interventions such as small amounts of fluids, ice chips, and good oral care.

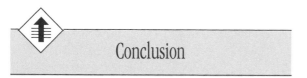

Conclusion

The major challenge regarding the appropriate provision of nutrition and hydration to patients with terminal illness is educational in nature. The physician must determine the goals of care set by patients and families, understand the therapeutic options available to meet those goals, and be able to explain the options in an understandable way to patients and families. It is the responsibility of the physician to strike a balance between the respect for patient autonomy and the obligation to recommend what is believed to be the best available treatment. Accurate assessment of the risks and benefits of an intervention based on critical reading of the clinical literature will usually result in a sound recommendation to the patient and family, allowing each patient and family to reach reasonable, informed decisions about how to best meet their needs.

The available data seem to indicate that unbiased assessment of risks and benefits has not been a routine part of clinical decision-making regarding nutrition for terminally ill patients. TPN and enteral nutrition by gastrointestinal intubation or forced oral nutrition appear to be rarely if ever indicated, based on lack of demonstrated benefits and significant potential side effects, even though they are sometimes used. Medications such as megestrol acetate and prednisone may have some appetite-stimulating properties, but early initiation of these drugs appears important, limiting their usefulness for patients with a prognosis of only several weeks. Nevertheless, these more fashionable therapeutic options are still often recommended to patients and families, while less exotic though highly effective interventions—such as mouth care and the modification of dietary intake to allow the patient to eat whatever they desire, on their own schedule—are often overlooked.

Similarly, there is little if any demonstrable benefit to providing artificial hydration at the end of life, and complications are documented. Still, the overwhelming desire to provide such treatment often precludes more useful interventions such as providing patients with sips of fluid, ice chips, and proper mouth care.

Even more distressing is the fact that, at least on an anecdotal basis, patients who either choose or are required by cultural or ethnic values to elect artificial nutrition and/or hydration at the end of life are not managed to avoid complications. Questions regarding the optimal fluid or calorie requirement for bedbound, inactive, dying patients have never been answered. While it may be very reasonable to provide artificial nutritional support or hydration to these patients based upon their individual needs, too often this therapy is administered based on fixed quantities, resulting in increased morbidity or premature mortality from fluid overload or aspiration of residual gastric contents.

In conclusion, the provision of artificial nutritional support and hydration to terminally ill patients, as with any other intervention, must be considered for each patient on an individual basis, taking into account the ethical principles of autonomy, beneficence, and nonmaleficence. Non-invasive interventions such as allowing ad lib oral intake, providing spoon feedings, and providing sips of fluid and ice chips, should be considered therapeutically on par with invasive interventions such as TPN, gastrointestinal intubation, and parenteral fluids. Paying attention to detail, considering correctable causes of decreased oral intake, and if artificial support is indicated, avoiding toxicity, are all vital to providing patients with high-quality, end-of-life care, which should be both the hope and goal of all therapy provided to patients who suffer from illnesses that limit life expectancy.

Bibliography

American College of Physicians: Parenteral nutrition in patients receiving cancer chemotherapy. *Ann Intern Med* 110:734, 1989.

Andrews M, Bell ER, Smith SA, et al: Dehydration in terminally ill patients. Is it appropriate palliative care? *Postgrad Med* 93:201, 1993.

Billings JA: Comfort measures for the terminally ill. Is dehydration painful? *J Am Geriatr Soc* 33:808, 1985.

Boyd KJ, Beeken L: Tube feeding in palliative care: Benefits and problems. *Palliat Med* 8:156, 1994.

Bruera E: Ambulatory infusion devices in the continuing care of patients with advanced diseases. *J Pain Symptom Manage* 5:287, 1990.

Bruera E, Breinneis C, Michaud M, et al: Use of the subcutaneous route for the administration of narcotics in patients with cancer pain. *Cancer* 62:407, 1988.

Bruera E, Legris MA, Kuehn N, Miller MJ: Hypodermoclysis for the administration of fluids and narcotic analgesics in patients with advanced cancer. *J Pain Symptom Manage* 5:218, 1990.

Bruera E, Macmillan K, Kuehn N, et al: A controlled trial of megestrol acetate on appetite, caloric intake, nutritional status, and other symptoms in patients with advanced cancer. *Cancer* 66:1279, 1990.

Burge FI: Dehydration symptoms of palliative care cancer patients. *J Pain Symptom Manage* 8:454, 1993.

Burge FI, King DB, Willison D: Intravenous fluids and the hospitalized dying: A medical last rite? *Can Fam Physician* 36:883, 1990.

Campbell-Taylor I, Fisher RH: The clinical case against tube feeding in palliative care in the elderly. *J Am Geriatr Soc* 35:1100, 1987.

Campos ACL, Butters M, Meguid MM: Home enteral nutrition via gastrostomy in advanced head and neck cancer patients. *Head Neck* 12:137, 1990.

Cimino JE: Medical ethics and the decision to feed or not to feed: A physician speaks. *Top Clin Nutr* 6:72, 1991.

Ciocon JO, Silverstone FA, Graver LM, Foley CJ: Tube feedings in elderly patients. Indications, benefits, and complications. *Arch Intern Med* 148:429, 1988.

Collaud T, Rapin CH: Dehydration in dying patients: Study with physicians in French-speaking Switzerland. *J Pain Symptom Manage* 6:230, 1991.

Conant M, Roy D, Shepard KV, Plasse TF: Dronabinol enhances appetite and controls weight loss in HIV patients. *Proc Am Soc Clin Oncol* 10:34, 1991.

Curran WJ: Defining appropriate medical care. Providing nutrients and hydration for the dying. *N Engl J Med* 313:940, 1985.

Dewys WD, Begg C, Lavin PT, et al: Prognostic effect of weight loss prior to chemotherapy in cancer patients. *Am J Med* 69:491, 1980.

Ethics Committee, American Nurses Association: ANA position statement on foregoing artificial nutrition and hydration. *Kentucky Nurse* 41:16, 1993.

Ettinger AB, Portenoy RK: The use of corticosteroids in the treatment of symptoms associated with cancer. *J Pain Symptom Manage* 3:99, 1988.

Evans WK, Nixon DW, Daly JM, et al: A randomized study of oral nutrition support versus ad lib nutritional intake during chemotherapy for advanced colorectal and non-small-cell lung cancer. *J Clin Oncol* 5:113, 1987.

Fansinger RL, MacEachern T, Miller MJ, et al: The use of hypodermoclysis for rehydration in terminally ill cancer patients. *J Pain Symptom Manage* 9:298, 1994.

Farr WC: The use of corticosteroids for symptom management in terminally ill patients. *Am J Hospice Care* 7:41, 1990.

Feuz A, Rapin, CH: An observational study of the role of pain control and food adaptation of elderly patients with terminal cancer. *J Am Dietetic Assoc* 94:767, 1994.

Finucane TE, Christmas C, Travis K: Tube feeding in patients with advanced dementia. A review of the evidence. *JAMA* 282:1365, 1999.

Gillick M: Sounding Board: Rethinking the role of tube feeding in patients with advanced dementia. *N Engl J Med* 342:206, 2000.

Grauer PA: Appetite stimulants in terminal care: Treatment of anorexia. *Hospice J* 9:73, 1993.

Grosvenor M, Bulcavage L, Chlebowski RT: Symptoms potentially influencing weight loss in a cancer population. *Cancer* 63:330, 1989.

Hanks GW, Trueman T, Twycross RG: Corticosteroids in terminal cancer. A prospective analysis of current practice. *Postgrad Med J* 59:702, 1983.

Heber D, Byerley LO, Chi J, et al: Pathophysiology of malnutrition in the adult cancer patient. *Cancer* 58:1867, 1986.

Holden C: Nutrition and hydration in the terminally ill cancer patient: The nurse's role in helping patients and families cope. *Hospice J* 9:15, 1993.

Kane RS: The death certificate. *J Am Geriatr Soc* 42:442, 1994.

Kardinal CG, Loprinzi CL, Schaid DJ, et al: A controlled trial of cyproheptadine in cancer patients with anorexia and/or cachexia. *Cancer* 63:2657, 1990.

Kaye P. *Notes on Symptom Control in Hospice and Palliative Care*. Essex, Hospice Education Institute, 1990, pp. 27–29.

King DG, Maillet JO: Position of the American Dietetic Association: Issues in feeding the terminally ill adult. *J Am Dietetic Assoc* 92:996, 1992.

Klein S: Clinical efficacy of nutritional support in patients with cancer. *Oncology* 7(suppl):87, 1993.

Klein S, Simes J, Blackburn GL: Total parenteral nutrition and cancer clinical trials. *Cancer* 58:1378, 1986.

Koch KA: Patient self-determination act. *J Florida Med Assoc* 79:240, 1992.

Lo B: Ethical issues in clinical medicine. In: Isselbacher KJ, Braunwald E, Wilson JD, et al, eds. *Harrison's Principles and Practice of Medicine,* 13th ed. New York, McGraw Hill, 1994, p. 6.

Loprinzi CL: Pharmacologic management of cancer anorexia/cachexia. *Oncology* 7(suppl):101, 1993.

Loprinzi CL, Ellison NM, Schaid DJ, et al: Controlled trial of megestrol acetate for the treatment of cancer anorexia and cachexia. *J Natl Cancer Inst* 82:1127, 1990.

Loprinzi CL, Michalak JC, Schaid DJ, et al: Phase III evaluation of four doses of megestrol acetate therapy for patients with cancer anorexia and/or cachexia. *J Clin Oncol* 11:762, 1993.

McCamish MA, Crocker NJ: Enteral and parenteral nutrition support of terminally ill patients: Practical and ethical perspectives. *Hospice J* 9:107, 1993.

McCann RM, Hall WJ, Groth-Juncker A: Comfort care for terminally ill patients. The appropriate use of nutrition and hydration. *JAMA* 272:1263, 1994.

McGeer AJ, Detsky AS, O'Rourke K: Parenteral nutrition in cancer patients undergoing chemotherapy: A meta-analysis. *Nutrition* 6:233, 1990.

Miller MG, McCarthy N, O'Boyle CA, Kearney MA: Continuous subcutaneous infusion of morphine vs. hydromorphone: A controlled trial. *J Pain Symptom Manage* 18:9, 1999.

Miller RJ, Albright PG: What is the role of nutritional support and hydration in terminal cancer patients? *Am J Hospice Care* 6:333, 1989.

Nelson KA, Walsh TD: Metoclopramide in anorexia caused by cancer-associated dyspepsia syndrome (CADS). *J Palliat Care* 9:14, 1993.

Nelson KA, Walsh D, Sheehan FA: The cancer anorexia–cachexia syndrome. *J Clin Oncol* 12:213, 1994.

O'Neill WM: Subcutaneous infusions—a medical last rite. *Palliat Med* 8:91, 1994.

Osoba D, Murray N, Gelmon K, et al: Phase II trial of megestrol in the supportive care of patients receiving dose-intensive chemotherapy. *Oncology* 8:43, 1994.

Ovesen L, Allingstrup L, Hannibal J, et al: Effect of dietary counseling on food intake, body weight, response rate, survival, and quality of life in cancer patients undergoing chemotherapy: A prospective, randomized study. *J Clin Oncol* 11:2043, 1993.

Park RHR, Allison MC, Land J, et al: Randomised comparison of percutaneous endoscopic gastrostomy and nasogastric tube feeding in patients with persisting neurological dysphagia. *Br Med J* 304:1406, 1992.

Parkash R, Burge F: The family's perspective on issues of hydration in terminal care. *J Palliat Care* 13:23, 1997.

Phillips PA, Rolls BJ, Ledingham JG, et al: Reduced thirst after water deprivation in healthy elderly men. *N Engl J Med* 311:753, 1984.

Printz LA: Terminal dehydration: a compassionate treatment. *Arch Intern Med* 152:697, 1992.

Schmitz P: The process of dying with and without feeding and fluids by tube. *Law Medicine Health Care* 19:23, 1991.

Scott AG: Nasogastric feeding in the management of severe dysphagia in motor neuron disease. *Palliat Med* 8:45, 1992.

Siebens H, Trupe E, Siebens A, et al: Correlates and consequences of eating dependency in institutionalized elderly. *J Am Geriatr Soc* 34:192, 1986.

Steiner N, Bruera E: Methods of hydration in palliative care patients. *J Palliat Care* 14:6, 1998.

Stiegmann GV, Goff JS, Silas D, et al: Endoscopic versus operative gastrostomy: Final results of a prospective randomized trial. *Gastrointest Endosc* 36:1, 1990.

Storey P, Hill HH, St. Louis RH, Tarver EE: Subcutaneous infusions for the control of cancer symptoms. *J Pain Symptom Manage* 5:33, 1990.

Stuart SP, Tiley EH, Boland JP: Feeding gastrostomy: A critical review of its indications and mortality rate. *South Med J* 86:169, 1993.

Sullivan DH, Patch GA, Walls RC, Lipschitz DA: Impact of nutrition status on morbidity and mortality in a select population of geriatric rehabilitation patients. *Am J Clin Nutr* 51:749, 1990.

Tchekmedyian NS, Hickman M, Siau J, et al: Treatment of cancer anorexia with megestrol acetate: Impact on quality of life. *Oncology* 4:184, 1990.

Terepka AR, Waterhouse C: Metabolic observations during the forced feeding of patients with cancer. *Am J Med* 20:225, 1956.

Viola RA, Wells GA, Peterson J: The effects of fluid status and fluid therapy on the dying: A systematic review. *J Palliat Care* 13:41, 1997.

Wall MG, Wellman NS, Curry KR, Johnson PM: Feeding the terminally ill: Dietitians' attitudes and beliefs. *J Am Dietetic Assoc* 91:549, 1991.

Waller A, Hershkowitz M, Adunsky A: The effect of intravenous fluid infusion on blood and urine parameters of hydration and on state of consciousness in terminal cancer patients. *Am J Hospice Palliat Care* 11:26, 1994.

Wasiljew BK, Ujiki CT, Beal JM: Feeding gastronomy. Complications and mortality. *Am J Surg* 143:194, 1982.

Ziegler TR, Young LS, Benfell K, et al: Clinical and metabolic efficacy of glutamine-supplemented parenteral nutrition after bone marrow transplantation. *Ann Intern Med* 116:821, 1992.

Neal J. Weinreb

Diagnostic Tests and Invasive Procedures

Introduction

A 77-year-old man with advanced pancreatic carcinoma and obstructive jaundice is admitted to a hospice program for terminal, palliative care. In addition to anorexia and fatigue, he suffers from intractable pruritus, which has not responded to pharmacologic intervention. The patient is so distressed that he is contemplating suicide. In discussion with the hospice interdisciplinary team, the medical director suggests endoscopic or radiologic biliary stenting. The hospice nurse appears uncomfortable and comments: "I thought that we don't do aggressive, invasive, life-prolonging procedures on hospice patients!" Nevertheless, after further explanation and discussion, the recommendation is presented to the patient and to his wife. To everyone's surprise and consternation, the patient categorically and repeatedly refuses the procedure, saying: "All I want is to die as quickly as possible. Doc, why can't you just put me to sleep?"

This anecdote highlights a strange and frustrating paradox in modern medicine. Palliative care is fast becoming accepted as a broadly desired area of clinical expertise, and its practitioners have access, when appropriate, to a rapidly growing armamentarium of technologically sophisticated, symptom-oriented interventions capable of substantial enhancement of comfort, even near the end of life. On the other hand, public support for the legalization of physician-assisted suicide appears to be substantial throughout the United States, suggesting that there continues to be deep-rooted disbelief in the ability and willingness of modern medicine and technology to address and alleviate pain and suffering. Furthermore, knowledge of which outcomes are truly important for terminal patients continues to be incomplete, and defining and analyzing symptom palliation for any given intervention can be deceptively difficult. Few trials define a standard of palliation based on aspects of onset, duration and degree of palliation, and symptom improvement, control, and prevention.

The balance between the benefits and burdens of intervention is often evaluated in terms of quality of life (QOL). However, even with validated tools for QOL measurement, QOL may correlate poorly with other indicators of health status. A number of patients with significant physical and/or psychological symptoms report good global quality of life, including 51 percent of patients with severe pain. Conversely, patients with less severe physical and psychological manifestations may describe their quality of life as poor. A new endpoint, the clinical benefit response, which uses disease symptoms as clinical endpoints, also may correlate poorly with subjective evaluations of QOL by patients and physicians, and criteria designed for use in one diagnosis or study may not be applicable in other circumstances.

Thus, patient attitudes towards "aggressive," invasive palliative interventions are likely to be highly variable and unpredictable. Studies suggest that some patients with advanced disease are willing to put up with significant, but time-limited, toxicity for interventions, such as palliative chemotherapy, intravenous antibiotics, and limited mechanical ventilation, in return for a modest benefit. Indeed, many patients, were they able, would not trade months of even debilitating illness for a single month of "quality time." However, other patients might well identify with the attitude of the patient (quoted at the start of the chapter) in eschewing any invasive intervention. Many more undoubtedly concur with the following instructions written by a physician in a model advance directive: "If there is little hope for recovery to my prior state of health, or if what hope exists requires prolonged and invasive medical treatments, I would prefer to receive care focused on my comfort rather than care focused on prolonging my life."

The purpose of this chapter is to identify various diagnostic procedures and invasive therapies that are potentially available to terminal patients; to examine the evidence that these interventions have palliative value near the end of life; and to consider the clinical circumstances in which these interventions can be appropriately recommended either to patients or to their health care surrogates. (Issues related to nutrition and hydration are discussed in Chapter 16.) These interventions will be examined from the viewpoint of end-of-life care as a whole, without raising issues regarding the Medicare Hospice Benefit (a prognosis of 6 months or less) and without any references to cost effectiveness or economic analysis.

General Principles

The usual goal of palliative care near the end of life, as defined by the World Health Organization, is achievement of the best possible quality of life for patients and their families. Control of pain, of other symptoms, and of psychological, social, and spiritual problems is paramount. This goal includes optimizing function and making the best of remaining time. It does not necessarily preclude other goals such as remission or even cure, and

some patients may wish to seek aggressive and/or experimental treatments for the primary terminal process until the very end. These patients are obviously no less entitled to optimal symptom management than those patients who are seeking comfort measures only, but their tolerance for risk and discomfort associated with invasive interventions may be considerably greater. For this reason, this discussion will be directed to those patients whose primary goal near the end of life is total symptom control and maximal functional capacity for as long as possible. In pursuit of this goal, it has been proposed that "palliative care must embrace all the high-tech, expensive, aggressive measures that can enhance patient and family care at the end-of-life" (Billings, 1998). Indeed, symptom control measures have expanded to include chemotherapy, radiation therapy, and other multimodal therapies.

The key factors in determining the appropriateness of end-of-life palliative interventions are summarized in Table 17–1 and discussed in the next sections.

Goal or Expected Outcome of the Proposed Intervention

Suppose, for example, that a patient with advanced metastatic carcinoma suffers a pathologic fracture

Table 17–1
Determining Appropriateness of Aggressive Palliative Interventions Near the End of Life

What is the goal or expected outcome of the proposed intervention?
Does the planned intervention have a high probability of efficacy?
How significant are potential toxicities, side effects, complications, and/or postintervention discomfort?
What is the patient's baseline level of function?
What is the life expectancy of the patient?
What does the patient want?

of the head of the femur. The proposed intervention is orthopedic stablilization via intramedullary rod fixation. Is the goal to restore ambulation, or purely to alleviate pain with turning and positioning? If the former, is the goal realistic? Will the patient be able to accomplish a postoperative rehabilitation program? If the latter, would a lesser procedure achieve the same outcome?

Probability of Efficacy

Efficacy needs to be defined in terms of rapidity of onset, degree of palliation, and the durability of the response. The assessment of efficacy must be applied towards the proposed intervention in general, as well as to the specific patient in particular. Thus, a chemotherapy drug reported in the literature to be 80 percent effective in alleviating bone pain would appear to be a reasonable palliative intervention. However, in a heavily pretreated patient with multiple drug resistance, such an agent might be considerably less effective, with the risk of toxicity outweighing any potential benefit, particularly if pain relief is incomplete and of only brief duration. Radiotherapy or spinal decompression can be effective modalities for preventing spinal cord compression, but they are essentially useless for that purpose in a patient who is already paraplegic.

Potential Toxicities, Side Effects, Complications, and Postintervention Discomfort

Clearly, adverse effects of treatment influence the patient's quality of life. The assessment of benefit versus risk requires a full understanding of the potential for undesired, negative, and even life-threatening consequences. For example, what are the chances that a patient with extensive bone metastases who has been heavily pretreated with chemotherapy and external radiotherapy will develop severe pancytopenia with symptomatic anemia and thrombocytopenia following proposed treatment with radiostrontium? What is the likeli-

hood of recurrent infection and sepsis following endoscopic stenting for biliary obstruction? In this regard, are metal stents better than plastic stents? What are the chances of perforating a viscus when performing a paracentesis to relieve discomfort caused by malignant ascites?

Patient's Baseline Level of Function

Invasive procedures and interventions that have high efficacy and low risk profiles may nonetheless be futile in improving the patient's overall well-being and quality of life. Consequently, such procedures would seem to be of little palliative value, particularly when the symptoms at which they are directed can be adequately controlled by less invasive means. For example, will a patient with metastatic breast carcinoma and severe dyspnea secondary to lymphangitic pulmonary carcinomatosis benefit from testing to confirm suspected hypercalcemia even though hypercalcemia can be easily treated? Should sclerotherapy for bleeding esophageal varices be advised for a patient with terminal cirrhosis and irreversible hepatic encephalopathy? Should a patient with far-advanced, terminal dementia and pneumonia be treated with intravenous antibiotics?

Life Expectancy

It would be illogical to initiate any therapeutic intervention unless there is a reasonable probability that the patient will survive for a sufficient time to realize a benefit from the procedure. Nonetheless, patients continue to be subjected to all kinds of aggressive therapies even within 1 to 2 days of death. In a study of 200 consecutive deaths at a large urban academic medical center, only 13 percent of the patients on mechanical ventilation and 19 percent of those on artificial nutrition and hydration underwent withdrawal of these interventions prior to death. In an Israeli ICU, no patient had antibiotics, nutrition, or fluids withheld. At a U.S. Veterans' Administration hospital, 27 percent of patients received ventilatory support and 18 percent were restrained during the last 48 hours of life. On the other hand, other studies indicate that for patients with metastatic cancer, antibiotics are commonly withheld at the very end of life, and interventive surgery for abdominal emergencies (obstruction, bleeding, dehiscence) is quite rare. Nevertheless, even here the majority of patients continued to receive blood transfusions and intravenous fluids.

As discussed at length in Chapter 1, predicting prognosis is never easy. However, with the judicious use of clinical guidelines and sound clinical judgment, physicians are getting more adept in predicting when life is coming to an end, as death approaches. By making these assessments, physicians can assist patients and families in making therapeutic decisions that will allow patients who have sufficiently long to live to benefit from indicated procedures, while avoiding such procedures in patients whose time is short.

Accurate prognostication is also critical in assessing the significance of potential delayed or late-onset adverse effects attributable to prior aggressive intervention. For example, many radiation oncologists continue to prescribe protracted, low-fractionation radiotherapy for end-stage cancer patients for fear of causing radiation toxicity, even though this toxicity would have a predicted time of onset long after the death of the patient.

Patient Wishes

The principle of autonomy allows competent patients to reject any proposed intervention no matter how beneficial that treatment is likely to be. The physician is ethically obligated to provide sufficient information to allow the patient to reach an informed decision, and professionally responsible to recommend and strongly espouse a course of action that is believed to be beneficial for the patient. However, a mature and understanding physician will accept a patient's final decision, and particularly in the context of end-of-life care, will be sure that the patient feels neither rejected

nor abandoned even if the physician's advice is not accepted. Nevertheless, a physician also has autonomous rights and professional integrity, and should feel no obligation to initiate or participate in patient-desired interventions that are medically ineffective or detrimental, or morally repugnant to the physician.

Diagnostic Tests

Diagnostic laboratory and imaging studies are appropriate and indicated in end-of-life care when the information obtained will assist in decision making about therapeutic interventions to control symptoms. On the other hand, routine testing for the purpose of monitoring the patient in anticipation of as-yet-nonexistent problems is generally not advisable.

For example, consider an alert, ambulatory patient with an unresectable gastric carcinoma, but no overt evidence of gastrointestinal bleeding, who complains of anorexia, weight loss, and chronic fatigue. The physician orders weekly CBCs with the thought that should the hemoglobin concentration decrease to less than 8 g/dL, a blood transfusion will be necessary. This type of testing, which fosters therapeutic interventions based on arbitrary laboratory values rather than on the patient's symptoms, makes little sense, particularly in the care of patients with end-stage disease. In contrast, should the same patient notice the passage of black stools, along with episodes of dizziness, palpitations, and increasing shortness of breath, measurement of hemoglobin concentration would be worthwhile to confirm the presence of severe anemia, provided, of course, that the patient would agree to interventions, such as a blood transfusion.

On occasions, patients thought to be near the end of life may need to undergo highly invasive procedures to clarify a suspected but previously unconfirmed diagnosis. Patients believed to have malignancies on the basis of abnormal imaging studies, suspicious needle aspirations, or other test results sometimes refuse to allow definitive biopsies or other procedures needed to obtain a tissue diagnosis, and elect a palliative approach. Should their illness not follow the expected course, these patients may be amenable to a new diagnostic evaluation including new imaging studies and even tissue sampling.

Diagnostic testing may have the most utility when there has been a sudden or acute change in the patient's status from the usual condition or level of function. In these circumstances, testing, as an adjunct to historical and physical assessment, may clarify not only the etiology of the change, but also indicate the potential for reversibility and restoration of the patient's usual status. The most common events that may require diagnostic studies in selected patients near the end of life are listed in Table 17–2 and will be discussed next.

Mental Status Changes

Acute and subacute changes in mental status of end-stage cancer patients, as well as in patients with terminal noncancer diagnoses, may be asso-

ciated with metabolic disorders, infection and sepsis, toxic drug reactions and interactions, primary central nervous system events including thrombotic and embolic infarction, bleeding, metastasis, and psychiatric disorders.

HYPERCALCEMIA

Hypercalcemia is the most common life-threatening, cancer-associated metabolic disorder. It occurs in 10 to 20 percent of all cancer patients, and when due to humoral mechanisms, may occur in the absence of bone metastases. When recognized, the symptoms of hypercalcemia are usually rapidly reversible with saline hydration and intravenous bisphosphonates such as pamidronate. Other active agents include calcitonin, corticosteroids, gallium nitrate, and plicamycin. With the exception of imminently dying patients, or patients with extremely poor performance status and refractory symptoms, serum calcium testing is reasonable for end-stage patients with the new onset or exacerbation of fatigue, lethargy, confusion, stupor, muscle weakness, and/or seizures, particularly in association with constipation, nausea, vomiting, ileus, anorexia, thirst, polyuria, weight loss, and pruritus.

Table 17–2
Potentially Useful Diagnostic Interventions in Palliative Care

SYMPTOM	ETIOLOGY	DIAGNOSTIC INTERVENTION
Acute or subacute change in mental status	Hypercalcemia	Serum calcium level
	Hyponatremia and other electrolyte abnormalities	Serum sodium and/or other electrolyte levels
	Hypothyroidism	Serum T-4 levels
	Medication toxicity	Serum drug levels
		Renal and liver function tests
	Brain metastases	CT scan of brain
New bone pain	Bone metastases and/or impending pathologic fracture	X-rays
		Bone scan
Back pain with/without neurologic symptoms	Spinal cord compression	MRI of spine
Dyspnea	Pleural effusion	Chest x-ray

HYPONATREMIA

Similar symptoms may be associated with other correctable metabolic disorders such as severe hyponatremia sometimes associated with the syndrome of inappropriate antidiuretic hormone secretion (SIADH). Hyponatremia near the end of life may also be caused by salt-wasting states associated with adrenal insufficiency (as in some patients with advanced AIDS) and chronic renal failure, cirrhosis and end-stage liver disease, hypothyroidism, and medications including diuretics, chlorpropamide, amitriptyline, Mellaril, vincristine, and cyclophosphamide. It should be remembered that when treating hyponatremia in end-stage patients, severe fluid restriction may not be accepted by the patient and family. In patients with SIADH, demeclocycline may ameliorate the symptoms associated with hyponatremia and allow more flexibility in fluid intake.

OTHER METABOLIC ABNORMALITIES

Additional, potentially reversible, symptomatic chemical abnormalities that may manifest as altered consciousness or mental function include disorders of potassium and magnesium metabolism, which are as likely to be iatrogenic in origin due to the primary terminal diagnosis or to co-existent morbidities. Testing for these, as well as for hypothyroidism, which is a fairly common late consequence of prior cancer treatment; azotemia caused by drug toxicity or obstructive uropathy; and hepatic encephalopathy; is indicated when therapeutic intervention is contemplated.

MEDICATION PROBLEMS

Changes in mentation and level of consciousness that are attributable to medications occur frequently towards the end of life. The need to control a multiplicity of symptoms nearly always provokes a proliferative pharmaceutical response with a resulting enhanced probablility of drug interactions. Declining hepatic and renal function may be associated with increasingly abnormal pharmacokinetics resulting in accumulation of a drug or its active metabolites to toxic levels. Empirical dose adjustments may sometimes be effective and adequate. This approach is commonly followed when titrating opioid analgesics. However, measurement of blood levels may sometimes be necessary to identify which of multiple drugs is responsible for the toxic side effects. When in doubt, blood level determinations may be essential before and after adjusting medications such as anticonvulsants, for which it is important to maintain a therapeutic range.

NEUROLOGIC ABNORMALITIES

The appearance or exacerbation of lethargy, weakness, confusion, headaches, memory loss, altered mental state, psychosis, focal neurologic deficits, seizures, nausea, and vomiting may indicate brain metastases, infectious encephalopathy, or cerebral infarction or hemorrhage. As will be discussed, radiotherapy and corticosteroids relieve clinical symptoms in 70 to 90 percent of patients with brain metastases, although the median survival is only 4 to 5 months from institution of treatment.

Because of the potential for meaningful palliative benefit and reversal of symptoms, imaging studies to confirm the diagnosis, and to rule out cerebral infarction or hemorrhage, can be considered even in end-stage patients with otherwise reasonable performance status. On the other hand, when imaging studies suggest the likelihood of carcinomatous meningitis; or, when, despite negative studies, the clinical index of suspicion is high, a confirmatory lumbar puncture is probably unnecessary in an end-stage patient because the response to palliative intrathecal therapy is generally poor.

Imaging studies can also be significant in evaluating neuropsychiatric dysfunction in patients with end-stage AIDS. Symptoms attributable to cerebral toxoplasmosis may decrease with systemic therapy, whereas the prognosis for even palliative improvement in patients with primary CNS lymphoma, progressive multifocal leukoencephalopathy, and AIDS dementia continues to be dismal.

INFECTIONS

Infections and sepsis are a common cause of altered mental status when patients are near the end of life. The issue of whether infections should be evaluated and treated will be discussed later.

Pain

Patients with advanced cancer and well-controlled symptoms who develop new onset of increasingly severe pain invariably have evidence for progressive parenchymal, soft-tissue, or neuroinvasive disease, or pathologic fracture in a site of pre-existent osseous metastasis. Most often, careful physical assessment will suffice to establish the etiology (e.g., painful hepatomegaly associated with progressive liver metastases). Sometimes, however, radiographic and/or radionuclide imaging (bone scan) will be necessary to identify and treat new sites of skeletal metastasis and impending or overt pathologic fracture.

Particular mention should be made of the ambulatory patient with refractory cancer who develops back pain that is often progressive, excrutiating, and unrelenting. Such a patient, unless actively dying, requires immediate evaluation for spinal cord compression. If one waits for the patient to develop evidence of motor, sensory, or autonomic dysfunction, the patient will probably be paraplegic for the rest of life. For those patients with spinal cord compression who are ambulatory at the time of diagnosis, 79 percent continue to be ambulatory on completion of radiotherapy. For those with weakness and who are unable to walk at the time of diagnosis, only 45 percent will be ambulatory on completion of treatment. (Treatment will be discussed in the section on radiotherapy.) In addition to physical and neurologic examination, patients with suspected spinal cord compression will usually also require some combination of plain spine radiographs, bone scan, magnetic resonance imaging, and, now less commonly, contrast myelography. Radiographic studies may also be indicated in patients with terminal noncancer diagnoses, especially for the detection and treatment of painful fractures caused by falls or osteoporosis.

Other Evaluations

Additional examples of diagnostic tests that may be appropriate in select patients near the end of life include chest radiographs for the diagnosis and treatment of symptomatic pleural effusions, echocardiography for constrictive pericardial effusions, electrocardiography for symptomatic supraventricular arrhythmias, Doppler venograms for deep vein thrombosis, prothrombin time/INR to monitor Coumadin anticoagulation, and abdominal radiography for possible mechanical small bowel obstruction. In fact, no test or study should be excluded per se, provided that, in each individual circumstance, it meets the test of therapeutic applicability for palliation of symptoms, and is acceptable to the patient.

Palliative Chemotherapy

Currently, there are more than 60 individual chemotherapeutic drugs approved by the U.S. Food and Drug Adminstration for use in the "war on cancer." These include cytotoxins of multiple biochemical classes, hormonally active agents, cytokines, vaccines, and monoclonal antibodies, as well as cytoprotective drugs to prevent or reduce toxicity, and adjunctive medications intended to boost the efficacy of the primary chemotherapeutic agents. Unfortunately, despite continued improvements in screening, locoregional control, and adjuvant therapy—which have translated into higher cure rates and greater survival—recurrent metastatic disease still occurs commonly, and usually with a fatal outcome.

Notwithstanding the extensive armamentarium described, for most cancers, patients with metastatic disease are essentially incurable, with disease progression leading to symptomatic morbidity and inevitable death. Consequently, with a few notable exceptions such as testicular carcinoma, Hodgkin's disease, and the acute leukemias, current treatments for metastatic cancer should be regarded as palliative therapy.

Patients with advanced metastatic malignancy usually experience multiple progressive symptoms including nociceptive and neuropathic pain, fatigue, anxiety, depression, malaise, anorexia, nausea, dysphagia, breathlessness, and cough. Curiously, however, as judged from the contents of most published reports, clinical trial design has traditionally ignored symptom relief as a therapeutic endpoint, concentrating instead on analyses of objective measurable tumor response or prolongation of life. In fact, although these latter endpoints are scientifically significant to physician investigators, they are less important to patients than the effect of treatment on symptoms and quality of life. For example, when given the choice between supportive care and chemotherapy in one study, 22 percent of patients chose chemotherapy for a survival benefit of 3 months, but 68 percent of patients chose chemotherapy if it substantially reduced symptoms without prolonging life.

In many randomized studies, the survival of patients in the treatment arm is compared to a matched cohort of patients who receive "best supportive care," a concept that usually includes antibiotics, analgesics, transfusions, corticosteroids, or any other symptomatic therapy including psychotherapy. Supportive care is generally defined as "the best care available as judged by the attending physician, according to institutional standards for each centre." However, few studies indicate how this supportive care is actually defined as "best." In light of published surveys in which even medical oncologists acknowledge that pain and symptom management in cancer patients continues to be suboptimal, it is disturbing to note how infrequently details of symptom management and response are provided for both treatment and "best supportive care" groups in published clinical trials. Furthermore, few trials, including those in which quality of life is assessed, control for the effect of adjunctive treatments such as antiemetics, corticosteroids, and hematopoietic growth factors that are commonly offered to chemotherapy patients and that may not necessarily be included as "best supportive care."

The emphasis on objective tumor response and survival analysis rather than on symptom improvement has created another paradox. To detect small,

but statistically significant differences in survival, and in an effort to minimize the incidence of life-threatening toxicity, most clinical trials in advanced metastatic disease exclude patients with poor performance status, those who are sickest, most symptomatic, and therefore, in greatest need of palliative intervention. For example, a study of irinotecan in patients with far-advanced colorectal carcinoma excluded patients with bulky liver or lung metastases, large abdominal masses, or unresolved bowel obstruction. Logically, one would anticipate that a truly effective palliative treatment would have the greatest effect on patients with the most severe symptoms. Obviously, the fear of causing toxic side effects that would negatively influence the quality of remaining life must be a valid and important concern in terminally ill patients, and analysis of toxicity is a vital component of any legitimate palliative study. However, arbitrary exclusion of patients with poor performance status and severe symptomatology creates the possibility that, in the future, patients with this profile will be denied access to a treatment shown in the trial to have palliative benefit and relatively low risk of toxicity, though never tested in that particular patient population.

Recently, outcomes related to symptom control and quality of life assessment are being incorporated into oncology clinical trials. It is generally assumed that unrelieved and increasing patient discomfort and disability translates into an ever-worsening quality of life. Conversely, symptom relief and functional improvement should logically be associated with higher quality of life scores. However, as previously pointed out, the correlation between symptomatology and quality of life is frequently weak or, on occasions, nonexistent. Therefore, good study design should incorporate both elements of symptom outcomes and quality of life measurement. One measure of symptomatic improvement is termed the "clinical benefit response" (Table 17–3). This is defined as a significant, sustained improvement in pain, performance status, weight, or other relevant symptom, with no deterioration in other symptoms. In assessing pain responses, decreasing opioid usage or a step-down on the WHO analgesic ladder is

Table 17–3

"Clinical Benefit" Response to Chemotherapy

> Sustained improvement in pain
>   Decreased pain with no change in analgesia
>   Same level of pain with less analgesia
> Improvement in performance status
> Stabilization or improvement in weight

often used as an important endpoint and scored as a significant success.

To the extent that decreased analgesic use correlates with decreased pain and increased function and well-being, this is a useful and significant outcome. However, decreased opioid use should not be the goal of and by itself, unless the patient has significant opioid side effects that are worse than the side effects of the new chemotherapy. Preoccupation with analgesic dose reduction as an independent endpoint may inadvertently contribute to refueling the "opiophobia" that has proven to be such an obstacle in achieving good pain management, particularly near the end of life.

A number of reports have been published demonstrating a clinical benefit for chemotherapy for patients with a variety of advanced, end-stage malignancies. Nevertheless, surveys indicate that a significant proportion of physicians recommend only supportive care for patients with widespread metastatic disease, expecting that patients will have a short but peaceful end to their life, protected from the side-effects of chemotherapy. Obviously, chemotherapy is not for every patient. Selection should be performed carefully to spare patients who have little chance to benefit from chemotherapy from exposure to side effects of ineffective treatments. However, as suggested by the following discussion, palliative chemotherapy may sometimes add significantly to patient comfort, even near the end of life.

Bronchogenic Carcinoma

Many symptoms and manifestations of advanced lung cancer are directly attributable to defined ana-

tomic metastases. Examples include somatic pain caused by discrete bone metastases or chest wall invasion, neuropathic pain associated with plexopathies, intractable coughing and hemoptysis attributable to endobronchial tumors, headache, changes in mentation caused by superior vena cava syndrome or brain metastases, and dyspnea caused by malignant pleural effusions. Because locoregional interventions such as radiotherapy are the procedures of choice for palliating such symptoms, systemic chemotherapy is rarely reported in terms of its success in alleviating specific manifestations of metastatic disease. Rather, palliative chemotherapy is usually described in terms of ability to improve quality of life, a parameter that does not always reference specific symptoms such as generalized pain, fatigue, dyspnea, anorexia, wasting, anxiety, and depression.

SMALL-CELL BRONCHOGENIC CARCINOMA

For patients with small-cell bronchogenic carcinoma, however—even in those with extensive disease—systemic chemotherapy may be of significant palliative benefit. With first-line therapy, well-documented response rates of greater than 50 percent have been observed in most studies, with improvement in symptoms and quality of life for most patients. Corresponding substantial increases in symptom-free survival suggest that most patients with small-cell lung cancer who are started on *de novo* chemotherapy should not be thought of, or regard themselves, as recipients of end-of-life care. On the other hand, when patients with small-cell lung cancer relapse after initial therapy, as unfortunately usually occurs, second-line chemotherapy is rarely of objective palliative benefit. However, when there has been an interval of at least several months between cessation of the primary treatment and relapse, reinstitution of the initial chemotherapy regimen, or treatment with oral etoposide, sometimes is associated with temporary tumor regression and improvement in symptoms.

NON-SMALL-CELL BRONCHOGENIC CARCINOMA

For the 75 percent of lung cancer patients who have non-small cell histology, chemotherapy trials with newer regimens incorporating agents such as cisplatin, carboplatin, gemcitabine, paclitaxel, docetaxel, vinorelbine, and irinotecan show 1-year survival rates of 35 to 40 percent in patients with stage IV disease. Is this modest increase in survival associated with sufficient clinical benefit to justify the side effects and toxicity of treatment? Many physicians, from a variety of specialties including primary care, pulmonary medicine, medical oncology, radiation oncology, and thoracic surgery, apparently continue to think not, and continue to recommend supportive care only for patients with stage IV disease.

Some studies suggest that the quality of life may be improved with chemotherapy for patients with metastatic disease as well as those with unresectable stage III disease. However, data supporting this proposition are sparse. A meta-analysis based on 11 randomized controlled trials involving 1190 patients published in 1997 reported that not one trial successfully measured quality of life using QOL assessment instruments (Lopez et al, 1997). However, several trials have documented relief of cancer-related symptoms such as pain, cough, and hemoptysis in approximately 70 percent of patients. Although in most of these trials, patients with poor performance status were excluded to spare them treatment-related toxicity, one study did demonstrate clinical benefit in some patients who were elderly and/or had poor prognostic factors.

Palliative weekly vinorelbine chemotherapy and palliative gemcitabine therapy have provided modest positive results, with about 25 to 40 percent of patients reporting improvements in either performance status or a variety of cancer-related symptoms such as cough, hemoptysis, dyspnea, and pain. In studies with both agents, more patients benefited from chemotherapy than was suggested by the objective response rate, suggesting that symptom palliation may not be dependent on demonstrated tumor regression.

In summary, with increasing attention being paid to symptom relief as a measured outcome in advanced bronchogenic non-small-cell carcinoma, there may be a role for chemotherapy as a valid, palliative intervention for selected patients near the end of life.

Breast and Prostate Carcinoma

Very prevalent, breast and prostate cancers share some characteristics that are of significance in end-of-life care. When patients with either of these malignancies present with advanced metastatic disease, many of them can achieve dramatic symptomatic relief, disease regression, and prolongation of life through the use of relatively nontoxic hormonal treatments.

Another shared characteristic is that patients with systemic breast and prostate carcinoma may have long, chronic courses, particularly when disease is restricted to osseous metastases. Effective palliative interventions, such as radiotherapy and bisphosphonates (see "Bone Pain" later in the chapter), are therefore frequently employed in both diseases even at a time well before the patient is close to the end of life, and their effects are well known and reliable for palliation of symptoms at the end-stage of disease as well.

Breast and prostate carcinoma differ, of course, in their sensitivity to currently available cytotoxic agents, which are usually regarded primarily as life-prolonging tools, and therefore their role purely for the purpose of symptom palliation is rarely reported.

BREAST CANCER

Multiple chemotherapies are active as single agents or in combination for the treatment of metastatic breast cancer. The most common "classic" combinations include cyclophosphamide, doxorubicin, and 5 FU (fluorouracil) (60 percent response rate), and cyclophosphamide, methotrexate, and 5 FU (40 percent response rate). Newer chemotherapeutic drugs have even greater activity both alone and in combinations. These include docetaxel, vinorelbine, paclitaxel, gemcitabine, epirubicin, cisplatin, mitoxantrone, ifosfamide, and an oral 5-FU analogue, capecitabine. Although most patients are treated with several sequential regimens before being judged to have chemotherapy-refractory disease, there is little information about how effective these treatments are in alleviating symptoms. There is a study, however, supporting a role for capeci-tabine as a palliative agent for patients with breast cancer who are refractory to anthracyclines and paclitaxel, demonstrating an overall clinical ben-efit response as positive in 20 percent of patients and stable in 30 percent.

PROSTATE CARCINOMA

In contrast to breast cancer, androgen-indepen-dent prostate carcinoma tends to be refractory to treatment. Second-line hormonal therapy, chemo-therapy (single agent or combination), or various investigational therapies such as monoclonal anti-bodies have not produced durable remissions. However, some chemotherapy regimens have been described as having palliative benefit. In a randomized trial comparing mitoxantrone/pred-nisone (M+P) to prednisone alone, 29 percent of patients receiving M+P had a positive response, defined as a two-point or greater decrease in pain intensity on a six-point pain scale, lasting for a minimum of 6 weeks. Twelve percent of the pa-tients treated with prednisone alone had a similar response ($P = 0.011$). Other patients had stable pain intensity, but were able to reduce their anal-gesic consumption by at least 50%. In a double-blind study, a noncytotoxic agent, suramin, in combination with hydrocortisone (S+H), was associated with a 43 percent pain response with a median duration of 240 days, compared with a placebo regimen (P+H) with a 28% pain response with a median duration of only 69 days. Despite the decrease in pain, performance status and qual-ity of life were similar in both treatment groups, raising the question as to whether there is any dif-ference with regard to total symptom palliation. These studies also do not indicate if there is any advantage for the mitoxantrone or suramin regi-mens compared to alternatives such as radiother-apy or radioisotopes.

Pancreatic Carcinoma

Until recently, chemotherapy was considered ineffective in pancreatic cancer. In recent years,

however, there are data suggesting that various chemotherapeutic agents may improve physical symptoms of patients with advanced disease.

In a single comparative study of patients with advanced pancreatic cancer, gemcitabine was found to be more effective than fluorouracil with respect to survival duration and general clinical status. More significantly, this investigation fos-tered the development of a new system for assess-ing clinical benefit for patients with advanced pancreatic cancer. This system has served as a model to be applied in other clinical trials seeking evidence of chemotherapy-mediated symptom palliation (Table 17–3). The outcome of gem-citabine therapy in more than 3000 patients with advanced pancreatic cancer (80 percent stage IV disease) has now been reported (Storniolo et al, 1999). In this study, which was funded by the drug manufacturer, after approximately 20 weeks the disease-related symptom improvement (de-fined in a fashion similar to clinical benefit) was 18.4 percent, compared to an objective tumor response rate of 12 percent. The median survival was 4.8 months and the 12-month survival was 15 percent. Treatment was discontinued in only 5% of patients due to adverse reactions. The investi-gators contend that these results indicate notable disease-related symptom improvement. The study lacked any control group, however, and did not address other symptoms or manifestations of pan-creatic carcinoma such as obstruction, jaundice, and pruritus. Based on this study, gemcitabine is approved by the United States Food and Drug Administration for the palliative treatment of ad-vanced pancreatic carcinoma.

Other agents reporting to have modest palliative activity in pancreatic carcinoma include a combina-tion of epirubicin, fluorouracil, and folinic acid, and the androgen receptor blocking agent, flutamide.

Colorectal Carcinoma

Conventional palliative chemotherapy for advanced colorectal cancer has been largely restricted to fluorouracil and related agents, often in combina-tion with leucovorin (folinic acid). This combination has been reported to lead to improved QOL in treated patients compared to those treated with "supportive care." Adding cisplatin to fluorouracil and leucovorin suggested that for some patients the quality of life "seemed to be better," while recent studies using irinotecan suggested that fluorouracil-refractory patients had a longer survival, fewer tumor-related symptoms, and a better quality of life than those treated with supportive care alone. Hepatic intra-arterial chemotherapy with 5-FUDR may alleviate discomfort in some patients with extensive liver metastases.

Of interest, there are now data indicating that fluorouracil-based therapy can also decrease QOL. In patients treated with weekly, high-dose 5-FU 24-hour infusions combined with folinic acid, interferon, or both modulators, QOL data revealed significant deterioration in physical functioning, social functioning, role functioning, and global QOL within 8 weeks, particularly in patients who were relatively symptom-free when beginning treatment. Anorexia, fatigue, nausea, vomiting, and diarrhea worsened in all arms of the study. Curiously, the QOL data were not included in the original report, which emphasized a positive tumor response of patients treated with this regimen. The correspondents who revealed the QOL data expressed regret that the patients' point of view was not taken into account in this report.

Other Malignancies

In gastric cancer, four small, randomized trials using combinations such as fluorouracil, leucovorin (folinic acid), and etoposide demonstrated survival and quality of life benefits for patients who received chemotherapy compared to those who received "best supportive care" (Ajani, 1998).

In patients with advanced transitional-cell carcinoma of the urinary tract who had previously received cisplatin, therapy with gemcitabine provided subjective symptomatic relief from pain, cystitis, dysuria, hematuria, and peripheral edema. Toxicity was reported as mild, and consisted of influenza-like symptoms and myelosuppression. The median survival was 5 months.

Gemcitabine is also reported to have activity in patients with refractory germ-cell tumors. However, the published reports have no information on symptom response or QOL.

Frail, elderly patients with refractory anemia with excess blasts in transformation or with overt acute myelocytic leukemia are extremely difficult to manage. Most of these patients do poorly with intensive induction chemotherapy. Aside from symptoms due to anemia, which can be managed with red blood cell transfusions, patients often suffer from recurrent infections and from bleeding complications. Life expectancy with supportive care only is usually 1 to 2 months. However, in one study, most patients who received a weekly regimen of low-dose cytosine arabinoside and thioguanine for at least 6 to 10 weeks became independent of platelet and red cell transfusions for periods of up to 2 years (Munshi and Tricot, 1997). The treatment was well tolerated and suitable for outpatient palliation.

Conclusions on the Role of Palliative Chemotherapy Near the End of Life

An objective assessment of the studies presented is admittedly somewhat deflating. Not a single study revealed a truly dramatic reversal in symptoms, although such an expectation is undoubtedly unrealistic for patients with such advanced disease. Nevertheless, as increased attention is concentrated on the effects of chemotherapy on palliation of symptoms, a clearer picture should emerge as to those circumstances in which it will contribute to overall patient comfort near the end of life. While one must remain cautious, the data suggest that chemotherapy may at times be an appropriate palliative intervention for specific patients with specific malignancies. It is incumbent upon the hospice and palliative care teams who offer such palliative chemotherapy to ensure that the goals of therapy are clearly defined, for themselves as well as for the patient and family. All concerned must also have the ability, resources, and willingness to treat toxic side effects in a manner consistent with the overall needs and desires of the patient.

Palliative Radiotherapy

Compared to chemotherapy, the role of radiation therapy in palliative, end-of-life care is well established, and associated with reproducible and highly effective outcomes. Pain, bleeding, and obstruction, particularly when attributable to localized primary, recurrent, or metastatic tumors, can often be alleviated with minimal toxicity with external-beam radiation or with brachytherapy. Furthermore, although endoscopic or surgical procedures are sometimes regarded as competing alternatives to radiotherapy for local disease manifestations, the option of multimodality treatment may offer even more effective and longer-lasting palliation. On occasion, symptoms attributable to disseminated disease, such as generalized pain associated with widespread skeletal metastases, may be alleviated with systemic radionuclides or hemibody radiation.

The key objective in administering palliative radiotherapy near the end of life is to achieve durable symptom relief consistent with the expected prognosis, by delivering a rapidly effective dose in as short a time possible, and while avoiding or minimizing short-term, toxic side effects. Protracted treatment schedules can be fatiguing and even debilitating for patients with advanced cancer, who sometimes will discontinue radiation treatments rather than complete a lengthy sequence of daily visits. For this reason, palliative care specialists increasingly advocate short fractionation schemes or even single-fraction treatments for patients with end-stage disease. On the other hand, many radiation oncologists continue to advocate higher-dose, long-fractionation protocols, for reasons of greater and longer-lasting efficacy, and for fear of late-onset side effects. In a survey of 2500 members of the American Society for Therapeutic Radiology and Oncology, long-fractionation schemes were advocated by 90 percent of the physicians. This tendency was most pronounced among older radiation oncologists and in nonacademic, private, community practice settings. Although data suggest that aggressive, protracted treatments may be advantageous for patients in whom the expected life-span is not short, the benefit shrinks to irrelevancy near the end of life, at which point effective, short-fractionation schemes seem to make more sense.

In patients with advanced cancer, clinical problems traditionally treated with radiotherapy are listed in Table 17–4, and will be discussed next.

Bone Pain

The pain from osseous metastases is one of the most common indications for palliative radiotherapy. Localized external-beam therapy will provide prompt pain relief in the treated area for 80 to 90 percent of treated individuals. Performance status may be a significant determinant of both the degree and duration of response. Patients with poor performance status often achieve less satisfactory and less durable pain relief than those with better performance scores. However, duration of response may be less important for patients whose life expectancy is limited to no more than several

Table 17–4

Indications for Palliative Radiotherapy

Bone pain secondary to osseous metasteses
   Impending pathologic fracture
   Back pain and impending spinal cord
     compression
Global and focal neurologic deficits associated
     with brain metastases
Pulmonary symptoms due to primary or
     metastatic disease to the lung
   Cough
   Hemoptysis
   Dyspnea
   Superior vena cava obstruction
Malignant dysphagia due to tumor obstruction
Painful hepatomegaly
Pelvic masses associated with pain and/or
     obstruction

weeks. It is unclear as to whether tumor type and histology is an independent variable influencing response rate. Some studies suggest that radiotherapy palliation is less successful for patients with bone metastases from non-small-cell lung cancer than for patients with either breast or prostate cancer. Other reports indicate no such difference.

EXTERNAL-BEAM RADIATION THERAPY

The optimum dose/fractionation schedule continues to be a matter of controversy. Since the initial large, randomized trial by the Radiation Therapy Oncology Group (RTOG) over 20 years ago (Tong, 1982; Hoegler, 1997), a number of studies confirm that low-dose, short-fractionation schedules can be less intrusive for the patient and clinically as effective for relief of bone pain as more protracted treatment programs. In one recent randomized trial (280 patients), a single 10-Gy treatment was as effective as a course of 22.5 Gy in five fractions in the management of painful bone metastases (Gaze et al, 1997). Another randomized trial showed that a single fraction of 8 Gy was as effective as 20 Gy in four fractions in relieving pain from bone metastases (Nielson et al, 1998). There was no significant difference in the duration of pain relief, number of new painful sites, or need for reirradiation. Toxicity was minor. Although single-fraction doses as low as 4 Gy can be effective in some patients, there is a dose–response effect, particularly regarding rapidity of pain relief and probability of pain relief after 4 weeks, suggesting that 8 Gy is probably the lowest optimal single fraction that should be recommended.

On the other hand, there are studies, including a reanalysis of the RTOG trial, suggesting that higher dose radiotherapy administered over longer time frames is more effective in achieving complete and durable relief of pain. Because of differences in study design, an evidence-based resolution to the dose/fractionation controversy is not yet apparent. In some trials, extent of pain relief is assessed by the treating physicians rather than by the patients. Other studies use variable patient pain assessment tools. Some investigations incorporate reduction in analgesic usage as a measured outcome. Other complicating factors include the development of new sites of pain outside the irradiated field, and the subsequent addition of systemic therapy following the initial radiotherapy. A reasonable conclusion at this time is that for patients near the end of life, low-dose, short schedules appear to offer the prospect of adequate pain relief within the expected survival time frame, while sparing the patient the discomfort and time expenditure associated with lengthy fractionation regimens. For patients with longer life expectancies, a more protracted course of radiotherapy may offer significant advantages.

End-stage patients with advanced malignancies and skeletal metastasis usually go on to develop multiple bone lesions and generalized pain. Occasionally, despite optimal use of opioids and adjuvant analgesic medications, bone pain may continue to be a major challenge. For some of these patients, systemic radiation treatment, either hemibody radiotherapy or injection of radionuclides, may provide effective palliation. Patients receiving hemibody radiotherapy usually receive 6 Gy to the upper half of the body and 8 Gy to the lower body. With this technique, approximately 70 percent of 168 patients in an RTOG study achieved some pain relief, and pain relief was complete in 20 percent. Half the patients had relief of pain within 48 hours, and 80 percent reported relief within 1 week, suggesting that this modality may be effective even in symptomatic patients with very short prognoses. Recurrent pain within the irradiated field was one fourth of that for conventional fractionated treatment. The main toxicities were nausea and vomiting, myelosuppression (severe in 10 percent of patients) and pneumonitis (which occurred infrequently when the dose to the upper body did not exceed 6 Gy). However, it should be anticipated that these and other toxicities can be significantly greater in patients who have been previously treated with chemotherapy and other radiopotentiating agents. Nausea and vomiting can usually be successfully controlled with ondansetron or similar antiemetic medication. Lower hemibody radiotherapy has also been reported to alleviate symptoms in platinum-refractory patients with ovarian carcinoma. Of 33 patients in one study, 70 percent obtained relief of symptoms for longer than 6 months, with a median duration of response of 11 months (Gelblum et al, 1998).

SYSTEMIC RADIOISOTOPES

Systemic radioisotopes are also effective for the management of painful osseous metastases. One major advantage is that selective absorption limits the exposure of normal tissue, thus reducing toxicity and theoretically increasing the therapeutic ratio. Systemic radionuclide therapy may therefore be suitable for patients who have had even extensive external-beam radiotherapy. However, there is risk of significant myelosupression, including severe thrombocytopenia, in patients who have been heavily treated with prior chemotherapy. Systemic radioisotopes are rarely effective for patients with predominantly lytic lesions and no radionuclide uptake on a bone scan. Therefore, a nuclear bone scan should be performed in assessing appropriateness of radionuclide therapy. Urinary incontinence, inability to follow radiation safety precautions, and severe renal insufficiency are also contraindications to radionuclide treatment.

Of the radioisotopes available, strontium-89 has been most extensively studied, particularly in patients with refractory prostate and breast carcinoma. Pain relief is achieved after administration of strontium-89 in about half the patients treated. Symptomatic relief rarely occurs within 4 weeks, and may not be manifested for up to 3 months. In fact, during the first several days after receiving radiostrontium, some patients may have a flare reaction similar to that experienced by patients starting hormonal therapy, with a resultant transient intensification of pain. Patients should be warned about this possible effect and receive additional analgesics in sufficient dosage to control the increased level of pain. Because of the relatively long time period before pain control is achieved with strontium-89, this intervention is

not appropriate for those patients whose life expectancy is less than 2 to 3 months.

There is no evidence that radiostrontium is more advantageous than conventional external beam radiotherapy. In a randomized trial comparing strontium-89 treatment with localized radiotherapy and hemibody radiotherapy, all treatments provided equally effective pain relief that was sustained for at least 3 months (Brundage et al, 1998). Orally administered phosphorus-32, which is considerably less expensive than strontium-89, has no greater toxicity and equal efficacy in terms of palliation of pain and duration of response as strontium-89, and may therefore represent a more cost effective alternative.

A more recently studied radioisotope, samarium-153, appears to have a more rapid onset of action than strontium-89. However, further experience is necessary to better understand the role of this agent in end-of-life care.

IMPENDING PATHOLOGIC FRACTURE

With regards to the prophylaxis and treatment of pathologic bone fractures, radiotherapy primarily plays an adjunctive role to surgical fixation (described later in the chapter). Painful lesions that involve at least 60 percent of the cortex are at risk for impending fracture. An improved prognostic system that combines four roentgenographic and clinical risk factors into a single score appears to reliably predict which patients can be safely managed with radiotherapy alone, and which patients will require orthopedic intervention. For high-risk patients, there is little evidence that radiotherapy alone is effective in preventing pathologic fractures, particularly in weight-bearing bones such as the femur. Rather, internal surgical fixation is an effective, generally preferred, palliative intervention that may benefit ambulatory patients even near the end of life, provided that death is not anticipated within a very short time period. Postoperative radiotherapy is usually recommended to forestall additional tumor-induced bone lysis, and to allow new bone synthesis. The usual dose is 20 Gy in five fractions, although single-dose radiotherapy may also be effective. In patients who are not surgical candidates because of poor performance status or short prognosis, single-fraction radiotherapy may alleviate pain, as described earlier, and the chance of fracture may be reduced through the use of weight-supporting devices or immobilization of the affected extremity.

BACK PAIN AND IMPENDING SPINAL CORD COMPRESSION

The vertebral column is the most common site for skeletal metastases. Spinal cord compression due to extradural tumor growth occurs in 5 percent of patients with cancer, and affects an estimated 20,000 patients per year in the United States alone. The most common primary tumors associated with spinal metastasis and cord compression are breast, lung, and prostate carcinoma, and lymphoma. As previously indicated, maintaining a high index of suspicion and early diagnosis is imperative to avert permanent neurologic damage.

The key alerting symptom is back pain which is typically progressive, unrelenting, and often described as excrutiating. The pain is usually worse with recumbency, may awaken the patient from sleep, and often persists despite even properly prescribed opioid analgesics. The pain can usually be localized with vertebral palpation. With progression, which may sometimes be dramatic and rapid, patients may evidence signs of motor weakness due to radiculopathy or plexopathy, sensory dysfunction including numbness, paresthesias, or loss of tactile sensation, and/or autonomic dysfunction including urinary or fecal incontinence. The probability for reversibility decreases with increasing neurologic impairment. A differential diagnosis includes epidural or subdural abscess or hematoma, herniated disk, carcinomatous meningitis, radiation or chemotherapy myelopathy, and the extremely rare intramedullary spinal cord metastasis.

The diagnostic work-up has already been discussed, and should include a complete physical and neurologic examination, plain spine radio-graphs, and most commonly, magnetic resonance imaging (MRI) of the entire vertebral column as there may be multiple levels of cord compression. When MRI is available, contrast myelography is rarely necessary.

Aggressive treatment may not be indicated for patients who are very near death. For patients who are already paraplegic, neurologic recovery is highly improbable, but they may nevertheless require treatment for pain relief. When spinal cord compression is first suspected, dexamethasone (10 mg IV initially followed by 4 mg orally every 6 hours) is usually initiated, and continued during the course of radiotherapy, which is currently the sole recommended treatment for most patients with spinal cord compression. On completion of radiation, dexamethasone should be tapered and discontinued, if possible, to avoid corticosteroid toxicity. Surgical decompression is generally not recommended, particularly in patients with refractory systemic disease who are near the end of life, except for extremely rare circumstances in which there is spinal instability, compression by bone, or failure of previous radiotherapy, and the patient's overall condition and prognosis justifies the morbidity of surgical intervention. Even then, it should be remembered that patients with poor performance status, as typically seen in hospice patients, have unfavorable outcomes and high surgical mortality.

With radiotherapy, nearly 80 percent of patients with spinal cord compression who are ambulatory at the time of diagnosis remain so on completion of treatment. Unfortunately, early intervention continues to be the exception rather than the rule. In one reported series, 78 percent of the patients were nonambulatory when initially seen by the radiation oncologist. The treatment volume should include 1 to 2 vertebrae above and below the level of the block. Because of concern for radiation myelopathy, most radiation oncologists prescribe treatment courses of 20 Gy in five fractions or 30 Gy in ten fractions. There are no data concerning the use of a single high dose of radiation in spinal cord compression, but it has been suggested that this might be a reasonable approach for patients with a prognosis of brief survival.

Global and Focal Neurologic Deficits Associated with Brain Metastases

Because of potentially dire ramifications for diminished mental status, functional abilities, and overall quality of life, the development of brain metastases can be devastating for patients and their caregivers, even in the face of otherwise extensive and refractory metastatic cancer. Typical symptoms, which may be attributable to tissue damage and/or increased intracranial pressure, include anorexia, nausea, vomiting, fatigue, weakness, lethargy, confusion, headaches, memory loss, altered mental state, psychosis, focal deficits, seizures, and coma. In patients with end-stage disease, brain metastases are more commonly multiple rather than solitary, but in any event the degree of disability is often disproportionate to the bulk of tumor.

For patients with new or recurrent solitary brain metastases and no or controlled extracranial disease, surgical resection or stereotaxic radiosurgery are sometimes options of choice. Because such conditions do not pertain to patients with refractory, end-stage disease, these modalities are inappropriate for end-of-life care. Indeed, it has been demonstrated that for patients with solitary brain metastasis and active extracranial disease, surgery plus radiotherapy offers no advantage over radiotherapy alone.

Whole-brain radiotherapy does effectively palliate clinical symptoms in 70 to 90 percent of patients with solitary or multiple brain metastases, with 75 to 80 percent of remaining survival time spent in an improved or stable neurologic state. A course of 20 Gy in five fractions is no less effective than a higher-dose, more protracted schedule. An ultrarapid schedule consisting of a single dose of 10 Gy was inferior in terms of rate of complete disappearance of neurologic symptoms and duration of symptom improvement, but might nonetheless be an option for some patients with advanced systemic disease.

Acute toxic effects of whole-brain radiotherapy are usually confined to erythema of the scalp, dry desquamation, and alopecia, provided that the patient is simultaneously treated with corticosteroids, as is traditional. The late side effects of cranial radiotherapy, including dementia, may be confidently discounted for patients receiving end-of-life care.

For some patients with brain metastases, manifestations of systemically advanced disease, and a brief anticipated life expectancy of only several weeks, the best palliative approach might be to avoid radiotherapy and use pharmacologic supportive measures such as corticosteroids and anticonvulsants for symptom management. In fact, patients with brain metastases whose symptoms fail to improve in response to corticosteroids probably have irreversible damage, and are unlikely to benefit from more aggressive measures such as radiotherapy.

Pulmonary Symptoms Due to Primary or Metastatic Lung Disease

In addition to complaints attributable to distant metastases, patients with advanced, end-stage bronchogenic carcinoma often present with a constellation of symptoms related to the primary intrathoracic tumor that may be palliated with external-beam radiotherapy or endoscopic brachytherapy.

Common symptoms related to the primary or metastatic intrathoracic tumors include chest pain, cough, hemoptysis, dyspnea, dysphagia, hoarseness, fatigue, anxiety, sleep difficulties, and a general sense of prostration. External-beam radiotherapy for symptom control is extensively used, although an optimal dosing schedule continues to be the subject of investigation. Studies tend to favor short-course radiotherapy in advanced disease, with a single 10-Gy dose sufficient for adequate palliation of patients with a poor performance status. For patients with better performance status, the 17-Gy dose in two weekly fractions appears to increase the durability of the palliative response.

Airway obstruction by endobronchial tumors is associated with distressing symptoms of cough, hemoptysis, and air hunger, and is often associated with atelectasis and postobstructive pneumonia. There is little evidence concerning the utility of external-beam radiotherapy in restoring airway patency and alleviating obstructive symptoms. However, external radiation may be a useful adjunctive technique following endoscopic interventions such as laser therapy, photodynamic therapy, and/or stent placement that can provide rapid symptomatic relief (discussed later).

Intraluminal brachytherapy, in which radioactive sources are placed endoscopically at the site of endobronchial obstruction, is quite effective in alleviating dyspnea, although only about one fourth of the patients will have complete relief. Cough, hemoptysis, and postobstructive pneumonia also generally improve. Intraluminal brachytherapy may be associated with acute hemoptysis, which may at times be massive and life threatening.

Patients with mass lesions in the chest may present with signs and symptoms of superior vena caval (SVC) compression, a complication that usually causes considerable discomfort. Depending on the duration of onset, symptoms attributable to mediastinal edema include dyspnea, orthopnea, cough, hoarseness, vocal cord paralysis, dysphagia, chest pain, and syncope. Coexistent cerebral hypertension may cause headache, visual disturbances, dizziness, somnolence, altered states of consciousness, and seizures. Typical physical findings include tachypnea and tachycardia; fixed dilatation of the neck and arm veins; dilatation of the thoracic collateral circulation; cyanosis; facial plethora; conjunctival, facial, and upper extremity edema; and increased intracranial pressure. Although SVC syndrome is traditionally regarded as a medical emergency, the onset is usually gradual and only rarely is the presentation rapid and life threatening. Rapid acuity of onset is, however, associated with a poorer response to treatment.

When SVC syndrome is the presenting manifestation of an undiagnosed malignancy, it is important to establish a histologic diagnosis, to identify patients with small-cell lung cancer or lymphoma who could benefit from systemic therapy. In end-of-life patients, however, in whom the diagnosis is known, and in whom systemic treatment is no longer relevant, there would seem to be no reason to delay the initiation of palliative radiotherapy. It should be remembered, however, that in 10 percent of cases, SVC syndrome in cancer patients may be from nonmalignant causes, increasingly from intravascular thrombosis associated with central venous catheters or other indwelling access devices. Patients in whom this etiology is suspected usually require anticoagulation and, sometimes, thrombolytic therapy.

Immediate measures for the management of SVC syndrome include administration of oxygen and diuretics and elevation of the head. Corticosteroids have traditionally been ordered routinely, but their use would seem indicated only where there is respiratory or central nervous system compromise. A brief course of radiotherapy to the thoracic inlet and mediastinum achieves good to excellent relief of symptoms as early as 3 to 4 days later in 80 percent of patients. Traditional treatment is 20 to 30 Gy in 5 to 10 fractions, but there is evidence that a single pulse dose may be sufficient for symptom relief. Following radiotherapy, SVC syndrome may recur in 10 to 15 percent of patients. Depending on their overall condition, such patients may be candidates for intravenous insertion of an expandable stent. Furthermore, recent experience suggests that percutaneous stent insertion may be preferable to radiotherapy even for the initial treatment of SVC obstruction (discussed later). With this alternative available, surgical bypass would be hard to justify in the context of end-of-life care.

Malignant Dysphagia

In addition to radiotherapy, potential palliative therapies for advanced esophageal cancer near the end of life include chemotherapy, endoscopic procedures (discussed later), and combinations of these. External beam radiotherapy (EBRT) is effective and non-invasive, but relief of dysphagia occurs only over a period of 4 to 6 weeks. Therefore, the major role for EBRT in patients with a short prognosis is as an adjunct to other palliative interventions. In one report, combination of EBRT and chemotherapy with fluorouracil/leucovorin rendered three patients free of symptoms of complete esophageal obstruction for 10 to 12 months until death. Brachytherapy offers more rapid symptomatic relief, and may be combined with EBRT for a more durable response in patients with a better outlook. For patients with a life expectancy of less than 3 months, brachytherapy alone is generally sufficient. EBRT also enhances the response to laser endoscopy for malignant dysphagia, and reduces the necessity for subsequent therapeutic endoscopy to maintain lifelong palliation. However, although the optimal palliative approach for malignant dysphagia is yet to be determined, it appears that insertion of a self-expanding metallic, membrane-coated stent may be the procedure of choice, with a prompt response and successful palliation of symptoms expected in more than 95 percent of cases.

Painful Hepatomegaly, Pelvic Soft-Tissue Masses, and Other Indications

Pain due to hepatic capsular distension from metastatic disease can be diminished in 75 to 90 percent of patients who complete a course of radiotherapy to the entire liver. Complete pain relief is achieved in about half of the patients within a median time of 10 to 12 days. Using a regimen of 10 fractions of 2 to 3 Gy, the median duration of response is approximately 3 months for patients with an expected survival of 4 to 6 months. Side effects are relatively minimal with about 20 percent of patients experiencing nausea and vomiting. Late hepatic toxicity, although theoretically possible, is essentially a nonconsideration for patients with a short life expectancy. There is no evidence that the use of concomitant chemotherapy or radiosensitizers enhances the palliative response.

Recurrent gynecologic and colorectal tumors often result in pelvic pain and vaginal or rectal

bleeding and/or foul discharge. Single doses of 10 Gy to the pelvis are often effective in relieving symptoms of pain or bleeding even in elderly patients with poor overall performance status. This approach is also effective for relief of pain and bleeding for patients with chemotherapy-refractory ovarian carcinoma. Toxic side effects are generally mild, consisting primarily of diarrhea.

Patients with advanced, refractory myeloproliferative and lymphoproliferative disorders may suffer from massive splenomegaly causing severe episodic abdominal pain, hypersplenism, portal hypertension, "crushed stomach" syndrome, and high-output cardiac failure. Splenic irradiation is effective in relieving pain for several months in approximately 90 percent of treated patients, and in decreasing splenomegaly in about 60 percent. Prior splenic infarctions and subsequent fibrosis often limit the response in terms of reduction in splenic size.

Patients with disseminated breast, lung, and prostate cancer may suffer visual loss secondary to uveal metastases. Because preservation of vision is a significant quality of life issue even near the end of life, uveal metastases should be treated with palliative radiotherapy. Most patients respond to a short, fractionated course of EBRT, administered with a technique that minimizes exposure of the lens, with improved or stabilized vision.

Surgical, Endoscopic, and Other Invasive Interventions

Although invasive interventions are generally looked upon as outside the scope of services that hospice and palliative care programs provide, carefully selected surgical, endoscopic, and other invasive interventions play a definite role in ensuring patients receive state-of-the-art end-of-life care. Potential invasive interventions are listed in Table 17–5, and discussed next.

Table 17–5

Surgical, Endoscopic, and Other Invasive Palliative Interventions

Palliative orthopedic surgery
Palliative amputation
Relief of bowel obstruction
Relief of biliary obstruction
Relief of upper tract obstructive uropathy
Relief of bronchial obstruction
Relief of vascular obstruction
Thoracentesis for pleural effusions
Paracentesis for ascites

Palliative Orthopedic Surgery

Aside from issues of pain management and potential neurologic injury as discussed, progressive osseous metastatic disease is oftentimes associated with ambulatory dysfunction, gait and postural instability, falling, and loss of functional independence, particularly when complicated by incipient or actual pathologic fracture. Moreover, the problem is not confined to advanced oncology patients. The incidence of severe osteopenia and osteomalacia is substantial in frail and elderly patients, particularly so in those with end-stage, chronic cardiovasular, pulmonary, renal, and neurologic illnesses, especially when compounded by nutritional compromise. The incidence of falling in such individuals approaches 80 percent on an annual basis. All too often, these falls result in fractures and other serious disabling injuries that accelerate dying, and materially detract from the quality of remaining life. Previously ambulatory patients often become bed-bound, and in the absence of a strong supportive service such as a hospice team, patients who live independently in their own homes may be placed in nursing homes or other similar facilities for the remainder of their lives. In appropriate circumstances, palliative orthopedic surgery can avert some of these dire outcomes, even for patients with very limited life expectancies.

Long-bone fractures are most common in the femur and humerus. The decision to perform surgery and the surgical technique must be individualized based on patient characteristics, the area of fracture, and the particular qualities of the bone involved. Pain and discomfort caused by humeral fractures can often be managed by immobilizing the involved extremity, especially in patients who are nonambulatory and in whom overall performance status is poor.

In the case of femoral fractures, underlying diagnosis, concurrent illnesses, mental status, performance status, anticipated life expectancy, prefracture ambulatory status, and patient/family goals and wishes are significant factors in the decision-making process. Patients with a short prognosis who were previously nonambulatory for reasons not directly attributable to pathology at the site of fracture probably should not be surgical candidates. Subsequent pain on turning or transferring may be managed with mechanical immobilization of the fractured limb and properly prescribed analgesics. A similar approach could be offered to formerly ambulatory patients whose life expectancy is estimated to be less than a month, recognizing that some of these patients might prefer an orthopedic intervention that could get them quickly back on their feet. These patients and families should be advised, however, that it is unusual for patients with such short life expectancies to be successfully discharged postoperatively.

Although cast immobilization is an excellent option in many cases for younger, non-tumor patients with femoral fractures who can afford to invest 8 to 10 weeks in the healing process, patients near the end of life rarely can afford that kind of time. Thus, for end-stage patients, regardless of the underlying diagnosis, internal medullary rod fixation for intertrochanteric and shaft fractures, and prosthetic reconstruction for fractures of the femoral head and neck, are often recommended. For patients with pathologic fractures, bone cement is commonly added for further stabilization, and postoperative radiotherapy may be offered depending on the overall prognosis. Fixation of long-bone fractures may be accomplished with minimal blood loss or morbidity, and patients can progress to immediate weight bearing the day after surgery. After internal fixation, 96 percent of patients experience good or excellent relief of pain.

In contrast, patients with acetabular fractures require extensive joint reconstruction, surgery has significant potential for morbidity and complications, and fewer patients experience good or excellent pain relief. These extensive procedures are rarely applicable to patients receiving end-of-life care.

Palliative Amputation

In caring for patients with terminal diseases, a recommendation to amputate an extremity is frequently a source of conflict for patients and family members, for patients/families and physicians, and among physicians with differing perceptions of how best to help the patient. This potential for disagreement is most pronounced in patients with end-stage, chronic, nonmalignant diseases, usually associated with multiple comorbidities, who develop vascular compromise and gangrene, and who were not perceived as imminently dying prior to the acute event. In these circumstances, many physicians believe that withholding surgical intervention in deference to a patient's wishes is a violation of their professional integrity as well the ethical principles of beneficence and nonmaleficence. There is also concern that amputation may be the most effective palliative intervention for controlling pain and foul drainage even in patients with a relatively short prognosis, although delineated "dry gangrene" is not invariably associated with severe pain or infection. It should also be recognized that very few end-of-life patients will be candidates for postamputation prostheses or rehabilitation.

As with all decision making, satisfactory conflict resolution depends on a careful and critical assessment of the patient's baseline physical, mental, and psychological function, and rigorous definition of the goals after amputation in the context of the overall prognosis and potential for restoration of function. There must also be a truthful informed consent process, and ultimately, respect for the patient's wishes as expressed either by an advance directive or by a properly delegated health care surrogate. Consultation with an experienced ethics committee is often useful and advisable in these circumstances.

For patients with locally advanced malignancies, even in the presence of extensive metastatic disease, palliative amputation may be necessary to control local pain, fungation, or the prospect of major bleeding. Although major amputations are often viewed as offering little to already compromised patients, they can dramatically improve the quality of life in carefully selected patients. Although so aggressive a palliative approach is probably not applicable to most end-stage patients with advanced metastatic cancer, amputation should at least be considered for patients in whom uncontrolled symptoms due to locally advanced disease are the key determinant in the shortened life expectancy.

Bowel Obstruction

Small bowel obstruction commonly occurs in patients with end-stage, refractory ovarian, colorectal, and gastric carcinoma, and less frequently in patients with metastatic breast cancer, lung cancer, and melanoma. In patients with extensive systemic disease, obstruction, which commonly fluctuates between partial and complete, is usually associated with multiple extraluminal metastatic implants. Consequently, surgery, even when technically feasible, rarely results in palliation of significant duration. In one series, only a bit more than half the patients survived more than 60 days postoperatively, and nearly half of these individuals had intermittent symptoms of obstruction until death. Clinical features predicting a poor surgical outcome include diffuse intraperitoneal carcinomatosis; palpable abdominal masses; recurrent ascites; cachexia, especially in elderly patients; poor nutritional status; hypoalbuminemia; malignant pleural effusions; and extensive hepatic or pulmonary metastases. Therefore, medical management including the use of octreotide, opioids, anticholinergic drugs, corticosteroids, antiemetics such as haloperidol, and (in the absence of colicky pain) motility enhancing agents, is generally the preferred approach near the end of life (see Chapter 8, Gastroinestinal Symptoms). Should intractable vomiting persist, a percutaneous venting gastrostomy is a superior technique to both nasogastric suctioning and operative gastrostomy.

For patients with unresectable or recurrent colorectal or gynecologic carcinomas, large bowel obstruction may be relieved with a diverting colostomy. However, this procedure rarely controls symptoms of pain, tenesmus, incontinence, and bleeding due to progressive local disease. Palliative surgery to address these complications is often associated with substantial morbidity, and mortality of greater than 10 percent.

Endoscopic procedures can provide effective palliation with less complications. Endoscopic laser photocoagulation allows effective palliation in 85 to 95 percent of the patients, with negligible mortality and treatment complications in less than 10 percent of patients so treated. Photodynamic therapy with a porfimer sodium laser may further enhance the response. For patients with left colonic obstruction, expandable metallic stents placed with fluoroscopic and endoscopic guidance effectively relieve symptoms of obstruction 80 to 90 percent of the time. Most patients are able to resume an oral diet within 24 hours. Although some series claim to encounter no complications, others report complications such as mild rectal bleeding, abdominal pain, pseudo-obstructive episodes due to fecal impaction, and occlusive tumor ingrowth into the stent lumen in about 5 to 10 percent of patients. The duration of effective stent function ranged from several weeks to more than 1 year, and almost always exceeded the patient's lifespan. Stent placement requires less inpatient time and appears to be more cost effective than a surgical colostomy. When appropriate, stent placement may be part of a multimodal palliative plan incorporating laser therapy and local radiotherapy or brachytherapy.

Malignant Dysphagia

As indicated, for palliation of the symptoms of malignant dysphagia, external radiotherapy and brachytherapy are most effective when used in conjunction with endoscopic interventions. A variety of techniques have proven effective including prosthetic stents, dilatation, laser therapy, and photodynmaic therapy. Treatment with self-expanding, membrane-coated metallic stents has a good and prompt effect on dysphagia, and has been perhaps the greatest recent advance in endoscopic palliation of malignant dysphagia and esophagorespiratory fistulas. Compared to radiotherapy and chemotherapy, in which dysphagia is relieved in about 50 percent of treated patients, 80 to 90 percent of patients treated with stent insertion are free of dysphagia. The membrane coating prevents or retards tumor ingrowth into the stent. Complications are unusual, but include bleeding, perforation, and mediastinitis.

Endoscopic palliation with Nd:YAG laser therapy appears to have a complementary role to other techniques including dilatation, stent placement and radiotherapy. As a solitary modality, laser therapy is usually administered at weekly intervals, with improvement in dysphagia observed after 3 to 4 weeks in 80 to 90 percent of patients. With the addition of external radiotherapy after initial laser treatment, the need for further endoscopy was substantially decreased. As a quality of life issue, rapid restoration of the ability to swallow both food and secretions renders endoscopic stent placement an appropriate palliative intervention for patients with even a very short life expectancy. On the other hand, mechanical dilatation, laser, photodynamic, and radiation therapy may have a complementary role for patients who are likely to survive long enough to benefit. These modalities also help in managing obstruction at the gastric cardia where stent placement may be technically difficult.

Biliary Obstruction

Biliary stenosis or obstruction in patients with pancreatic carcinoma, cholangiocarcinoma, or extensive liver metastases is almost always accompanied by extremely distressing symptoms of jaundice, pruritus, anorexia, indigestion, nausea, vomiting, and wasting. With the exception of patients with a very short life expectancy, alleviation of these symptoms by endoscopic, percutaneous, or surgical bypass procedures often results in tangible improvement in both physical and psychological well-being. Currently, surgical bypass is generally performed only in those patients undergoing laparotomy with intention to cure who are subsequently found to have unresectable disease. Cholecystoenteric and choledochoenteric bypass appear equally effective. Significantly for patients with advanced, end-stage disease, both are associated with considerable morbidity, and some patients never regain their preoperative performance status. Endoscopic stenting provides at least equivalent duration of survival at reduced cost and shorter hospital stay. Thus, for all intents and purposes, obstructive jaundice in patients near the end of life is treated either endoscopically or percutaneously. For patients with coexistent gastric outlet obstruction, laparoscopic gastrojejunostomy appears to be an excellent alternative to classical surgery, providing a good functional result with only minimal impairment of the quality of life.

Endoscopic stenting involves retrograde cannulation of the common bile duct, performance of a sphincterotomy, and placement of either a plastic or metallic endoprosthesis. On occasions, the procedure may be technically difficult, time consuming, and exhausting for the patient. Successful stent placement is considerably greater with this technique (95%) when the obstructing lesion involves the distal common bile duct, as typically seen in patients with pancreatic carcinoma. When the site of obstruction is more proximal and closer to the hilum of the liver, success rates decline to only 50 percent, and morbidity and mortality increase. For these lesions, percutaneous internal–external drainage may be more prudent, with a higher success rate, albeit a greater incidence of immediate serious complications. The most common long-term complication is clogging, which typically occurs after 3 to 4 months with plastic prostheses. Although patency duration may be substantially greater with metallic stents,

there appears to be little reason to incur the added expense of these devices in patients with a life expectancy of less than 6 months. The two most important independent risk factors for predicting prognosis are tumor size and presence of distant metastatic disease. For patients with tumors exceeding 3 cm in size, the median survival is 3.2 months, compared to 6.6 months for those with smaller tumors. The median survival for patients with metastatic disease is 2.5 months compared to 9 months for those without metastases. Other than clogging, additional causes for recurrent jaundice include tumor overgrowth or ingrowth, duodenal obstruction due to tumor invasion, and stent impaction into the bile duct wall. Cholangitis occurs in 20 percent of patients, sometimes with consequent sepsis. The responsible bacteria often have a high frequency of antibiotic resistance. As with all other end-of-life crises, a decision as to how aggressively to treat either clogging or infection depends on a careful appraisal of the patient's overall condition, prognosis, and desires.

Upper Tract Obstructive Uropathy

The inevitable endpoint of bilateral ureteral obstruction is renal failure and uremia. The clinical manifestations of untreated uremia include increasing fatigue, anorexia, dulling of the sensorium, and eventual coma, presumably associated with decreasing perception of pain and suffering, culminating in a "peaceful" death. Because this clinical cascade has traditionally been regarded as a blessing for the patient with far advanced, symptomatic cancer—much as pneumonia was identified as the "friend" of the senile elderly—there has been little fervor for aggressive intervention for upper urinary tract obstruction in patients with end-stage disease. The older, and largely outdated technique of open nephrostomy had a 50 percent rate of major, life-threatening complications, more than 40 percent of patients never left the hospital, and 30 percent died within 52 days of surgery. The overall median survival was 3.3 months. Studies suggest that in patients with end-stage malignancy the results are little different using modern techniques of cystoscopic ureteral stenting and percutaneous nephrostomy. In a study of approximately 100 patients with advanced malignancy (mean age 68), the median survival after palliative endourologic urinary diversion was 3.5 months, of which 1.5 months was spent in the hospital. Thus, it appears that even modern urinary diversion procedures offer little in terms of symptom palliation in patients with end-stage cancer, and are therefore difficult to recommend as appropriate for most patients near the end of life.

Bronchial Obstruction

In addition to radiotherapy (discussed earlier), endoscopic management of symptomatic tracheobronchial airway stenosis can provide significant palliation for patients with malignant airway complications. Multimodality therapy including combinations of laser therapy, radiation therapy, and expandable metallic stent placement can improve survival and quality of life for patients with complete malignant bronchial obstruction. Metallic stents can even alleviate obstruction in the area of the carinal bifurcation with little evidence of complications directly attributable to the stent. Photodynamic therapy (PDT) with porfimer sodium was recently approved for palliation of symptoms for patients with completely or partially obstructing endobronchial non-small-cell lung cancer. At 1 month or later, PDT alleviated symptoms of dyspnea and cough in about 25 percent of treated patients, and hemoptysis in nearly 80 percent. PDT appeared more effective than Nd:YAG laser therapy, particularly regarding hemoptysis. PDT cannot be used concurrently with radiotherapy, but may be used sequentially. It is contraindicated in patients with respiratory–esophageal fistulas or with tumors eroding into major vessels. Patients will be photosensitive for at least 30 days, and must avoid direct sunlight or even bright indoor light without skin and eye protection. Some patients may experience severe chest pain after PDT.

Vascular Obstruction

Aside from their established use in the management of occlusive coronary and peripheral vascular disease, expandable metallic shunts are increasingly employed for the management of vascular occlusive disease associated with malignancy such as superior vena cava (SVC) syndrome. In a series of 12 patients with SVC syndrome, most of whom had advanced bronchogenic carcinoma, 11 patients had immediate relief of obstruction after radiologically controlled placement of self-expanding metal stents (Shah et al, 1996). There were no major complications. SVC obstruction recurred in only one patient after 3 months. The other patients survived without relapse for 1 to 10 months. In a larger series of 76 patients with SVC syndrome in which stent insertion was compared to radiotherapy, stenting provided faster relief of symptoms and significantly greater improvement in symptoms than radiation therapy (Nicholson et al, 1997). Significantly fewer patients developed recurrent symptoms after stent insertion than with radiotherapy, and there were three times as many complications in patients treated with radiation therapy alone compared to those who were stented. It was therefore suggested that percutaneous stent insertion should be the palliative procedure of first choice for malignant SVC obstruction.

Expandable stents can also alleviate symptoms caused by portal hypertension in patients with locally advanced biliary cancer or with liver metastases. With the transjugular intrahepatic portosystemic stent-shunt technique, symptoms of portal hypertension—including tense ascites, mesenteric congestion, and variceal bleeding—disappeared after the procedure. There was a significant improvement of the patients' performance status allowing early ambulation.

Thoracentesis for Pleural Effusions

Compared to pericardial effusions, malignant pleural effusions are commonly encountered in patients with end-stage malignancy. Typical symptoms include progressive dyspnea, orthopnea, persistent coughing, and chest pain. Because these symptoms can materially compromise the quality of an even severely limited life, and treatment is generally successful in alleviating symptoms, palliative intervention is nearly always justified. Classical treatment usually consists of sequential thoracenteses or large bore tube thoracostomy, usually with sclerotherapy. For patients with an overall estimated life expectancy of very short duration, placement of a small, indwelling pleural catheter can be used successfully to drain the pleural space, even in a home setting. This procedure has considerably less morbidity than either repeated thoracentesis or tube thoracostomy, and an incidence of pnuemothorax below 5 percent.

For patients with a somewhat longer life expectancy, tube thoracostomy and sclerotherapy are usually recommended. Traditional large-bore tube thoracostomy with chest tubes connected to continuous wall suction and underwater drainage requires inpatient care, limits patient mobility, often causes considerable patient discomfort, and is expensive. Studies suggest that ambulatory pleural drainage with a small-bore catheter connected to a closed gravity drainage bag system, is a safe, effective, and more patient-friendly alternative. In one series, half the patients treated with small-bore catheters and sclerotherapy had a complete response of at least 30 days duration. In a randomized study comparing large and small-bore catheters (18 patients), all patients found the large catheter somewhat or very unpleasant, whereas this was the case for only 2 patients with the small catheter (Clementsen et al, 1998). Regarding the need for subsequent thoracentesis, the small catheter was no less effective than the large one. Based on this admittedly preliminary evidence, increased use of small-bore catheters seems reasonable, particularly in the context of end-of-life care.

An ideal sclerosing agent is not yet available. Tetracycline has been studied most extensively, but it is no longer available in the United States for intrapleural administration. Doxycycline (500 mg) is highly effective, with 92 percent of patients in one trial free of recurrent pleural effusion for at least 3 months from instillation (Pulsiripunya et al, 1996). Side effects include pain in the majority of patients, fever, and sometimes troublesome cough. Patients should be pretreated with opioid analgesics prior to sclerotherapy with doxycycline. Intrapleural bleomycin (60 units) can also be used as a sclerosing agent. It is not painful, but can cause transient fever, and is expensive. Dose adjustments are advisable in elderly patients and in those with renal insufficiency in order to avoid systemic toxicity (alopecia, mucositis, and skin ulcers). Talc powder in the form of a slurry may also be instilled via a chest tube, with a reported efficacy of 80 to 90 percent. Talc is inexpensive, but requires knowledge of special sterile technique by the pharmacist and is associated with significant pain, fever, and on occasions, respiratory distress syndrome. Talc also may solidify, especially in small-bore chest tubes, leading to residual loculated effusions. Talc may also be administered by insufflation (poudrage) via videothoracoscopy. This minimally invasive approach may be justified in end-stage patients with longer life expectancies who have failed to respond to conventional tube thoracostomy. This technique may also be valuable in patients with often refractory chylous effusions. Patients with persistent pleural drainage who cannot be sclerosed, or those with a persistent air leak, can be successfully managed as outpatients or at home via chest tube with a Heimlich valve.

Paracentesis for Ascites

Management of massive, tense ascites is a problem in end-of-life care in two types of patients with differing pathophysiology: (1) end-stage cancer patients (usually gynecologic, breast, or colorectal cancer) and (2) end-stage liver disease patients (usually associated with cirrhosis). In nonmalignant ascites, sodium retention, mediated by neural and humoral mechanisms, causes an increase in total body sodium and water with ascitic fluid in equilibrium with total body fluid. In contrast, malignant ascites, usually caused by some combination of fluid secretion by tumor implants and interference with normal venous and lymphatic drainage, accumulates independently from total body volume. The clinical significance of this distinction is that whereas dietary water and salt restriction and judicious use of diuretics are integral to the management of nonmalignant ascites, they are of little value and sometimes contraindicated in a patient with malignant ascites.

The only goal in treating ascites near the end of life is to alleviate the typical symptoms of abdominal distension, early satiety, anorexia, indigestion, reflux, nausea, immobility, and respiratory distress. There is no advantage to treating asymptomatic patients.

NONMALIGNANT ASCITES

For patients with nonmalignant, end-stage liver disease, the combination of salt and water restriction, and prescription of diuretics (usually spironolactone or amiloride) is effective in controlling fluid overload in 90 percent of patients. It should be pointed out, however, that overly aggressive diuretic therapy can exacerbate fatigue due to electrolyte imbalance, lead to falls due to orthostatic hypotension, and add to patient discomfort by causing sleep deprivation due to frequent nocturia and embarrassing episodes of urinary incontinence.

For patients who continue to be symptomatic, large-volume paracentesis is generally safe and effective, with removal of up to 5 liters of fluid at a single session. Non-edematous, hypoalbuminemic patients may sometimes require concurrent infusion of plasma volume expanders during paracentesis to avoid symptomatic hypotension. For patients whose life expectancy exceeds more than a few weeks, an indwelling catheter may promote greater comfort, although with some increased risk of infection. Radiologically placed nephrostomy-type tubes may be a satisfactory alternative to surgical placement of a Tenckhoff peritoneal dialysis catheter. Peritoneovenous shunts are rarely indicated in end-of-life care, especially in patients with terminal liver disease in whom their use is sometimes complicated by an increased risk of sepsis, disseminated intravascular coagulation, and shunt occlusion, and a significant incidence (10 to 20 percent) of perioperative death.

MALIGNANT ASCITES

As indicated, fluid restriction and diuretics are rarely effective in controlling malignant ascites, and may promote symptomatic intravascular volume depletion. Paracentesis is the most commonly used means of managing malignant ascites, and is recognized as being highly effective. The use of plasma volume expanders is generally not necessary after paracentesis for malignant ascites. Sclerotherapy with bleomycin or doxycycline may retard fluid reaccumulation in only about 30% of patients, and is of dubious value, especially in patients with short life expectancies. Similarly, intraperitoneal infusion of radioisotopes or chemotherapy such as cisplatin is probably neither necessary nor warranted for symptom management near the end of life. There are ongoing investigations of the use of intraperitoneal tumor necrosis factor and metalloproteinase inhibitors, but these are currently inapplicable to the routine management of malignant ascites. Although peritoneovenous shunts are also ill advised in patients in whom death is anticipated within several weeks, a beneficial effect was reported in 19 patients with malignant ascites in whom predicted life expectancy was several months (Wickremesekera and Stubbs, 1997). All had a prior unsatisfactory experience with repeated paracentesis and diuretics. The shunts were inserted under general anesthesia, and were associated with an average hospital stay of 6 days; 16 patients had excellent shunt function with resolution of ascites and associated symptoms. Late shunt occlusion occurred in 5 patients with recurrence of ascites, but patency was reaccomplished in 4 of the 5. The median survival was 5.5 months, and 14 patients were free of ascites at the time of their deaths.

Pericardiocentesis for Pericardial Effusions

Pericardial metastasis and malignant effusion are not infrequent, especially for patients with cancers of the breast and lung and with lymphoma, but the majority of patients never have signs and symptoms directly related to this complication.

When symptomatic, patients most commonly complain of dyspnea with exertion or at rest, coughing, and chest pain or heaviness. The severity of the symptoms is related to the rate at which the effusion accumulates. Manifestations of pericardial tamponade may therefore occur early with a relatively small volume, rapidly accumulating effusion, or later in the course, when the volume of fluid relative to pericardial distensibility is so great as to increase intrapericardial pressure and impair diastolic ventricular filling. Signs and symptoms of tamponade include neck vein distension, hypotension, resting tachycardia, and pulsus paradoxicus. Peripheral edema occurs less commonly, but, when present, can lead the physician to err in prescribing diuretics that may worsen the underlying pathophysiology.

Patients with pericardial tamponade are usually critically ill at the time of presentation. However, even patients with refractory, end-stage disease who, at the onset of tamponade, are not so debilitated due to other cancer manifestations as to cause imminent death, are likely to have increased comfort and a better quality of remaining life as a result of therapeutic intervention. The procedure of choice is echocardiographically guided pericardiocentesis and attempted intrapericardial sclerosis with either doxycycline or bleomycin. Success in controlling recurrence is generally achieved 70 to 80 percent of the time with minimal toxicity. With doxycycline, multiple instillations may be necessary. The experience with bleomycin is still quite limited. There are also anecdotal reports of success with interleukin-2 and interferon alpha-2b, but there is no evidence that these agents are more advantageous than the traditional ones. For hemodynamically compromised patients with a better overall performance status and a life expectancy of greater than 3 to 4 months, pericardiocentesis followed by subxiphoid pericardiectomy (pericardial "window") is a more durable palliative approach. This discussion, of course, presupposes refractoriness to chemotherapy. However, for patients with longer prognoses, radiosenstitive malignancies, and no prior irradiation of the chest and mediastinum, radiation therapy may also be considered.

Home Inotropic Therapy for Patients with End-Stage Congestive Heart Failure

As hospice and nonhospice palliative care programs care for increasing numbers of patient with refractory congestive heart failure (CHF), questions have arisen about the palliative nature of home infusional inotropic support. To date, the data are inadequate. Dobutamine is currently the preferred intravenous inotropic agent, with amrinone and milrinone as potential alternatives. Optimal infusion schedules have not been clearly defined. Dobutamine infusion may improve the functional status and quality of life of some patients, but intermittent therapy (dobutamine "holiday") has been associated with increased risk of sudden death. There is in fact no indication that inotropic therapy prolongs survival. Pending further evidence, individualized efficacy trials in which the patient is his or her own control, and the endpoint is symptom palliation, could be appropriate, especially in end-of-life programs with an interest in clinical investigation.

Continuous or Intermittent Positive Airway Pressure in Patients with Chronic Obstructive Pulmonary Disease

Much as with CHF, questions have been raised as to whether the efficacy of more aggressive interventions in COPD such as continuous or intermittent positive airway pressure has a significant impact on patient comfort near the end of life.

Home nasal continuous or intermittent positive airway pressure ventilation (NPPV) has been of major benefit to patients with obstructive sleep apnea. There are suggestions that this technique may also ameliorate symptoms of respiratory distress for some patients with advanced COPD and CHF. In one study, 14 hypercapneic COPD patients in stable clinical condition were evaluated after 6 months of NPPV plus long term oxygen therapy (Perrin et al, 1997). Significant improvements were noted in objectively scored physical mobility, energy, emotional well-being, and quality of life, as well as in arterial blood oxygenation and, possibly, in life expectancy. However, it is important to remember that this experience may not be translatable to the end-of-life setting, for which there is as yet no clear outcome information. Furthermore, NPPV may be associated with deleterious effects, particularly among patients with concurrent atrial fibrillation, and patient tolerance and acceptability may be poor. There are numerous learning needs, requiring expert nursing and respiratory therapy involvement to assist patients and families with NPPV machine management, cardiovascular complications, and depressive symptoms. Thus, NPPV, at this point, should not be regarded as a standard component of end-of-life care for COPD or CHF, and its indications should always be subject to careful assessment.

Antibiotics for Sepsis and Intercurrent Infection

Sepsis is a common sentinel event in both elderly and debilitated patients with end-stage disease. In addition to fever, symptoms of sepsis include altered mental status and delerium, dyspnea, pain, and lassitude. Multiple studies indicate that, with the possible exception of patients with far-advanced metastatic cancer, even actively dying patients continue to receive intravenous antibiotics almost up to the moment of death. At one palliative care unit, although 72 percent of known infections were treated with antibiotics, the majority of the patients died nonetheless during the same admission. Thus, in many patients at the end-stage of their disease, it may often be eminently reasonable and entirely proper to regard the devel-

opment of infection as a signal terminal event and recommend withholding antibiotic therapy.

When sepsis is related to an infected or occluded catheter, central line device, or stent, or attributable to a drainable collection or associated with painful cellulitis, more aggressive intervention may be warranted, depending on the patient's premorbid condition and level of function. Intervention may also be appropriate when a patient develops an intercurrent localized infection, such as a urinary tract infection. Under these circumstances, appropriate cultures and imaging studies may be reasonable, even in the context of end-of-life care. Although one might argue that antibiotic treatment could be entirely empirical in terminal patients, the continuing and growing problem of antibiotic resistance suggests that the rules for proper selection of antibiotics should not be relaxed even near the end of life.

Transfusions and Hematopoietic Growth Factor

Anemia

Regardless of the terminal diagnosis, anemia that is sufficiently severe to cause symptoms can be a significant problem in end-of-life care. Contributing factors include concurrent debility and nutritional inadequacy, blood loss, renal or hepatic insufficiency, and bone marrow suppression associated with prior chemotherapy and radiotherapy or the anemia of "chronic disease." Current treatment options include transfusion of red blood cells and administration of subcutaneous erythropoietin.

Red cell transfusions are generally well tolerated, and with appropriate arrangements with a blood bank, can be safely administered in a home setting. However, there are potential significant complications including severe allergic reactions and possible fluid overloading. Furthermore, in terminally ill patients, symptoms such as marked fatigue, breathlessness, palpitations, and dizziness may be due to multiple etiologies other than anemia, and may not improve significantly even after transfusion. A recommendation for red cell transfusion should never be triggered by some arbitrarily predetermined value of hemoglobin concentration or hematocrit. Rather, the decision should be based on a critical assessment of the symptoms, the patient's ambulatory and functional status, and the history of response to prior transfusions.

There are few indications for the use of erythropoietin in end-of-life care. The main virtue of erythropoietin is that, when effective, patients have fewer fluctuations in hemoglobin concentrations compared to those treated with intermittent transfusions, and the risk of transfusion reactions is obviated. Erythropoietin can be continued in end-stage patients with refractory anemia previously shown to be responsive and benefiting from treatment. It might be initiated in patients with a life expectancy greater than 2 to 3 months who cannot be safely transfused, or in whom anemia may be exacerbated by other, concurrent palliative treatments (e.g., chemotherapy, systemic radiotherapy, gancyclovir for prophylaxis of CMV retinitis in patients with advanced AIDS). Under all circumstances, it is important to make early clinical decisions regarding dose adjustment or drug withdrawal, as some patients do not respond to erythropoietin therapy. For optimal response, some patients may require supplemental oral iron. Because of gastrointestinal intolerance, this may not always be acceptable to debilitated patients with terminal diseases.

Granulocytopenia and Thrombocytopenia

Granulocytopenia and thrombocytopenia become issues in end-of-life care primarily in patients with end-stage hematologic illnesses or AIDS. Granulocytopenia may be a significant side effect of various antibiotics and antiviral agents used to treat or prevent opportunistic infections in AIDS. Although definitive antiretroviral treatment should not be within the purview of end-of-life programs, aggressive prophylaxis of quality of life threaten-

ing opportunistic infections in patients with refractory disease is a proper goal of palliative care. Granulocyte colony-stimulating factor (G-CSF) is often prescribed in conjunction with these treatments in order to minimize the risk of concurrent granulocytopenia. However, it has not been clearly demonstrated that G-CSF reduces the rate of severe infection or mortality from infection when given prophylactically, and therefore, it should not represent "routine" care for end-stage patients.

With regards to severe thrombocytopenia, patients with terminal hematologic disease (leukemia or myelodysplasia) or bone marrow failure due to other causes are almost invariably refractory to transfused platelets by the time they are referred for end-of-life care. Consequently, except in unusual circumstances, platelet transfusions are unlikely to have significant palliative benefit, and should be discouraged. Similarly, intravenous gamma globulin, which is sometimes indicated for the treatment of immune thrombocytopenia in patients with AIDS, is generally not applicable in patients with end-stage disease. Thrombopoietin has not yet been approved for use in the United States, and its role, if any, in end-of-life care is yet to be defined.

Conclusion

You think it's beautiful to die for your country. The first bombardment taught us better. Actually, it's better not to have to die at all!

Erich Maria Remarque,
All Quiet on the Western Front

It seems paradoxical to depict techniques for alleviation of suffering as "invasive" or "aggressive," terms that evoke images of carnage and destruction. Although many people reluctantly come to accept the inevitability of death, everyone who has given the matter any thought wishes his or her death to be a "good" one. Few individuals equate this desire with the experience of medical trench warfare, where they are cut off from the "home front" and subject to continual bombardment with ostensibly "friendly fire." As palliative soldiers, what attitude ensures that as we choose and deploy our weapons, we never forget the overall interests and aspirations of the population we are trying to liberate?

I chose the discussion of the palliative use of blood products as the concluding section of this chapter with that question in mind. On multiple occasions, the Bible identifies the blood as synonymous with *nefesh,* sometimes rendered as soul, but best translated as the "essence of life." If we focus only on specific symptoms and lose sight of the global suffering of our patients, then despite our most effective invasive interventions, we are likely to be regarded, as were our English predecessors of the 19th century, not as healers but as no more than body snatchers. On the other hand, when we make the effort to penetrate the patient's *nefesh,* to recognize and alleviate not only physical but also emotional and spiritual distress, the most aggressive palliative maneuvers will be accepted as life-restoring, even if not life-prolonging. In the words of Maimonides: "In the sufferer, let me see ever the human being."

References

General Introduction

Alpert HR, Emanuel L: Comparing utilization of life-sustaining treatments with patient and public preferences. *J Gen Intern Med* 13:175, 1998.

Altwein J, Ekman P, Barry M, et al: How is quality of life in prostate cancer patients influenced by modern treatment? The Wallenberg symposium. *Urology* 49(suppl):66, 1997.

Berger A, Portenoy RK, Weissman DE, eds: *Principles and Practice of Supportive Oncology.* Philadephia, Lippincott-Raven, 1998.

Berger JT, Majerovitz D: Stability of preferences for treatment among nursing home residents. *Gerontologist* 38:217, 1998.

Billings JA: Palliative care: definitions and controversy. *Princ Pract Support Oncol* 1:1, 1998.

Bonnefoi H, A'Hern RP, Fisher C, et al. Natural history of stage IV epithelial ovarian cancer. *J Clin Oncol* 17:767, 1999.

Braddock CH 3rd, Edwards KA, Hasenberg NM, et al: Informed decision making in outpatient practice: Time to get back to basics. *JAMA* 282:2313, 1999.

Brown NK, Thompson DJ, Prentice RL: Nontreatment and aggressive narcotic therapy among hospitalized pancreatic cancer patients. *J Am Geriatr Soc* 46:839, 1998.

Council on Ethical and Judicial Affairs, AMA: Medical futility in end-of-life care. *JAMA* 281:937, 1999.

Covinsky KE, Wu AW, Landefeld S, et al: Health status versus quality of life in older patients: Does the distinction matter? *Am J Med* 106:435, 1999.

Doyle D, Hanks GWC, Macdonald N, eds: *Oxford Textbook of Palliative Medicine,* 2nd ed. Oxford, Oxford University Press, 1998.

Dunn GP: Surgery and palliative medicine: New horizons. *J Palliat Med* 1:215, 1998.

Eidelman LA, Jakobson DJ, Pizov R, et al: Foregoing life-sustaining treatment in an Israeli ICU. *Intensive Care Med* 24:162, 1998.

Emanuel EJ, Fairclough DL, Slutsman J, Emanuel LL. Understanding economic and other burdens of terminal illness: The experience of patients and their caregivers. *Ann Intern Med* 132:451, 2000.

Fins JJ, Miller FG, Acres CA, et al: End-of-life-decision making in the hospital: Current practice and future prospects. *J Pain Symptom Manage* 17:6, 1999.

Goodlin SJ, Winzelberg GS, Teno JM, et al: Death in the hospital. *Arch Intern Med* 158:1570, 1998.

Groeger JS, White P Jr, Nierman DM, et al: Outcome for cancer patients requiring mechanical ventilation. *J Clin Oncol* 17:991, 1999.

Hoffman K, Glimelius B: Evaluation of clinical benefit of chemotherapy in patients with upper gastrointestinal cancer. *Acta Oncol* 37:651, 1998.

Karlawish JHT, Quill T, Meier DE, for the ACP-ASIM end-of-life care consensus panel: A consensus-based approach to providing palliative care to patients who lack decision-making capacity. *Ann Intern Med* 130:835, 1999.

Kinzbrunner BM: The terminally ill patient. In: Abeloff MD, Armitage JO, Lichter AS, Niederhuber JE, eds. *Clinical Oncology,* 2nd ed. New York, Churchill Livingstone, 2000.

Klastersky J: Supportive care in oncology. *Bull Mem Acad R Med Belg* 152:10, 1997.

Leland JY, Schonwetter RS: Advances in hospice care. *Clin Geriatr Med* 13:381, 1997.

Maltoni M, Nanni O, Pirovano M, et al: Successful validation of the palliative prognostic score in terminally ill cancer patients. *J Pain Symptom Manage* 17:240, 1999.

Miner TJ, Jaques DP, Tavaf-Motamen H, Shriver CD: Decision making on surgical palliation based on patient outcome data. *Am J Surg* 177:150, 1999.

Patmaik A, Doyle C, Oza AM: Palliative therapy in advanced ovarian cancer: balancing patient expectations, quality of life and cost. *Anticancer Drugs* 9:869, 1998.

Pirovano M, Maltoni M, Nanni O, et al: A new palliative prognostic score: A first step for the staging of terminally ill cancer patients. Italian multicenter and study group on palliative care. *J Pain Symptom Manage* 17:231, 1999.

Razavi D: Quality of life: A new end point in patients treated with chemotherapy for advanced cancer. *Topics Support Care* 28:2, 1998.

Sabbatini P, Larson SM, Kremer A, et al: Prognostic significance of extent of disease in bone in patients with androgen-independent prostate cancer. *J Clin Oncol* 17:948, 1999.

Scott CB. Issues in quality of life assessment during cancer therapy. *Semin Radiat Oncol* 8(suppl 1):5, 1998.

Stephens RJ, Hopwood P, Girling DJ: Defining and analysing symptom palliation in cancer clinical trials: A deceptively difficult exercise. *Br J Cancer* 79:538, 1999.

Weeks J: Evaluating palliative therapies for hormone-refractory prostate cancer: Clinical trials and clinical care. In: Perry MC, ed. *American Society of Clincal Oncology 1998 Fall Educational Book*. Philadelphia, WB Saunders, 1998, pp. 157–158.

Chemotherapy

Ajani JA: Chemotherapy for gastic carcinoma: New and old options. *Oncology (Huntingt)* 12(suppl 7):44, 1998.

American Society of Clinical Oncology: Clinical practice guidelines for the treatment of unresectable non-small cell lung cancer: Adopted on May 16, 1997 by the American Society of Clinical Oncology. *J Clin Oncol* 15:2996, 1997.

Blum JL, Jones SE, Buzdar AU, et al: Multi-center phase II study of capecitabine in paclitaxel-refractory metastatic breast cancer. *J Clin Oncol* 17:485, 1999.

Bunn PA Jr, Vokes EE, Langer CJ, Schiller JH: An update on North American randomized studies in non-small cell lung cancer. *Semin Oncol* 1998; 25(suppl 9):2, 1998.

Conroy T, Guillemin F: Quality of life in advanced colorectal cancer. *J Clin Oncol* 17:1644, 1999. Letter.

Cunningham D, Pyrhonen S, James RD, et al: Randomised trial of irinotecan plus supportive care versus supportive care alone after fluorouracil failure for patients with metastatic colorectal cancer. *Lancet* 352:1413, 1998.

Einhorn LH, Stender MJ, Williams SD: Phase II trial of gemcitabine in refractory germ cell tumors. *J Clin Oncol* 17:509, 1999.

Elderly lung cancer vinorelbine Italian study group: Effects of vinorelbine on quality of life and survival of elderly patients with advanced non-small cell lung cancer. *J Natl Cancer Inst* 91:66, 1999.

Ellis PA, Smith IE, Hardy JR, et al: Symptom relief with MVP (mitomycin C, vinblastine and cisplatin) chemotherapy in advanced non-small cell lung cancer. *Br J Cancer* 71:366, 1995.

Glimelius B, Ekstrom K, Hoffman K, et al: Randomized comparison between chemotherapy plus best supportive care with best supportive care in advanced gastric cancer. *Ann Oncol* 8:163, 1997.

Graziano F, Cataano G, Cascinu S: Chemotherapy for advanced pancreatic cancer: The history is changing. *Tumori* 84:308, 1998.

Greenway BA: Effect of flutamide on survival in patients with pancreatic cancer: Results of a prospective, randomised, double-blind, placebo-controlled trial. *BMJ* 316:1935, 1998.

Gridelli C, Perrone F, Gallo C, et al: Vinorelbine is well tolerated and active in the treatment of elderly patients with advanced non-small cell lung cancer. A two-stage phase II study. *Eur J Cancer* 33:392, 1997.

Hernandez-Boluda JC, Sierra J, Esteve J, et al: Treatment of elderly patients with AML: Results of an individualized approach. *Haematologica* 83:34, 1998.

Hickish TF, Smith IE, OBrien ME, et al: Clinical benefit from palliative chemotherapy in non-small cell lung cancer extends to the elderly and those with poor prognostic factors. *Br J Cancer* 78:28, 1998.

Lara PN JR, Meyers FJ: Treatment options in androgen-independent prostate cancer. *Cancer Invest* 17:137, 1999.

Lopez PG, Stewart DJ, Newman TE, Evans WK: Chemotherapy in stage IV (metastatic) non-small cell lung cancer. Provincial lung disease site group. *Cancer Prev Control* 1:18, 1997.

Lorusso V, Pollera CF, Antimi M, et al: A phase II study of gemcitabine in patients with transitional cell carcinoma of the urinary tract previously treated with platinum. *Eur J Cancer* 34:1208, 1998.

Munshi NC, Tricot GJ: Single weekly cytosine arabinoside and oral 6-thioguanine in patients with myelodydplastic syndrome and acute myeloid leukemia. *Ann Hematol* 74:111, 1997.

Noble S, Goa KL: Gemcitabine. A review of its pharmacology and clinical potential in non-small cell lung cancer and pancreatic cancer. *Drugs* 54:447, 1997.

Otto T, Krege S, Otto B, et al: Therapy with mitomycin C, folic acid and r-fluorouracil in treatment of metastatic, refractory urinary bladder carcinoma—phase II study. *Urologe A* 36:243, 1997 (German).

Scheithauer W, Rosen H, Kornek GV, et al: Randomised comparison of combination chemotherapy plus supportive care with supportive care alone in patients with metastatic colorectal cancer. *BMJ* 306: 752, 1993.

Shepherd FA: Chemotherapy for non-small cell lung cancer: Have we reached a new plateau? *Semin Oncol* 26(suppl 4):3, 1999.

Silvestri G, Pritchard R, Welch HG: Preferences for chemotherapy in patients with advanced non-small cell lung cancer: Descriptive study based on scripted interviews. *BMJ* 317:771, 1998.

Small EJ, Marshall ME, Reyno L, et al: Superiority of suramin + hydrocortisone (S+H) over placebo + hydrocortisone (P + H): Results of a multi-center double-blind phase III study in patients with hormone refractory prostate cancer (abstract). *Proc Am Soc Clin Oncology* 17:1187a, 1998.

Souhami RL, Spiro SG, Rudd RM, et al: Five-day oral etoposide treatment for advanced small-cell lung cancer: Randomized comparison with intravenous chemotherapy. *J Natl Cancer Inst*, 89:577, 1997.

Storniolo AM, Enas NH, Brown CA, et al: An investigational new drug treatment program for patients with gemcitabine: Results for over 3000 patients with pancreatic carcinoma. *Cancer* 85:1261, 1999.

Tannock IF, Osoba D, Stockler MR, et al: Chemotherapy with mitoxantrone plus prednisone or prednisone alone for symptomatic hormone-resistant prostate cancer: A Canadian randomized trial with palliative end points. *J Clin Oncol* 14:1756, 1996.

Thatcher N, Hopwood P, Anderson H: Improving quality of life in patients with non-small-cell lung cancer: research experience with gemcitabine. *Eur J Cancer* 1997; 33(suppl 1):S8, 1997.

Thatcher N, Jayson G, Bradley B, et al: Gemcitabine: Symptomatic benefit in advanced non-small cell lung cancer. *Semin Oncol* 24 (suppl 8):S8, 1997.

Tsavaris N, Tentas K, Tzivras M, et al: Combined epirubicin, 5-fluorouracil and folinic acid vs no treatment for patients with advanced pancreatic cancer: A prospective comparative study. *J Chemother* 10:331, 1998.

Radiotherapy

Arcangeli G, Giovinazzo G, Saracino B, et al: Radiation therapy in the management of symptomatic bone metastases: The effect of total dose and histology on pain relief and response duration. *Int J Radiat Oncol Biol Phys* 42:1119, 1998.

Ben Josef E, Shamsa F, Williams AO, Porter AT: Radiotherapeutic management of osseous metastases: A survey of current patterns of care. *Int J Radiat Oncol Biol Phys* 40:915, 1998.

Brundage MD, Crook JM, Lukka H: Use of strontium-89 in endocrine-refractory prostate cancer metastatic to bone. Provincial genitourinary cancer disease site group. *Cancer Prev Control* 2:79, 1998.

Catton CN, Gospodarowicz MK: Palliative radiotherapy in prostate cancer. *Semin Urol Oncol* 15:65, 1997.

Corn BW, Donahue BR, Rosenstock JG, et al: Palliation of AIDS-related primary lymphoma of the brain: Observations from a multi-institutional database. *Int J Radiat Oncol Biol Phys* 38:601, 1997.

Gaspar LE, Nag S, Herskovic A, et al: American Brachytherapy Society (ABS) consensus guidelines for brachytherapy of esophageal cancer. *Int J Radiat Oncol Biol Phys* 38:127, 1997.

Gava A, Bertossi L, Zorat PL, et al: Radiotherapy in the elderly with lung carcinoma: The experience of the Italian Geriatric Radiation Oncology Group. *Rays* 22(suppl):61, 1997.

Gaze MN, Kelly CG, Kerr GR, et al: Pain relief and quality of life following radiotherapy for bone metastases: A randomised trial of two fractionation schedules. *Radiother Oncol* 45:109, 1997.

Gelblum D, Mychalczak B, Almadrones L, et al: Palliative benefit of external-beam radiation in the management of platinum refractory epithelial ovarian carcinoma. *Gynecol Oncol* 69:36, 1998.

Hellman RS, Krasnow AZ: Radionuclide therapy for palliation of pain due to osteoblastic metastases. *J Palliat Med* 1:277, 1998.

Hoegler D: Radiotherapy for palliation of symptoms in incurable cancer. *Curr Probl Cancer* 21:135, 1997.

Janjan NA: Radiation for bone metastases: Conventional techniques and the role of systemic radiopharmaceuticals. *Cancer* 80(suppl):1628, 1997.

Jeremic B, Shibamoto Y, Acimovic L, et al: A randomized trial of three single-dose radiation therapy regimens in the treatment of metastatic bone pain. *Int J Radiat Oncol Biol Phys* 42:161, 1998.

Lingareddy V, Ahmad NR, Mohiuddin M: Palliative reirradiation for recurrent rectal cancer. *Int J Radiat Oncol Biol Phys* 38:785, 1997.

Lutz ST, Huang DT, Ferguson CL, et al: A retrospective quality of life analysis using the lung cancer symptom scale in patients treated with palliative radiotherapy for advanced non-small cell lung cancer. *Int J Radiat Oncol Biol Phys* 37:117, 1997.

Mercadante S: Malignant bone pain: Pathophysiology and treatment. *Pain* 69:1, 1997.

Mertens WC, Filipczak LA, Ben-Josef E, et al: Systemic bone-seeking radionuclides for palliation of painful osseous metastases: current concepts. *CA* 48:361, 1998.

Mirels H: Metastatic disease in long bones. A proposed scoring system for diagnosing impending pathological fractures. *Clin Orthop* 249:256, 1989.

Nair N: Relative efficacy of 32P and 89 Sr in palliation in skeletal metastases. *J Nucl Med* 40:256, 1999.

Nielson OS, Bentzen SM, Sandberg E, et al: Randomized trial of single dose versus fractionated palliative radiotherapy of bone metastases. *Radiother Oncol* 47:233, 1998.

Oneschuk D, Bruera E: Palliative management of brain metastases. *Support Care Cancer* 6:365, 1998.

Paulino AC, Reddy SP: Splenic irradiation in the palliation of patients with lymphoproliferative and myeloproliferative disorders. *Am J Hosp Palliat Care* 13:32, 1996.

Pignon T, Scalliet P: Radiotherapy in the elderly. *Eur J Surg Oncol* 24:407, 1998.

Pons F, Herranz R, Garcia A, et al: Strontium-89 for palliation of pain from bone metastases in patients with prostate and breast cancer. *Eur J Nucl Med* 24:1210, 1997.

Prie L, Lagarde P, Palussiere J, et al: Radiotherapy of spinal metastases in breast cancer. Apropos of a series of 108 patients. *Cancer Radiother* 1:234, 1997.

Resche I, Chatal JF, Pecking A, et al: A dose-controlled study of 153 Sm-ethylenediaminetetramethylenephosphonate (EDTMP) in the treatment of patients with painful bone metastases. *Eur J Cancer* 33:1583, 1997.

Sawyer EJ, Timothy AR: Low dose palliative radiotherapy in low grade non-Hodgkin's lymphoma. *Radiother Oncol* 42:49, 1997.

Serafini AN, Houston SJ, Resche I, et al: Palliation of pain associated with metastatic bone cancer using samarium-153-lexidronam: A double-blind

placebo-controlled clinical trial. *J Clin Oncol* 16: 1574, 1998.

Speden D, Nicklason F, Francis H, Ward J: The use of pamidronate in hypertrophic pulmonary osteoarthropathy. *Aust NZ J Med* 27:307, 1997.

Sykes AJ, Kiltie AE, Stewart AL: Odansetron versus a chlorpromazine and dexamethasone combination for the prevention of nausea and vomiting: A prospective, randomised study to assess efficacy, cost effectiveness and quality of life following single-fraction radiotherapy. *Support Care Cancer* 5:500, 1997.

Tan R, Young A: The role of chemoradiotherapy in maintaining quality of life for advanced esophageal cancer. *Am J Hosp Palliat Care* 15:29, 1998.

Tong D, Gillick L, Henderickson FR: The palliation of symptomatic osseous metastasis: Final results of the study by the Radiation Therapy Oncology Group. *Cancer* 50:893, 1982.

Vyas RK, Suryanarayana U, Dixit S, et al: Inoperable non-small cell lung cancer: Palliative radiotherapy with two weekly fractions. *Indian J Chest Dis Allied Sci* 40:171, 1998.

Surgery, Endoscopy, and Other Invasive Interventions

Abdel-Wahab M, Gad-Elhak N, Denewer A, et al: Endoscopic laser treatment of progressive dysphagia in patients with advanced esophageal carcinoma. *Hepatogastroenterology* 45:1509, 1998.

Arnell T, Stamos MJ, Takahashi P, et al: Colonic stents in colorectal obstruction. *Am Surg* 64:986, 1998.

Baron TH, Dean PA, Yates MR 3rd, et al: Expandable metal stents for the treatment of colonic obstruction: Techniques and outcomes. *Gastrointest Endosc* 47:277, 1998.

Beattie GJ, Smyth JF: Phase I study of intraperitoneal metalloproteinase inhibitor BB94 in patients with malignant ascites. *Clin Cancer Res* 4:1899, 1998.

Binkert CA, Ledermann H, Jost R, et al: Acute colonic obstruction: clinical aspects and cost-effectiveness of preoperative and palliative treatment with self-expanding metallic stents—a preliminary report. *Radiology* 206:199, 1998.

Brune IB, Feussner H, Neuhaus H, et al: Laparoscopic gastrojejunostomy and endoscopic biliary stent placement for palliation of incurable gastric outlet obstruction with cholestasis. *Surg Endosc* 11:834, 1997.

Burger JA, Ochs A, Wirth K, et al: The transjugular stent implantation for the treatment of malignant portal and hepatic vein obstruction in cancer patients. *Ann Oncol* 8:200, 1997.

Clementsen P, Evald T, Grode G, et al: Treatment of malignant pleural effusion: pleurodesis using a small percutaneous catheter. A prospective randomized study. *Respir Med* 92:593, 1998.

Cwikiel M, Cwikiel W, Albertsson M: Palliation of dysphagia in pateints with malignant esophageal strictures. Comparison of results of radiotherapy, chemotherapy and esophageal stent treatment. *Acta Oncol* 35:75, 1996.

De Gregorii MA, Mainar A, Tejero E, et al: Acute colorectal obstruction: Stent placement for palliative treatment—results of a multicenter study. *Radiology* 209:117, 1998.

Dohmoto M, Hunerbein M, Schlag PM: Palliative endoscopic therapy of rectal carcinoma. *Eur J Cancer* 32A: 25, 1996.

Doyle JJ, Hnatluk OW, Torrington KG, et al: Necessity of routine chest roentgenography after thoracentesis. *Ann Intern Med* 124:816, 1996.

Feretis C, Benakis P, Dimopoulos C, et al: Palliation of large-bowel obstruction due to recurrent rectosigmoid tumor using self-expandable endoprostheses. *Endoscopy* 28:319, 1996.

Fiocco M, Krasna MJ: The management of malignant pleural and pericardial effusions. *Hematol Oncol Clin North Am* 11:253, 1997.

Gross CM, Kramer J, Waigand J, et al: Stent implantation in patients with superior vena cava syndrome. *AJR Am J Roentgenol* 169:429, 1997.

Katayama A, Konishi T, Hiraishi M, et al: A combination of laser therapy, radiation therapy, and stent placement for the palliation of complete malignant bronchial obstruction. *Surg Endosc* 12:1419, 1998.

Lec BH, Choe DH, Lee JH, et al: Metallic stents in malignant biliary obstruction: Prospective long-term clinical results. *AJR Am J Roentgenol* 168:741, 1997.

Lee CW, Bociek G, Faught W: A survey of practice in management of malignant ascites. *J Pain Symptom Manage* 16:96, 1998.

Malawer MM, Buch RG, Thompson WE, Sugarbaker PH: Major amputations done with palliative intent in the treatment of local bony complications associated with advanced cancer. *J Surg Oncol* 47:121, 1991.

Mares DC, Mathur PN: Medical thorascopic talc pleurodesis for chylothorax due to lymphoma: A case series. *Chest* 114:731, 1998.

McNamara P, Sharma K: Surgery or palliation for hip fractures in patients with advanced malignancy? *Age Ageing* 26:471, 1997.

Nicholson AA, Ettles DF, Arnold A, et al: Treatment of malignant superior vena cava obstruction: Metal stents or radiation therapy? *J Vasc Interv Radiol* 8:781, 1997.

O'Sullivan GJ, Grundy A: Palliation of malignant dysphagia with expanding metallic stents. *J Vasc Interv Radiol* 10:346, 1999.

Patz EF Jr: Malignant pleaural effusions: Recent advances and ambulatory sclerotherapy. *Chest* 113 (suppl): 74S, 1998.

Pereira-Lima JC, Jakobs R, Maier M, et al: Endoscopic biliary stenting for the palliation of pancreatic cancer: Results, survival predictive factors, and comparison of 10-French with 11.5 French gauge stents. *Am J Gastroenterol* 91:2179, 1996.

Ponec RJ, Kimmey MB: Endoscopic therapy of esophageal cancer. *Surg Clin North Am* 77:1197, 1997.

Ponn RB, Silverman HJ, Federico JA: Outpatient chest tube management. *Ann Thorac Surg* 64:1437, 1997.

Prat F, Chapat O, Ducot B, et al: Predictive factors for survival of patients with inoperable malignant distal biliary strictures: A practical management guideline. *Gut* 42:76, 1998.

Prat F, Chapat O, Ducot B, et al: A randomized trial of endoscopic drainage methods for inoperable malignant strictures of the common bile duct. *Gastrointest Endosc* 47:1, 1998.

Pulsiripunya C, Youngchaiyud P, Pushpakon R, et al: The efficacy of doxycycline as a pleural sclerosing agent in malignant pleural effusion: A prospective study. *Respirology* 1:69, 1996.

Raikar GV, Melin MM, Ress A, et al: Cost-effective analysis of surgical versus endoscopic stenting in the management of unresectable pancreatic cancer. *Ann Surg Oncol* 3:470, 1996.

Rogan M: Porfimer sodium phototherapy for obstructing endobronchial non-small cell lung cancer. *Photofrin Prescribing Information*. New York, Sanofi Pharmaceutical, 1999.

Runyon BA: Treatment of patients with cirrhosis and ascites. *Semin Liver Dis* 17:249, 1997.

Ryan JM, Hahn PF, Mueller PR: *AJR Am J Roentgenol* 171:1003, 1998.

Sargeant IR, Tobias JS, Blackman G, et al: Radiotherapy enhances laser palliation of malignant dysphagia: A randomised study. *Gut* 40:362, 1997.

Segreti EM, Morris M, Levenback C, et al: Transverse colon urinary diversion in gynecologic oncology. *Gynecol Oncol* 63:66, 1996.

Shah R, Sabanathan S, Lowe RA, Mearns AJ: Stenting in malignant obstruction of superior vena cava. *J Thorac Cardiovasc Surg* 112:335, 1996.

Shekarriz B, Shekarriz H, Upadhyay J, et al: Outcome of palliative urinary diversion in the treatment of advanced malignancies. *Cancer* 85:998, 1999.

Shiraishi T, Kawahara K, Shirakusa T, et al: Stenting for airway obstruction in the carinal region. *Ann Thorac Surg* 66:1925, 1998.

Shumate CR, Baron TH: Palliative procedures for pancreatic cancer: When and which one? *South Med J* 89:27, 1996.

Siersema PD, Dees, van Blankenstein M: Palliation of malignant dysphagia from oesophageal cancer. Rotterdam oesophageal tumor study group. *Scand J Gastroenterol* 225(suppl):75, 1998.

Smith GS, Barnard GF: Massive volume paracentesis (up to 41 liters) for the outpatient management of ascites. *J Clin Gastroenterol* 25:402, 1997.

Sonett JR: Endobronchial stents: Primary and adjuvant therapy for endobronchial airway obstruction. *Md Med J* 47:260, 1998.

Tham TC, Carr-Locke DL, Vandervoort J, et al: Management of occluded biliary Wallstents. *Gut* 42:703, 1998.

Tsang TS, Freeman WK, Sinak LJ, Seward JB: Echocardiographically guided pericardiocentesis: Evolution and state-of-the-art technique. *Mayo Clin Proc* 73:647, 1998.

Wickremesekera SK, Stubbs RS: Peritoneovenous shunting for malignant ascites. *NZ Med J* 110:33, 1997.

Wilkins HE 3rd, Cacioppo J, Connolly MM, et al: Intrapericardial interferon in the management of malignant pericardial effusion. *Chest* 114:330, 1998.

Wilkinson SP: Treatment options for cirrhotic ascites. *Eur J Gastorenterol Hepatol* 10:1, 1998.

CHF and COPD

Celli BR: Standards for the optimal management of COPD: A summary. *Chest* 113(suppl):283S, 1998.

Dormans TP, Gerlag PG, Russel FG, Smits P: Combination diuretic therapy in severe congestive heart failure. *Drugs* 55:165, 1998.

Havranek EP, Abrams F, Stevens E, Parker K: Determinants of mortality in elderly patients with heart failure: The role of angiotensin-converting enzyme inhibitors. *Arch Intern Med* 158:2024, 1998.

McCloskey WW: Use of intravenous inotropic therapy in the home. *Am J Health Syst Pharm* 55:930, 1998.

Parmar MS, Kanya-Forstner N: N-CPAP in the prevention for recurrent intubations and hospitalizations in a patient with refractory congestive heart failure. *Can J Cardiol* 14:1405, 1998.

Perrin C, El Far Y, Vandenbos F, et al: Domiciliary nasal intermittent positive pressure ventilation in severe COPD: Effects of lung function and quality of life. *Eur Respir J* 10:2835, 1997.

Petty TL: Supportive therapy in COPD. *Chest* 113(suppl): 256S, 1998.

Simonds AK: Nasal ventilation. *Postgrad Med J* 74:343, 1998.

Smith CE, Mayer LS, Metsker C, et al: Continuous positive airway pressure: patients' and caregivers' learning needs and barriers to use. *Heart Lung* 27:99, 1998.

Antibiotics

Grossman RF: The value of antibiotics and the outcomes of antibiotic therapy in exacerbations of COPD. *Chest* 113(suppl 4):249S, 1998.

Pereira J, Watanabe S, Wolch G: A retrospective review of the frequency of infections and patterns of antibiotic utilization on a palliative care unit. *J Pain Symptom Manage* 16:374, 1998.

Robinson WM, Ravilly S, Berde C, Wohl ME: End-of-life care in cystic fibrosis. *Pediatrics* 100:205, 1997.

Palliative Hematology: Transfusions and Growth Factors

Adamson JW: Epoietin alfa: Into the new millennium. *Semin Oncol* 25(Suppl 7):76, 1998.

Coyle TE: Hematologic complications of human immunodeficiency virus infection and the acquired immunodeficiency syndrome. *Med Clin North Am* 81:449, 1997.

Geissler RG, Schulte P, Ganser A: Clinical use of hematopoietic growth factors in patients with myelodysplastic syndromes. *Int J Hematol* 65:339, 1997.

Griggs JJ, Blumberg N: Recombinant erythropoietin and blood transfusions in cancer chemotherapy-induced anemia. *Anticancer Drugs* 9:925, 1998.

Herter J: Hematopoietic supportive care. *Clin Cancer Res* 3:2666, 1997.

Stockelberg D, Lehtola P, Noren I: Palliative treatment at home for patients with haematological disorders. *Support Care Cancer* 5:506, 1997.

Richard Fife
Richard A. Shapiro
Neal J. Weinreb

Chapter

18

Physician-Assisted Suicide and Euthanasia

Introduction

The development and routine application of advanced, life-prolonging technology, especially in chronic, irreversible, incapacitating illnesses, has raised difficult clinical, ethical, legal, and political issues for the practice of medicine. With attention increasingly directed at the quality, rather than merely the duration, of life, and with a shift in the doctor–patient relationship away from professional paternalism and towards absolute patient self-determination, the question "whose life is it anyway?" has been extended to include ending life on patient demand. Consequently, physician-assisted suicide (PAS) and euthanasia have been in the forefront of medical-ethical issues, and continue to be the focus of intense public debate in the United States.

Within the medical community, interest and controversy about physician-assisted suicide were sparked by the anonymous article "It's Over, Debbie" (*JAMA*, 1988) and by the thoughtful case presentations and subsequent writings by proponents such as Dr. Timothy Quill. The participation by Dr. Jack Kevorkian in assisted suicides in Michigan graphically brought the subject before the public and the courts. Although Kevorkian's actions appeared to violate statutory law, jurors repeatedly refused to convict him to the extent that he claimed his participation was restricted to assisting in suicide. However, when he carried his activity to the point of videotaping and publicizing a "mercy killing," a Michigan jury found him guilty of murder. This suggests that the public continues to maintain a clear distinction between euthanasia, still considered unacceptable, and assisted suicide, for which there appears to be an undercurrent of popular support.

The organized medical community, as represented by national organizations such as the AMA, regards PAS with disfavor. Surveys suggest that only 15 to 20 percent of physicians would agree to participate in PAS, even if the practice were legal. Nevertheless, 50 to 60 percent of oncologists report having been asked by patients to help them end their lives because of concerns about pain and suffering, worries about being a burden, and as a means of exerting continued independence and control.

Although the justices of the United States Supreme Court ruled unanimously in 1997 that there is no constitutional right to assistance in committing suicide, the court clearly indicated that state legislatures were empowered to address the issue, and that the individual states would be appropriate "laboratories" in which the ramifications of PAS might be explored. Nonetheless, proposed legislation to allow PAS was defeated in 26 states in 1997 and 1998, and voters rejected state ballot initiatives to legalize PAS in California, Michigan, and Washington state, although a significant minority (30 to 40 percent) favored these proposals. Oregon voters, however, approved the Oregon Death with Dignity Act in 1996 by a 60 percent majority. Opponents of the Oregon legalization of PAS sought to circumvent the state law by threatening physician participants with penalties specified in the federal Controlled Substance Act. This approach was rejected by the United States Attorney General. The controversial so-called Pain Relief Promotion Act of 1999, whose purpose is to render PAS illegal in all states while emphasizing access to expert pain and symptom management, is still pending congressional action.

Regardless of judicial, legislative, and political positions, physicians continue to play a part in individual decisions of life extension and termination. They will continue to be asked to make judgments and recommendations regarding the extension of the length of life, assessment of the quality of life, and defining options for the relief of pain and suffering. The possibility of further legalization of PAS will place an even greater responsibility and burden on health care professionals, and a challenge to the traditional concepts of the physician's mission.

The purpose of this chapter is to assist physicians with an interest in end-of-life care in grappling with the issue as to whether, and under what circumstances, assisted suicide might be considered as a therapeutic option in the management of patients with terminal disease.

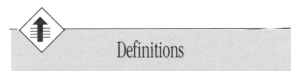

Definitions

Physician-Assisted Suicide

With physician-assisted suicide (PAS), following a patient-initiated request, a physician provides the means for the patient to end his or her life. Typically, the physician offers counseling, information, and instruction; prescribes (and sometimes delivers) the requisite medication; but does not otherwise participate in the final act. The presence of the physician during the suicide process is sometimes encouraged, but remains a matter of patient and physician preference. (Guidelines and legal requirements in Oregon and the Netherlands, where PAS is either legal or legally tolerated, will be discussed later.) "Assisted dying" is a somewhat evasive and less satisfactory terminology that could just as easily be applied to hospice and palliative care as to assisted suicide.

Euthanasia

The term "euthanasia" is derived from the Greek *Eu* (good) and *Thanatos* (death). Although helping a terminally ill patient achieve a "good death" is the goal of everyone involved in hospice medicine and end-of-life care, in modern usage, euthanasia is a direct action taken by a physician or other third party with the intention of ending a patient's life as a response to unmitigated pain and suffering.

The term "voluntary euthanasia" refers to the action of a physician and a competent patient who jointly agree, via a process of informed consent, to terminate the patient's life. Involuntary euthanasia

is a commonly practiced veterinary procedure ("putting an animal down"), but could be conceivably applied (with trepidation) to the act of ending the life of a terminally ill, suffering patient lacking decision-making capacity at the request of a legally authorized health care surrogate. Rare episodes reported in the Netherlands notwithstanding, independent action by the physician or other third party (e.g., husband shooting a severely demented wife), even if felt to be in the patient's best interest, is not euthanasia, and could be legally considered to be murder. Euthanasia implies an active role for the physician. "Passive euthanasia," which has been used synonymously with withholding or withdrawing treatment on the patient's instruction, tends to blur the distinction between these separate end-of-life issues, and is a term best avoided.

Terminal or Total Sedation

For a relatively small number of terminally ill patients near the natural end of life, alleviation of discomfort due to pain, dyspnea, bleeding, or other symptoms may not be achieved with conventional means. Because such patients experience not only marked physical but also severe emotional and spiritual distress often associated with agitation, the physician, with appropriate consent from the patient or family, may prescribe high-dose medication sufficient to sedate and keep the patient unconscious until death ensues. This is commonly termed "terminal or total sedation." (The actual medical indications and techniques for using terminal sedation as a therapeutic intervention near the end of life are discussed in Chapter 12.)

Because death from PAS as commonly practiced by administration of barbiturates is not instantaneous and occasionally may not ensue for as much as 24 hours, there is a legitimate question as to the difference between PAS and total sedation. It is classically argued that with PAS, the intention of the physician is to help to bring death for the purpose of relieving pain and suffering. With total sedation, the intention of the physician, as reflected in the choice and dosage of medication, is to alleviate pain and suffering rather than to hasten death, although the latter outcome frequently occurs and may often be welcomed by the patient's family and the doctor. The ethical justification for this distinction is the principle of double effect.

Double Effect

The principle of double effect refers to an action that may have two distinct effects, one planned and desired, and another anticipated but unwanted or unneeded. An example is the administration of chemotherapy to a patient with cancer. The desired effect is tumor regression and prolongation of life. The potential undesired side effects include neutropenia and fatal septicemia. The principle of double effect teaches that if the primary goal of the action is to cause a desired effect, and the patient is informed and aware of the potential adverse consequences, assuming there is no negligence, no moral culpability is attached should the unfavorable outcome occur.

Although the formulation of the principle of double effect is often attributed to medieval scholastics, its origins date to late antiquity, as it is repeatedly applied in Talmudic reasoning and jurisprudence. The proper application of the principle depends not only on the actor's intent, but also on the proximate inevitability of the undesired effect, and on an assessment as to whether the action chosen is proportionate to the severity of the problem to be addressed and is the best or only alternative. For example, one cannot cut off the head of a squawking chicken in an attempt at noise abatement and then deny accountability for the chicken's death on the basis of double effect!

The application of the doctrine of double effect to end-of-life care has been criticized by some medical ethicists, who argue that "at best, it is often claimed disingenuously or, at worst, it has become a [shallow] meaningless mantra recited by . . . surreptitious practitioners of euthanasia cloaked as palliative care clinicians" (Cherny, 2000).

Intent

Human intentions are usually complex, sometimes ambiguous, frequently inconstant, often difficult to pin down, and easily subject to manipulation. For this reason, it has been suggested that "appeal to intention offers no basis for a clear moral distinction between [such closely similar actions as] withdrawing life sustaining treatment and PAS" (Miller, et al, 2000). Dr. Marcia Angell (1999) has argued that whereas intent is important in criminal law (e.g., differentiating murder from manslaughter), "the situation is different for compassionate doctors caring for the terminally ill, [who] want to relieve their patients' suffering, . . . sometimes in whatever way possible." Others would argue, however, that assessment of intent is not only a linchpin of all legal/justice systems, but is critical for even the most rudimentary social interactions (e.g., is the lion out for a postprandial stroll or on a preprandial prowl? Might its intention change unpredictably, and is it worth trying to know?).

Because virtually all human action can be invested with moral significance, and because ends do not necessarily justify means, intent, although often difficult to evaluate, should not be easily dismissed. Even nonverbalized intent may sometimes have ethical and even legal significance. It stands to reason, therefore, that when dealing with emotionally charged end-of-life issues, the prudent physician will document with even greater care than usual the full details of doctor–patient interactions, so as to leave the least possible doubt about the intentions of all parties involved.

Professional Integrity

Just as the patient's autonomy and right to self-determination must be respected, so too the physician is entitled to take "professional actions that are consistent with one's ethical and moral beliefs, and [to avoid] actions that are contrary to one's beliefs" (Oregon Death with Dignity Act). This right, also referred to as conscientious practice or conscientious objection, allows a clinician to withdraw from a patient relationship when the patient's wishes conflict with the clinician's own moral beliefs. The application of this principle is contingent on nonabandonment of the patient's continuing needs and sufficient notice to effect the transfer of care to another physician.

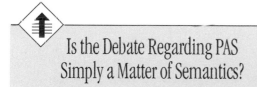

Is the Debate Regarding PAS Simply a Matter of Semantics?

Among both proponents and opponents of legalized PAS, there are those who contend that the debate is nothing more than a question of semantics. Some argue that there is no essential ethical difference between withholding life-prolonging treatment at the instruction of an informed, competent patient and honoring the request of that patient for a supply of medication sufficient for a successful suicide. In the case of an incompetent patient with a properly executed advance directive, why distinguish between withdrawal of life-sustaining equipment on instruction of a designated health care surrogate and the request of that same surrogate that the doctor administer a lethal injection? Is a living will that abjures aggressive, life-prolonging treatment anything other than a predated, highly contingent, promissory suicide note? What about the competent patient who determines to hasten death by refusing food and drink, or the physician whose prescription of heavy sedation to alleviate pain, dyspnea, or other symptoms inevitably, although allegedly without intention, accelerates the end of life?

Although seemingly irrational and possibly hypocritical, our society currently sanctions all of the above activities except PAS and euthanasia. Rigorous attention to the logical implications of our language suggests that we do not really disapprove of PAS and euthanasia except when they are performed intentionally as actions called PAS or euthanasia. In reality, we accept the basic premise of PAS and euthanasia provided we give them a

different name and justify their use as interventions meant to prevent futile treatment or prolongation of the dying process. We are already positioned on that dreaded slippery slope that opponents of PAS insist we must avoid. This slope may be so steep that, regardless of whether our current moral status is deemed high or low, the effect on the patient's situation is essentially negligible! Our system approves the goals of PAS. Logical hairsplitting and subtle nuances offer no moral comfort and promote only confusion.

The justices of the Second Circuit United States Court of Appeals advanced this very argument when overturning New York State legislation prohibiting PAS. However, the thinking of the Second Circuit was rejected by the United States Supreme Court, which firmly espoused a strong legal distinction between refusing unwanted treatment and PAS. Although nuance of language is subject to the same logical criticism as assessment of intention, it is similarly essential to a functional legal system and indeed to all social intercourse. The formulation of arbitrary distinctions may sometimes be the sole mechanism to achieve compromise and consensus in a diverse, pluralistic community.

General support for patient self-determination, including refusal of undesired treatment, which is not easily accepted by all ethnic and religious groups, might be jeopardized if the distinction from suicide is blurred or removed. Furthermore, the distinction between withholding/withdrawal of treatment and PAS may not necessarily be totally arbitrary. Refusal of food, drink, and treatment can constitute the autonomous actions of patients or their representatives, and are subject only to a physician's advice, but not to his or her consent. Although a doctor who disagrees with the patient's decision may withdraw and transfer care to a colleague, were no alternative physician available, the doctor would have no choice but to comply with the patient's wishes.

Assisted suicide, on the other hand, presupposes the voluntary compliance of the physician, who based on the principle of professional integrity and conscientious practice, has no ethical or legal obligation to participate. Absent physician involvement, the patient still has recourse to other means of committing suicide. All these might be seen as sufficient grounds to argue that the distinction between refusal of treatment and PAS/euthanasia is substantive, and not merely semantic.

History and Background

Ancient Greece and Rome

Episodes of assisted suicide and euthanasia are recorded in the classical literary and historical sources of antiquity. There is abundant evidence that these actions were in common use in ancient Greece and Rome. Antiquity, of course, does not automatically confer moral legitimacy on these procedures, as abhorrent practices such as human sacrifice and infanticide for population control were also practiced in ancient civilizations. Consider the following examples: "There must be a law that no imperfect or maimed child shall be brought up, and to avoid an excess of population, some children must be exposed, for a limit must be fixed to the population of the state" (Aristotle, *Politics* VII). "Children also, if weak and deformed we drown, not through anger, but through the wisdom of preferring the sound to the useless" (Seneca, *Concerning Anger*).

The Bible

Of greater relevance to the current debate are case reports describing withdrawal of treatment, assisted suicide, and euthanasia in texts such as the Bible and Talmud, which are the basis of the Judeo-Christian-Islamic life-affirming traditions that have largely shaped the American ethos. Saul, the first king of Israel, defeated in battle, surrounded by the enemy, and anticipating capture, humiliation, and a tortured death, asked his armor-bearer to kill him with his own sword. The armor-bearer con-

scientiously objected and refused, whereupon Saul, as soldiers have done even in modern times, fell on his sword and died. Whether this suicide was condemnable or laudatory to avoid desecration of God's name has been debated by Biblical commentators, but it has been emulated by generations of martyrs who chose suicide rather than being forced to violate cardinal principles of faith.

The epilogue of the Saul story is also relevant to this chapter. A messenger, looking to curry favor with David, Saul's rival and successor, brought news of the king's death. Possibly embellishing the details, he related how he had found Saul dying of his self-inflicted wounds, and, in the spirit of mercy killing, finished him off. To his undoubted dismay, David did not take kindly to the deed and ordered the messenger's execution. It is not clear whether this represented a rejection of the concept of euthanasia or merely concern about *lese majesté*.

The Talmud

The Talmud relates a number of episodes suggesting that natural death is preferable to prolonged physical or emotional suffering. Furthermore, there is a suggestion that life-prolonging maneuvers may be withheld or withdrawn from dying, suffering patients in the story of Rabbi Judah the Prince, whose maid was praised for interrupting the prayers of his colleagues and students, which she perceived as an impediment to a beneficent death.

Euthanasia is mentioned and endorsed in association with the martyrdom of Rabbi Hananiah ben Tradyon, who was burned at the stake by Romans. One of the guards, knowing that death was inevitable, and wishing to prevent further cruelty, removed a sponge that was tortuously damping the flames, thus mercifully hastening the Rabbi's death and gaining himself a guaranteed ticket to paradise.

Finally, there is an episode of euthanasia by proxy that may be of relevance to assisted suicide. Rabbi Ulla, on a journey from Babylon to Israel, camped with two men who quarreled. The situation turned violent and one man slit the throat of the other. With the victim exsanguinating on the ground, the perpetrator asked Ulla whether he had done the right thing. Ulla, fearing for his own life, assented, and secretly hoping to spare the dying victim prolonged agony, suggested that the incision be extended to transect the trachea, thus causing immediate death. Troubled as to whether he might be an accessory to murder, he later reviewed the case with his teacher, Rabbi Yochanan, who justified Ulla's action as necessary for self-preservation. Because it was not condemned as unnecessary or excessive, one might presume that the "assisted euthanasia" was approved, or even expected, behavior.

Of course, these anecdotes relate to unusual circumstances and may not necessarily be applicable to everyday life. As a general rule, Western religious tradition emphasizes the sanctity of life and despite a strong belief in an afterlife with few exceptions emphasizes the importance of prolonging life in this world. Consequently, suicide and euthanasia are anathema to these major world religions. Furthermore, from a religious viewpoint, the doctor is conceived of as a divinely authorized healer and a restorer of life. Therefore, physician participation in suicide or euthanasia is doubly problematical. Secularists, on the other hand, also regard "life" as one of the inalienable rights of humankind, but coupled to "liberty" (autonomy) and conceivably modified by "the pursuit of happiness." The position that these three basic rights are coequal in importance, as contrasted with the religious outlook which regards the latter two as not absolute, creates the philosophical gradient that moves the controversy about euthanasia and PAS.

The United States and the United Kingdom

In 1994, Ezekiel Emmanuel reviewed the history of euthanasia in the United States and in the United Kingdom. The first reference to euthanasia in the English language is found in Sir Thomas More's *Utopia* (1516): "They console the incurably ill by sitting and talking with them and by alleviating whatever pain they can. Should life become unbearable for these incurables, the

magistrates and priests do not hesitate to prescribe euthanasia . . . ."

In the late 18th century, the framers of the United States Constitution rejected the age-old concept that inflicting painful suffering had instructive, deterrent, or redemptive value by prohibiting cruel and unusual punishment. Although the morality and social utility of capital punishment continues to be hotly debated, there has been an inexorable movement towards insuring that even the most reprehensible criminal is entitled to protection from physical pain and suffering. The trend to medicalize executions by using lethal injection has parenthetically focused attention on why we appear to treat condemned criminals with greater compassion than we treat victims of the ravages of terminal illness.

After 1846, as anesthesia with ether and chloroform was increasingly applied to surgical procedures, suggestions were offered that these agents might also be useful in alleviating terminal suffering. In 1870, Samuel Williams proposed using morphine in conjunction with general anesthetics to intentionally end a patient's life. Debates about the ethics of euthanasia continued for the next 35 years, further fueled by controversy linked to emerging Darwinian theories such as "survival of the fittest" as applied to social utilitarianism. In 1906, a bill to legalize euthanasia was introduced and eventually defeated in the Ohio legislature. For much of the 20th century, euthanasia and PAS continued to be illegal throughout the United States and in most of the rest of the world.

Nazi Germany

A notable exception was Nazi Germany, where state-sanctioned euthanasia was promoted to advance that regime's perverted concepts of racism, eugenics, and purification of society. Even today, it seems easy to be taken in by the diabolically upbeat Nazi propaganda films designed to convince the German people that culling the physically and mentally disabled was not only crucial for the protection and development of the fatherland, but was also a humane benefit and favor for the victims themselves. The moral depravity of this approach, and its indelible association with the Nazi program of barbarous medical experimentation and mass genocide, continues to influence the current debate over PAS and euthanasia for patients with devastating terminal illness.

Today

Public awareness and interest in PAS and euthanasia appear to have paradoxically increased in direct proportion to advances in medical knowledge and the resultant substantial gains in expected longevity over the past 50 years. The routine application of technologically advanced, artificial, life-prolonging devices and techniques regardless of clinical appropriateness has supplanted the experience of a natural death, shifted the process of dying away from home and family to the hospital and health care professionals, and altered the definition of death itself.

Increased longevity has seen a shift in the prevalence of terminal disease states away from infectious illnesses and towards malignancies and chronic, irreversible degenerative organ failure disorders. Many physicians, sometimes under pressure from patients and their families, continue to overemphasize ephemeral hopes for curative success and ignore or minimize existent symptoms and side effects of life-prolonging treatment.

On the other hand, the public, although increasingly conditioned to expect medical miracles, is well aware that, with the progression of chronic illness, the level of independent function and quality of life inexorably decrease, and the symptoms of disease become ever more distressing. The heightened emphasis on quality, and not only quantity, of life is reflected in a growing sentiment that control of the management of terminal illness needs to be recaptured from the health care profession and asserted by individual patients and their loved ones. This change in the public attitude towards end-of-life care has contributed to both the development and growth of hospice and pal-

liative medicine and also increased pressure to consider the ending of an undesired life as a therapeutic option.

The debate over PAS and euthanasia has intensified during the past decade, particularly after the publication of two articles in which physicians described personal participation in hastening a patient's death in response to perceived pain and suffering. The first paper entitled "It's Over, Debbie" was published anonymously in *JAMA,* and purportedly related the clinical relationship between a young resident on call and a 20-year-old woman with terminal ovarian carcinoma. The patient, who weighed only 80 pounds and appeared much older than her 20 years, was cachectic and suffering relentless pain and intractable vomiting. The resident described the situation as a "gallows scene" and stated that her only words to him were "let's get this over with." He proceeded to administer a lethal dose of morphine with the clear intention of causing a death that quickly ensued.

The second paper, in the *New England Journal of Medicine,* was written by Dr. Timothy Quill, an internist and hospice medical director. It described the story of his long-time patient, Diane, who presented with acute myelomonocytic leukemia. Although Diane was young and a good candidate for aggressive induction chemotherapy with a 25 percent chance for long-term survival, after discussing her options with her family and physician, she decided to forego an attempt at curative treatment in favor of a palliative approach. She availed herself of hospice services, but increasingly stated neither her family nor the hospice seemed to be able to deal adequately with the emotional pain and suffering, as well as the growing bone pain, and sense of dependence and isolation. She requested help from her physician to end her pain and suffering, and, after considerable soul-searching and detailed discussions with Diane, Quill prescribed medication and helped Diane understand how to take a lethal dose.

The response of the medical community to "It's Over, Debbie" was generally unfavorable. The resident had a brief and apparently shallow professional relationship with his patient, appeared to have had no contact or input from her family, and left no indication he had considered or proposed other options such as hospice, or sought additional consultation before acting unilaterally. Indeed, there was even speculation that the entire story was fictional and written for the purpose of stimulating discussion. In contrast, Quill, whose candid disclosure potentially jeopardized his medical career, had a deep and professionally intimate knowledge of his patient's mind-set and family situation. After many detailed and emotionally charged discussions with the patient, he could in good conscience conclude that he had come to know, respect, and admire Diane's desire for independence and her decision to stay in control of her own life. Nevertheless, although there has been widespread recognition of Quill's personal and professional integrity and intellectual acumen, his assertion that PAS is a constitutional right and his advocacy of the legalization of PAS are not currently supported by a majority of physicians in the United States. In fact, serial surveys indicate that whereas support for legalizing PAS has increased somewhat among the general public, it has progressively decreased among physicians. Although this trend may partly reflect an element of wariness related to the emergence of patient-unfriendly managed-care providers, it has undoubtedly been influenced by the literature concerning PAS and euthanasia as practiced in the Netherlands.

PAS in the Netherlands

The Netherlands has a population of approximately 16 million, of which 14 percent are older than 65 years. With a death rate of 8.69/1000 population, there are an estimated 139,000 total annual deaths. Currently in the Netherlands, there are about 9700 explicit requests for euthanasia or PAS each year. Approximately 3600 reports are granted, accounting for 2.6 percent of all deaths, an increase from 2.1 percent in 1990.

In contrast to attitudes of American physicians, physician-assisted death is supported by a majority of Dutch physicians. Most Dutch pharmacists are also supportive of euthanasia and PAS and are prepared to fill prescriptions written for these purposes.

Although euthanasia is officially a crime in Holland, it has been accepted there for over 20 years, and in fact is supported by guidelines issued by the Royal Dutch Medical Association in 1984 and endorsed by a government-appointed commission. These guidelines stipulate that four conditions must be met before euthanasia is performed (Table 18–1): (1) the patient must be a mentally competent adult; (2) the patient must request euthanasia voluntarily, consistently, and repeatedly over a reasonable time, and the request must be documented; (3) the patient must be suffering intolerably, with no prospect of relief, although the disease need not be terminal; and (4) the doctor must consult with another physician not involved in the case.

Seven years after the guidelines were developed, a study headed by the Dutch attorney general found that the above guidelines appeared to have been met in about two thirds of the cases, although only 486 of an estimated 3700 physician-assisted deaths were reported as such. In 1000 deaths, in clear violation of the guidelines, the patient was not competent when euthanasia was performed. Consultation took place in 63 percent of the cases, but in only 37 percent of those deaths that were unreported. In almost half of the unreported cases, the decision had been discussed less formally with at least one colleague, but only 7 percent of general practitioners met all criteria for a good consultation. It is not clear to what extent alternatives to euthanasia were discussed. Ten years ago, hospice and palliative care services were apparently not widely available in the Netherlands, and only now, partly in response to criticism in the United Kingdom and other European countries, is further development of palliative care as an alternative to euthanasia part of official national health care policy. On the other hand, euthanasia was performed in fewer than one third of the patients who requested it,

Table 18–1

Guidelines for PAS/Euthanasia: Comparison of the Netherlands and Oregon

GUIDELINE	NETHERLANDS	OREGON
Physician action	Euthanasia/PAS	PAS only
Conscientious objection	Yes	Yes
Age requirement	Adult	Adult
Legal residency		Oregon only (prior waiting period)
Mentally capable	Yes	Yes (physician certified)
Voluntary only	Yes	Yes
Multiple requests	Yes (repeated, consistent, and documented)	Yes (oral × 2; 15-day interval) witnessed (written)
Indication	Intolerable suffering	Terminal disease
Mandatory consultation	Yes	No
Coexistent psychiatric illness	Counseling optional	Counseling mandatory
Psychiatric illness	Yes	No
Offer alternative options	Not required	Mandatory
Mandatory reporting	Yes	Yes
Legality	Technically illegal	Legal
Immunity from prosecution	Highly probable	Yes

and the prognosis for natural death was estimated as one week or less in 87 percent of patients on whom euthanasia was performed, and one month or less in an additional 12 percent.

Following this study from the Dutch attorney general, a new procedure for reporting and reviewing cases of euthanasia was formulated and enacted into law in 1994. In studies reported in 1996, the fraction of physician-assisted deaths that were reported increased from 18 percent in 1990 to 41 percent in 1995, but physicians complained that the new reporting procedure was burdensome. Euthanasia increased somewhat between 1990 and 1995, but continued to largely be confined to terminally ill patients with very short life expectancies. The incidence and quality of second-opinion consultation increased compared to 1990 (64 percent met all criteria for good consultation), but still left room for improvement. Psychiatric consultation for medical patients who request physician-assisted death was relatively rare. The ending of life without the patient's explicit consent appar-

ently decreased slightly, but still accounted for 0.7 percent of all deaths. Some 58 percent of Dutch nursing homes had written guidelines for euthanasia, but in only 65 percent were all official requirements for prudent practice included. Euthanasia was reported to be acceptable under specific conditions in 90 percent of Dutch nursing homes; only 10 percent banned it completely.

In 1994, the Dutch Supreme Court ruled that in exceptional circumstances, physician-assisted death might be justifiable for patients with unbearable mental suffering but no physical illness. Subsequently, guidelines were published for euthanasia of the mentally ill. As expected, euthanasia for hopelessly depressed or demoralized patients is even more controversial than euthanasia for patients with terminal physical illnesses. The new guidelines have been condemned in other countries as having the potential to dangerously alter the practice of psychiatry and further erode the value and sanctity of life. In a 1996 survey of Dutch psychiatrists (552/667 responding), 205 (37 percent) had received at least one explicit, persistent request for physician-assisted death, and 12 had complied. Sixty-four percent of the respondents thought that euthanasia because of a mental disorder could be acceptable. In practice, however, requests for physician-assisted death were rarely granted, with an incidence of 2 to 5 actual deaths resulting from an estimated 320 requests.

In the Netherlands, the drugs most frequently dispensed for the purpose of accomplishing physician-assisted death include barbiturates, sometimes alone (10 percent), but usually in combination with various muscle relaxants (69 percent). Combinations of muscle relaxants and benzodiazepines are prescribed less frequently. Potassium chloride was administered in only 2 percent of the euthanasia cases. Because experience indicated that the oral route was less reliable and too slow, and overt physician intervention was required in 15 percent of cases initially planned as PAS, lethal injection is now preferred to oral ingestion. Pretreatment with antiemetic agents is sometimes offered as well. The use of additional drugs, such as opioids (13 percent) or antidepressants, apparently increased the likelihood of complications.

Contrary to the assumption that physician-assisted death is a technically simple and straightforward procedure, clinical problems with the performance of euthanasia, and particularly PAS, were common. Technical problems included poor venous access in some euthanasia cases, and difficulties in administering the oral medication for PAS due to difficulties in swallowing or irritation of the throat. Clinical complications included spasm, myoclonus, nausea, vomiting, and a longer than expected interval between the administration of medications and death, and failure to induce coma and death. Consequently, the Royal Dutch Medical Association now recommends that the physician should be present when euthanasia or PAS is carried out. Two thirds of general practitioners and nursing home physicians in the Netherlands endorse the statement that a physician who provides assistance with suicide should be present and prepared to administer a lethal drug if the suicide attempt fails.

Some of the reported complications of euthanasia and PAS have been attributed to a "learning curve" phenomenon. In earlier years, many Dutch physicians lacked knowledge about the optimal use of lethal drugs and protocol recommendations were not always followed. The Royal Dutch Association of Pharmacy now regularly updates its guidelines on the use and preparation of relevant drugs. Following the most recent update of 1998, it is asserted that the incidence of complications has significantly decreased, particularly if one discounts the longer and unpredictable time to death with PAS as inherent in the procedure itself. Nevertheless, because even minor complications and unintended effects can be stressful and burdensome to the patient and to attendant loved ones, the Dutch reviewers emphasize that physicians need to be aware of the possible, although exceptional, complications and should be trained to handle them properly. This suggestion has been endorsed by American supporters of physician-assisted death as a therapeutic option of last resort; it is particularly applicable to the state of Oregon and in any other similar models yet to come, in which PAS, but not euthanasia, is both legal and practiced.

PAS in the United States: The Oregon Experience

Although the population of Oregon (3.3 million) is only one fifth that of the Netherlands, the death rate of 8.8 per 1000 and the percentage of elderly people (13.2 percent) is nearly identical to that of the Netherlands. Nevertheless, when expressed as the percentage of total deaths, PAS-induced mortality in Oregon during 1999 was only 3 percent of that associated with physician-assisted death in the Netherlands.

PAS was legalized in Oregon in October 1997 with the passage of the Death with Dignity Act. Under this statute, eligibility for PAS is restricted to patients older than 18 years of age, who are residents of Oregon, terminally ill (life expectancy of less than 6 months), mentally "capable" of making and communicating decisions about their health care, and on their own volition make two oral requests for PAS and one written, witnessed request over a period of 15 days (Table 18–1). The patient's primary physician and a consultant are required to confirm the terminal diagnosis and prognosis and determine that the patient is capable. If either physician believes the patient's judgment is impaired due to depression or some other psychiatric or psychological disorder, the patient must be referred for counseling. The physician must inform the patient of all feasible alternative options, including pain control and hospice and palliative care, and review the risks and results of ingesting the lethal dose of medication. Physicians must report all prescriptions for lethal medications that are actually given to the patient. Physicians are not compelled to participate in PAS in violation of their own moral convictions, and are protected from criminal prosecution when they adhere to the requirements of the legislation.

During 1998, the first year of legalized PAS, 23 patients received prescriptions for lethal medications and 15 died after taking the prescribed medications (barbiturates in all cases, usually with antiemetics). Of the 8 patients not choosing to take their own lives, 7 died of their terminal illnesses, and 1 committed suicide during 1999. Thirteen of the 15 patients had cancer, and 8 were older than 69 years of age. Although not so stated, one has the impression that death was not as imminent in these patients as in the Dutch patients described earlier. The time from ingestion to unconsciousness ranged from 3 to 20 minutes, and the time from ingestion to death ranged from 15 minutes to 11.5 hours. No vomiting or seizures were reported. Eight patients who received prescriptions did not use them, with 6 having died of their underlying illnesses. Of the two who remained alive in January 1999, one subsequently died of the underlying illness and the second committed suicide during 1999. The frequency with which physicians were present during the act of suicide was not reported.

Oregon ranks third nationally in the rate of hospice admissions and is among the top five states in per-capita use of morphine for medical purposes. Seventy-one percent of the patients who elected PAS were being cared for on hospice programs. Thus, lack of access to excellent palliative care was not likely a factor in patient requests for PAS. Rather the decision to request and use a prescription for lethal medication was associated with concern about loss of autonomy or control of bodily functions, not with fear of intractable pain or concern about financial loss. The choice of PAS was not associated with level of education or health insurance coverage. Compared to all terminal patients, those who elected PAS did not inordinately express concern about being a burden to family and friends. However, retrospective bereavement surveys suggested that loved ones often perceived or imagined this concern as a significant motif in the decision to request PAS.

During 1999, 33 patients received prescriptions after a request for PAS and 26 patients died after taking the lethal medications. Physicians granted 1 in 6 requests for a prescription, and 1 in 10 requests actually resulted in suicide. Many patients who sought assistance with suicide had to ask more than one physician for a prescription for lethal medication. As in 1998, the patients were mostly elderly and suffering from terminal cancer, although amyotrophic lateral sclerosis was the terminal diagnosis in 4 patients, and chronic obstructive pulmonary disease in 4 others. Seventy-eight percent were enrolled in a hospice program before they died. The median interval between the first request for PAS and death was 83 days, as compared with 22 days in 1998. The longest interval between ingestion and death was 26 hours, but 24 patients died within 4 hours. As in 1998, no significant complications were reported. Interviews with physicians and family members indicated that the main reasons for requesting PAS were concern about loss of autonomy and control of bodily functions, an inability to participate in activities that make life enjoyable, physical suffering with particular reference to dyspnea and dysphagia as well as pain, and a determination to control the manner of death.

Concern has been raised as to whether depression was underrecognized or underreported among Oregonians requesting PAS with the result that potentially treatable patients were instead allowed to kill themselves. In prior studies of terminally ill patients, the rates of depression have ranged from 59 to 100 percent, whereas only 20 percent of the patients who requested PAS were reported or diagnosed as depressed. In answer, it was noted that a total of 28 patients who requested PAS received medications for depression or anxiety or were evaluated by a mental health professional. Only 3 of the 28 changed their minds about obtaining a prescription for a lethal medication. Nevertheless, it is conceded that the magnitude of the role of depression in requests for PAS requires further well-designed studies, pending which all patients requesting assistance with suicide should undertake a mental health consultation and be offered referral to a hospice program.

As previously noted, hospice and palliative care services, the quality of which was undocumented, was sometimes not perceived as a substitute or deterrent for PAS. However, patients for whom palliative interventions were made were significantly more likely to change their minds about assisted suicide than those for whom interventions were not made. Parenthetically, since enactment of the Death with Dignity Act, total hospice referrals have increased in Oregon by 20 percent.

The Disputation: Arguments Pro and Con

In the United States, legitimization and legalization of physician-assisted suicide as a therapeutic option is the most controversial current issue in end-of-life care. Profound differences over fundamental ethical questions and societal values have resulted in seemingly irreconcilable positions with little evidence for the existence of any middle ground. There is little disagreement about the clin-

ical concerns that have motivated those who have put the issue of PAS "into play" in the arena of public opinion. The controversy swirls around the issue as to whether PAS violates professional and societal ground rules sufficiently so as to make it totally inadmissible.

In Favor of PAS

The proponents of PAS as a therapeutic option in end-of-life care have offered four major reasons as compelling justifications for their position (Table 18–2). A clearer understanding of the relative significance of each, from the perspective of the patient and family, has emerged from the experience with PAS in Oregon (discussed earlier).

INADEQUATE OR UNAVAILABLE PAIN AND SYMPTOM MANAGEMENT

One of the most haunting and disturbing images in American literature is Thomas Wolfe's description of the death of his own brother as depicted by Ben Gant in the novel *Look Homeward Angel:* "Ben's thin lips were lifted in a constant grimace of torture and strangulation, [and the] sound of his gasping—loud, hoarse, unbelievable, filling the room and orchestrating every moment of it—

Table 18–2

Conditions Promoting Consideration of Physician-Assisted Suicide

CONDITION	MANIFESTATION
Physical suffering	Inadequate or unavailable pain and symptom management
Emotional suffering	Irreversible loss of control and independence
Social suffering	Intractable socioeconomic burdens of terminal illness
Existential suffering	Hopelessly worsening quality of life

gave to the scene its final note of horror." Although written 70 years ago, this could be a contemporaneous description of a dying, undertreated patient with AIDS, COPD, or cancer. A number of studies indicate a high prevalence of uncontrolled pain and dyspnea, among other symptoms in dying patients. It is hardly surprising that some patients would elect to accelerate their own death rather than undergo protracted, unrelenting physical suffering, even if only contemplated and not yet experienced. Under such circumstances, if a rational person chooses to die rather than to live miserably, should society have the right to say no?

AUTONOMY AND PRIVACY: THE PATIENT'S RIGHT TO CHOOSE

Even when adequate symptom palliation is achieved, the Oregon experience indicates that dying patients assign particular importance to control of their bodily functions and right to self-determination. Autonomy is a hallmark principle of clinical ethics. The right to refuse unwanted treatment and the constitutional right to privacy were key elements in the precedent-setting 1976 Quinlan decision regarding unwanted artificial ventilation, and in the Cruzan decision involving the right to remove a feeding tube from a patient in a persistent vegetative state. The courts have extended the right to refuse treatment even to patients with non-terminal conditions. The 1986 opinion in *Bouvia v. Superior Court (CA)* stated: "The right to die is an integral part of our right to control our own destinies so long as the rights of others are not affected." Today, a patient can refuse any life-sustaining procedure or treatment, and unassisted suicide is not generally illegal. That being so, why should a person not be free to choose any mode of "final exit" that does not endanger others, even if the cooperation of another party such as a physician is necessary?

PERCEPTION OF BEING A BURDEN

As patients with terminal illnesses progressively lose physical independence, they often suffer from erosion of their self-image and a loss of self-worth. They are also usually aware of the invariably onerous financial burden imposed on others by their deteriorating condition, not only in terms of medical expenses but also in terms of the investment of time, effort, and money by family and friends. One study of attitudes towards euthanasia and PAS in the United States indicated that 60 percent of the respondents chose "economic burden" as a reason for PAS as opposed to only 20 percent who chose "avoiding pain." Although the Oregon results indicated that patients who requested PAS were not at greater economic disadvantage than those who did not, it is uncertain that this finding is applicable to other areas of the country or the world in general in which economic disparity may be more pronounced. In any event, in as much as there appears to be little immediate prospect that affordable, universal health care and long-term care will be instituted in the United States, does society have the right to refuse PAS to those terminally ill patients who regard it as the best option for alleviating what has been termed "social suffering"?

EXISTENTIAL SUFFERING

Even if the patient is not suffering physically and is not a financial burden, emotional pain and distress cannot be ignored. Is it possible that the patient's perceived quality of life can be so low that it is unethical to force the individual to continue that life? Is such an emotional state necessarily synonymous with a syndrome of pathologic depression that would render the patient incompetent to make life decisions? Consider the case of a 42-year-old psychologist whose disability and weakness progressed to complete quadriplegia and total dependence on others. "She was imposing on her family as they were forced to watch her dying slowly . . . her pain was adequately controlled, but this existential suffering remained profound." She requested assistance in dying, but was told that was illegal. Rather, she was offered total sedation. "In the doctor's mind, this approach was justified by the inability to relieve her psychological and existential distress while maintaining a wakeful state."

Is this approach truly different or better from an ethical viewpoint than PAS?

In Opposition to PAS

The counterarguments to legalization of PAS are summarized in Table 18–3, and also should be examined with reference to the published reports from Oregon that were described earlier.

IMPROVED ACCESS TO ADEQUATE HOSPICE AND PALLIATIVE CARE OBVIATES NEED FOR PAS

PAS need not be and ought not to be a subject for controversy because a model for quality end-of-life care for the terminally ill is already available. The real debate should be about improved access to hospice and palliative care programs. Although there are more than 3000 hospice providers in the United States, the quality of hospice care is variable, and there are millions of people in this country who do not have access to hospice services. Funding restrictions and overly restrictive and rigid interpretation of the Medicare rule mandating a life expectancy of 6 months or less have placed restraints on the ability of many hospices to respond appropriately to need, and have resulted in a majority of patients being referred to hospice less than 2 weeks before death. With education and legislative changes, hospice palliative care could mark-

Table 18–3

Arguments Against Legalization of Physician-Assisted Suicide

> Improved access to hospice and palliative care obviates need for PAS.
> Individual patient autonomy rights must yield to the overall societal concern for the sanctity of human life.
> PAS is a "slippery slope" leading to social injustice and depravity.
> PAS is incompatible with the role of the physician as healer and protector of life.

edly reduce suffering in almost all terminally ill patients, rendering PAS unnecessary. Of course, there would still be the rare, exceptional case where suffering was intractable and resistant. And, it should also be noted that 75 percent of the Oregon patients who elected PAS were enrolled on hospice programs!

PATIENT AUTONOMY IS NOT LIMITLESS

The Bouvia decision (discussed earlier) emphasized the right to control one's destiny provided that the rights of others are not affected. Daniel Callahan reasons that because PAS requires assistance by another person, it is no longer a private act but a form of communal action (Hendin, 1998). Although the individual physician who opposes PAS may abstain on the basis of conscientious objection, it is argued that PAS threatens the very fabric of society by cheapening and denigrating the perceived value of human life. There is a solid core of opinion, usually but not always religiously based, that life is sacred and infinitely precious no matter its "quality," and that this belief is key to preserving our moral status. Because society has an overriding responsibility to protect the sanctity of life, individual freedom of action, such as to allow PAS, should be abrogated in favor of the overall good.

PAS IS A "SLIPPERY SLOPE" LEADING INEVITABLY TO SOCIAL DEPRAVITY

Some advocates for PAS also support euthanasia for sick patients who cannot kill themselves. "[This] comes as no surprise to opponents of PAS [who] predicted long ago that if assisted suicide is permitted, euthanasia would not be far behind" (Manning, 2000). Reacting in part to the Dutch experience, opponents of PAS foresee euthanasia without consent, euthanasia for mental illness, and eventually, euthanasia for the physically handicapped, elderly, demented, homeless, and anyone else deemed socially useless or undesirable. For those who are skeptical that highly cultured societies would never countenance such behavior, "slippery slope" debaters justifiably introduce Adolph Hitler, Joseph Goebbels, Joseph Mengele, and their followers into evidence. Closer to home, there is already sufficient concern in this country about abusive, self-serving managed care practices that have caused politicians of all stripes to recognize the need for some type of "patient bill of rights." Can we be truly sure that were PAS to be broadly legalized, patients might not come under subtle pressure to make the request? There seems to be no evidence for this in Oregon to date, but can we afford to be complacent?

PAS Is a Violation of the Hippocratic Oath

PAS is antithetical to the role of the physician as a healer and protector of life whose most basic obligation is *primum non nocere,* "first, do no harm." As deliberately killing a patient is regarded as harm *par excellence,* this maxim would appear to clearly apply to any action by a physician that serves to hasten death. Advocates for PAS such as Dr. Sherwin Nuland prefer to treat the Hippocratic Oath and similar formulations as ancient, perhaps occasionally relevant guidelines, which should be interpreted and modified as necessary in accordance with the doctor's appraisal of a patient's needs and desires, and in accordance with the physician's individual conscience. "To seek refuge in ancient aphorisms is to turn away from the unique needs of each of our patients who have entrusted themselves to our care." The observation that a strong and increasing majority of American physicians oppose legalization of PAS and would refuse to participate even if legally able suggests that *primum non nocere* continues as a significant component of the professional psyche of most physicians.

Conclusion

The ultimate resolution of this debate is unclear. It seems likely that, given the undercurrent of public support, assisting terminally ill patients in sui-

Table 18–4

Suggested Physician Responses to a Request for Physician-Assisted Suicide

1. Identify, acknowledge, and clarify the request.
2. Explore the patient's concerns and address total suffering.
3. Achieve a shared understanding of the goals of treatment.
4. If treatment goals cannot be achieved, search for acceptable alternatives to PAS.
5. If the patient insists on suicide, clarify the level of participation expected and conscientiously acceptable to the physician.
6. Offer all information relevant to informed consent, including realistic options.
7. Do not hesitate to seek emotional support from colleagues.

Source: Adapted from Tulsky JA, Ciampa R, Rosen EJ: Responding to legal requests for physician-assisted suicide. *Ann Intern Med* 132:494, 2000.

cide will be more and more a reality in our society. In addition to guidance from an individual 's conscience, and religious beliefs if present, what advice should a physician seek in responding to a legal request for PAS? The Assisted Suicide Consensus Panel of the University of Pennsylvania Center for Bioethics offered the following paraphrased suggestions in a paper in *Annals of Internal Medicine,* which are also listed in Table 18–4 (Tulsky et al, 2000).

Identify, acknowledge, and clarify the request. Using open-ended questions (see Chapter 3), encourage patients to feel comfortable in sharing their ideas and feelings. If it is evident that a patient is seeking PAS, address the issue head on. If the patient appears to be skirting the issue, probe cautiously to find out whether PAS is indeed under consideration. In the absence of some patient initiative, do not recommend PAS as a therapeutic option.

Explore the patient's concerns and address total suffering. Try to identify the elements of suffering that are fueling the patient's desire to hasten death. As indicated, these most often involve concern about loss of independence, loss of control of bodily functions, worsening and unrelenting symptoms, and fear of being a burden to family and friends. After an in-depth discussion, the patient may agree to consider alternate approaches other than suicide.

Achieve a shared understanding of the goals of treatment. When palliative treatment is proposed, the physician and patient should agree on realistic goals and endpoints of response. A key component of all palliative care is restoration of hope that continued living will be meaningful. Oftentimes, by focusing attention on particularly significant life events or milestones, even a short-term treatment plan may assure patients that they are back in control of their lives.

If treatment goals cannot be achieved, search for acceptable alternatives to PAS. Seek additional expert consultation if treatment outcomes are suboptimal. In the rare circumstance when all standard and unconventional options for palliation of suffering are exhausted, and the patient reasserts an interest in PAS, discuss other relevant and more universally acceptable options. These may include withdrawal of life-sustaining treatment such as dialysis, total sedation, or voluntary cessation of eating and drinking.

If the patient insists on suicide, clarify the level of participation expected and that is conscientiously acceptable for the physician. Despite the best efforts of the attending physician and consultant experts, some patients will persist in requesting PAS. This is the time when the issue can no longer be avoided and each physician must decide how to respond based on personal belief and conviction. The principle of conscientious practice guarantees the physician's right to withdraw from the care of a patient who chooses a treatment that is morally objectionable for the clinician. It would seem that right would extend even to abstaining from a direct referral to a colleague who would be prepared to participate in PAS. However, the physi-

cian should be most careful not to abandon other necessary and appropriate care of the patient, unless specifically asked to withdraw.

Offer all information relevant to informed consent including realistic options. Patients must be fully informed about their legal options as well as all the details of the PAS procedure, including potential complications. There should be agreement as to the physician's attendance during the suicide and the physician's role if events do not go smoothly. The patient and family need to be aware that the time from ingestion of lethal medication to death may be variable, occasionally extending for many hours. There should be a plan as to what to do if the attempted suicide fails or if patients change their minds midstream. Family members should be integrated into the discussion as they are likely to play an active role in assisting the suicide, and must face the emotional consequences thereafter.

Do not hesitate to seek emotional support from colleagues. Many physicians will experience feelings of frustration, failure, emptiness, and abandonment when receiving a request for assisted dying, and more so should a patient actually commit suicide. Physicians and other health care professionals need to take care of each other, and the support of colleagues can be critical in affirming the physician's own sense of self-worth and continued mission as a healer.

The debate about PAS is more subtle and sensitive than committed proponents and opponents are sometimes willing to acknowledge. Competent physicians caring for terminal patients have always been positioned somewhere on that notorious ethical slippery slope. The real conundrum is to define where on that slope we are willing to take a stand—a muddy and ambiguous task that subjects us to high levels of stress and to potential abuse.

Ultimately, what has to inform the physician's decision-making, regarding PAS or any other aspect of the doctor–patient relationship, is nothing more than as much wisdom and kindness as his or her education, character and faith will permit. The challenge is well described in the words of Dr. Walter J. Kade (2000), the pseudonym of a physician who himself participated in PAS: "Although we have accepted our roles as comforters in end-of-life care, we have not struggled with or found solutions to active roles in accomplishing their deaths. I am grateful for the great disruption in my emotional stability that this experience precipitated. This act should never be easy, never routine. It should be among the most difficult and disquieting acts we embark upon." Based largely on the Dutch experience, the question is: Will Dr. Kade write those same words after PAS number 2, or number 5, or number 20? Writing in September 2000, we must, at this time, leave this question hanging and unanswered.

References

Abramson N, Stokes J, Weinreb N, Clark WS: Euthanasia and doctor-assisted suicide: responses by oncologists and non-oncologists. *South Med J* 91:637, 1998.

Angell M. Caring for the dying—Congressional mischief. *N Engl J Med* 341:1923, 1999. Editorial. (See correspondence *N Engl J Med* 342: 1049, 2000.)

Angell M: The Supreme Court and physician-assisted suicide—The ultimate right. *N Engl J Med* 336:50, 1973. Editorial.

Angell M: Euthanasia in the Netherlands—Good news or bad? *N Engl J Med* 335:1676, 1996. Editorial.

Anonymous: A piece of my mind. It's over, Debbie. *JAMA* 259:272, 1988.

Binstock RH: Long-term care for older people: Moral and political challenges of access. In: Monagle JF, Thomasma DC, eds. *Health Care Ethics: Critical Issues*. Silver Spring, MD, Aspen, 1994.

Blendon RJ, Szalay US, Knox RA: Should physicians aid their patients in dying? The public perspective. *JAMA* 267:2658, 1992.

Burt RA: The Supreme Court speaks: not assisted suicide but a constitutional right of palliative care. *N Engl J Med* 337:1234, 1997.

Caplan AL, Snyder L, Faber-Langendoen K: The role of guidelines in the practice of physician-assisted suicide. *Ann Intern Med* 132:476, 2000.

Cherny NI: The use of sedation in the management of refractory pain. *Princ Pract Support Oncol* 3:1, 2000.

Chin AE, Hedberg K, Higginson GK, Fleming DW: Legalized physician-assisted suicide in Oregon—The first year's experience. *N Engl J Med* 340:577, 1999.

Churchill LR, King NM: Physician-assisted suicide, euthanasia and withdrawal of treatment. *BMJ* 315: 137, 1997.

Dworkin G, Frey RG, Bok S: *Euthanasia and Physician-Assisted Suicide (For and Against)*. New York, Cambridge University Press, 1998.

Emmanuel EJ: The history of euthanasia debates in the United States and Britain. *Ann Intern Med* 121:793, 1994.

Emanuel EJ, Daniels ER, Fairclough DL, Clarridge BR: The practice of euthanasia and physician-assisted suicide in the United States: Adherence to proposed safeguards and effects on physicians. *JAMA* 280:507, 1998.

Emanuel EJ, Fairclough DL, Slutsman J, Emanuel LL: Understanding economic and other burdens of terminal illness: The experience of patients and their caregivers. *Ann Intern Med* 132:451, 2000.

Faber-Langendoen K, Karlawish JHT: Should assisted suicide be only physician assisted? *Ann Intern Med* 132:482, 2000.

Field MJ, Cassel CK, eds: *Approaching Death: Improving Care at the End of Life*. Washington, DC, National Academy Press, 1997.

Fohr SA: The double effect of pain medication: Separating myth from reality. *J Palliat Med* 1:315, 1998.

Ganzini L, Nelson HD, Schmidt TA, et al: Physicians' experiences with the Oregon Death with Dignity Act. *N Engl J Med* 342:557, 2000. (See correspondence *N Engl J Med* 343:150, 2000.)

Gordijn B, Janssens R: The prevention of euthanasia through palliative care: New developments in the Netherlands. *Patient Educ Couns* 41:35, 2000.

Groenewoud JH, van der Heide A, Onwuteaka-Philipsen BD, et al: Clinical problems with the performance of euthanasia and physician-assisted suicide in the Netherlands. *N Eng J Med* 342:551, 2000.

Groenewoud JH, van der Maas PJ, van der Wal G, et al: Physician-assisted death in psychiatric practice in the Netherlands. *N Engl J Med* 336:1795, 1997.

Haley K, Lee MA, eds: *The Oregon Death with Dignity Act—A Guidebook for Health Care Providers*, 1st ed. Portland, The Center for Ethics in Health Care, 1998.

Haverkate I, Muller MT, Cappetti M, et al: Prevalence and content analysis of guidelines on handling requests for euthanasia or assisted suicide in Dutch nursing homes. *Arch Intern Med* 160:317, 2000.

Hendin H: *Seduced by Death: Doctors, Patients, and Assisted Suicide.* New York, Norton, 1998.

Jecker NS: Physician-assisted death in the Netherlands and in the United States: Ethical and cultural aspects of health policy development. *J Am Geriatr Soc* 42:672, 1994.

Kade WJ: On being a doctor. Death with dignity: A case study. *Ann Intern Med* 132:504, 2000.

Kissane DW, Kelly BJ: Demoralisation, depression and desire for death: Problems with the Dutch guidelines for euthanasia of the mentally ill. *Aust NZ J Psychiatry* 34:325, 2000.

Lau HS, Riezebos J, Abas V, et al: A nation-wide study on the practice of euthanasia and physician-assisted suicide in community and hospital pharmacies in the Netherlands. *Pharm World Sci* 22:3, 2000.

Manning MT: Letter to the Editor. *N Engl J Med* 343:152, 2000.

Miller FG, Fins JJ, Snyder L: Assisted suicide compared with refusal of treatment: A valid distinction? *Ann Intern Med* 132:470, 2000.

More T: *Utopia and Other Writings.* New York, New American Library, 1984.

Muller MT, Van der Wal G, Van Eijk JT, Ribbe MW: Voluntary active euthanasia and physician-assisted suicide in Dutch nursing homes: Are the requirements for prudent practice properly met? *J Am Geriatr Soc* 42:624, 1994.

Nuland SB: Physician-assisted suicide and euthanasia in practice. *N Engl J Med* 342:583, 2000. Editorial. (See correspondence *N Engl J Med* 343:150, 2000.)

Onwuteaka-Philipsen BD, van der Wal G, Kostense PJ, van der Maas PJ: Consultation with another physician on euthanasia and assisted suicide in the Netherlands. *Soc Sci Med* 51:429, 2000.

Peck MS: *Denial of the Soul.* New York, Random House, 1997.

Quill TE: *Death and Dignity: Making Choices and Taking Charge.* New York, Norton, 1993.

Quill TE: Doctor, I want to die. Will you help me? *JAMA* 270:870, 1993.

Quill TE: Death and dignity: A case of individualized decision making. *N Engl J Med* 324:691, 1991.

Quill TE, Coombs Lee B, Nunn S. Palliative treatments of last resort: Choosing the least harmful alternative. *Ann Intern Med* 132:488, 2000.

Quill TE, Dresser R, Brock DW: The rule of double effect—A critique of its role in end-of-life decision making. *N Engl J Med* 337:1768, 1997.

Quill TE, Lo B, Brock DW: Palliative options of last resort: A comparison of voluntarily stopping eating and drinking, terminal sedation, physician-assisted suicide, and voluntary active euthanasia. *JAMA* 278:2099, 1997.

Shaiova L: Case presentation: Terminal sedation and existential distress. *J Pain Symptom Manage* 16:403, 1998.

Snyder L, Caplan AL: Assisted suicide: Finding common ground. *Ann Intern Med* 132:468, 2000.

Sullivan AD, Hedberg K, Fleming DW: Legalized physician-assisted suicide in Oregon—The second year. *N Engl J Med* 342:598, 2000. (See correspondence *N Engl J Med* 343:150, 2000.)

Swarte NB, Heintz AP: Euthanasia and physician-assisted suicide. *Ann Med* 31:364, 1999.

Tulsky JA, Ciampa R, Rosen EJ: Responding to legal requests for physician-assisted suicide. *Ann Intern Med* 132:494, 2000.

Van der Maas PJ, van der Wal G, Haverkate I, et al: Euthanasia, physician-assisted suicide, and other medical practices involving the end of life in the Netherlands, 1990–1995. *N Eng J Med* 335:1699, 1996.

Willems DL, Daniels ER, van der Wal G, et al: Attitudes and practices concerning the end of life: A comparison between physicians from the United States and from the Netherlands. *Arch Intern Med* 160:63, 2000.

Wolfe J, Fairclough DL, Clarridge BR, et al: Stability of attitudes regarding physician-assisted suicide and euthanasia among oncology patients, physicians, and the general public. *J Clin Oncol* 17:1274, 1999.

Wolfe T: *Look Homeward, Angel.* New York, Scribners, 1947, p. 574.

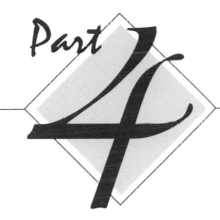

Part 4

Special Groups

Michael Wohlfeiler

End-of-Life Care for Patients with AIDS

Introduction

Patients with AIDS often need hospice and end-of-life care and they represent a unique population for several reasons. First, precise prognostic determinations can be difficult because most deaths occur from opportunistic infections that are, at least to some extent, treatable. Second, continual improvements in antiretroviral therapy and opportunistic disease prophylaxis and treatment have continually increased the interval between AIDS diagnosis and death. Third, patients with AIDS also present significant psychosocial and socioeconomic challenges that must be dealt with.

Those infected with the AIDS virus are mostly younger people in their second through fourth decades of life. The existence of a large group of young adults afflicted with a terminal disease has meant that end-of-life care programs have had to learn to deal with psychosocial problems that were substantially different from those seen in their more typical, predominantly elderly patient population. Further complicating the psychosocial care of terminal AIDS patients is the fact that there has been enormous fear and stigmatization accompanying a diagnosis of HIV or AIDS, as many persons infected with the disease tended to be from groups already marginalized by society—gays, minorities, immigrants, and intravenous drug users.

Determining Prognosis in AIDS

One of the greatest challenges in providing end-of-life care for AIDS patients has always been the difficulty in determining which patients are appropriate for hospice and end-of-life care. The very nature of HIV disease has made these determinations very difficult. Because most of the morbidity and mortality of AIDS results from opportunistic infections that are to some extent treatable and temporarily reversible, each patient may not always follow an inexorably progressive and fatal course. Additionally, as treatment modalities have improved, the interval between diagnosis with AIDS and death has lengthened. Less than a decade ago, the average survival after a first episode of PCP was approximately 10 months. With the development of antiretroviral therapy, followed later by highly active antiretroviral therapy (HAART) and improvement in opportunistic infection prophylaxis, that period has steadily increased and may now conceivably be indefinite. This constantly changing prognosis in AIDS makes it difficult for clinicians to determine which AIDS patients have progressed to a stage of disease that makes it appropriate for them to receive end-of-life care.

Despite these challenges, the National Hospice Organization's Medical Guidelines Task Force, in 1996, published medical guidelines for determining prognosis in selected noncancer diseases, including AIDS. These guidelines are discussed in Chapter 1 (Table 1–14) and, for completeness, are reprinted here as Table 19–1.

It is important to note that the factors delineated by the task force represent guidelines rather than absolute criteria for determining prognosis. The task force acknowledged that HIV mortality is a dynamic variable that is affected by a number of factors—new and changing therapies, the practitioner's skill and experience in management of HIV disease, and the individual patient's ability to tolerate treatment. Because of the waxing and waning clinical course that can be so characteristic of AIDS, it was suggested that the clinical course over the previous months might be more reflective of the patient's prognosis.

Antiretroviral Therapy Near the End of Life

The NHO Medical Guidelines Task Force noted that patients receiving antiretroviral therapy may have a greatly lengthened prognosis and therefore generally might not be appropriate to receive hospice or end-of-life care. In fact, one

Table 19–1

Guidelines for Determining a Prognosis of 6 Months or less for Patients with AIDS

CD4+ count < 25 cells/µL in periods free of acute illness

Or

HIV RNA (viral load) > 100,000 copies on a persistent basis

HIV RNA (viral load) < 100,000 copies in the presence of:
    Patient refusal to receive antiretroviral or prophylactic medications
    Declining functional status
    One or more "other factors" listed below

HIV-related opportunistic illnesses

Disease	*Prognosis for Survival*
CNS lymphoma	2.5 months
Progressive multifocal leukoencephalopathy	4 months
Cryptosporidiosis	5 months
AIDS wasting syndrome (loss of 1/3 lean body mass)	< 6 months
MAC bacteremia, untreated	< 6 months
Visceral Kaposi's sarcoma, unresponsive to treatment	50% 6-month mortality
Renal failure, refuses dialysis	< 6 months
Advanced AIDS dementia complex	6 months
Toxoplasmosis	6 months

Other factors associated with a poor prognosis for patients with AIDS
    Chronic persistent diarrhea for 1 year
    Persistent serum albumin < 2.5 g/dL
    Concomitant substance abuse
    Age > 50
    Decision to forego antiretroviral therapy, chemotherapy, and prophylactic drug therapy related
        to HIV disease and related illnesses
    Congestive heart failure, symptomatic at rest

SOURCE: Reprinted with permission from Stuart B, Connor S, Kinzbrunner BM, et al: *Medical Guidelines for Determining Prognosis in Selected Non-Cancer Diseases.* Arlington, National Hospice Organization, 1st ed, 1995; 2nd ed, 1996.

could conclude that by the time a patient with AIDS transitions to palliative care, there is probably little if any benefit to continuing antiretroviral therapy. The fact that the patient is now in the terminal stages of the disease can be considered *a priori* evidence that antiretroviral therapy is no longer effective, most likely due to the development of antiretroviral resistance. Because of the toxicities and lack of palliative benefit of antiretrovirals, hospices may require termination of those medications prior to admission to their programs. Despite that, it may be psychologically very difficult for the patient to give up the only therapy that is directed at the underlying HIV infection. An alternative approach for those patients may be to allow them to enter a palliative care program while on antiretrovirals and then use the spiritual and psychosocial resources of hospice to guide them until they can accept termination of those therapies.

Palliative Care of Patients with AIDS

Palliative care in AIDS can be conceptualized as a continuum consisting of specific therapy directed at AIDS-related illnesses such as infection and malignancy, as well as treatments focused primarily on providing comfort and symptom control near the very end of life.

Specific treatments directed at AIDS-related infection or malignancy are not generally perceived as part and parcel of end-of-life care. However, efforts to have patients access hospice and palliative care services earlier in the course of AIDS dictates that end-of-life care providers be willing to provide such care when indicated, based on the patient's overall clinical condition and quality of life concerns. For example, a terminally ill AIDS patient with CMV retinitis who is still well enough to read or interact with family and friends, may be treated with ganciclovir while on a hospice program, as quality of life concerns would dictate that this patient should not be allowed to go blind. If, however, the patient's underlying AIDS has progressed to the point that he or she is comatose or severely encephalopathic, then continuing intravenous therapies for CMV is unlikely to enhance quality of life. At that stage, it is more likely that the discomfort and toxicities associated with drug treatment would outweigh benefit for the patient's quality of life.

Likewise, with regard to primary or secondary prophylaxis against opportunistic infection, each prophylactic regimen should be evaluated by weighing the likely benefit of that regimen on the patient's quality of life against the toxicities and discomfort likely to be associated with it. As the patient's clinical status declines, a point will inevitably be reached at which the balance shifts away from continuing such therapies and warrants discontinuation of all opportunistic infection prophylaxis.

Therefore, as treatment and prophylaxis of common AIDS-related opportunistic infections and malignancies seen near the end of life are discussed in the next section, it is important to keep these principles in mind.

Opportunistic Infection Treatment and Prophylaxis Near the End of Life

Symptoms in AIDS are often a direct consequence of specific opportunistic infections (OIs). Because most OIs respond partially or completely to appropriate therapy, symptoms may at times be palliated most effectively by prevention and/or treatment of the underlying infection. Therefore, in an end-of-life care setting, the primary purpose of prophylaxis and treatment of OIs must be relief of symptoms rather than restorative or curative care. The most common OIs that are seen in AIDS patients near the end of life are *Pneumocystis carinii* pneumonia (PCP), cytomegalovirus (CMV) retinitis, and *Mycobacterium avium intracelluare* (MAC). Table 19–2 summarizes each OI's symptoms and recommended treatments for AIDS patients near the end of life.

PNEUMOCYSTIS CARINII PNEUMONIA

Pneumocystis carinii (PCP) is the most common of all OIs. The primary symptoms of PCP are typically fever, cough, and profound dyspnea. In the palliative care setting, treatment of acute PCP should be considered for patients who, though terminal, are not imminently dying and still have an acceptable quality of life. It is preferable to administer PCP treatment as oral therapy using trimethoprim sulfamethoxazole (TMP-SMX), trimethoprim plus dapsone, or trimethoprim plus atovaquone. If a patient refuses therapy or cannot tolerate toxicities associated with therapy, management should be based purely on symptom control. The patient should receive supplemental oxygen and morphine to relieve dyspnea. Corticosteroids are often a useful adjunctive therapy to improve dyspnea and hypoxemia. (See Chapter 7 for a full discussion of the treatment of dyspnea at the end of life.) Corticosteroids or nonsteroidal anti-inflammatory drugs (NSAIDs) may also be effective in reducing the fever and generalized discomfort of PCP.

PCP occurs in about 80 percent of patients who do not receive prophylaxis. Therefore, it is reasonable, even near the end of life, to treat all patients who tolerate oral TMP-SMX with a dose of one double-strength tablet daily or every other day as primary or secondary prophylaxis for PCP infection.

CYTOMEGALOVIRUS RETINITIS

Cytomegalovirus (CMV) can cause disease in a wide variety of sites, though by far the most common is the retina of the eye. If left untreated, CMV

Table 19–2

Common Opportunistic Infections in Patients Near the End of Life with AIDS

INFECTION	COMMON SYMPTOMS	TREATMENT	DOSE
PCP	Fever, cough, dyspnea	Prophylaxis: TMP − SMX	1 DS tablet daily or every other day
		Treatment: TMP − SMX	2 DS tablets q 8 h × 21 days
		TMP + dapsone	TMP: 5 mg/kg PO tid + Dap: 100 mg PO qd for 21 days
		TMP + atovaquone	TMP: 5 mg/kg PO tid + Ata: 750 mg PO bid for 21 days
CMV Retinitis	Blindness	Primary prophylaxis: Not recommended near the end of life	
		Treatment: ganciclovir	IV: Induction: 5 mg/kg q 12 h × 14–21 days Maintenance: 5 mg/kg qd Oral: 1000 mg PO tid (after induction, for maintenance only) Intravitreal implant
MAC complex	Fever, night sweats, weight loss, diarrhea, fatigue, cytopenias	Treatment should be symptomatic only near the end of life Toxicity of prophylaxis and primary treatment of infection outweigh potential benefits in terminally ill patients	NSAIDs, steroids (dexamethasone 2 mg PO qd), analgesics, anti-diarrheals

retinitis can progress rapidly to blindness. Preservation of sight is an obvious quality of life issue, and as such, treatment of active CMV disease or secondary prophylaxis for previous infections should be considered part of palliative care.

There are three approved therapies for treatment and suppression of CMV retinitis: ganciclovir, foscarnet, and cidofovir. Ganciclovir is probably the most frequently used in the hospice setting. Intravenous ganciclovir is used for the treatment of active CMV while either the oral form or an intravitreal implant can be used for maintenance therapy. However, it should be noted that the oral form is associated with a risk of more rapid rate of CMV progression. Both the intravenous and oral forms of ganciclovir can cause significant bone marrow suppression (primarily neutropenia), which can be problematic and should be monitored.

Cidofovir is only administered every 2 weeks (after the induction dosing of weekly for 2 weeks), which would seem to make it ideal for a hospice setting. Unfortunately, it has significant nephrotoxicity, making it a difficult agent to use near the end of life. Foscarnet has similar nephrotoxicity to cidofovir and maintenance therapy requires daily infusions, making it even more problematic.

Regarding prophylaxis, whereas PCP will occur in almost 80 percent of AIDS patients who are not receiving prophylactic therapy, CMV retinitis occurs in only about 25 percent of patients not treated prophylactically. Suspicion of CMV retinitis is usually raised by the patient's report of symptoms and is then readily detectable by ophthalmologic examination. Once diagnosed, CMV retinitis generally responds rapidly to treatment. Therefore, primary prophylaxis to prevent CMV retinitis is not indicated in the palliative care setting.

MYCOBACTERIUM AVIUM COMPLEX

Mycobacterium avium complex (MAC) can develop in AIDS patients with CD4 counts of less than 75/mm³. Disseminated disease causes fever, night sweats, weight loss, diarrhea, fatigue, and cytopenias. Treatment of disseminated MAC disease requires the administration of multiple antibiotics, including ethambutol, rifabutin, and erythromycin, which although reducing certain symptoms in some patients, cause significant side effects that most often outweigh their benefit in a palliative care setting. Therefore, with rare exception, MAC treatment should not be continued in patients who are near the end of life.

Rather, the focus of care should shift to pure symptom management. Symptoms such as diarrhea and fever should be treated with standard symptom management approaches (described later). One study has found that for patients who were unable to tolerate MAC therapy or who were symptomatic despite therapy, dexamethasone at a dose of 2 mg daily will significantly alleviate a number of symptoms (Wormser et al, 1994).

As with primary therapy, the toxicity of agents used to provide prophylaxis against MAC infection, such as rifabutin and clarithromycin, dictates against their routine use in AIDS patients near the end of life.

Treatment of HIV-Associated Malignancies Near the End of Life

Assessment of the efficacy of palliative care for HIV-associated malignancies should take into account medication side effects, ease of drug administration, and effectiveness of symptom relief and patient acceptability. The two most common cancers seen in AIDS patients are Kaposi's sarcoma (KS) and lymphoma, although the prevalence of other neoplasms such as rectal carcinoma is increasing.

KAPOSI'S SARCOMA

Kaposi's sarcoma (KS) in patients with HIV is a different entity than the classic form of the disease seen predominantly in older white males of Mediterranean and northern and eastern European extraction. In the setting of HIV infection, KS affects primarily homosexual and bisexual men and is a much more aggressive neoplasm. KS is now known to be caused by human herpesvirus 8 (HHV-8). KS manifests as mucocutaneous and visceral lesions. It can be seen in early HIV infection when the CD4 count is still relatively intact, and in that setting KS is usually slow growing and indolent. As the immune system declines, however, KS may become fulminant and disseminated.

Mucocutaneous KS may cause pain due to the location and size of the lesions. It also often causes edema secondary to lymphatic obstruction. Visceral lesions will cause pain and other symptoms that vary with the organ or organs involved. For example, KS of the gastrointestinal tract (the most common extracutaneous site) will often cause abdominal pain, melena, hematochezia, anemia, diarrhea, or weight loss. Pulmonary involvement may present with dyspnea and/or hemoptysis.

Palliation of symptoms may be best achieved by using standard KS treatments, such as chemotherapy and radiation therapy, to reduce the size of the lesions. With the development of newer forms of chemotherapy such as liposomal doxorubicin, treatments have become less toxic and can be administered less frequently. As with all therapies, an appropriate risk–benefit assessment must be made, and the therapy should be continued only as long as the palliative benefit outweighs the side effects. For patients for whom chemotherapy or radiation therapy is not appropriate, standard symptom management principles apply.

LYMPHOMA

The two types of lymphoma most commonly seen in AIDS patients are non-Hodgkins lymphoma (NHL) and primary central nervous system lymphoma (PCNSL). Either form of lymphoma is generally aggressive and poorly responsive to treatment. In addition, the very substantial toxicities of the available treatments generally preclude their use in a palliative care setting. As such, lymphomas should be palliated with traditional measures such as corticosteroids, analgesics, and other symptom management interventions.

Symptom Management of Patients with AIDS Near the End of Life

AIDS patients near the end of life, whether or not they are candidates for prophylaxis or treatment of AIDS-related infections or neoplasms, require direct management of their symptoms. As with all patients, it should be stressed that symptom management must be individualized. All decisions regarding the appropriateness of interventions should be made using the same weighting of benefits and toxicities already discussed.

FEVER

The evaluation of fever in patients with advanced AIDS is presented in Table 19–3. The first step is to assess the patient for obvious sources of infection such as infected intravenous lines, catheters, and decubiti. The clinician should consider the possibility that previous infections for which the patient has been receiving secondary prophylaxis (e.g., MAC, CMV, or PCP) have reactivated. If that seems probable, appropriate empiric therapy should be initiated if such therapy is likely to maintain or improve the patient's quality of life. The possibility of noninfectious causes of fever, such as drug or tumor fever, should also be considered. If those are thought to be likely, the offending drug should be withdrawn or, for tumor fever, nonsteroidal anti-inflammatory medications should be administered. If the etiology of the fever remains unclear, it may be appropriate to initiate a limited workup aimed at detecting readily reversible conditions. This may include such diagnostic procedures as a chest radiograph, routine laboratory studies, and urinalysis. A trial of empiric broad-spectrum antibiotic therapy can be initiated but should be discontinued after 3 to 5 days if there is no response. If the fever persists despite

Table 19–3

Evaluation of Fever in Patients with Advanced AIDS

POTENTIAL SOURCE	RECOMMENDED INTERVENTION
IV line or indwelling catheter	Remove and/or replace
Decubiti	Treat (see Chapter 10)
Reactivation of opportunistic infection (PCP, CMV, MAC)	Empiric treatment if appropriate (see Table 19–2)
Medication	Discontinue potentially offending agent
Tumor fever	NSAID
If above ruled out:	
Patient with good performance status	Limited evaluation followed by 3–5 days of empiric antibiotics
Patient with poor performance status or no response to empiric antibiotic	Symptomatic treatment with NSAID or dexamethasone 2–4 mg/day

antibiotics and the etiology remains unknown, it should be treated symptomatically with antipyretics. For more refractory fevers, steroids such as dexamethasone (2 to 4 mg/day) may be appropriate.

GASTROINTESTINAL SYMPTOMS

Patients with AIDS suffer from a variety of gastrointestinal disorders, most commonly related to opportunistic infections or medications. A full discussion of gastrointestinal symptoms and treatments near the end of life is given in Chapter 8; information unique to patients with HIV will be discussed next.

DYSPHAGIA, ODYNOPHAGIA, AND HICCUPS Dysphagia, odynophagia (painful swallowing), and hiccups can be relatively common in late-stage AIDS and are usually the result of esophagitis. The most frequent cause of esophagitis is *Candida* infection. Other etiologies include CMV, herpes simplex infection, and aphthous ulcerations. Dysphagia and odynophagia can also occur as a result of neoplastic processes such as Kaposi's sarcoma and lymphoma. Even if the patient has a preserved appetite, esophageal symptoms can prevent the patient from eating or drinking. If the pain or obstruction is severe enough, the patient may not even be able to swallow normal oral secretions.

Esophageal symptoms should be evaluated by first obtaining a good history. Most patients will complain of odynophagia or dysphagia with both liquids and solids. Physical examination will frequently, but not always, reveal oropharyngeal candidiasis. Since candidiasis is by far the most common cause of esophageal symptoms, empiric treatment should be initiated with a systemic antifungal agent, especially since locally acting antifungals will only be effective against oropharyngeal disease. The antifungal drug of choice is fluconazole given as a 200-mg loading dose followed by 100 mg daily for at least 14 days. Other systemic antifungals such as ketoconazole may also be effective, but the risk of hepatotoxicity and drug–drug interactions is greater.

If the symptoms do not improve with antifungal therapy, other causes such as ulcerative disease should be considered. Unfortunately a definitive diagnosis of ulcerative disease and its etiology requires invasive diagnostic procedures such as endoscopy with biopsy. If CMV or herpes is thought to be likely, it is reasonable to consider an empiric trial of ganciclovir or other antiherpes treatment. If there is no improvement in symptoms after 7 to 10 days, therapy should be discontinued and other diagnoses considered. For aphthous ulcerations, oral corticosteroids (e.g., prednisone 40 to 60 mg daily) can be effective. Alternatively, thalidomide (100 to

300 mg daily) can be used. Though the FDA approved thalidomide in 1998 for treatment of erythema nodosum leprosum, numerous studies have demonstrated its effectiveness in treating oral and esophageal aphthous ulcerations.

Hiccups can have a variety of causes including central nervous system lesion or infection, diaphragmatic irritation due to tumor or inflammation, metabolic derangement, and systemic infection. Nonetheless, in HIV-infected patients, esophagitis is usually the most common predisposing condition. When esophagitis results from gastroesophageal reflux disease, treatment with H_2-antagonists such as ranitidine or proton pump inhibitors such as omeprazole is indicated. For symptomatic treatment, chlorpromazine (Thorazine) is most commonly used. Though this is the only FDA-approved drug for the treatment of hiccups, there are anecdotal reports of successful treatment with other medications such as baclofen.

NAUSEA AND VOMITING   The patient's current medications should be evaluated as a possible cause of the nausea and vomiting and any nonessential medications should be eliminated or changed. Conditions such as pancreatitis, gastritis, peptic ulcer disease, and gastroparesis are frequent causes of nausea and vomiting in patients with AIDS and these causes should be considered.

Pharmacologic therapy should be directed both at specific suspected diseases (e.g., H_2-antagonists for gastritis, metoclopramide for gastroparesis) and at symptom control with antiemetics. The most commonly used antiemetics are the phenothiazines and include prochlorperazine and promethazine. The use of adjunctive medications such as steroids (dexamethasone), benzodiazepines, antihistamines (diphenhydramine, hydroxyzine), or anticholinergics may enhance the effectiveness of antiemetics. Other interventions that can be tried include changing the patient's diet or giving the patient smaller, more frequent meals until symptoms are under adequate control. If the vomiting is so severe that the patient is unable to take oral medications, the antiemetics should be administered parenterally or by suppository. Chronic nausea may respond

to dronabinol, 2.5 to 5 mg twice a day. Finally, appropriate precautions, such as elevation of the head of the bed, must always be taken to minimize the patient's risk of aspiration during episodes of vomiting.

DIARRHEA   An attempt should first be made to determine the etiology of the diarrhea and whether it is acute or chronic in onset. If acute, one must consider whether it may be due to infection, such as cryptosporidiosis or giardiasis, or whether it is secondary to medication side effects, as may occur with antiretroviral agents or antibiotics. Therefore, medications should be carefully reviewed as a possible cause of the diarrhea and suspect medications should be discontinued.

In some patients, a brief trial of an antiparasitic agent such as metronidazole or paromomycin may be indicated. Antimotility agents such as loperamide or diphenoxylate or bulk supplements like psyllium, should be tried initially for symptom control. Severe, chronic diarrhea, which may be secondary to changes in the intestinal wall due to the HIV virus itself, may respond only to opioids such as oral tincture of opium. The usual starting dose is 6 drops (0.6 mL) in 2 ounces of water every 4 hours. The dose should then be titrated until symptom control is achieved. There is no maximum dose for tincture of opium. With any of these agents, the patient must always be monitored for the development of constipation or fecal impaction, especially when fluid intake is inadequate.

Octreotide is a synthetic somatostatin analogue that is approved for treatment of profuse water diarrhea caused by to vasoactive intestinal peptide tumors and carcinoid tumors. It has shown variable effectiveness in treating diarrhea in AIDS patients. Its major disadvantages are its high cost and the fact that it needs to be administered subcutaneously on a regular basis.

DYSPNEA AND RESPIRATORY DISTRESS

A full discussion of dyspnea and respiratory distress can be found in Chapter 7. Causes of dyspnea in end-stage AIDS patients include acute pneumothorax and pneumonia from either community-acquired or opportunistic pathogens. The etiology of dyspnea may become apparent through a thorough physical examination and history. Simple blood tests such as a CBC may be necessary to rule out conditions such as anemia. Diagnostic aids such as a chest radiograph and oxygen saturation measurement can be obtained, but only if they are likely to be of benefit in managing the patient's condition. Initiation of empiric therapy such as antibiotics for suspected bacterial pneumonia or PCP may be appropriate. Supplemental oxygen, opioids, and anxiolytics can be used to decrease respiratory distress and increase patient comfort.

ALTERATION IN MENTAL STATUS, SEIZURES

A full discussion of neurologic symptoms near the end of life can be found in Chapter 9. Alterations in mental status can occur due to a variety of reasons. Evaluation to determine the etiology of the change in mental status or the new onset of seizures should be limited to patients whose quality of life and prognosis have previously been of an acceptable degree and who have now undergone an acute change. Focused laboratory studies may, for example, rule out potentially correctable electrolyte abnormalities or other metabolic disturbances. Nuclear or radiographic diagnostic imaging may be helpful in selected circumstances when there is a high index of suspicion that the patient suffers from an easily treatable condition that will restore the person's quality of life (e.g., cerebral toxoplasmosis). However, it would be equally acceptable to avoid the imaging study and treat such patients with a limited course of empiric therapy for the suspected reversible condition (e.g., toxoplasmosis) and monitor the patient for a response to the treatment.

With regard to therapies focused purely on symptom management, antiepileptics such as phenytoin and carbamazepine are generally used as seizure prophylaxis. Active seizures can be treated with benzodiazepines such as lorazepam and diazepam. For HIV encephalopathy (also known as AIDS dementia complex), the patient can be considered for a trial of psychostimulants such as methylphenidate. If the patient develops agitation or psychosis, phenothizines such as haloperidol or chlorpromazine may be beneficial.

ASTHENIA

A full discussion of asthenia can be found in Chapter 11. Asthenia, or chronic debilitating fatigue, is a common symptom in AIDS patients that is often associated with impaired physical functioning. Though fatigue may be considered by some to be an unavoidable sequella of advanced HIV disease, its significant effect on quality of life makes it a particularly distressing symptom for many patients. Estimates of the prevalence of fatigue among patients with AIDS range from 40 to 50 percent. Some studies have shown a higher prevalence of fatigue among HIV-infected women compared to HIV-infected men. Other variables that appear to be correlated with fatigue include more advanced disease (as indicated by greater numbers of physical symptoms and treatment for AIDS-related medical conditions) and high levels of psychological distress. It is important to keep in mind that fatigue is often a symptom of depression. Differentiating between medical and psychological etiologies of fatigue can be very difficult in clinical practice. Further complicating the assessment is the fact that the medical and psychological factors are often multifactorial and frequently coexist. Treatment of asthenia in patients with end-stage AIDS may include steroids (prednisone 20 mg once or twice a day, or dexamethasone 2 to 4 mg two to four times a day), as well as heavy doses of reassurance and support.

DEPRESSION

A full discussion of depression can be found in Chapter 11. Not surprisingly, depression is a common comorbid condition in end-stage AIDS. Depression not only negatively affects the patient's quality of life, but may also exaggerate pain and other symptoms. As such, it is exceedingly important to recognize and treat depression. The class of antidepressants known as selective serotonin re-uptake inhibitors (SSRIs) should be the first choice in treating depression. The SSRIs are taken only once daily, have generally mild and manageable side effects, and tend to be very effective. There are multiple SSRIs available and the choice of a particular one should be individualized to the patient.

PAIN MANAGEMENT

A full discussion of the treatment of pain near the end of life can be found in Chapter 6. Pain is extremely common in late-stage AIDS. Several studies have shown it to be the most common symptom, affecting 75 to 80 percent of patients. Studies have also shown pain to be underreported and undertreated.

Neuropathic pain is the major challenge in managing the pain of patients with AIDS. It may result from a toxic peripheral neuropathy secondary to drugs such as the nucleoside analogs d4T (Zerit), ddI (Videx) or ddC (Hivid), or it may be due to the HIV infection itself. Neuropathic pain can be disabling if severe. It usually presents first in the feet and may progress up the legs or to other parts of the body.

Neuropathic pain unfortunately does not respond well to opioids alone. Traditionally, tricyclic antidepressants such as amitriptyline have been the drugs of choice for first-line treatment of peripheral neuropathy. These drugs are of limited benefit in reducing neuropathic pain in AIDS patients, however, and dose-related side effects such as somnolence and orthostatic hypotension further limit their usefulness. Another class of drugs that has been used to treat neuropathic pain is the anticonvulsants. Increasingly it appears that gabapentin may be significantly more beneficial than TCAs. There is anecdotal evidence that another anticonvulsant, lamotrigine, may also be effective in reducing AIDS-related neuropathic pain. Clinical studies looking at lamotrigine as therapy for AIDS-related peripheral neuropathy are currently ongoing.

Largely due to the lack of consistently effective treatments for peripheral neuropathy, many HIV patients seek out nontraditional approaches including massage and acupuncture, prescription and nonprescription medications, vitamins and supplements, and exercise. The reported effectiveness of these interventions varies, and until more definitive studies are performed, needs to be evaluated on a case-by-case basis based on the outcome of symptomatic benefit.

Conclusion

The care of patients with AIDS has changed markedly since the disease was initially described in the early 1980s. Primarily affecting younger people, and once a rapidly fatal disease, AIDS has now become a chronic and controllable illness, with the inevitability of death postponed for significant and meaningful periods of time. Unfortunately, patients with AIDS all too often still face the prospects of a premature death, challenging those who provide hospice and palliative care to patients near the end of life to meet their unique needs. It is hoped that the information presented will assist in that process.

References

Breitbart W, McDonald MV, et al: Fatigue in ambulatory AIDS patients. *J Pain Symptom Manage* 15:159, 1998.

Broder S, Merigan TC, Bolognesi D: *Textbook of AIDS Medicine*. Baltimore, Williams & Wilkins, 1994.

Chaisson RE, Benson CA, et al: Clarithromycin therapy for bacteremic *Mycobacterium avium* complex disease. A randomized, double-blind dose-ranging study in patients with AIDS. AIDS clinical trials group protocol 17 study team. *Ann Intern Med* 121:905, 1994.

Chin DP, et al: Impact of *Mycobacterium avium* complex bacteremia and its treatment on survival of AIDS patients: A prospective study. *J Infect Dis* 170:578, 1994.

Chin DP, Reingold AL, et al: The impact of *Mycobacterium avium* complex bacteremia and its treatment on survival of AIDS patients—A prospective study. *J Infect Dis* 170:578, 1994.

Hogg RS, Strathdee SA, et al: Lower socioeconomic status and shorter survival following HIV infection. *Lancet* 344:1120, 1994.

Kinzbrunner BM: *Vitas Pain Management Formulary.* Miami, Vitas Healthcare, 1995.

Mellors JW, Rinaldo CR Jr, Gupta P, et al: Prognosis in HIV-1 infection predicted by the quantity of virus in plasma. *Science* 272:1167, 1996.

Mills GD, Jones PD: Relationship between CD4 lymphocyte count and AIDS mortality, 1986–1991. *AIDS* 7:1383, 1993.

Moore RD, Chaisson, RE: Natural history of opportunistic disease in an HIV-infected urban clinical cohort. *Ann Int Med* 124:633, 1996.

Neaton JD, Wentworth DN, et al: Considerations in choice of a clinical endpoint for AIDS clinical trials. Terry Beirn Community Programs for Clinical Research on AIDS (CPCRA). *Stat Med* 13:2107, 1994.

Nicholas P: *Self-Care for Peripheral Neuropathy in HIV Disease.* 13th International AIDS Conference, Durban, South Africa, July 2000. Abstract ThPeB5250.

Reiter GS, Kudler NR: Palliative Care and HIV. *AIDS Clinical Care* 3: 21-26, 1996.

Reiter GS, Kudler NR: Palliative Care and HIV. *AIDS Clinical Care* 4: 27-36, 1996.

Saag MS, Holodniy M, Kuritzkes DR, et al: HIV viral load markers in clinical practice. *Nat Med* 2:625, 1996.

Schofferman J, Brody R: Pain in far advanced AIDS. In: Foley KM, Bonica JJ, Ventafridda V, et al, eds. *Advances in Pain Research and Therapy,* vol. 16. New York, Raven, 1990, pp. 379–386.

Spector SA, McKinley G, Lalezari JP, et al, for the Roche cooperative ganciclovir study group: Oral ganciclovir for the prevention of cytomegalovirus disease in persons with AIDS. *N Engl J Med* 334:1491, 1996.

Stuart B, Connor S, Kinzbrunner BM, et al: *Medical Guidelines for Determining Prognosis in Selected Non-Cancer Diseases,* 2nd ed. Arlington, National Hospice Organization, 1996.

Wormser, GP, Horowitz H, Dworkin B: Low-dose dexamethasone as adjunctive therapy for disseminated *Mycobacterium avium* complex infections in AIDS patients. *Antimicrob Agents Chemother* 38:2215, 1994.

Judith Ann Haythorne Macurda

Care of Children Near the End of Life

Children receiving hospice care can be compared to snowflakes. No two snowflakes are alike, and we can only enjoy their beauty for a short time.

Diane Majeski, hospice nurse

Introduction

Children are not supposed to die, but unfortunately they do. Children with life-threatening conditions present multiple challenges to providers of medical care who generally focus on life and conquering disease. These providers may feel a sense of failure when they cannot "save" a child. Children with terminal illnesses also present challenges to their parents and family members. These individuals may feel powerless that they cannot do more to improve the quality or the length of their child's life. Dying children present challenges to their classmates, friends, and neighbors, all of whom are affected. Dying children present challenges to the health care system in general as their needs cannot always be met within the existing structure of our health care system. Finally, children who die present challenges even after their death. The ongoing life of the family and others may be affected by prolonged and unresolved grief.

Improvement in end-of-life care for adults has occurred over the past 20 years since the institution of hospice care in the United States. Now approximately 50 percent of adults dying of cancer receive hospice care where "comfort care" and quality of life are emphasized. Children, however, are often among those receiving inadequate care near the end of their lives. In 1995, there were more than 3000 hospice organizations in the United States. Only 500 of these hospices admitted children, and there were only 22 that specialized in palliative care for children. Today most of the over 3000 hospices will consider admitting children, but only 1 percent of children needing hospice care actually receive it.

In 1997, approximately 100,000 children and adolescents under the age of 19 died in the United States. Thirty-six percent of these deaths were due

to accidents, and most of these children die while undergoing acute care therapy and would not be appropriate for palliative or hospice care. The remaining 64 percent die from congenital and genetic syndromes and other anomalies, malignancies, diseases of the heart, neurodegenerative and other inherited progressive diseases, and AIDS. Many of these children are appropriate candidates for palliative or hospice care from the time of diagnosis, because only supportive care is possible.

Of the 12,400 children diagnosed with cancer each year in the United States, 30 percent will die. Unfortunately, improvement in symptom management associated with end-of-life care in children with malignancies has not advanced at the same rate as curative therapies. As stated in a recent editorial in the *New England Journal of Medicine* (Morgan & Murphy, 2000):

> Children are not just "little adults," and caregivers skilled in the care of dying adults generally lack the expertise to deal with the unique medical and psychosocial needs of children. The overwhelming success of programs for the treatment of childhood cancer and the tremendous stakes involved in saving the life of a child make both parents and caregivers reluctant to abandon a curative approach. Thus, the continuation of the aggressive care is encouraged even if there is little or no realistic hope of a favorable outcome. The push for a cure means that less attention is often given to controlling symptoms. Commonly, aggressive treatments are not abandoned until shortly before death. Thus, there is little or no time for patients, family members or caregivers to address emotions, anticipatory grieving or to participate in decisions about care.

Comparison of Adult and Pediatric Hospice Care

The needs of some children and their families under hospice or palliative care are markedly different from those of adults (Table 20–1). One basic difference is that the child has not achieved a "full

Table 20–1

Differences Between Hospice Care of Children and Adults

CHILDREN	ADULTS
PATIENT ISSUES	
Not legally competent	Mentally competent, possible advance directives
Child in a developmental process that affects understanding of life and death, sickness and health, God, etc.	Understanding more complete
Has not achieved a "full and complete life"	Often advanced in age
Lack of verbal skills to describe needs, feelings	Verbal skills may be good
Child protects parents and significant others at own expense	
Child often in a highly technical medical environment	Frequently at home
FAMILY ISSUES	
Protection of the child from information about his or her health	Diagnosis known
Desire to do everything possible to save the child	Realistic expectations
Potential difficulty dealing with siblings	
Financial stress	Financial stress
Fear that care at home is not as good as in the hospital	Home care frequently chosen
Grandparents feel helpless in dealing with their children and grandchildren	
Family needs relief from burden of care	Respite may be necessary
CAREGIVER ISSUES	
Desire to protect children, parents, siblings	
Feeling a sense of failure in not saving the child	Prognosis accepted
Lack understanding of children's cognitive level	
Feeling sense of "ownership" of children, even at the expense of parents	
Out-of-date ideas about pain in children, especially infants	
Lack of knowledge about children's disease processes	
Influence of "unfinished business" on style of care	
INSTITUTIONAL/AGENCY ISSUES	
Less reimbursement or none for children's hospice/home care	Medicare, Medicaid, private insurance
High staff intensity caring for children at home	
Ongoing staff support necessary	
Children's services have immediate appeal to public	
Special competencies are needed in pediatric care	
No established admission criteria	Established admission policies
Unusual bereavement needs for family members	

SOURCE: Adapted from Children's Hospice International 2000 Informational Overview, with permission

and complete life," and consequently the family and caregivers want to do everything possible to save the child and thus prolong his or her life. Another major difference is that the child is in a developmental process and is not considered legally competent. This is in sharp contrast to adults, who can make their own decisions regarding aggressive therapy and may have delineated advance directives that instruct and bind their families and medical care providers to follow their wishes. Yet another difference is that medical caregivers, especially those who care primarily for adults, may not be adequately trained in assessing and treating pain and symptoms occurring in children. Medical caregivers focused on curative modalities may not pay adequate attention to symptom control or focus on important psychospiritual aspects of care. Parents are often poorly prepared for the death of their child because the focus has been only on curative approaches.

Pediatric and Adult Hospice Care in the United States

Since the passage of the Medicare Hospice Benefit legislation in the United States, hospice care has been functionally defined as appropriate for people with 6 months or less to live and who are seeking palliative (comfort) care. Medicaid and most private insurance providers have adopted a similar restrictive scope for their benefits. Many children, especially those with malignancies, may undergo aggressive therapy aimed at cure until the very end of their lives. Consequently, they are not considered eligible for hospice care under the current definition. Further, because the aggressive treatment might be successful, it is also difficult to firmly establish a prognosis of 6 months or less.

Pediatric hospices in the United States have generally developed programs that are not as restrictive as the traditionally defined hospice. Their funding is more "creative," often depending heavily on fund raising and charity, and their admission criteria are more lenient to better meet the needs of the children and their families. Pediatric hospitals are also becoming more sensitive to the psychosocial needs of their patients and families and are improving in symptom control. A partnership between hospice care and pediatric oncologist needs to be further explored and developed, because research has shown that when hospice care is introduced earlier, children are more likely to be described as calm and peaceful near the end of their lives.

There are marked differences between hospice care in the United States and in Europe, where different medical care systems are in place. In a study reported from Boston, 49 percent of the children with cancer in the study who died, did so in the hospital, with about half of these deaths occurring in the intensive care unit (Wolf, et al, 2000). In the Netherlands, 31 percent of children terminally ill with cancer died in the hospital and 69 percent died at home. In the United Kingdom, where pediatric oncology centers have oncology outreach programs, 70 to 80 percent of children with progressive malignant disease die at home.

Finally, terminally ill children served within the traditional hospice system in the United States have a different diagnosis mix when compared to their adult counterparts. While cancers remain the dominant terminal illnesses in all age groups, adults served by hospice care also suffer from chronic debilitating illnesses such as dementia, end-stage cardiac disease, and degenerative diseases like amyotrophic lateral sclerosis (ALS). In contrast, children in hospice care with diagnoses other than cancer tend to have congenital syndromes and anomalies, progressive neurodegenerative diseases, neuromuscular disorders, disorders of mucopolysaccharide metabolism, congenital cardiac conditions, cystic fibrosis, and AIDS.

Pediatric Pain Management

It has been estimated that 89 percent of children with cancer suffer from pain. Historically, pain has been undertreated in children, even to the point where neonates have undergone surgery without anesthesia. Although pain management has greatly improved in recent years, children are still frequently undermedicated for pain. This undermedication results from physician lack of knowledge about pharmacalogic and nonpharmacologic practices as applied to children and from misconceptions and myths suggesting that young children do not perceive pain in the same way as adults.

In response to the widespread undertreatment of children with pain, many medical institutions and organizations, including the World Health Organization, have made pain control and palliative care in children a priority over the past several years. This has resulted in a increase in awareness of the problem and some improvement in the treatment of pain in children. A recent study found that based on parental report on a group of terminally ill children, pain was the most commonly treated symptom (Wolf, et al, 2000). However, of the 76 percent of the study children treated for pain, the treatment was successful in fewer than 30 percent of the children. Thus there is still a great need for improvement.

A thorough discussion of the management of pain near the end of life can be found in Chapter 6, and the reader is referred to this chapter for a detailed review of the principles of pain management of patients near the end of life. The discussion that follows will be confined to pain management issues unique to terminally ill children.

Physiology of Pain

There are two main types of physical pain, nociceptive and neuropathic. Nociceptive pain includes somatic pain and visceral pain. Somatic pain is a direct result of peripheral tissue damage in bones, joints, muscle, skin, or connective tissue. It is usually described as aching or throbbing and is well localized. This type of pain responds to both opioids and, especially in the case of bone pain, nonsteroidal anti-inflammatory agents (NSAIDs). Visceral pain arises from organs such as the stomach, gall bladder, and pancreas. The two main mechanisms of visceral pain arise from either tumor invasion of the organ capsule, which results in aching and fairly well-localized pain; or obstruction of a hollow viscus, which results in cramping and

poorly localized pain. Both types of nociceptive pain usually respond to nonopioids and opioids.

Neuropathic pain is caused by stimulation of either the peripheral or the central nervous system. It is generally described as burning or stabbing in nature. Neuropathic pain generally responds to adjuvant analgesics such as anticonvulsants or tricyclic antidepressants.

Nociceptive systems in children have been described as "plastic," in that they can perceive pain from a given amount of tissue damage in various ways. The amount of pain perceived by the child can be influenced by emotional factors such as anxiety and fear, behavioral factors such as social activities and physical restraint, and cognitive factors such as expectations and understanding. Consequently, to adequately control children's pain requires not only the pharmacologic administration of appropriate analgesics but also nonpharmacologic techniques.

Misconceptions and Fears Regarding Pain Control in Children

Multiple barriers to adequate pain management exist in children as well as adults. Some of these barriers are similar, including but not limited to the fear of addiction, fear that the need for analgesia means the illness is progressing, and fear of respiratory depression due to opioid toxicity. There are also several myths about pain and pain management unique to children. These are outlined in Table 20–2 and discussed next.

Table 20–2

Myths That Create Barriers to Effective Pain Management Specific to Children

Infants do not feel pain
Children tolerate pain better than adults
Children are unable to communicate appropriately about their pain
Children will tell caregivers when they are having pain

Figure 20–1

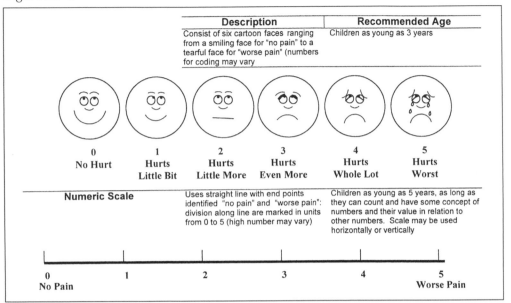

	Description	Recommended Age
	Consist of six cartoon faces ranging from a smiling face for "no pain" to a tearful face for "worse pain" (numbers for coding may vary)	Children as young as 3 years

0	1	2	3	4	5
No Hurt	Hurts Little Bit	Hurts Little More	Hurts Even More	Hurts Whole Lot	Hurts Worst

Numeric Scale	Uses straight line with end points identified "no pain" and "worse pain": division along line are marked in units from 0 to 5 (high number may vary)	Children as young as 5 years, as long as they can count and have some concept of numbers and their value in relation to other numbers. Scale may be used horizontally or vertically

0	1	2	3	4	5
No Pain					Worse Pain

Pain rating scale for children
SOURCE: From Whaley LF and Wong DL: *Nursing Care of Infants and Children*, 3rd ed. St. Louis, Mosby. Copyright 1987 Mosby. Reprinted with permission.

INFANTS DO NOT FEEL PAIN

Historically it was believed that young infants do not feel pain. It has been shown, however, that the central nervous system of a 26-week-old fetus has the structural and neurochemical ability to experience pain.

CHILDREN TOLERATE PAIN BETTER THAN ADULTS

There is a serious misconception that children have a higher tolerance to pain than adults. In fact, children's ability to tolerate pain increases with age; older children experience less pain with procedures than younger children. Children do not become accustomed to pain or painful procedures. Rather, they often experience increased anxiety and perception of pain with repeated procedures.

CHILDREN ARE UNABLE TO COMMUNICATE APPROPRIATELY ABOUT THEIR PAIN

Children are in fact able to communicate where and how much they hurt. Children as young as 3 years old have been taught to use appropriate pain scales, such as the faces pain scale (Fig. 20–1), and can localize pain by pointing to an area of their body. What is true is that special assessment skills are necessary to properly evaluate children's pain.

CHILDREN WILL TELL CAREGIVERS WHEN THEY ARE HAVING PAIN

Although children can usually share information about their pain, they may not always do so. Younger children may have inadequate communication skills, and older children may not report pain because they may fear the treatment (injections) or they may have adjusted to chronic pain. The level of activity of a child may or may not reflect the pain level. A child may elect to watch TV rather than play outside, and may use distracting activity such as playing with puzzles to cope with pain.

Pain Assessment

Pain in children can be consistently and objectively assessed by the use of pediatric assessment tools

Table 20–3

QUEST: Assessment of Pain in the Pediatric Patient

> **Q**uestion the child
> **U**se pain-rating scales
> **E**valuate behavior and physiologic changes
> **S**ecure parents' involvement
> **T**ake action and evaluate the results

SOURCE: Baker CM, Wong DI: QUEST: A process of pain assessment in children. *Orthop Nurse* 6:11, 1987.

and pain rating scales. The assessment should include not only physical factors, but also social and emotional factors as well. One useful acronym is the QUEST approach to pediatric pain assessment (Table 20–3). It promotes the use of multiple sources for a systematic pain assessment and promotes a complete pain assessment.

Parents and family members should be empowered by requesting and believing in their input regarding pain levels and treatments they feel are most effective. A complete pain assessment includes a report based on the patient's and the parents' description of the pain. The most valuable information is received from the children themselves, but parental input should also be sought because parents know their child better than anyone else (Table 20–4). Specific words used by the child to describe pain should be used (e.g., hurt, "owie," "boo-boo") in order to establish proper lines of communication. As with adults, physical examination, behavioral observations, and physiologic measures are the other components of a pain assessment.

Multiple behavioral pain assessment scales for young children have been developed (Fig. 20–1 and Table 20–5). To obtain reliability and validity in assessing pain, the same observer should evaluate the child over time whenever possible. Therefore, especially in home patients, parents should be trained in the use of the chosen scale so that they can report to hospice nurses or other clinical personnel in a common language.

Table 20–4

Pain Experience History

CHILD FORM	PARENT FORM
Tell me what pain is.	What word(s) does your child use in regard to pain?
Tell me about the hurt you have had before.	Describe the pain experiences your child has had before.
Do you tell others when you hurt? If yes, who?	Does your child tell you or others when he/she is hurting?
What do you do for yourself when you are hurting?	How do you know when your child is in pain?
What do you want others to do for you when you hurt?	How does your child usually react to pain?
What don't you want others to do for you when you hurt?	What do you do for your child when he/she is hurting?
What helps the most to take your hurt away?	What does your child do for him/herself when he/she is hurting?
	What works best to decrease or take away your child's pain?
Is there anything special that you want me to know about you when you hurt? (If yes, have the child describe.)	Is there anything special that you would like me to know about your child and pain? (If yes, describe.)

SOURCE: From Joyce BA, Schade JG, Keck JF, et al: Reliability and validity of preverbal pain assessment tools. *Issues Comp Pediatr Nurs* 17:121, 1994. Copyright 1994 Hemisphire Pub. Corp., adapted with permission.

Table 20–5

Behavioral Pain Assessment Scales for Young Children

FLACC SCALE SCORING			
CATEGORIES[a]	0	1	2
Face	No particular expression or smile	Occasional grimace or frown, withdrawn, disinterested	Frequent to constant quivering chin, clenched jaw
Legs	Normal position or relaxed	Uneasy, restless, tense	Kicking or legs drawn up
Activity	Lying quietly, normal position, moves easily	Squirming, shifting back and forth, tense	Arched, rigid or jerking
Cry	No cry (awake or asleep)	Moans or whimpers; occasional complaint	Crying steadily, screams or sobs, frequent complaints
Consolability	Content, relaxed	Reassured by occasional touching, hugging, or being talked to; distractable	Difficult to console or comfort

RILEY INFANT PAIN SCALE ASSESSMENT TOOL				
BEHAVIOR/CATEGORY	0	1	2	3
Facial	Neutral/smiling	Frowning/grimacing	Clenched teeth	Full cry expression
Body movement	Calm, relaxed	Restless/fidgeting	Moderate agitation or moderate mobility	Thrashing, flailing, incessant agitation or strong voluntary immobility
Sleep	Sleeping quietly with easy respiration	Restless while asleep	Sleeps intermittently (sleep/awake)	Sleeping for prolonged periods of time interrupted by jerky movements or unable to sleep
Verbal/voice	No cry	Whimpering, complaining	Pain crying	Screaming, high-pitched cry
Consolability	Neutral	Easy to console	Not easy to console	Inconsolable
Response to movement/touch	Moves easily	Winces when touched/moved	Cries out when moved/touched	High-pitched cry or scream when touched or moved

[a] Each of the five categories (F)face; (L) Legs; (A) Activity; (C) Cry; (C) Consolability is scored from 0 to 2, which results in a total score between 0 and 10.
SOURCE: Merkeland S, et al: The FLACC: A behavioral scale for scoring postoperative pain in young children. *Pediatr Nurse* 23:293,1997; Slade JG, Joyce BA, Gerkensmeyer J, Keck JF: Comparison of three preverbal scales for postoperative pain assessment in a diverse pediatric sample. *J Pain Symptom Manage* 12:348, 1996.

The pain assessment scale being used for a child should be clearly recorded in the chart. It should be used, and the results recorded, on routine visits, during exacerbation of pain, and within an hour following new interventions. It is important for the child to become familiar with the scale as early in the disease process as possible for best results. The faces scale has been successfully used by children as young as 3 years old. Another useful method for determining pain is with five red poker chips. The chips are placed on a table in front of the child, who is instructed to take away chips to the level of pain he or she is experiencing. In addition to the type of scales used, goals for pain control should be delineated and discussed with the family and patient when appropriate.

Nonpharmacologic Pain Interventions

Nonpharmacologic interventions are frequently effective in the pediatric population for improving pain control. They have been categorized primarily as physical, behavioral, or cognitive. Physical interventions include thermal stimulation, massage, and touch in general. Examples of behavioral interventions include relaxation therapy and behavioral modification. Cognitive interventions include distraction, such as looking at books or blowing bubbles, and guided imagery. When a child's attention is completely absorbed by one of these techniques, the neuronal responses caused by tissue damage are actually reduced. The child is not simply ignoring the pain; it is actually reduced.

Pharmacologic Management of Pain in Children

Use of appropriate analgesic medications will relieve pain in most children. As in adults, and as expressed by the World Health Organization, the four main concepts behind adequate pain control are by the ladder, by the clock, by the appropriate route, and by the child.

BY THE LADDER

The basis of pharmacologic pain management in children, like adults, is the World Health Organization's analgesic ladder. It presents a three-step approach to pain management based on mild, moderate, or severe pain with appropriate analgesic choices for each step. The first step for controlling mild pain is a nonopioid analgesic. Acetaminophen is the drug of choice if the child can take oral medication. If the pain is not controlled with acetaminophen alone, a mild opioid, usually codeine, is added, and the Tylenol or a nonsteroidal anti-inflammatory drug (NSAID) is continued. If the pain persists, then a strong opioid, preferably morphine, should be added. At this point the Tylenol or NSAID should be continued but the weak opioid discontinued. Tables 20–6 and 20–7 show commonly used nonopioid and opioid drugs and the recommended doses in pediatric patients.

BY THE CLOCK

Medication should be administered "by the clock" on a regular schedule to prevent pain rather than on an as-needed basis to treat recurrent pain. This relieves the caregiver of continually having to access the child for routine pain medication and leads to better pain control. Additional "rescue" doses of a short-acting medication should be available for intermittent or breakthrough pain.

BY THE APPROPRIATE ROUTE

Medications should be taken by the appropriate route—the route that is simplest, most effective, and least painful for the child. If the child can tolerate oral medications, either liquids or pills, that is the preferred route. At times the subcutaneous or intravenous route may be necessary for rapid pain control or titration or if the child is unable to tolerate oral medications. Both of these methods are compatible with patient-controlled analgesia (PCA) pumps, which can be controlled either by the child or the primary caregiver if the child is too young or otherwise not able to self-

Table 20–6

Starting Oral Doses for Nonopioid Drugs

MEDICATION	ADMINISTRATION	COMMENTS
Acetaminophen	10–15 mg/kg/dose q4h to max of 650 mg/dose	Nongastric ulcergenic, does not inhibit platelet function, not anti-inflammatory
Choline magnesium (trisalicylate)	7.5–25 mg/kg/dose bid-tid: max single dose 1500 mg	Does not interfere with platelet aggregation
Ibuprofen	10 mg/kg/dose to max single dose of 800 mg q6–8h	Antiinflammatory activity but may have gastrointestinal and hematologic effect
Naproxen	5–7.5 mg/kg/dose to a max of 500 mg/dose	Antiinflammatory activity but may have gastrointestinal and hematologic effect

SOURCE: Adapted with permission from World Health Organization: *Cancer Pain Relief and Palliative Care in Children*. London, World Health Organization, 1998.

medicate. The subcutaneous route is especially useful in the home setting because it avoids the need for an IV line.

Intramuscular injections are to be avoided, because they are painful and drug absorption is irregular. The rectal route is generally disliked by children and also results in inconsistent absorption. However, if there is transient vomiting or if the child is comatose, it may be necessary to use the rectal route.

BY THE CHILD

All medications should be adjusted "by the child" based on what the needs are at any given time. There is no single dose that should be appropriate for all children. Strong opioids do not have a ceiling dose and must be titrated to the patient's comfort. If unacceptable side effects develop, such as persistent severe myoclonus or uncontrollable vomiting, an alternative opioid should be selected. Because opioids have incomplete cross-tolerance, the new medication should be started at 50 percent of the equianalgesic dose of the "old" medication, and titrated to effectiveness.

PEDIATRIC USE OF SPECIFIC OPIOIDS

MORPHINE   Morphine is the recommended strong opioid of choice for controlling severe pain in children. It is the "gold standard" to which other opioids are compaired. The recommended starting dose is 0.2 to 0.4 mg/kg orally, every 4 hours, and it can be titrated until the pain is relieved. Because the aqueous solutions of morphine are bitter, children generally prefer the drug mixed in a flavored syrup.

In infants less than 6 months old, the pharmacokinetics of morphine are different. The starting dose of morphine in infants should be between one quarter and one third of the initial dose for older children, based on mg/kg. Morphine should be administered to infants where observation and interventions are available in the case of respiratory depression. If oral administration is not possible, subcutaneous or intravenous infusion starting at 0.03 mg/kg/hr should be initiated, or if the child has been on oral morphine, an appropriate conversion should be made.

HYDROMORPHONE   Hydromorphone is similiar to morphine in its pharmacokinetics and effectiveness. Children tolerate the liquid form of hydromorphone better than morphine. At this time there is no long-acting oral form of hydromorphone, although a concentrated solution is available for subcutaneous or intravenous infusion. Hydromorphone can be useful if morphine causes intolerable side effects. The starting dose of hydromorphone is 0.03 to 0.08 mg/kg per dose every 4

Table 20–7

Starting Oral Doses for Opioid Drugs

MEDICATION	ADMINISTRATION	COMMENTS	STARTING DOSES IV	IV TO PO
Codeine	0.5–1 mg/kg/dose q 4 to 6 h; max: 60 mg/dose	Tablet as sulfate: 30 mg Liquid: 3 mg/mL.	N/A	N/A
Acetaminophen and codeine	0.5–1 mg/kg/dose of codeine q 4 to 6 h; max: 2 tablets/dose; 15 mL/dose	Elixir: acetaminophen 24 mg and codeine 2.4 mg/mL with alcohol 7% Suspension: acetaminophen 24 mg and codein 2.4 mg/mL alcohol free Tablet: #3: acetaminophen 300 mg and codeine 30 mg	N/A	N/A
Hydrocodone and acetaminophen	3–6 years: 5 mL 3 or 4 times/day 7–12 years: 10 mL 3 or 4 times a day >12 years: 1 to 2 tablets q 4 to 6 h; max: 8 tablets a day	Tablet: hydrocodone 5 mg and acetaminophen 500 mg Oral solution: 0.5 mg hydrocodone and 33.4 mg/mL acetaminophen	N/A	N/A
Oxycodone	Instant release 0.05–0.15 mg/kg/dose up to 5 mg/dose/4 to 6 hr Sustained release can administer 10 mg q 12 h	Instant release: 5 mg Concentrated solution: 0 mg/mL Sustained release: 10 mg, 20 mg, 40 mg, 80 mg	N/A	N/A
Morphine	0.2–0.5 mg/kg/dose every 4 to 6 hr prn for solution or instant release tablets 0.3–0.6 mg/kg/dose every 12 hr for sustained release	Solution: 2 mg/mL Concentrated solution: 20 mg/mL Tablet (instant release): 15 mg Tablet (sustained release): 15 mg, 30 mg, 60 mg, 100 mg, 200 mg	0.1 mg/kg/dose, 0.1 to 0.2 mg/kg/ dose q 2 to 4 hr: max 15 mg/dose	10 mg IV s= 30 mg PO
Fentanyl	Lozenge: < 15 kg: contraindicated >2 years (15–40 kg): 5–15 µg/kg: max dose: 400 µg > 40 kg: 5 µg/kg; max dose 400 µg Transdermal patch: >18 years	Lozenge: 100 µg, 200 µg, 300 µg Patch: 25 µg/hr, 50 µg/hr, 75µg/hr, 100 µg/hr	1 to 2 µg/kg/ dose; max: 50 µg/dose Continuous I infusion: 1 µg/kg/hr	N/A

(continued)

Table 20–7 (continued)

Starting Oral Doses for Opioid Drugs

MEDICATION	ADMINISTRATION	COMMENTS	STARTING DOSES IV	IV TO PO
Hydro-morphone	0.03–0.08 mg/kg/dose, PO q 4 to 6 h; max: 5 mg/dose	Injection: 1,2,3, and 4 mg/mL Tablet 2 mg, 4 mg Syrup: Hydromorphone 1 mg and guaifenesen 100 mg/5 mL Suppository: 3 mg	15 μg/kg IV q 4 to 6 h; max: 2 mg/dose	1.5 mg IV = 7.5 mg PO
Methadone	0.1–0.2 mg/kg q 4 to 12 h; max: 10 mg/dose	Tablet: 5 mg, 10 mg Solution 1 mg/mL Concentrate: 10 mg/mL	0.1 mg/kg IV q4 to 12h; max 10 mg	10 mg IV = 20 mg PO

SOURCE: Adapted from Hockenberry-Eaton M, Barrera P, Brown M, et al: *Pain Management in Children with Cancer.* Houston, Texas Cancer Council, 1999, with permission.

to 6 hours as necessary. Hydromorphone should be used with caution in infants and young children, and should not be used in neonates due to potential CNS effects.

OXYCODONE Oxycodone is considered a strong opioid and is available in immediate and sustained-release forms in addition to combination products with Tylenol. At this time there are no parenteral preparations available. The initial dose is 0.05 to 0.15 mg/kg per dose every 4 to 6 hours. Oxycodone can be titrated in the same way as morphine and does not have a ceiling limit.

METHADONE Methadone is recommended for children who are unable to tolerate morphine or hydromorphone due to side effects of nausea or sedation. It is a synthetic long-acting opioid analgesic with a prolonged half-life (19 hours in children and 35 hours in adults) that requires careful dosage adjustments. The initial dose is 0.2 mg/kg PO (maximum dose, 10 mg per dose), but should be given on an every 4 hours as needed (prn) schedule initially rather than routinely every 8 to 12 hours as other long-acting opioids. Due to its long half-life, methadone ac-

cumulates slowly and may lead to symptoms of overdosage over several days even in a child who appears to be doing well initially. Methadone may cause respiratory depression, sedation, increased intracranial pressure, hypotension, and bradycardia. The respiratory effects last longer than analgesia and lower dosages should be used in children with renal or hepatic impairment. Oral duration of action is 6 to 8 hours initially and 24 to 48 hours after repeated doses. Not until after 48 hours or more of methadone administration should a routine schedule be initiated.

FENTANYL Fentanyl is available in a patch form for transdermal absorption and in the form of oral lozenges for short-acting, immediate-release medication. The patches are recommended only in children over 12 years, or greater than 50 kg, and the safety and efficacy are still being established in pediatrics. They are not recommended for acute pain because 12 to 16 hours are required from application of the patch to achieve steady blood levels. They may be useful in older patients with stable chronic pain where analgesic requirements have already been determined.

The doses for fentanyl lozenges for children over 2 years of age are listed in Table 20–7. They are not recommended in children under 2 years or weighing less than 15 kg.

NEONATAL DOSING CONSIDERATIONS

Special dosing consideration should be given to neonates and infants due to differences in their pharmacokinetics and pharmacodynamics. Only acetaminophen can be administered at the regular recommended dose (10 to 15 mg/kg) for short periods of time without danger of hepatotoxicity. Because the rate of absorption is slower and the half-life of acetaminophen is prolonged in infants, the dosage schedule should be every 6 hours rather than every 4 hours.

Opioids should be used for severe pain in neonates. The starting doses in infants under 6 months should be one quarter to one half of the suggested doses. Generally, the pharmacokinetics of opioids in infants above 6 months and children are similar to those in adults, but neonates show reduced clearance of most opioids. This increased sensitivity to morphine and other opioids is probably the result of a combination of factors including smaller volume of distribution, decreased clearance, and possible increased permeability into the brain. These factors in combination with the newborn's immature responses to hypoxia and hypercarbia may result in respiratory depression at relatively low doses of morphine. This depression can be reversed with naloxone. The recommended dose of naloxone is 10 µg/kg up to a total dose of 100 µg/kg. Monitoring of infants for respiratory depression should continue for at least 24 hours after morphine is discontinued.

OPIOID SIDE EFFECTS

Although all opioids have similar side effects in both adults and children, recommended medications are slightly different for children than those frequently used for adults. Some of the side effects such as vomiting and sedation may improve in days to a week, while others will need to be treated. Assessment of possible side effects should be performed with both the parent and the child because children may not spontaneously volunteer information. The most common side effects are constipation and nausea and vomiting which are frequently transient and are discussed in the subsequent section on symptom management.

ADJUVANT MEDICATIONS

Direct involvement of the nerves by tumor invasion or as a side effect of chemotherapy may result in neuropathic pain. This type of pain is frequently described as shooting, burning, or stabbing. It usually responds well to tricyclic antidepressants and anticonvulsants. Tricyclic antidepressants are classically used for burning-type pain; however, many clinicians use them as first-line medications for all neuropathic pain.

Amitriptyline and nortriptyline are the most commonly used medications. They should be started at 0.1 to 1.2 mg/kg at bedtime. The dose may be increased by 50 percent every 2 to 3 days up to 0.5 to 2.5 mg/kg at bedtime, although many patients will not tolerate the larger doses.

Anticonvulsants are useful for the treatment of neuropathic pain that is described as shooting or stabbing. Carbamazepine or phenytoin are the most commonly used anticonvulsants for neuropathic pain. Gabapentin is increasingly being used for neuropathic pain; the dose of gabapentin is 5 mg/kg PO at bedtime. It may be increased to bid on day 2 and tid on day 3. The maximum dose is 300 mg/day. Adjuvant analgesic drugs and their dosages are listed in Table 20–8.

Symptom Management

Constipation

Constipation is an expected side effect of opioid analgesic use. Although increased fiber, fluid, and bulk in the diet may help treat constipation, medications are often necessary. A stool softener such

Table 20–8

Adjuvant Analgesic Drugs

DRUG CATEGORY	DRUG DOSE	INDICATIONS	COMMENTS
Antidepressants	• Amitriptyline, 0.2–0.5 mg/kg. Escalate by 25% every 2–3 days up to 1–2 mg/kg if needed. • Alternatives doxepin, imipramine, nortriptyline	• Neuropathic pain (vincristine-induced, radiation plexopathy, tumor invasion) • Insomnia	• Usually, improved sleep and pain relief within 3–5 days • Anticholinergic side effects are dose limiting. Use with caution for children with increased risk for cardiac dysfunction
Anticonvulsants	• Carbamazepine, 2 mg/kg PO every 12 hr • Phenytoin, 2.5 mg/kg PO every 12 hr • Clonazepam, 0.01 mg/kg every 12 hr	• Neuropathic pain, especially shooting, stabbing pain	• Monitoring for hematologic, hepatic, and allergic reactions. Side effects: gastrointestinal upset, ataxia, disorientation, somnolence
Neuroleptics	• Chlorpromazine, 0.5 mg/kg IV/PO every 4–6 hr • Promethazine, 0.5–1 mg/kg IV/PO every 4–6 hr • Haloperidol, 0.01–0.1 mg/kg PO every 8 hr	• Nausea confused child, psychosis, acute agitation • Enhancement of opioid analgesia	• Consider concurrent use of antihistamine (e.g., diphenhydramine) to avoid dystonic reaction if high doses or prolonged course is used
Sedatives, hypnotics, anxiolytics	• Diazepam, 0.05–0.1 mg/kg PO every 4–6 hr • Lorazepam, 0.02–0.04 mg/kg PO/IV every 4–6 hr • Midazolam, 0.05 mg/kg IV every 5 min prior to procedure; 0.3–0.5 mg/kg PO every 30–45 min prior to procedure	• Acute anxiety, muscle spasm, premedication for painful procedures	• Sedative effect may limit opioid use. Other side effects include depression and dependence with prolonged use
Antihistamines	• Hydroxyzine, 0.05–1 mg/kg every 4–6 hr • Diphenhydramine, 0.5–1 mg/kg every 4–6 hr	• Opioid-induced pruritus, anxiety, nausea	• Sedative side effects may be helpful
Psychostimulants	• Dextroamphetamine, methylphenidate, 0.1–0.2 mg/kg twice a day.	• Opioid-induced somnolence, potentiation of opioid analgesia	• Side effects include agitation, sleep disturbance, and anorexia

(continued)

Table 20–8 (continued)
Adjuvant Analgesic Drugs

DRUG CATEGORY	DRUG DOSE	INDICATIONS	COMMENTS
Psychostimulants *(continued)*	Escalate to 0.3–0.5 as needed		Administer second dose in early afternoon to avoid sleep disturbances
Corticosteroids	• Prednisone, prednisolone, and dexamethasone dosage depends on clinical situation (e.g. dexamethasone 6–12 mg/m²/day	• Headache from raised intracranial pressure, spinal or nerve compression; widespread metastases	• Side-effects include oedema, dyspeptic symptoms, and occasional gastrointestinal bleeding

SOURCE: Adapted with permission from World Health Organization: *Cancer Pain Relief and Palliative Care in Children.* London, World Health Organization, 1998.

as docusate sodium should also be administered in combination with a stimulant such as senna. Recommended dosages based on age can be found in Table 20–9.

Nausea and Emesis

The etiology of the nausea and/or emesis should first be determined to permit institution of effective therapy. (See Chapter 8 for a full discussion of the causes of nausea and emesis.) Opioid analgesics and other medications frequently induce nausea and emesis, although opioid-induced nausea is usually not very severe. Changing or discontinu-

ing the offending agent is generally preferred, but if the suspect medication is medically indicated and necessary, antiemetics will be required. A list of antiemetics, and their dosage schedules in pediatric patients, may be found in Table 20–10.

Phenothiazines are among the most commonly used agents for nausea, and they work by depressing emetogenic activity at the chemoreceptor trigger zone (CTZ) in the brainstem. However, phenothiazines may cause extrapyramidal symptoms (EPS), and this can be a particularly troublesome complication in children. Therefore, despite the overall wide usage of phenothiazines, some pediatric experts recommend that these agents should only

Table 20–9
Treatment of Constipation in Children

MEDICATION	AGE	DOSE
Docusate sodium	< 3 years	10–40 mg/24 hrs
	3–6 years	20–60 mg/24 hrs
	6–12 years	50–500 mg/24 hrs
Senna	All ages	10–20 mg/kg/dose
	Or	Or
	1 month to 1 year	55–109 mg qhs (max 218 mg/24 hr)
	1–5 years	109–218 mg qhs (max 436 mg/24 hr)
	5–15 years	218–436 mg qhs (max 872 mg/24 hr)

be used after other antiemetic agents have proven unsuccessful in controlling a child's symptoms. Prochlorperazine, promethazine, and chlorpromazine are the most commonly used phenothiazines.

Other medications utilized to treat nausea and emesis include metoclopramide, antihistamines, and agents that reduce gastric acid secretion. Metoclopramide works both centrally by inhibiting the CTZ and peripherally by accelerating gastric emptying. It too can cause extrapyramidal

symptoms, which can be prevented or reversed by the use of the antihistamine diphenhydramine. Antihistamines also work on the CTZ, possibly by blocking labyrinthine impulses. Vomiting due to gastritis should be treated by a combination of antacids and a histamine (H_2) blocker such as ranitidine (Zantac).

Vomiting that is due to intermittent or partial bowel obstruction may be improved by the use of steroids or sublingual atropine. Belladonna and

Table 20–10
Medications for Nausea and Vomiting

MEDICATION	DOSAGE	COMMENTS
Promethazine	0.25–1 mg/kg/dose q4–6 hr prn	Extrapyramidal symptoms (reversed by diphenhydramine) or hypotension may occur. Use only in prolonged vomiting of known etiology
Chlorpromazine	>6 mo: PO: 2.5–6 mg/kg/24 hr in 4–6 hr doses PR: 1mg/kg/dose q6–8 h	Similar to above
Prochlorperazine	>10 kg or >2 yr: 0.4 mg/kg/24 hr ÷ tid-qid	Similar to above
Dexamethasone	Loading dose: 1–2 mg/kg/dose PO, IV, IM Maintenance dose: 1–2 mg/kg/ 24 hours	Use a 4 to 6-hour dosage schedule
Diphenhydramine	5 mg/kg/24 hr given q 6 h Maximum dose: 300 mg/24 hr	Contraindicated with MAO inhibitor use; not for use in neonates due to potential CNS effects; use with caution in infants and young children
Metoclopramide	1–2 mg/kg/dose q2–6 h IV/IM/PO	Premedicate with diphenhydramine to reduce extrapyramidal symptoms
Ondansetron	Dose based on body surface area <0.3 m²: 1 mg tid prn 0.3–0.6 m²: 2 mg tid prn 0.6–1.0 m²: 3 mg tid prn >1.0 m²: 4–8 mg tid prn 4–11 years old: 4 mg tid prn Over 12 years old: 8 mg tid prn	
Granisetron	Over 2 years old: 10–20 10–20 mg/kg/dose	Give dose 15–60 minutes before chemotherapy. The same dose may be repeated 2 or 3 times within the 24 hours following chemotherapy

SOURCE: Drug dosages from Hirshfeld AB, Getachew A, Sesions J: Drug doses. In: Sibery GK, Iannone R, eds. *The Harriet Lane Handbook*, 15th ed. St. Louis, Mosby, 2000, pp. 599–892.

opium suppositories are useful for lower gastro-intestinal cramping and pain. Some children may need a nasogastric tube placed for decompression. If vomiting is refractory, two or more classes of medications may be combined to increase effectiveness. Although benzodiazapines such as lorazepam (Ativan) do not have specific antiemetic effects, they are frequently given in combination with the above medications.

Projectile emesis, usually accompanied by little or no nausea, is often associated with increased intracranial pressure from primary or secondary malignant lesions in the central nervous system. Projectile emesis may be effectively treated with high doses of steroids, such as dexamethasone.

Nausea and vomiting from certain chemotherapeutic agents may respond well to ondansetron or granisetron. Although these agents are very effective for this application, they are not very effective in preventing nausea from other causes.

Nonpharmacologic interventions that may help with nausea and vomiting include changing the child's diet to include foods such as clear liquids (ginger ale and other sodas, apple juice, and jello). Popsicles, sherbet, ice chips, yogurt, and other cold foods may also appeal to children. Room-temperature foods are frequently tolerated better than hot foods. Generally, foods that are greasy, spicy hot, or characterized by a strong odor should be avoided. Multiple small meals or snacks are tolerated better than larger servings. Distraction with television or games may also help.

Agitation

Hypoxia frequently causes agitation and restlessness, due to apparent shortness of breath. Opioids and oxygen are the treatments of choice. Morphine may be used at the rate of 0.3 mg/kg per dose PO every 3 to 4 hours and titrated as necessary. Benzodiazepines such as diazepam at the rate of 0.12 to 0.8 mg/kg per day in three divided doses, or lorazepam given 0.03 to 0.04 mg/kg per day in 3 or 4 divided doses, may also be useful. Haloperidol 0.01 to 0.03 mg/kg per 24 hours may also be

useful for controlling agitation and hallucinations. It may also be useful in controlling nightmares that frequently occur in the preterminal child.

Excess Secretions

Excess oral secretions are frequently apparent when the child can no longer swallow. The noisy sounds made as the child breathes can be extremely upsetting to family members. It is caused by a thin layer of secretions over the glottis. Excess secretions are best treated by sublingual atropine (6 µg/kg per dose PO 3 or 4 times a day to a maximum of 300 µg/dose). Scopolamine patches placed behind the ear can be used for children over 12 years old.

Sleep Disturbances

Sleep disturbances are common in pediatric patients who are near death. Often the child will sleep on and off during the day and be awake at night. This sleep pattern creates difficulty for caregivers, who generally need to sleep at night. If the child's insomnia has an identifiable cause, such as pain, depression, anxiety, or medication side effect, appropriate treatment should be initiated. If the insomnia is related to depression, amitriptyline 0.5 to 2 mg/kg at bedtime, or nortriptyline 1 to 3 mg/kg per day may be helpful.

If chronic opioid administration results in excessive sleepiness, then methylphenidate may be helpful. The dose is 0.3 mg/kg per dose up to 10 to 15 mg PO 2 or 3 times a day.

Nonpharmacologic interventions as guided imagery, distraction, and relaxation techniques may also be helpful. For nonspecific insomnia, the medications and pediatric doses are listed in Table 20–11.

Anxiety

Anxiety is a common occurrence in terminally ill children. In younger children it may be difficult to

Table 20–11
Medications for Insomnia

MEDICATION	DOSAGE
Hydroxyzine	0.5–2.0 mg/kg PO at bedtime
Diphenhydramine	0.5–1.0 mg/kg PO at bedtime
Chloral hydrate	50–75 mg/kg PO at bedtime
Diazepam	0.5 mg/kg PO at bedtime
Pentobarbital	2–6 mg/kg PO at bedtime

SOURCE: Adapted from Meek RS, Belasco JB, Noll RB: Terminal care for children with cancer: In: Ablin AR, et al, eds. *Supportive Care of Children with Cancer,* 2nd ed. Baltimore, Johns Hopkins University Press, 1997.

differentiate pain from anxiety or fear. Nonpharmacologic measures such as emotional and spiritual support and strong family relationships, in addition to support from the hospice team, may help to allay a child's anxiety. If pharmacologic interventions are necessary, benzodiazepines are the preferred agents. If these medications are not successful, phenothiazines may be useful.

Seizures

Since the occurrence of a seizure may be extremely distressing to the family and caregivers, the possibility of a seizure occurring and the appropriate management should be discussed in advance. It should be emphasized that seizures are usually self-limiting, and appropriate first-aid measures should be reviewed. Maintenance anticonvulsant therapy should be continued as long as possible. If seizures, especially status epilepticus, are anticipated, appropriate medications and dosages should be available in the home. Phenobarbital suppositories are helpful for anticonvulsant therapy after the child can no longer swallow. Valium suppositories may also be useful. A full discussion of seizure disorders near the end of life can be found in Chapter 9.

End-of-Life Care at Home

End-of-life care for children in the United States, whether provided by a hospice or a nonhospice palliative care program, is generally provided in the child's home. There are many issues to consider when choosing to have end-of-life care provided in the home. First, while children overwhelmingly prefer to be cared for at home, the family needs to have the commitment to have the child at home, cope with the stress, and share tasks.

Generally the mother is the primary caregiver and the parents are actually able to provide more attention and support to the siblings when the child is cared for at home. When the terminally ill child is cared for in the hospital, usually the parents are there with him or her to the detriment of the siblings, who may know little of their sibling's status.

With the child at home, brothers and sisters can assist in his or her care and entertainment to the best of their abilities. This can lead to enhanced communication between the family members and the child. It increases the control of the parents and decreases the isolation of the dying child. Studies have shown that with this "normalization" of family life, children are more peaceful in death, and that bereavement is less complicated for the surviving parents and siblings.

Staffing Issues

Due to the complex issues associated with terminally ill children, the entire end-of-life care team must be actively involved in the care plan. The team should consist of, at minimum, a physician, nurse, social worker, and chaplain, who all have experience in caring for terminally ill children. Although home health aid services may be offered, the mother or primary caregiver frequently prefers to provide the child's personal care.

If possible the physician who cared for the child in the acute care setting should continue to care for the child during hospice care. It may be difficult, however, for these physicians to stop curative therapy and to change to the palliative care model. Nevertheless, studies have shown that the medical relationship between the child, family, and physician should be maintained, because it aids in a smooth transition to hospice care. However, when the child is receiving palliative care at home, the pediatrician or family physician usually resumes primary care responsibilities. If this physician is unfamiliar with pain and symptom management in terminally ill children, the hospice or palliative care medical director should become involved. Every effort should be made to assure that the child and his or her family receive the most effective care possible.

The child and his or her family will frequently form a relationship with one particular member of the hospice team—often a nurse. If this individual is not available to make a home visit, usually a telephone call from that individual will often be more effective than a home visit from a substitute nurse. Such "broken" relationships may have lasting negative effects on the acceptance of care and the quality of life of the dying child.

Family Communication Regarding the Terminally Ill Child

One of the most sensitive issues in pediatric end-of-life care relates to the child's family members and their communication with the child about his or her condition. Children, even young ones, generally are aware of the fact that they are dying. However, because parents frequently want to protect their children from information about their health, and children want to protect their parents from worry that the child may die, the result is a lack of meaningful communication about the child's death. The child may thus be isolated at a time when he or she most needs love and support. The child may feel guilty and alone, and the parents and siblings undergo psychological stress. Medical personnel may also continue this charade. This situation is illustrated by the following case:

Timmy was a 10-year-old boy who was dying from cancer. His family had felt strongly that he should not be told of his terminal status and continually avoided discussing the issue with him. Because he had some difficulty with nausea, Timmy was on a bland diet. One day Timmy decided he really wanted a taco to eat. His mother told him this was not possible due to his diet, to which Timmy replied: "For heaven's sake, I'm dying! Let me have the taco!" At last the subject was broached and meaningful communication followed.

When discussing death with children, adults need to follow the child's lead regarding the timing and extent of the conversation. Communication may be brief, but the child should determine the timing. The conversation should be specific and literal. Expressions comparing death to a trip or a long sleep can be confusing to a child and should be avoided. Sometimes nonverbal communication through art, music, and puppets is the easiest way for both adults and children to communicate.

It is important to acknowledge the completeness of the child's life and to give him or her a sense of accomplishment by acknowledging his or her impact on the family and community. Both children and adults need to know it is normal to experience a wide range of emotions when facing death. Older children need to be part of the discussions and decision making regarding their own death, and their wishes should be respected as much as possible. All children need to be reassured of continuing love and physical closeness in addition to adequate symptom control. Lastly, it is necessary to realize when children need to be alone and honor when they do not want to communicate.

Children's Understanding of Death

As children grow and develop they assimilate the concepts relating to death of irreversibility, universality, nonfunctionality, and causality. Irreversibility refers to the understanding that dead things do not become alive again. With universality, it is understood that all living things will die at some time. Nonfunctionality refers to the ending of all life functions. Causality relates to why people die. These concepts must be integrated with the child's developmental level and age (Table 20–12).

Table 20–12

Children's Understanding of Death Related to Age

AGE	LEVEL OF UNDERSTANDING
Birth to 3 years old	Unable to differentiate temporary separation from abandonment
3–6 years old	Recognizes death, but not its irreversibility
6–12 years old	Develops concrete understanding of death and its concepts

Children from birth to age 3 are unable to differentiate temporary separation from abandonment, but by the age of 3 are able to recognize death as an entity. Children from 3 to 6 may recognize death but not that it is irreversible. Children in this age group may use fantasy and "magical thinking." Using "magical thinking," the child may think he or she can cause death by thoughts, and consequently may suffer from misplaced guilt. By age 7 most children understand all the death concepts of irreversibility, universality, nonfunctionality, and causality.

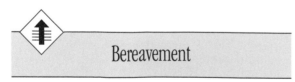

Bereavement

A full discussion of bereavement is found in Chapter 14. However, the grief felt by families following the death of a child is unlike any other. Therefore, no discussion about pediatric end-of-life care would be complete without a discussion of the specific bereavement issues related to the loss of a child.

The pain and loss are immeasurable. Nothing changes the lives of family members as much as the death of a child. Hospice staffs need to understand the basis of this difficult grieving if they are to intervene and assist the family.

There is great stress on the parents due to the death of the child being "out of order." Parents are not supposed to outlive their children. They frequently ask themselves questions like "Why my child?" "Why not me?" and "How can I ever go on?" The death of their child can challenge their belief system and spirituality.

Guilt

Guilt is a frequent factor for bereaved parents. It has been suggested that there are five different types of guilt that bereaved parents may experience. The first is cultural guilt, in that parents are supposed to take care of their children and that they have failed, or the child would not have died. The second type of guilt is causal guilt, especially prominent in familial or inherited disorders, when the parent feels responsible for transmitting the disease or condition to the child. In other diseases the parents may blame themselves for real or imagined negligence. Moral guilt occurs when parents feel they are being punished for some prior action. In survival guilt, the parent feels he or she should have died instead of the child. For example, survival guilt often occurs when the parent survives an auto accident but the child is killed. And, finally, there is recovery guilt, which occurs when parents feel guilty as they move through their grief and start to get on with their lives.

Blame

Bereaved parents often want to blame someone for the death of their child. At times this blame is placed on their spouse or on another child, and this blaming can lead to more stress on the family system. The primary caregiver may also experience the loss of an accustomed role and activities, especially if the child's illness was prolonged. The mother's full attention may have been devoted to the child and his or her needs, doctor's appointments, and even visits from the hospice staff. When the child dies, she has to redefine her life.

Stress

It can easily be seen how profound stress is placed on a relationship under these circumstances. This stress can be further aggravated by different or incompatible grieving styles between the partners. For example, women may want to talk about their grief in detail, while men often want to submerge themselves in work and not talk about grief at all. Partners need to understand each other's grieving style to have the relationship survive intact. Although there is conflicting research, the divorce rate appears to be higher following the death of a child.

Unaddressed Grief

The parents may choose to cope with their grief by not addressing it, but unaddressed grief also leads to difficulties. This type of grief may be portrayed by never mentioning the child's name; siblings may not know much about the circumstances of the death or how the parents are feeling. There may be no familial discussion about the death or its effect on the family members. Unaddressed grief may also lead to difficulties for the surviving children in regard to death, and may lead to a delayed grief reaction released with a future death. It has been suggested that with unaddressed grief, surviving family members may have difficulty forming intimate relationships due to a fear of being abandoned after being in this situation.

Grieving has a marked social component. For grieving to progress, the parent needs to talk about what has happened. Support groups, such as those sponsored by the Society of Compassionate Friends or other community resources, can facilitate moving through the tasks of mourning. In these groups, parents can share their thoughts and feelings with others who have also lost a child.

Ideally, bereavement interventions start before the death of the child. The hospice team first needs to help the family stay connected with the child until death. Usually this is not a problem if the child is at home and the family members are the primary caregivers. At times however, parents may have difficulty seeing and accepting their child's decline and want to distance themselves from this painful situation. This may lead to guilt after the death and complicate bereavement.

Hospice teams need to facilitate communication not only between the patient and family but also between family members themselves. Helping the family members say meaningful things before death increases the peacefulness of the child and avoids regrets after the death. The hospice staff and family can also encourage the creation of videos, photos, and other momentos that can be cherished in the future. One hospice program has the children stamp handprints placed like a hug on tee-shirts for the parents so they can always have their "hug" shirt. Having the child make handprints or footprints on a plaster of paris plaque is therapeutic for the child and also gives the parents a memento for the future.

Respite Care

Respite care is important to have available to the primary caregiver. Often the mother is the primary caregiver and is hesitant to leave the child's bedside. A hospice volunteer can help by being with the child so the mother can take a break. In England, "hospice houses," such as Helen House, have been developed to care for the child and provide the caregiver a respite.

Planning for Death

Parents also need to be encouraged to plan for the death, by including the wishes of the child, if possible. One 16-year-old boy wanted to have a pizza party with his friends as his death approached. Although he was only able to eat a couple of bites, he enjoyed the event and the normalcy it brought to his life. The friends also benefited from the party because they were able to be there "for" and with him.

Preplanning the funeral may be a beneficial activity for some children and their families. It can be especially beneficial for siblings to be involved in planning a service that reflects the uniqueness of their brother or sister. Kathy, a 17-year-old girl dying from Hodgkin's lymphoma, wanted to choose what her siblings would wear to her funeral. She had them try on various outfits and they selected one together for the occasion. Her wishes were followed.

Mourning

After death the interventions center around what W.J. Worden has called the "tasks of mourning." The first task is "accepting the reality of the loss." Even after a prolonged illness, death may seem unreal. It is helpful if the parents see the body and are able to have a commemorative service.

The second task of mourning is "processing the pain of the loss." The strong feelings and grief that are associated with death need to be expressed or emotional or physical difficulties may arise in the future. Most bereaved parents have some anger. It may even be anger at the child for having died and leaving them alone. Anger is often displaced on other people, with health care providers being frequent targets. The parent needs to be helped to find an expression of the anger that will bring it to a conclusion.

Adjusting to an environment where the deceased is missing is the third task of mourning. Finally, survivors need "to emotionally relocate the deceased so that one can move on with life." This latter action is the last task.

To assist the parents and family with the tasks of mourning, bereavement services should be made available to the parents and siblings of the deceased child. These may take the form of individual grief counseling, couples counseling, family counseling, bereavement support groups, and social support groups.

Assessment of Grieving Potential

The end-of-life care team should assess the grieving potential of the family at or as soon after admission to the hospice or palliative care program as possible. The situation should be reassessed prior to the time of the death of the child. Bereave-

ment risk must also be assessed for all surviving family members, including parents, grandparents, and siblings.

Sibling Grief

A child's death markedly affects surviving siblings. Siblings spend the most time together of any family subgroup and exert great influences on the development of each other's identity. Studies have shown that siblings of dying children have about twice the risk of developing psychological disturbances as the general population. This increased incidence is related to family dynamics, demographic characteristics, and the characteristics of the disease.

Children definitely do grieve. How children grieve, however, is dependent on their age, developmental level, and the individual situation. Even within that framework, all children are individuals and each will grieve in his or her own way.

Generally, the parents are the best people to tell the other children of the death. Upon hearing the news, younger children may want to return to the familiar safe activity of playing, while older children may seek solitude to gain control. Depending on their age and developmental level, they may experience any of the types of guilt described earlier. Younger children may have "magical thinking," where they believe they may have caused the death or illness of their sibling by their thoughts or unrelated actions. Nonverbal means of communication such as art, music, and play therapy may be the best way to help these children.

In the short term following the death, children may exhibit reactions similar to adult grief reactions. They may have frequent headaches, stomachaches, and other physical problems. They may have sleeping difficulties and fear the dark or resist going to bed. They may be anxious about new activities, or they may become irritable and argumentative. Other children may become sad, lonely, and withdrawn. Age regression is not unusual following the death of a sibling. Most children have decreased ability to concentrate and their school grades may go down.

Because the parents may be consumed by their own grief, it may be helpful to have a trusted adult (aunt, uncle, or friend) to care specifically for each sibling. The hospice team, especially the social workers, can also offer grief support and further resources for the child's grief care.

Siblings who experience the death of a brother or sister in childhood may have long-term effects. Feelings of loneliness and sadness can persist for years in siblings. Even up to 30 years later siblings have reported that the death has continued to have an impact on their lives. It often serves as a reminder of the value of life.

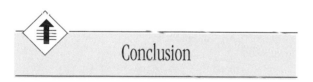

Conclusion

Pediatric hospice care as we know it can and does make a difference. Hospice facilitates the inclu-sion of the patient and family in the decision-making process. It allows the child to remain at home in familiar surroundings with loving care-givers. In addition to providing good pain and symptom relief and leading to a more peaceful death for the child, hospice also facilitates be-reavement for the parents and siblings.

Although nothing can remove the pain associ-ated with a child's death, hospice care can miti-gate bereavement for the parents and siblings. Unfortunately, only 1 percent of children who could benefit from hospice services actually re-ceive it. In response to the continuing challenges involved in pediatric palliative and end-of-life care, the American Academy of Pediatrics' Committee on Bioethics has recently issued the policy rec-ommendations, given in Table 20–13.

Although the recommendations in Table 20–13 have not been widely implemented, the list of recommendations provides a clear roadmap of how to achieve integrated and consistently good care of dying children. What remains now is to

Table 20–13

American Academy of Pediatrics' Committee on Bioethics Recommendations for Pediatric End-of-Life Care

1. Palliative care and respite programs need to be developed and widely available to provide intensive symptom management and promote the welfare of children living with a life-threatening or terminal conditions.
2. At the diagnosis of a life-threatening or terminal condition, it is important to offer an integrated model of palliative care that continues throughout the course of the illness, regardless of the outcome.
3. Changes in the regulation and reimbursement of palliative care and hospice services are necessary to improve access for children and families in need of these services. Modifications in current regulations should include broader eligibility criteria concerning the length of expected survival; the provision of respite care and other therapies beyond those allowed by a narrow definition of "medically indicated." Adequate reimbursement should accompany these regulatory changes.
4. All general and subspecialty pediatricians, family physicians, pain specialists and pediatric surgeons need to become familiar and comfortable with the provision of palliative care to children. Residency, fellowship training and continuing education programs should include topics such as palliative medicine, communication skills, grief and loss, managing prognostic uncertainty, and decisions to forgo life-sustaining medical treatment, spiritual dimensions of life and illness, and alternative medicine. Pediatric board and sub-board certifying examinations should include questions on palliative care.
5. An increase in support for research into effective pediatric palliative care programming, regulation and reimbursement, pain and symptom management, and grief and bereavement counseling is necessary.

American Academy of Pediatrics: Policy statement: Palliative care for children (RE0007), 106:351, 2000.

enlarge upon the hospice and palliative care model so more children and their families can be served and achieve optimal care near the end of their lives.

Bibliography

Anand KJ: Clinical importance of pain and stress in preterm neonates. *Biol Neonate* 73:1, 1998.

Baker CM, Wong DL: QUEST: A process of pain assessment in children. *Orthop Nurse* 6:11, 1987.

Brenner P: *2000 Overview*. Alexandria, VA, Children's Hospice International, 2000.

Brenner PR: The volunteer component. In: Armstrong-Dailey A, Goltzer SZ, eds. *Hospice Care for Children*. New York, Oxford University Press, 1993, p. 184–197.

Davies B: After a child dies: Helping the sibling. In: Armstrong-Dailey A, Goltzer SZ, eds. *Hospice Care for Children*. New York, Oxford University Press, 1993, pp. 140–153.

Davies B, Dorninica F, Stevens M, et al: The development of paediatric palliative care. In: Doyle D, Goeffrey WCH, MacDonald N, eds. *Oxford Textbook of Palliative Medicine*. Oxford, Oxford University Press, 1996, pp. 1087–1106.

Davies B, Eng B: Special issues in bereavement and staff support. In: Doyle D, Goeffrey WCH, MacDonald N, eds. *Oxford Textbook of Palliative Medicine*. Oxford, Oxford University Press, 1996, pp. 1085–1095.

Davies B, Howell D: Special services for children. In: Doyle D, Goeffrey WCH, MacDonald N, eds. *Oxford Textbook of Palliative Medicine*. Oxford, Oxford University Press, 1996, pp. 1077–1084.

Faulkner KW: Children's understanding of death. In: Armstrong-Dailey A, Goltzer SZ, eds. *Hospice Care for Children*. New York, Oxford University Press, 1993, pp. 9–21.

Foley KM: Controlling the pain of cancer. *Sci Amer* 275930:164, 1996.

Gemke RJ, Zwaan CM, Revesz T: *N Engl J Med* 342: 1997, 2000. Letter.

Gibbons MB: Psychosocial aspects of serious illness in childhood and adolescence. In: Armstrong-Dailey A, Goltzer SZ, eds. *Hospice Care for Children*. New York, Oxford University Press, 1993; pp. 60–84.

Goldman A: *N Engl J Med* 342:1997, 2000. Letter.

Goldman A: Life threatening illnesses and symptom control in children. In: Doyle D, Goeffrey WCH, MacDonald N, eds. *Oxford Textbook of Palliative Medicine*. Oxford, Oxford University Press, 1996, pp. 1033–1043.

Goldman A, ed. *Care of the Dying Child*. Oxford, Oxford University Press, 1994.

Gorther E: Lessons in grief: A practical look at school programs. In: Armstrong-Dailey A, Goltzer SZ, eds. *Hospice Care for Children*. New York, Oxford University Press, 1993, pp. 122–139.

Harper BC: Staff support. In: Armstrong-Dailey A, Goltzer SZ, eds. *Hospice Care for Children*. New York, Oxford University Press, 1993, pp. 184–197.

Hirshfeld AB, Getachew A, Sesions J: Drug doses. In: Sibery GK, Iannone R, eds. *The Harriet Lane Handbook,* 15th ed. St. Louis, Mosby, 2000, pp. 599–892.

Hockenberry-Eaton M, Barrera P, Brown M, et al: *Pain Management in Children with Cancer*. Houston, Texas Cancer Council, 1999.

Levetown M, Carter MA: Child-centered care in terminal illness: An ethical framework. In: Doyle D, Goeffrey WCH, MacDonald N, eds. *Oxford Textbook of Palliative Medicine*. Oxford, Oxford University Press, 1996, pp. 1108–1117.

Martinson I: A home care program. In: Armstrong-Dailey A, Goltzer SZ, eds. *Hospice Care for Children*. New York, Oxford University Press, 1993, pp. 219–230.

McGrath PA: Pain control. In: Doyle D, Goeffrey WCH, MacDonald N, eds. *Oxford Textbook of Palliative Medicine*. Oxford, Oxford University Press, 1996, pp. 1013–1031.

Milch RA, Freeman A, Clark E: *Palliative Pain and Symptom Management for Children and Adolescents*. Washington, DC, Division of Maternal and Child Health, U.S. Department of Health and Human Services, 1989.

Miles MS, Demi AS: Toward the development of a theory of bereavement guilt: Sources of guilt in bereaved parents. *Omega* 12:299, 1984.

Miser JS, Miser AW: Pain and symptom control. In: Armstrong-Dailey A, Goltzer SZ, eds. *Hospice Care for Children*. New York, Oxford University Press, 1993, p. 22–59.

Morgan ER, Murphy SB: Care of children who are dying of cancer. *N Engl J Med* 342:347, 2000. Editorial.

Policy Statement: Palliative care for children (RE0007). *Am Acad Pediatr* 106:351, 2000.

Robin B: Analgesia and sedation. In: Sibery GK, Iannone R, eds. *The Harriet Lane Handbook,* 15th ed. St. Louis, Mosby, 2000; pp. 893–902.

Sahler OJZ, Frager G, Levetown M, et al: Medical education about end-of-life care in the pediatric setting: Principles, challenges, and opportunities. *Pediatrics* 105:575, 2000.

Sligh JS: An early model of care. In: Armstrong-Dailey A, Goltzer SZ, eds. *Hospice Care for Children*. New York, Oxford University Press, 1993, pp. 219–230.

Stevens MM: Care of the dying child and adolescent: Family adjustment and support. In: Doyle D, Goeffrey WCH, MacDonald N, eds. *Oxford Textbook of Palliative Medicine*. Oxford, Oxford University Press, 1996, pp. 1057–1075.

Stevens MM: Psychological adaptation of the dying child. In: Doyle D, Goeffrey WCH, MacDonald N, eds. *Oxford Textbook of Palliative Medicine*. Oxford, Oxford University Press, 1996, pp. 1014–1055.

Wolfe J, Grier HE, Klar N, et al: Symptoms and suffering at the end of life in children with cancer. *N Engl J Med* 342:326, 2000.

Wong DL, Backer C: Pain in children: Comparison of assessment scales. *Pediatr Nurs* 14:9, .

Worden JW: *Grief Counseling and Grief Therapy: A Handbook for the Mental Health Practitioner*, 2nd ed. New York, Springer, 1991.

Worden JW, Monahan JR: Caring for bereaved parents. In: Armstrong-Dailey A, Goltzer SZ, eds. *Hospice Care for Children*. New York, Oxford University Press, 1993, pp. 122–139.

World Health Organization: *Cancer Pain Relief and Palliative Care in Children*. London, World Health Organization, 1998.

Index

Pages followed by f indicate figure. Pages followed by t indicate table.